Studies in Medieval Science

STUDIES IN MEDIEVAL SCIENCE
Alchemy, Astrology, Mathematics and Medicine

PEARL KIBRE

THE HAMBLEDON
PRESS

The Hambledon Press 1984
35 Gloucester Avenue, London NW1 7AX

History Series 19

ISBN 0 907628 21 4

British Library Cataloguing in Publication Data

Kibre, Pearl
Studies in medieval science.
– (History series; 19)
1. Science – Europe – History
I. Title
501 Q127.E8

This book contains 376 pages.

Printed and bound by Redwood Burn Ltd.,
Trowbridge, Wiltshire.

CONTENTS

Contents		v
Acknowledgements		vii
Preface		ix
Select Bibliography of Pearl Kibre		xi
I	The *Quadrivium* in the Thirteenth Century Universities (with Special Reference to Paris)	175-91
II	The Boethian *De Institutione Arithmetica* and the *Quadrivium* in the Thirteenth Century University Milieu at Paris	67-80
III	Albertus Magnus on Alchemy	187-202
IV	The *Alkimia Minor* Ascribed to Albertus Magnus	267-300
V	The *De Occultis Naturae* Attributed to Albertus Magnus	23-39
VI	Albertus Magnus, *De Occultis Naturae*: Latin Text	157-83
VII	Alchemical Writings Ascribed to Albertus Magnus	499-518
VIII	An Alchemical Tract Attributed to Albertus Magnus	303-16
IX	Further Manuscripts Containing Alchemical Tracts Attributed to Albertus Magnus	238-47
X	Two Alchemical Miscellanies: Vatican Latin MSS. 4091, 4092	167-76
XI	A Fourteenth Century Scholastic Miscellany	261-71
XII	Arts and Medicine in the Universities in the Later Middle Ages	213-27
XIII	The Faculty of Medicine at Paris, Charlatanism and Unlicensed Medical Practices in the Later Middle Ages	1-20
XIV	"Astronomia" or "Astrologia Ypocratis"	133-56
XV	Lewis of Caerleon, Doctor of Medicine, Astronomer and Mathematician († 1494?)	100-108
XVI	Hitherto Unnoted Medical Writings of Dominicus of Ragusa (1424-1425 A.D.)	990-5
XVII	Dominicus de Ragusa, Bolognese Doctor of Arts and Medicine	383-6
XVIII	Cristoforo Barzizza: Professor of Medicine at Padua	389-98
XIX	Giovanni Garzoni of Bologna (1419-1505), Professor of Medicine and Defender of Astrology	504-14
XX	The Intellectual Interests Reflected in Libraries of the Fourteenth and Fifteenth Centuries	257-97
Index		1-15

ACKNOWLEDGEMENTS

The articles collected here first appeared in the following places and are reprinted by the kind permission of the original publishers.

I	*Arts Libéraux et Philosophie au Moyen Age: Actes du Quatrième Congrès International de Philosophie Médiévale, Université de Montréal* (Paris, 1969).
II	*Boethius and the Liberal Arts: A Collection of Essays*, ed. M. Masi (Berne, 1981).
III	*Albertus Magnus and the Sciences: Commemorative Essays, 1980*, ed. J.A. Weisheipl (Pontifical Institute of Mediaeval Studies, Toronto, 1980).
IV	*Isis*, xxxii, pt. 2, No. 86 (June 1949).
V	*Osiris*, xi (1954).
VI	*Osiris*, xiii (1958).
VII	*Speculum*, xvii, no. 4 (October 1942).
VIII	*Isis*, xxxv, pt. 4, No. 102 (1944).
IX	*Speculum*, xxxiv, No. 2 (April 1959).
X	*Ambix*, viii, No. 3 (October 1960).
XI	*The New Scholasticism*, 15 (1941).
XII	*Les Universités à la Fin du Moyen Age: Actes du Congrès International de Louvain, 26-30 Mai 1975*, ed. Jacques Paquet and Jozef Ijsewijn (Institut d'Études Médiévales, Louvain, 1978).
XIII	*Bulletin of the History of Medicine*, xxvii, No. 1 (1953).
XIV	*Science and History: Studies in Honor of Edward Rosen, Studia Copernica, xvi* (Ossolineum, 1978).
XV	*Isis*, 43, pt. 2, No. 132 (July 1952).
XVI	*Bulletin of the History of Medicine*, vii, No. 4 (1939).
XVII	*Bulletin of the History of Medicine*, xlv, No. 4 (1971).
XVIII	*Bulletin of the History of Medicine*, xi, No. 4 (1942).
XIX	*Isis*, 58, pt. 4, No. 194 (1968).
XX	Reprinted from the *Journal of the History of Ideas* (with permission of its editors), Vol. vii, No. 3 (June 1946).

PREFACE

The following collection of essays or articles, prepared largely from manuscript sources and published in various periodicals and books over a number of years, illustrate aspects of medieval intellectual and scientific endeavor. The essays cover such subjects as the study and application of the seven liberal arts, particularly the quadrivial arts, the nature of the universe, alchemy, which in the words of Albertus Magnus, 'best imitates nature', and the science of the stars, particularly in its relation to man. They also cover the study and practice of medicine as an art, distinguished by Plato in his dialogues from an empirical knack by virtue of its considered concern for rational procedure or the relation of cause and effect. Also included are accounts of some noteworthy bibliophiles and the nature of their collections in the late thirteenth, fourteenth and fifteenth centuries.

I am grateful indeed for the opportunity provided by Mr. Martin Sheppard to present these studies in the hope that they may both interest their readers and inspire further investigation into an ever fascinating and engrossing area of human intellectual endeavor and development. I wish also to take this opportunity to thank my assistant, Mr. Irving A. Kelter, for his help in preparing the collection.

Pearl Kibre
Professor of History Emeritus
The Graduate Center
City University of New York

BIBLIOGRAPHY OF PEARL KIBRE

1936

The Library of Pico della Mirandola, New York: Columbia University Press, 1936

1937

With Lynn Thorndike, *A Catalogue of Incipits of Mediaeval Scientific Writings in Latin*. Cambridge, Mass.: The Mediaeval Academy of America, 1937.

1938

Review of *G. Pico della Mirandola, sincretismo religioso-filosofica, 1463-1494* by Eugenio Anagine. *The American Historical Review*, 43 (1938), 683-684.

1939

"Descriptions and Brief Analyses of Some Incunabula now in the Library of the New York Academy of Medicine." New York, 1939. (Typescript.)

"Hitherto Unnoted Medical Writings by Dominicus de Ragusa (1424-1425 A.D.)." *Bulletin of the History of Medicine*, 7 (1939), 990-995.

1940

Review of *The Medieval Library*, by James Westfall Thompson. *The American Historical Review*, 45 (1940), 615-616.

1941

"The *Alkimia minor* Ascribed to Albertus Magnus." *Isis*, 32 (1941), 267-300. "A Fourteenth Century Scholastic Miscellany." *The New Scholasticism*, 15 (1941), 261-271.

Review of *Catalogue des manuscrits alchimiques latins*, Volume 1: *Manuscrits des bibliothèques publiques de Paris antérieurs au xviie siècle,* described by James Corbett. *The American Historical Review*, 46 (1941), 451-452.

Review of *Princeps Concordiae: Pico della Mirandola and the Scholastic Tradition,* by Avery Dulles. *Isis*, 33 (1941), 532-534.

1942

"Alchemical Writings Ascribed to Albertus Magnus." *Speculum*, 17 (1942), 499-518.

"Cristoforo Barzizza, Professor of Medicine at Padua." *Bulletin of the History of Medicine*, 11 (1942), 389-398.

With Lynn Thorndike. "More Incipits of Mediaeval Scientific Writings in Latin." *Speculum*, 17 (1942), 342-366.

1944

"An Alchemical Tract Attributed to Albertus Magnus." *Isis*, 35 (1944), 303-316.

1945

"Hippocratic Writings in the Middle Ages." *Bulletin of the History of Medicine*, 18 (1945), 371-412.

Review of *The Christian Interpretation of the Cabala in the Renaissance,* by Joseph Leon Blau. *Journal of Religion*, 25 (1945), 143-144.

Review of *The Comet of 1577: Its Place in the History of Astronomy*, by C. Doris Hellman. *Speculum*, 20 (1945), 354-355.

1946

"The Intellectual Interests Reflected in Libraries of the Fourteenth and Fifteenth Centuries." *Journal of the History of Ideas,* 7 (1946), 257-297.

Review of *La Révélation d'Hermès Trismégiste. Volume 1: L'astrologie et les sciences occultes*, by A. Festugière. *Speculum*, 21 (1946), 253-255.

1948

The Nations in the Mediaeval Universities. Cambridge, Mass.: Mediaeval Academy of America, 1948.

1950

Review of *Aspects de l'Université de Paris. Speculum*, 25 (1950), 123.

1952

"Lewis of Caerleon, Doctor of Medicine, Astronomer, and Mathematician (d. 1494?)." *Isis*, 43 (1952), 100-108.

Review of *Catalogue des manuscrits alchimiques latins*, Volume 2: *Manuscrits des bibliothèques publiques de Paris, antérieurs au xvii*e *siècle*, described by James Corbett, *Catholic Historical Review*, 38 (1952), 206-208.

1953

"The Faculty of Medicine at Paris, Charlatanism and Unlicensed Medical Practices in the Later Middle Ages." *Bulletin of the History of Medicine*, 27 (1953), 1-20.

Review of *Roger Bacon and his Search for a Universal Science: A reconsideration of the life and work of Roger Bacon in the light of his own stated purposes*, by Stewart C. Easton. *The American Historical Review*, 58 (1953), 595-596.

1954

"Albertus magnus." *New Century Cyclopedia of Names*, Volume 1. New York, 1954.

"The De Occultis Naturae Atrributed to Albertus Magnus." *Osiris Volumen Undecim. Dedicated to Lynn Thorndike* (1954), 23-29.

"List of Subscribers [to *Osiris* with note of appreciation for 'the continued co-operation and good will of all scholars toward *Osiris*'] *Osiris Volumen Undecim. Dedicated to Lynn Thorndike* (1954), 530-533.

"Lynn Thorndike (with bibliography and portrait.)" *Osiris Volumen Undecim. Dedicated to Lynn Thorndike* (1954), 5-22.

"Scholarly Privileges: Their Roman Origins and Medieval Expression." *The American Historical Review*, 59 (1954), 543-567.

"The University of Paris and the Stationarii in the Thirteenth and Fourteenth Centuries." *Columbia University Columns*, 4 (1954), 13-18.

Review of *The Domesday Geography of Eastern England*, by H. C. Darby. *Isis*, 45 (1954), 115-117.

Review of *Ioannes Picus Mirandulanus Comes Concordiae, Oratio de Hominis Dignitate. Church History*, 23 (1954), 281-282.

1955

"Academic Oaths at the University of Paris in the Middle Ages." In *Essays in medieval life and thought*,pp. 123-138. Ed. John H. Mundy, Richard W. Emery and Benjamin N. Nelson. Essays in honour of Austin Patterson Evans. New York, 1955.

Review of *Augustine to Galileo: The History of Science A.D. 400-1650*, by A. C. Crombie. *Scripta Mathematica*, 21 (1955), 177-178.

1956

Review of *L'Enseignement de l'écriture aux universités médiévales, by* István Hajnal' *Speculum*, 31 (1956) 514-516.

Review of *The Metalogicon of John of Salisbury: A Twelfth Century Defense of the Verbal and Logical Arts of the Trivium* by Daniel D. McGarry. *The American Historical Review*, 61 (1956), 685.

1957

"Albertus Magnus, *De Occultis Nature*." *Osiris*, 13 (1957), 157-183.
Review of *Guillelmi de Ockham: Opera Politica,* Volume 3, ed. H. S. Offler. *The American Historical Review*, 62 (1957), 664.
Review of *Student Life in Ave Maria College, Medieval Paris: History and Chartulary of the College*, by Astrik L. Gabriel. *Speculum*, 32 (1957), 835-838.

1958

Foreword to *Libellus de alchimia ascribed to Albertus Magnus*, tr. by Sister Virginia Heines. Berkeley and Los Angeles, 1958.
Review of *The Age of Dante: A concise History of Italian Culture*, by Domenico Vittorini. *The American Historical Review*, 63 (1958), 647-648.

1959

"Further Manuscripts Containing Alchemical Tracts Attributed to Albertus Magnus." *Speculum*, 34 (1959), 238-247.

1960

"Two Alchemical Miscellanies: Vatican Latin MSS 4091, 4092." *Ambix*, 8 (1960), 167-176.
Review of *The University of Toulouse in the Middle Ages: Its Origins and Growth to 1500 A.D.*, by Cyril E. Smith. *Speculum*, 35 (1960), 148-151.

1961

Scholarly Privileges in the Middle Ages: The Rights, Privileges, and Immunities of Scholars and Universities at Bologna, Padua, Paris and Oxford. London: Mediaeval Academy of America, 1961.
"Cardinal Domenico Grimani, 'Questio de intentione et remissione qualitatis'; A Commentary on the Tractate of that title by Richard Suiseth (Calculator)," *Didascaliae: Studies in honor of Anselm M. Albareda*, pp. 149-203. Ed. Sesto Prete. New York, 1961.
Foreword to *The Medieval University 1200-1400*, by Lowrie J. Daly. New York, 1961.

1962

The Nations in the Mediaeval Universities. Reprint edition, Cambridge, Mass.: The Mediaeval Academy of America, 1962.
Scholarly Privileges in the Middle Ages: the Rights, Privileges, and Immunities of Scholars and Universities at Bologna, Padua, Paris and Oxford. Cambridge, Mass.: Mediaeval Academy of America, 1962.

Review of *Skara House at the Medieval University of Paris*, by A. L. Gabriel. *Speculum*, 37 (1962), 278-279.

1963

With Lynn Thorndike, *A Catalogue of Incipits of Mediaeval Scientific Writings in Latin*. Revised and augmented edition, Cambridge, Mass.: Mediaeval Academy of America, 1963.

1964

Review of *Manuscrits scientifiques médiévaux de l'Université de Salamanque et de ses "Colegios Mayores"*, by Guy Beaujouan. *Speculum*, 39 (1964), 690-692.

1965

"The Christian: Augustine." In *The Educated Man: Studies in the History of Educational Thought*, pp. 97-112. Ed. Paul Nash et al. New York, 1965.

Review of *Isidore of Seville: The Medical Writings*, ed. and tr. W. D. Sharpe. *Speculum*, 40 (1965), 754-756.

1966

The Library of Pico della Mirandola. Reprint edition, New York: AMS Press, 1966.

With Marshall Clagett and Gaines Post. "Lynn Thorndike." *Speculum*, 41 (1966), 598-599.

Review of *Liber Receptorum Nationis Anglicanae (Alemanniae) in Universitate Parisiensi ab anno MCCCCXXV ad annum MCCCCXCIV*, ed. A. L. Gabriel and G. C. Boyce. *Speculum*, 41 (1966), 127-128.

1967

"Giovanni Garzoni of Bologna (1419-1505) Professor of Medicine and Defender of Astrology." *Isis*, 58 (1967), 504-514.

New Catholic Encyclopedia. New York, 1967. Articles on: "Heloise," "Paris, University of [Origin and Early Development before 1500]," "Peter of Vinea," "Richard of Wallingford," "Saint-Denis-en-France, Abbey of," "Serlo of Bayeux," "Simon Bredon," "Tempier, Etienne," "Turpin of Reims."

"Thorndike, Lynn (1882-1965) In Memoriam." *Archives internationales d'histoire des sciences*, 20 (1967), 285-288.

Review of *The Mediaeval Statutes of the Faculty of the University of Freiburg im Breisgau*, ed. H. Ott and J. M. Fletcher. *Speculum*, 42 (1967), 181-182.

1968

"Further Addenda and Corrigenda to the Revised Edition of Lynn Thorndike and Pearl Kibre. A Catalogue of Incipits of Mediaeval Scientific Writings in Latin, 1963." *Speculum*, 43 (1968), 78-114.

1969

"The Quadrivium in 13th-Century Universities (with Special Reference to Paris)." In *Arts libéraux et philosophie au Moyen Age. Actes du quatrième Congrès International de Philosophie Médiévale, Université de Montréal, Canada, 27 août-2 Septembre, 1967*. Montreal, 1969, pp. 175-191.

Review of *Commentaires de la Faculté de médicine de l'Université de Paris (1516-1560)*, by Marie-Louise Concasty. *Bulletin of the History of Medicine*, 43 (1969), 591-593.

Review of *Paris and Oxford Universities in the Thirteenth and Fourteenth Centuries: An Institutional and Intellectual History*, by Gordon Leff. *Speculum*, 44 (1969), 642-646.

1970

Dictionary of Scientific Biography. New York, 1970. Articles on: "Adam of Bodenstein," Vol. 1, and "Bernard of Trevisan," Vol. 2.

Review of *Garlandia: Studies in the History of the Medieval University*, by Astrik L. Gabriel. *The American Historical Review*, 75 (1970), 2025-2026.

1971

"Dominicus de Ragusa, Bolognese Doctor of Arts and Medicine." *Bulletin of the History of Medicine*, 45 (1971), 383-86.

Review of *Acta Facultatis Artium Universitatis Vindobonensis, 1385-1416*, ed. Paul Uiblein. *Speculum*, 46 (1971), 398-400.

1972

With Gray C. Boyce and Astrik L. Gabriel. "Eugene Cardinal Tisserant." *Speculum*, 47 (1972), 603-604.

New Century Italian Renaissance Encyclopedia. New York, 1972. Articles on: "Academies," "Astrology and Magic," "Universities."

"Raymond de Roover." *The American Historical Review*, 77 (1972), 1202-1203.

1973

Review of *Chaucer's Physician: Medicine and Literature in Fourteenth-Century England*, by Huling E. Ussery. *The American Historical Review*, 78 (1973), 668-669.

Review of *Les Universités du Languedoc au XIIIe siècle.* (Cahiers de Fanjeaux, V). *Speculum,* 48 (1973), 422-427.

Review of *Universities in Politics: Case Studies from the Late Middle Ages and Early Modern Period*, ed. John W. Baldwin and Richard A. Goldthwaite. *The American Historical Review,* 78 (1973), 1433-1434.

1974

Review of *La Faculté des arts et ses maîtres au XIIIe siècle,* by Palémon Glorieux. *Speculum*, 31 (1974), 734-735.

1975

Review of *English Schools in the Middle Ages*, by Nicholas Orme. *The American Historical Review*, 80 (1975), 92-93.

"Hippocrates latinus: Repertorium of Hippocratic Writings in the Latin Middle Ages," [Fasc. I]. *Traditio*, 31 (1975), 99-126.

"Matheolus of Perugia's Commentary on the Preface to the *Aphorisms* of Hippocrates." *Bulletin of the History of Medicine,* 49 (1975), 405-428. With Nancy G. Siraisi.

1976

"Hippocrates Latinus. Fasc. II." *Traditio*, 32 (1976), 257-292.

1977

"Hippocrates Latinus. Fasc. III." *Traditio*, 33 (1977), 253-295.

"The Faculty of Medicine at Paris; Charlatanism, and Unlicensed Medical Practices in the Later Middle Ages." Reprinted in *Legacies in Law and Medicine*, ed. C. R. Burns (New York: Science History Publications, 1977), 52-71.

"Introduction" to *Alchemy and the Occult: A Catalogus of Books and Manuscripts from the Collection of Paul and Mary Mellon given to Yale University Library*, Volume III: *Manuscripts 1225-1671,* compiled by Laurence C. Witten and Richard Pachella (New Haven: Yale University Library, 1977).

1978

"Hippocrates Latinus. Fasc. IV." *Traditio*, 34 (1978), 193-226.

"Arts and Medicine in the Universities of the Later Middle Ages." in *Les Universités A La Fin Du Moyen Age,* ed. by J. Paquet and J. Ijsewijn (Louvain: Institut d'Etudes Médiévales U.C.L., 1978), 213-227.

"Astronomia or *Astrologia* Ypocratis." in *Science and History Studies in Honor of Edward Rosen, Studia Copernicana XVI (Wroclaw:* Ossolineum, 1978; New York: Science History Publications, 1978), 133-156.

1979

"Hippocrates Latinus. Fasc. V." *Traditio*, 35 (1979), 273-302.

1980

"Hippocrates Latinus. Fasc. VI." *Traditio*, 36 (1980), 347-372.

"Albertus Magnus on Alchemy." in *Albertus Magnus and the Sciences: Commemorative Essays 1980*, ed. by J. A. Weisheipl, O. P. (Toronto: Pontifical Institute of Mediaeval Studies, 1980), 187-202.

1981

"Hippocrates Latinus. Fasc. VII." *Traditio*, 37 (1981), 267-289.

"The Boethian *De Institutione Arithmetica* and the *Quadrivium* in the Thirteenth Century University Milieu at Paris." in *Boethius and the Liberal Arts*, ed. by M. Masi (Berne: Peter Lang, 1981), 67-80.

1982

"Hippocrates Latinus. Fasc. VIII: Conclusion and Indexes of Treatises, Translators and Commentators." *Traditio*, 38 (1982), in press.

I

THE *QUADRIVIUM* IN THE THIRTEENTH CENTURY UNIVERSITIES (WITH SPECIAL REFERENCE TO PARIS)

The transmission and development from Antiquity to the Middle Ages of the framework of the seven liberal arts and especially of the *Quadrivium* or four mathematical arts, arithmetic, geometry, music and astronomy, is a well known aspect of medieval culture. Yet the extent to which this framework was carried over into the curriculum of the faculties of arts of the newly established university associations in the thirteenth century, is still somewhat obscure and ill-defined.[1] This is in all probability due to the fact that the thirteenth century university statutes that have come down to us are fragmentary and summary in nature. For Paris as well as for Oxford, the two universities with which this account will be concerned, with particular emphasis on Paris, little information other than that relating to the newly translated Aristotelian writings is to be gleaned from the thirteenth century university statutes. Judging indeed from the statute provisions alone, the time-worn division into *Trivium* and *Quadrivium* had been abandoned and the subjects particularly of the *Quadrivium* crowded out by the Aristotelian texts in natural and moral philosophy. The only reference to the *Quadrivium* in the Paris statutes is in the curriculum outlined in 1215 for the faculty of arts by the papal legate Robert de Curzon. It is there asserted that "no books other than those of the philosophers, rhetoricians and *quadriviales*, might be lectured on in feast days."[2] In the case of Oxford, the thirteenth century statutes contain no mention of the *Quadrivium*. However, the term is used in letters patent of Edward I for 30 December, 1274, relating to the chancellor and university.[3] For the other thirteenth century universities statutory materials are either lacking or are equally uninformative.

1. Cf. Hastings RASHDALL, *Universities of Europe,* edited by F. M. POWICKE and A. B. EMDEN, 3 vols., Oxford University Press, 1936, I, p. 35 et seq.; 441-443, 447, 450, 474; III, 152, 480-482; and see also *Munimenta academica,* or *Documents Illustrative of Academical Life and Studies at Oxford,* Pt. I: *Libri cancellarii et procuratorum,* edited by Rev. Henry ANSTEY, London, 1868, I, p. 34, for the year 1267, where the Aristotelian works are listed; also *Statuta antiqua universitatis oxoniensis,* ed. S. GIBSON, Oxford, 1931, p. xcii-cxviii.

2. "Non legant in festivis diebus nisi philosophos et rhetoricas, et quadruvialia . . . " *CUP,* I, no 20 (cf. no 201).

3. "Cancellarius et universitas ville nostre Oxonie ubi suum posuerunt trivium et quadrivium fundamenta." Cited by S. GIBSON, Introduction to *Statuta antiqua,* p. xciv; *Medieval Archives of the University of Oxford,* ed. by H. E. SALTER, Oxford Historical Society, 2 vols., 1917-1919, I, p. 34.

Yet, despite the lacunae in the statutes, the conclusion that this connotes the abandonment by the universities named of the teaching of the subjects of the *Quadrivium* is not borne out by other available sources of information. On the contrary, there is ample evidence that the mathematical arts, although not in the time honored quadrivial framework, were carried over into the university arts curriculum and were being taught or lectured on in the thirteenth century alongside the newly translated texts of Aristotle. This is evident especially when we turn our attention to the writings of scholars associated with the universities, as well as to the collections of *Quodlibeta* and *Questiones disputatae*, still largely in manuscript,[4] and to guides or manuals. Among the last named group, the most informative is the summary in the form of questions on subjects and texts, prepared by an anonymous master of arts of the University of Paris, for candidates taking the examination for the baccalaureate or for the license in arts, in the first half of the thirteenth century.[5] Another manual prepared for students in which the quadrivial arts noted is the pseudo-Boethian *De disciplina scholarium*, which has been assigned to the second quarter of the thirteenth century,[6] together with the equally spurious commentary on it attributed to St. Thomas Aquinas,[7] but, since it cites him, belonging to the late thirteenth century. Further evidence is also provided by the extant thirteenth century manuscript texts relating to the subjects of the *Quadrivium*, as well as by inventories and catalogues of manuscripts.[8] In the following summary account of the quadrivial arts, especially in the University of Paris and to some extent in Oxford, some use has been made of all the above sources. They should all also well repay further study and more detailed consideration than has been possible here.

Before turning to the individual disciplines of the *Quadrivium*, it may be of interest to take note of the expressed views of some prominent scholars of Paris and Oxford on the mathematical arts as a whole. In this regard the opinions of Robert Grosseteste and his disciple Roger Bacon, who were associated with both Universities, have pertinency. Both wrote extensively on mathematical subjects

4. On this subject, see especially P. GLORIEUX, *La littérature quodlibétique de 1260 à 1320,* in *BibTh,* V (1925) and XXI (1935).

5. *Barcelona, Archivo de la Corona de Aragon, Ripoll 109,* fol. 134v-158v, of which fol. 134r-137r relate specifically to the arts of the *Quadrivium.* I have obtained a microfilm of the text which has alfeady been described at some length by Mgr. GRABMANN who discovered it, *Eine für Examinazwecke abgefasste Quästionensammlung der Pariser Artistenfakultät aus der ersten Hälfte des 13. Jahrhunderts* in *MAG,* II, p. 188-99; by R. M. MARTIN, O.P., *Travaux récents relatifs à la faculté des arts aux XIIIe – XIVe siècles,* in *RHE,* XXXI (1935), p. 359-368; and by Canon Fernand VAN STEENBERGHEN, *Aristotle in the West,* Louvain, 1955, p. 95 et seg. The text has been dated between 1230 and 1240.

6. *PL,* LXIV, 1223-38. On the work see Paul LEHMANN, *Pseudo-Antike Literatur des Mittelalters,* Leipzig and Berlin, 1927, reprinted Darmstadt, 1964, p. 27-28, and 101; also C.H. HASKINS, *Studies in Mediaeval Culture,* Clarendon Press, 1929, reprinted Frederick Ungar Publishing Co., New York (n.d.), p. 73 seq.

7. THOMAS AQUINAS, *Opera omnia,* ed. S. E. FRETTE, Paris, 1875, XXVI, especially p. 591 seq.; and see M. GRABMANN, *Die echten Schriften des hl. Thomas von Aquin,* in *BGPMA,* XXII (1920), p. 9.

8. In this regard, see the observation by M.-D. CHENU, O.P., regarding the means for reconstructing the intellectual life of the University of Paris in the thirteenth century, in *PIEM,* I (1932), p. 12. Of catalogues of manuscripts, attention might be called particularly to Léopold DELISLE, *Inventaire des MSS Latins de la Sorbonne* (MSS de la *Bibliothèque Impériale, nos. 15176-16718),* in *Bibliothèque de l'École des Chartes,* Paris, XXXI (1871), p. 1-50, 135-161, where a number of XIIIth century manuscripts are listed; also L. DELISLE, *Le cabinet des manuscrits,* III, p. 8-114.

and on natural science.[9] And both maintained that the mathematical arts provide the gateway and key to all other sciences.[10] Roger Bacon particularly in his *Opus maius* asserted that anyone who knows the four mathematical sciences can make progress without undue labor and difficulty in acquiring knowledge of both human and divine science. And contrariwise, he argued, those who are ignorant of these disciplines cannot know the other sciences. And also they cannot become conversant with the affairs and occupations of this world. Moreover, what was even worse, in his opinion, those who are ignorant of mathematics are unable to perceive their own ignorance and are therefore unable to seek a remedy.[11] Bacon went on to demonstrate the truth of his assertion by pointing to particular men of science of his day who by means of their excellent knowledge of mathematics had learned all the sciences. And chief among these very illustrious persons, he named Bishop Robert of Lincoln (Grosseteste) and Friar Adam Marsh (de Marisco).[12]

Roger Bacon's view of the end toward which the mathematical arts are directed did not coincide precisely with the Augustinian precept that training in the liberal arts was intended to sharpen the faculties of the mind so that they might penetrate the words of Scripture and cope with theological truth.[13] Nor was it wholly encompassed in the explanation given by the twelfth century savants of Chartres, "in the words of the Book of Wisdom," that, just "As the world . . . is ordered according to number, measure, and weight," just so are "the sciences of the *Quadrivium* – arithmetic and geometry, music and astronomy," cultivated as "the instruments which the human mind has at its disposal for recognizing the art of the Creator."[14] Bacon, it is true, as well as other scholars of his time, did

9. On bibliography relating to the careers of both Robert Grosseteste and Roger Bacon, in relation to Oxford and Paris, see H. RASHDALL, *Universities of Europe*, edited by F. M. POWICKE and A. B. EMDEN, 1936, III, p. 238 seq. Also on Grosseteste, the excellent studies of A.C. CROMBIE and the late Rev. D. CALLUS, O.P., listed in the following note. See also D. E. SHARP, *Franciscan Philosophy at Oxford in the Thirteenth Century*, 1930, reprinted New York, Russell and Russell Incorp., 1964, p. 12 et seq.; also VAN STEENBERGHEN, p. 136 et seq. For a survey of Bacon's mathematical works and a summary of the mathematics of his time, see D. E. SMITH, *The Place of Roger Bacon in the History of Mathematics*, in *Roger Bacon Essays*, collected and edited by A. G. LITTLE, Oxford, 1914, p. 153-83.

10. ROBERT GROSSETESTE, *De artibus liberalibus*, ed. L. BAUR, 1912, p. 1; A. C. CROMBIE, *Robert Grosseteste and the Origins of Experimental Science*, Oxford, 1953; also in *Robert Grosseteste, Essays in Commemoration*, edited by D. A. CALLUS, O.P., Oxford 1955, p. 59; ROGER BACON, *Opus maius*, Part IV, Dist. 1, chap. 1-3, edited by J. H. BRIDGES, Oxford, Clarendon Press, 1897, Vol. 1, especially p. 97, 103-104; English translation by R. B. BURKE, Philadelphia, University of Pennsylvania Press, 1928, p. 116, 121-122. See also ROGERI BACONIS *Moralis philosophia*, ed. Eugenio MASSA, Turici, In aedibus Thesauri mundi, 1953, pars prima, p. 3; also *Communia mathematica*, partes prima et secunda, nunc primum edidit R. STEELE, Oxford, Clarendon Press, London, 1940 (*Opera hactenus inedita Rogeri Baconi*, Fasc. xvi), p. 3.

11. *Opus maius*, IV, Dist. 1, chap. 1, BRIDGES ed., p. 97; BURKE trans., p. 116.

12. *Ibid.*, IV, Dist. 1, chap. 3, BRIDGES ed., p. 108; BURKE trans., p. 125-26. For Friar Adam de Marisco or Adam of Marsh, see H. RASHDALL, *Universities*, 1936, III, p. 248, note 4; also D. E. SHARP, *Franciscan Philosophy at Oxford*, 1964, especially p. 118-19.

13. For Augustine's views on the arts, see É. GILSON, *Introduction à l'étude de Saint Augustin*, in *EPM*, XI, 2nd ed., 1943; also my essay on Augustine in *The Educated Man*, edited by Paul NASH, Andreas M. KAZAMIAS, and H. J. PERKINSON, New York, John Wiley and Sons Inc., 1965, p. 98 seq. Bacon was, however, well aware of the earlier views which he summarized. See *Opus maius*, Part. II, chap. 3, BRIDGES ed., I, 36-37; BURKE trans., I, 40-41.

14. Raymond KLIBANSKY, *The School of Chartres*, in *Twelfth Century Europe and the Foundations of Modern Society*, edited by M. CLAGETT, Gaines POST and Robert REYNOLDS, Madison, The University of Wisconsin Press, 1961, p. 9.

recognize the importance of the mathematical arts for theology and the need for the theologian to know them. The theologian, he asserted, should have ample knowledge of numeration, so that he might know all the algoristic methods for both whole numbers and fractions. "He should know how to compute, add, subtract, halve, multiply, divide, and extract roots."[15] However, in accord with his mentor Robert Grosseteste, Bacon emphasized also the essential importance of the mathematical arts for the investigation of the natural world as well as for the world of affairs.[16]

Roger Bacon argued further on the basis of the authority of Ptolemy and Boethius that mathematics was necessary to every discipline and science, since according to Aristotle,[17] the essential parts of philosophy, both natural and divine, are mathematical. He then went on to demonstrate that even grammar and logic, since they are according to Alpharabi, in his book on Sciences, the accidental parts of philosophy, "cannot be known without mathematics." Grammar, in particular, Bacon asserted, is dependent on the mathematical art, music, since the latter is the science that must consider the nature of tones. And among the varieties and parts of music associated with grammar, Bacon noted that one relates to prose, another to meter, a third is concerned with rhythm and a fourth with song. Logic also, Bacon asserted, depends on music, in accordance with the views of Alpharabi in his aforementioned book on Sciences, and of both Aristotle and Averroes. Furthermore, Bacon continued, mathematics is required by logic because its central core is based on the *Posterior Analytics* which teaches the mathematical art of demonstration. Similarly, since logic begins with the *Book of Categories*, "it is clear that the category of quantity cannot be known without mathematics."[18] Indeed, there is no question in Bacon's mind but that mathematics is needed in every science. This, he affirmed, is further attested in the sixth book, 22nd proposition of Euclid's *Elements.* And this necessity extends to all four parts of mathematics, namely to geometry, arithmetic, music and astronomy. These were all founded when the human race began. Hence Bacon placed them first among the arts that should be studied, since through them one may advance to other sciences.[19]

In thus placing mathematics before logic in the program of studies, Roger Bacon differed from other of his contemporaries. For example, Robert Grosseteste apparently had himself developed his methodological approach to science from his prior study of the *Posterior Analytics.*[20] And Thomas Aquinas specifically asserted that the appropriate course of education was instruction in logical topics first, since logic teaches method for all philosophy or scientific inquiry. Mathematical training should then be second, physical or natural philosophy third. And this, in turn, should be followed by moral science, and finally by instruction in

15. *Opus maius*, Part II, chap. 3; part IV, chap. 16; BRIDGES ed., I, 219 seq.; BURKE trans., I, 242-247.

16. *Ibid.*, IV, Dist. I, chap. 1; *Opus tertium*, chap. 6; A. C. CROMBIE, *Robert Grosseteste*, p. 50 et seq.; also D. E. SHARP, *Franciscan Philosophy at Oxford*, p. 119 and 120; and for a corrective on Bacon's position in relation to his contemporaries, BAUR, *Die Philosophie des Robert Grosseteste,* in *BGPMA,* XVIII, 4-6, p. 16 et seq.

17. *Opus maius*, IV, Dist. I, chap. 2.

18. *Ibid.*, BRIDGES ed., p. 99-101; BURKE trans., p. 118-120.

19. *Ibid.*, IV, Dist. I, chap. 3.

20. A. C. CROMBIE, *Robert Grosseteste and the Origins of Experimental Science*, Oxford, 1953, p. 46 et seq.

divine wisdom or theology.[21] Bacon, however, continued to maintain that the illustrious men of science of his own time, whom he had named earlier, depended primarily upon their knowledge of mathematics to further their studies on the rainbow, on comets, on the generation of heat, and their investigations of localities of the earth and other matters of which both theology and philosophy treat. He specifically denied that other sciences could be known or understood by means of dialectical and sophistical arguments as commonly maintained. They could, he argued, be made understandable rather by means of mathematical demonstration, which enters into the truths and activities of other sciences and regulates them. Without such mathematical demonstration, other sciences cannot be clearly understood, nor can they enter into the thought process and be learned.[22]

Roger Bacon's plea for mathematical studies was perhaps the more vehement since, in his opinion, the actual status of the mathematical arts in the universities was far different from that which he advocated. Mathematical studies, he pointed out, had been neglected for about thirty or forty years, and this neglect had practically destroyed Latin studies in the sciences.[23] He noted specifically that students knew only three or four propositions of Euclid at most. And the science of perspective, he reported, was lectured on only twice in Oxford before 1267.[24] However, at Paris, he added, these works were not lectured on at all until much later.[25]

To what extent Bacon's appraisal of the situation is accurate it is not possible to determine with certitude. Yet one may venture to suggest that since he appears to have been of a highly irascible and critical turn of mind,[26] he may have been exaggerating the actual neglect. This assumption is supported by other evidence, that points to the continued teaching of the quadrivial arts at both Oxford and Paris. For example, in accounts of the careers of three men associated with Oxford and Paris at the close of the twelfth and the beginning of the thirteenth century, namely "Hugues" the physician, Alexander Neckam, and St. Edmund (Edmund of Abingdon), Archbishop of Canterbury, note is taken of the fact that they studied and possibly taught the arts of the *Quadrivium*. "Hugues", according to his epitaph, "a clever physician" (d. 1199), reportedly "taught the *Quadrivium*" in the University of Paris.[27] Alexander Neckam (d. 1217), who apparently divided his student and teaching career between Paris and Oxford, included a discussion of the arts of the *Quadrivium* in both his *De*

21. ST. THOMAS, *In VI Eth.*, lect. 7, in *Opera omnia*, Paris, 1875, Vol. XXV, p. 503. See also *St. Thomas Aquinas Philosophical Texts*, selected and translated with an introduction by Thomas GILBY, Oxford University Press, 1951, p. 10-11.

22. *Opus maius*, IV, Dist. I, chap. 3; BRIDGES ed., I, p. 108; BURKE trans., I, p. 126-27.

23. *Opus maius*, IV, Dist. I, chap. 1; *Opus tertium*, chap. 6.

24. BACON, *Epistola ad Opus minus ad Clementem IV*, ed. J. S. BREWER, *Opera hactenus inedita*, London, 1859, p. 323; also *Opus minus, loc.cit.*, p. 327.

25. *Ibid.*, p. 327: "Studium parisiense adhuc non habuit usum istarum quinque scientiarum," i.e., mathematics, perspective, experimental science and alchemy.

26. See the brief appraisal of Roger Bacon in H. RASHDALL, *Medieval Universities*, III, p. 242 seq.; also Lynn THORNDIKE, *A History of Magic and Experimental Science during the First Thirteen Centuries of our Era*, 2 vols., New York, 1923, II, Chap. LXI, especially p. 634 et seq.

27. E. LESNE, *Histoire de la propriété ecclésiastique en France (*Facultés catholiques de Lille. *Mémoires et travaux*, fasc. 50, tom. V: *Les écoles de la fin du VIIIe siècle à la fin du XIIe*), V, Lille, 1940, p. 252. His epitaph is reproduced by C. E. DU BOULAY, *Historia*

natura rerum and in the versified or metrical paraphrase of that work, *De laudibus divinae sapientiae*.[28] He especially satirized the manner in which the mathematical disciplines of the *Quadrivium* (he does not use the term), that is, arithmetic, music, geometry, and astronomy, were taught by members of the University of Paris. They took cognizance, he affirmed, of one point of view only, the positive, except when the demonstrator used the argument of reducing to an impossibility. He also went on to show the correspondence between the seven arts and the seven planets, and concluded that "Just as the latter give light to the world, just so do the seven arts adorn and fortify the intellective arts (*artes ingenuae*)."[29] The third witness to the continuity of the *Quadrivium*, St. Edmund of Abingdon, Archbishop of Canterbury, 1233, is said to have studied both at Paris and Oxford and to have lectured on the *Quadrivium* at Oxford in the first quarter of the thirteenth century, before he obeyed the admonition from heaven to devote himself without reservation to theology.[30]

Still other evidence is provided by the two guides or manuals mentioned earlier, which also attest to the presence of the quadrivial arts as a part of the curriculum of the University of Paris in the first half of the thirteenth century century. The pseudo-Boethius and his commentator instructed students not to omit the quadrivial arts, arithmetic, geometry, astrology (*sic* in the words of the commentator), and music.[31] Furthermore, the summary or guide prepared probably between 1230 and 1240 by an anonymous master of arts at Paris for candidates taking the examinations for the baccalaureate and the license in arts,[32] included the quadrivial or mathematical arts, astronomy, geometry, arithmetic, and music. However, these arts are now classified as a subdivision of natural philosophy, one of the three philosophies into which the subject matter taught was divided, the other two comprising rational (grammar, rhetoric and logic) and moral philosophy. The mathematical arts, all of them concerned with quantity, as here indicated, made up only one of the three divisions of natural philosophy, the other two being metaphysics and physics.[33]

As the tract by the anonymous master of arts indicates, the quadrivial arts together with those of the *Trivium* no longer constituted the sole offerings in the arts curriculum. Attention to this fundamental change was also drawn by St. Thomas Aquinas. He asserted that the old divisions into *Trivium* and *Quadrivium* were no longer adequate to encompass the whole of speculative philosophy.[34]

universitatis parisiensis, 6 vols., Paris, 1665-1673, II, p. 749:

Physicus excellens. . .
Quadrivium docuit, ac totum scire reliquos
anno millesimo bis centum, sed minus uno.

28. ALEXANDER NECKAM, *De naturis rerum libri duo*, with the Poem of the same author, *De laudibus divinae sapientiae*, edited, with a long introduction, by Thomas WRIGHT, in *RBMAS*, 34 (1863), chap. 173, p. 283 et seq. On Alexander Neckam, see L. THORNDIKE, *History of Magic and Experimental Science*, II, chap. XLIII; also RASHDALL, *Medieval Universities*, III, 28 and note.

29. ALEXANDER NECKAM, *De natura rerum*, p. 283-284, 293 et seq. for the mathematical arts; also p. 362-65; and the *De laudibus*, p. 497-503.

30. D. KNOWLES in *Lexikon für Theologie und Kirche*, Freiburg, 1959, III, p. 662-63; *Histoire littéraire de la France*, XVI; DU BOULAY, *Historia*, III, p. 101; H. RASHDALL, *Medieval Universities*, III, p. 238-39, and notes.

31. *PL*, LXIV, 1223-1238; THOMAS AQUINAS, *Opera omnia* 1875, XXVI, p. 591.

32. *Ripoll 109*, fol. 134r-137v; GRABMANN, *loc.cit.*, 1936, II, p. 188-199.

33. *Ibid.*, II, p. 188-199; *Ripoll 109*, fol. 134r-137v.

34. THOMAS AQUINAS, *In lib. Boetii De trinitate*, Quaest. V, art. 1, ad primum. . . ad tertium, *Opera omnia*, Paris, 1875, XXVIII, p. 525 et seq.

For St. Thomas Aquinas, whose classification differs from that of the anonymous master, speculative philosophy comprised a threefold division into mathematical, natural, and divine. Hence the *Quadrivium*, as the mathematical section, constituted only one third of speculative philosophy. In his program of studies, as indicated earlier, mathematical arts follow those of the *Trivium*, and especially logic. They should precede studies in natural philosophy or physics which require experience (*experimentum*), since, in St. Thomas' opinion, the mathematical arts would prepare the mind, or open the way, for the apprehension and understanding of the other physical or natural disciplines.[35]

Before turning for additional evidence to the materials relating to the individual mathematical arts, it may be of interest to note that there were carried over from Antiquity two major groupings or, as Baur pointed out, orders of succession. The first is the Nichomachean: arithmetic, music, geometry (or the variant geometry, music), and astronomy; the second, the Varronean: geometry, arithmetic, astronomy and music. This latter or Varronean type was carried over from Antiquity by Martianus Capella. It also appears in the variant: music, arithmetic, geometry, and astronomy.[36] Roger Bacon makes use of the Varronean type: geometry, arithmetic, astronomy and music; whereas St. Thomas Aquinas follows the Nichomachean order of arithmetic first. And we shall follow his lead and consider first the status in the universities of arithmetic, the science of numbers and a species of quantity.

The importance of arithmetic in the university curriculum, regardless of where it was placed in the listing of the quadrivial arts, appears to have been generally accepted.[37] St. Thomas pointed out that arithmetic formed the principal part of mathematics and preceded geometry, including perspective, as well as astrology and music.[38] Roger Bacon similarly attested the importance of arithmetic. Although he placed it second among the mathematical arts, he was careful to call attention to the fact that geometry and astronomy or astrology both make use of what arithmetic teaches.[39] Arithmetic at Paris was apparently taught from earlier texts of Greek and Moslem origin, in Latin translation, as well as from contemporary works based on these two traditions. The principal text of Greek origin was the arithmetic of Boethius, that is his paraphrase or translation of the work of Nichomachus of Gerasia (*fl.*100 A.D.). This work was named as the text in arithmetic by the anonymous master of arts in his summary for students in arts at Paris. He there designated the author of the work as Nichomachus and Boethius as the translator, and thus, as Mgr. Grabmann has pointed out, clearly registered his judgment (which coincides with that of modern scholarship) regarding the authorship of the *Institutio arithmeticae.*[40] This treatise, as the work of

35. *Ibid.*; also *In VI Eth.*, lect. 7, *Opera omnia*, XXV, p. 503.

36. BAUR, XVIII, p. 17-18.

37. For the whole question of teaching of arithmetic in the University, see the excellent summary and bibliography provided by Guy BEAUJOUAN, *L'enseignement de l'arithmétique élémentaire à l'Université de Paris aux XIIIe et XIVe siècles. De l'abaque à l'algorisme*, in *Homenaje à Millás-Vallicrosa*, I, Consejo superior de investigaciones cientificas, Barcelona, 1954, p. 93-124.

38. ST. THOMAS AQUINAS, *In XII libros Metaphysicorum*, in *Opera omnia*, Paris, 1875, XXIV, p. 468b.

39. ROGER BACON, *Opus maius*, IV, BRIDGES ed., I, p. 222-23; BURKE trans., I, p. 245.

40. GRABMANN, *MAG*, 1936, II, 189; *Ripoll 109*, fol. 134v. For various commentaries and texts on the arithmetic of Boethius, see L. THORNDIKE and P. KIBRE, *A Catalogue of*

Boethius, had constituted the standard medieval textbook for mathematical instruction in the pre-university schools.[41] In content it relates to theory of numbers as distinguished from the more elementary and practical abacus arithmetics and the books of calculation by means of *calculi* (pebbles), as well as from the later *algorismus.* In addition, there are extant a number of thirteenth century manuscripts containing tracts on the abacus and commentaries on them by such well known earlier medieval scholars as Bede, Gerbert, and others. But it is somewhat difficult to correlate these works with university teaching.[42]

Although the anonymous master of the first half of the thirteenth century made no mention of other arithmetical works than that of the Nichomachus-Boethian *Arithmetic*, it appears probable that in the second half of the century lectures incorporating the Hindu art of reckoning or the so-called Arabic numerals were already being used. A century had elapsed since the translations by Robert of Chester and possibly also by Gerard of Cremona of Abu' Abdallah Mohammed ibn Musa Al Khowarismi's systematic tract on algebra and also since the translations, possibly by Adelard of Bath and by John of Seville, of his arithmetic, from which the term Algorism was derived.[43] And in 1202 there had appeared the *Liber abaci* by Leonardo Fibonacci di Pisa, incorporating the Hindu numerals. However it is not possible to connect Leonardo Fibonacci di Pisa[44] with the northern universities. On the other hand, there is a strong likelihood that the works of another author, Jordanus Nemorarius,[45] on the Hindu numerals were being utilized for instruction in the universities of both Paris and Oxford in the later thirteenth century. The survival of a number of thirteenth century manuscripts of his works at Paris strongly supports this possibility.[46] Also Roger Bacon cited him on triangles and on weights, and was apparently acquainted with his other works.[47] These comprise an *Algorismus demonstratus,* an elementary tract on practical computations which explained the Arabic nu-

Incipits of Mediaeval Scientific Writings in Latin, new and augmented edition, Cambridge, Mass., Mediaeval Academy of America, 1963, Index; and for thirteenth century commentaries especially cols. 416, 682, 1587.

41. See further F. L. HEIBERG, *Geschichte der Mathematik und Naturwissenschaften in Altertum*, Munich, 1925, p. 49.

42. HALLIWELL, *Rara arithmetica*, 1841, p. 5-7, 27-28. For MSS of the authors named see THORNDIKE and KIBRE, *Catalogue of Incipits*, 1963, Index.

43. See ROBERT OF CHESTER's *Latin translation of the Algebra of al-Khowarizmi*, with an introduction, critical notes and an English translation by L. C. KARPINSKI, New York, The Macmillan Co., 1915; also L. C. KARPINSKI, *The History of Arithmetic*, 1925, reissued, New York, Russell and Russell Inc., 1965, p. 53 et seq.; and MOHAMMED IBN MUSA ALCHWARIZIMI's *Algorismus*, edited by Kurt VOGEL, Aalen, Otto Zeller Verlagsbuchhandlung, 1963. For other Latin translations, see THORNDIKE and KIBRE, *Catalogue of Incipits*, 1963, col. 624, and 1601.

44. *Ibid.*, col. 300, 302, 1414, for MSS and editions of this work; also M. CANTOR, *Vorlesungen über Geschichte d. Mathematik*, Leipzig, 1894, II, p. 3-35, 167, 205.

45. It is not clear that he was the same as Jordanus of Saxony, a member of the Dominican Order who was master of arts at Paris and author of a number of ecclesiastical writings as well as of a commentary on *Priscian minor*. For recent bibliography, see G. GERATHS, *Lexikon für Theologie und Kirchengeschichte*, V, Freiburg, 1960, 1120-22.

46. BEAUJOUAN, *loc. cit.*, p. 93; Beaujouan also notes that the library of Richard of Fournival, many of whose books could be traced back to the Sorbonne in 1271, included in addition to a *Liber algorismi*, the *Algorismus demonstratus*, the *Elementa arithmeticae*, and *De numeris datis* of JORDANUS NEMORARIUS as well as problems on progression. *Ibid.*, p. 104. For a long list of manuscripts of Jordanus Nemorarius' works, see especially CANTOR, II, 20.

47. ROGER BACON, *Opus maius*, BRIDGES ed., I, p. 158, 169 and notes; BURKE trans., I, p. 179, 190-95.

merals and the various methods of operation;[48] also an *Arithmetica demonstratus* on the theory of numbers, which treats progressively of proportions of numbers and although depending largely on Boethius, makes use of letters as general symbols instead of particular numbers.[49] In addition, a further treatise by Nemorarius on algebra, *De numeris datis,* made use of general symbols,[50] and he also composed others related to fractions, proportion and triangles.[51] However, the two manuals on Hindu numerals that apparently served university needs best, judging from the extent to which they were copied and recopied, were composed by scholars closely associated with the University of Paris. The first of these was the versified *Carmen de algorismo* composed by Alexander de Villedieu (c. 1203 or c. 1220),[52] who is also well known for his widely adopted new grammar, the *Doctrinale.* And the second, in prose, was the *Algorismus vulgaris* by John Halifax or Sacrobosco (c. 1230-40),[53] who was similarly represented in the university curriculum by another textbook, namely his work on astronomy, the *Sphaera.* Although of English origin, Sacrobosco's association with the University of Paris in the thirteenth century is supported, the late Professor Lynn Thorndike noted, by a number of manuscripts of his works dating from this time, and by the fact that he is mentioned by a contemporary thirteenth century scholar as at Paris. There is also extant a detailed and extended commentary, embodying the substance of his lectures on the work of Sacrobosco, by Peter of Dacia, which appeared at Paris in 1291.[54]

The study in the universities of the second mathematical art, that of geometry, described by Alexander Neckam and others as the science dealing with continuous immobile quantity,[55] was based primarily on Euclid's *Elements.* An analysis of the fifteen books of this work was provided by the anonymous master of arts at Paris, who named it as the textbook in use there.[56] The *Elementa geometriae,* known in the earlier Middle Ages in the Boethian

48. A brief analysis of this and the following works is given by Paul ABELSON, *The Seven Liberal Arts*, New York, 1939, reprinted New York, Russell and Russell Inc., 1965, p. 104 et seq. For editions and MSS, see THORNDIKE and KIBRE, *Catalogue of Incipits*, 1963, col. 237, 431, 958.

49. *Ibid.*, col. 812, 1030, 1600; also ABELSON, p. 105.

50. *Ibid.*, p. 105. THORNDIKE and KIBRE, *Catalogue of Incipits*, 1963, col. 959, 1455.

51. *Ibid.*, col. 398, 875, 1247; 1139; 260, 700 respectively.

52. *Ibid.*, col. 597, and for commentaries on it, see *ibid.*, Index; HALLIWELL, *Rara arithmetica*, 1841, p. 73; *Histoire littéraire*, XVI, p. 113. BEAUJOUAN, *loc.cit.*, p. 97, 106, notes that this work, which puts into verse the rules of al-Khowarizmi, was written between 1200 and 1203.

53. *Ibid.*, p. 16; the date of composition for Sacrobosco's work is here given as *ca.* 1250. See also L. C. KARPINSKI's introduction to his edition of ROBERT OF CHESTER's *Latin Translation of the Algebra of al-Khowarizmi*, New York, 1915, p. 16. Karpinski suggests *ca.* 1220 for the date of composition of Alexander's work.

54. THORNDIKE and KIBRE, *Catalogue of Incipits*, 1963, Index, under Sacrobosco; and *The Sphere of Sacrobosco and its Commentators*, edited and translated with introduction by Lynn THORNDIKE, Chicago, Illinois, University of Chicago Press, 1949, especially p. 2 et seq., 59. BEAUJOUAN, *loc. cit.*, p. 106, suggests that the *Sphere* was composed *ca.* 1230-1245.

55. "Geometria quae circa immobilem magnitudinem versatur". ALEXANDER NECKAM, p. 284. For the earlier enumerated threefold importance of geometry for technology, medicine or health and for the soul or philosophy, see H. M. KLINKENBERG, *Der Verfall des Quadriviums in frühen Mittelalter*, in *Artes liberales*, edited by Josef KOCH, Leiden-Köln, E. J. Brill, 1959, p. 5 et seq.

56. *Ripoll Ms. 109*, fol. 134r-v; GRABMANN, *MAG*, 1936, II, p. 189.

version,[57] had been translated in the twelfth century by Adelard of Bath,[58] and it was apparently also translated[59] and/or commented on in the thirteenth century by Campanus of Novara, a protégé of Urban IV.[60] The *Elementa* was the subject of further commentaries by Albertus Magnus and Roger Bacon.[61] In addition, there may have been utilized in the Universities of Paris and Oxford the *Practica geometriae* ascribed to Hugh (of St. Victor), composed in the twelfth century,[62] as well as the work of the same title by Leonardo Pisano.[63]

The concentration on geometry along with logic at the close of the twelfth and the beginning of the thirteenth century had aroused some contemporary comment. Pierre of Blois complained that students concerned themselves with reasoning on the point, line, and surface before they learned grammar.[64] Alain de Lille (d. 1202) defined the straight line, the curve, the circumflex, the triangle, the tetragon, and so on, and drew attention to the discussions and explanations of the *Elementa* of Euclid by masters of the university.[65]

The declared purpose of the study of geometry in thirteenth century university circles appears to have undergone an important change from that enunciated earlier. It was no longer deemed useful primarily as an instrument for land measurement, for medicine, or for philosophy, as had been previously asserted.[66] Rather, on the one hand, it was held to be a valuable tool for the study, understanding, and demonstration of theological truth. It was to this end, for example, that Alexander of Hales made use of Euclid's *Elements.*[67] And Roger Bacon went so far also as to maintain that the spiritual sense of Scripture could not be comprehended unless the literal sense was known. And this, in his opinion, could not be understood without knowing the significance of the terms and of the things signified, all of which could best be acquired through a study of geometry. No one, he held, could represent or describe these unless he was well

57. THORNDIKE and KIBRE, *Catalogue of Incipits*, 1963, col. 584, 870, 1126, 1216, 1234, 1258, 1591 and cf. 1692, for manuscripts and printed editions of the Boethian version.

58. *Ibid.*, 268, 584, 586, 726, 1123, 1152, for Adelard of Bath's translation.

59. For MSS incorporating this version, see *Salamanca 221*, 14th cent., fol. 1-177 (G. BEAUJOUAN, *Manuscrits scientifiques médiévaux de l'Université de Salamanque*, Bordeaux, Féret et fils, 1962, p. 66); and *Paris, Bibliothèque nationale 7292*, fol. 188r-245v.

60. THORNDIKE and KIBRE, *Catalogue of Incipits*, 1963, col. 1152, 1391-92 for CAMPANUS OF NOVARA's commentary on EUCLID'S *Elementa geometriae.* See also *Histoire littéraire de la France*, XVI, p. 114; and RASHDALL, III, p. 249 and notes.

61. THORNDIKE and KIBRE, *Catalogue of Incipits*, 1963, col. 1499 and 1574 respectively.

62. *Ibid.*, 1080, for manuscripts and editions of this work. Further manuscripts not named there are: *Cambridge, Gonville and Caius 413 (630)*, 12th-14th cent., fol. 2-8v; and, without name of author, *Paris, Bibliothèque nationale 14056*, fol. 247; *15362*, fol. 201, and *Mazarin 433 (717)*, fol. 1. It is not clear whether this *Practica geometriae* is the same as the copies of the *Practica geometriae* donated to St. Augustine's Abbey, Canterbury, by John of London, who has been identified with Roger Bacon's friend, friar John. See M. R. JAMES, *Ancient Libraries of Canterbury and Dover*, Cambridge University Press, 1903, p. 320. The library also had a number of other copies of EUCLID's *Geometry* with commentaries (*loc. cit.*).

63. THORNDIKE and KIBRE, *Catalogue of Incipits*, 1963, col. 1152, 1362, 1477.

64. PIERRE DE BLOIS, *Epist. 103*, as reported by *Histoire littéraire*, XVI, p. 115.

65. *Histoire littéraire*, XVI, p. 115, citing *Anti-Claud.*, III, c. 6 and 7.

66. H. M. KLINKENBERG, *Der Verfall des Quadriviums im frühen Mittelalter*, in *Artes liberales*, ed. by Josef KOCH, Leiden and Köln, 1959, p. 5.

67. ALEXANDER OF HALES, *Questio III de simplicitate divinae essentiae*: ". . . est exemplum hic de puncto: video enim punctum totum, quae non habet partem. . ." *Summa theologica*, ed. R. P. B. KLUMPE, O.F.M., Quaracchi, 1924, I, p. 51, b, n.

acquainted with Euclid's *Elements* and the works of Theodosius, Milleius and other geometricians.[68] Bacon gave as examples for the need for geometry to explain scripture, the ark of Noah and the temple of Solomon. He also compared the infusion of grace through the multiplication of light to the corporeal multiplication of light; and he noted the use of the triangle as the illustration of the Trinity. "Therefore," he affirmed, "I count nothing more fitting for a man diligent in the study of God's wisdom than the exhibition of geometrical forms . . . before his eyes."[69]

Bacon went on then to assert that "without doubt the whole truth of things in the world lies in the literal sense, . . . and especially of things relating to geometry, because we can understand nothing fully unless its form is presented before our eyes, and therefore in the Scripture of God, the whole knowledge of things to be defined by geometrical forms is contained and far better than mere philosophy could express it."[70]

On the other hand, aside from the avowed importance of geometry in the demonstration of theological truth, there was emphasized in thirteenth century university writings, if we so classify the works of Grosseteste and Roger Bacon, the particular importance of mathematics, and specifically of geometry in the study of nature or natural phenomena. Robert Grosseteste in his tract *On Lines, Angles, and Figures,* asserted that the study of geometry is of the greatest value, since it is impossible to know natural philosophy without it. Also since geometric lines, angles, and figures rule the universe, man cannot achieve a scientific understanding of nature without mathematics and especially geometry.[71] Furthermore, according to Grosseteste, and as pointed out by Crombie, mathematical science and geometry in particular could often provide the reason (*propter quid*) for factual knowledge acquired through the physical sciences.[72] And this line of thought is similarly developed by Roger Bacon in his tract entitled *De multiplicatione specierum* as well as in the *Opus tertium.*[73]

On the third of the quadrivial arts, namely music, although the university statutes are mute, other evidence similarly attests the continuing concern with this subject as one of the mathematical arts, in university circles in the thirteenth century. The anonymous master of arts again provides the essential information

68. BACON, *Opus maius*, BRIDGES ed., I, p. 211, and note; BURKE trans., I, p. 233. In regard to Theodosius it is of interest to note that a catalogue of books of the Sorbonne in 1290 contains a Latin translation, made probably from the Arabic, of the geometry of Theodosius: *Histoire littéraire*, XXIV, p. 478-79. As there noted, there are listed in addition several Latin tracts on *planimetria* and *stereometria* with commentaries, as well as a *Practica geometria* in both Latin and French. See also for THEODOSIUS, *De sphaera,* translated by GERARD OF CREMONA, THORNDIKE and KIBRE, *Catalogue of Incipits,* 1963, col. 1523 and for MILLEIUS or MENELAOS, *Libri de figuris sphericis,* also translated by GERARD OF CREMONA, *ibid,,* col. 397.

For manuscripts of the *planimetria*, *ibid*., 1545; and *stereometria*, *ibid*., 26, 34, etc. (see Index). However, the MSS are all of the 14th-15th centuries.

69. ROGER BACON, *Opus maius*, BRIDGES ed., I, p. 210-12; BURKE trans., I, p. 232-33; 234, for the quotation.

70. *Ibid*., BRIDGES ed., I, 212; BURKE trans., I, 234, for the quotation.

71. GROSSETESTE, *De lineis, angulis, et figuris seu de fractionibus et reflexionibus radiorum*, edited by L. BAUR, in *BGPMA*, IX (1912), p. 5 et seq., 59-60, 65-66. See also BAUR, *BGPMA,* XVIII, p. 98; A. C. CROMBIE, *Grosseteste and Experimental Science,* 1953, p. 50; and the recent stimulating study by Olaf PEDERSEN, *Du quadrivium à la physique*, in *Artes liberales*, ed. Josef KOCH, Leiden-Köln, E. J. Brill, 1959, especially p. 120 et seq.

72. CROMBIE, p. 51-52; BAUR, *BGPMA,* IX (1912), p. 59 et seq.

73. BAUR, *ibid*, XVII, 4-6 (1917), p. 98 et seq.

on music as a part of the curriculum and of the textbook in use, namely the *De musica* of Boethius.[74] And the pseudo-Boethius, together with his commentator, confirmed the presence of music as one of the quadrivial arts that should not be omitted or bypassed by the student.[75] To what extent the *De musica* of Boethius was supplemented in the instruction on the subject by other, more contemporary, writings, it is not possible to determine. Of the several authors of such works composed in the thirteenth century, the *Histoire littéraire* lists a French priest Elias Salomon author of *De scientia artis musicae,* dedicated to Gregory IX;[76] Marchetus of Padua, who composed an *Ars musicae* and a tract entitled *Musicae mensuratae*, as well as a commentary on the work of Franco of Cologne;[77] also Engelbert of Admont,[78] Jerome de Moravia, and so on.[79] As the *Histoire littéraire* further notes, these works attempted to explain the relation between sounds, the rules of chant and of musical composition.

The attachment to music and its significance as one of the important mathematical arts is further explained by Robert Grosseteste and Roger Bacon. In his definition of music, Grosseteste generally followed the lead of Hugh of St. Victor, who lived a century earlier,[80] and he divided music into three parts, that is, music of the universe, man-made music, and instrumental. He noted also that music comprises harmony and rhythm;[81] and his view is concurred in by Roger Bacon.[82] Grosseteste further brought music into a consideration with medicine, particularly in regard to the medical significance of music and its influence on health.[83] He cited Haly, *De regimine regali,* in his discussion of the necessity of a knowledge of music for the physician, as did Roger Bacon who makes a like assertion.[84] On the relation further of music and medicine, Grosseteste also pointed out that the concern is not with the organ affected by the bodily motions produced by music but with the moderation produced through these motions.[85]

The effect of music on mind and body and in arousing men to action apparently also entered into the university discussions on the subject. Alexander Neckam in relating the planets with each of the seven liberal arts had associated Mars with music, and had thus emphasized the potency of instrumental music in calling armed men into battle.[86] And this aspect of music was included in the

74. *Ripoll 109* fol. 135; GRABMANN, *MAG*, 1936, II, p. 189-90. For manuscripts and editions of this work, see THORNDIKE and KIBRE, *Catalogue of Incipits*, 1963, col. 897, 1006, 1126, 1297; analysis and commentaries, 36, 188, 542, 687, 950, 1160, 1183; extracts, 1226.

75. PS-BOETHIUS, *PL*, LXIV, 1234; THOMAS AQUINAS, *Opera omnia*, Paris, 1875, XXVI, p. 591; see also *Histoire littéraire*, XVI, p. 258.

76. *Ibid*., XVI, p. 267-68; XXI, 503-5.

77. THORNDIKE and KIBRE, *Catalogue of Incipits*, 1963, col. 442, 1291; and for the commentary on Franco of Cologne, *ibid*., col. 310, 1083.

78. *Ibid*., col. 896, 1143.

79. *Ibid*., col. 896, 1308, 1703.

80. HUGH OF ST. VICTOR, *Didascalicon*, II, 12; ed. H. BUTTIMER, 1939, p. 32.

81. BAUR, *BGPMA*, XVIII, p. 18-21.

82. R. BACON, *Op. tert*., ep. 60, BREWER ed., p. 232. Baur indicates that this view is based on the *De ortu scientiarum* and on ST. AUGUSTINE, *De musica*. See also BACON, *Opus maius*, BRIDGES ed., I, p. 214 et seq.; BURKE trans., I, p. 236 et seq.

83. BAUR, *BGPMA*, XVIII, p. 18-22, 25.

84. *Ibid*., XVIII, 22; ROGER BACON, *Opus tert*., ep. 60, BREWER ed., p. 232.

85. GROSSETESTE, *De artibus liberalibus*, text ed. BAUR, *BGPMA*, XVIII, p. 2-4.

86. ALEXANDER NECKAM, p. 284.

study of harmony which generally stressed the mathematical side of music. The specific role of harmony in arousing the passions or in elevating moral virtues was a topic of disputation as the titles of two *Quodlibeta* on these topics by Pierre d'Auvergne, professor of theology at Paris between 1296 and 1302, indicate.[87]

The question, too, of which was preferable, instrumental or vocal music, in regard to the effects produced was also discussed. St. Thomas Aquinas noted on this question that although both instrumental music and songs are found in the Old Testament, the church preferred the second because they are of greater moral worth. The first or instrumental music, in St. Thomas' opinion, since it leads to bodily pleasure or enjoyment, is against wisdom.[88] In this regard he differed greatly from Roger Bacon, who particularly stressed the part that music plays in providing the relaxation necessary to the health of mind and body. "The prophet Elijah," Bacon noted, "bade the lute be brought, in order that his soul, stirred by the delight of physical harmony, might be caught up to contemplate divine things."[89]

The importance of the study of music for the theologian was especially emphasized by Roger Bacon. He did not claim, however, that the study of music is necessarily essential for an understanding of Scripture. However, he did hold that the theologian should have a practical acquaintance with singing, with instruments, and with other musical things, including the dance. He should have an understanding of their composition and their use in a mystical sense, as well as knowledge of the theory underlying them. He should derive this knowledge, Bacon asserted, from the various writings on the subject in conjunction with a consideration of the practical and theoretical nature of the materials. The theologian, Bacon went on to explain, needs such information because Scripture is full of musical terms like rejoice, shout for joy, and so on; as well as with the names of such musical instruments as the cithara, cymbals, and the like. Finally, Bacon added, the theologian should derive from his study of the musical art an understanding of the theories underlying the accents, melody, and meters of the sacred text, even though grammar provides the practical rules for them.[90]

On the university teaching of astronomy, the fourth of the mathematical arts, there is evidence similar to that for the other arts. The commentator on the pseudo-Boethius placed astrology or astronomy first among the quadrivial arts, and the anonymous master indicated Ptolemy as the principal author utilized at Paris.[91] However, other than the *Almagest,* which is named, it is not clear what other works were lectured on or taught by the university professors.[92] Ptolemy's *Almagest* was, to be sure, one of the most important sources of astronomical

87. CROMBIE, *Robert Grosseteste*, p. 92; PIERRE D'AUVERGNE, *Quodlibeta*, VI (1301 Christmas), in *BibTh,* V (1925), p. 257, 263: 15. "Utrum harmoniae musicales sint excitativae passionum, puta raptus vel aliorum huiusmodi". 16. "Utrum harmoniae musicae ad mores valeant seu virtutes".

88. THOMAS AQUINAS, *Summa theologica,* IIa-IIae, q. 91, 2, 4-5, in *Opera omnia*, 1875, IV, p. 76.

89. BACON, *Opus maius*, Moral philos., Pt. III, chap. 21, BRIDGES ed., I, p. 365; BURKE translation, II, p. 786, which I here quote.

90. *Ibid.*, BRIDGES ed., I, p. 236, and note 2; BURKE trans., I, p. 259-260.

91. *Ripoll ms 109*, fol. 134r-v (GRABMANN, *loc.cit.*, 1936, p. 186); *PL,* LXIV, 1229; THOMAS AQUINAS, *Opera omnia*, 1875, XXVI, p. 601.

92. As indicated by GRABMANN, *loc.cit.*, 1936, p. 186 et seq., the information on textbooks in the *Ripoll MS* is unclear.

knowledge transmitted by Antiquity. It had become available for use by western scholars in the Latin translations from both Greek and Arabic made in the course of the twelfth century,[93] and it apparently provided the chief subject for disputations in astronomy by university professors at Paris as elsewhere. However, there is evidence that there were a goodly number of other works on astronomy available for university use in the thirteenth century. In this connection it is of interest to note that the anonymous list of textbooks dating from the close of the twelfth and the early thirteenth centuries, which Professor Haskins associated with Paris, does not mention the *Almagest.* It names only Ptolemy's *Canons,* and the astronomical works of Alfraganus which had also been translated in the course of the twelfth century.[94] Materials on the science of the stars, it need scarcely be asserted, had been greatly augmented in the twelfth and thirteenth centuries by the translations not only of the *Almagest* but also of the works of a number of Moslem astronomers as well as by the introduction of astronomical manuals and tables from Spain.[95] From the return of Adelard of Bath from Cordova in the twelfth century, bringing with him to England and France the rudiments of Moslem astronomical learning,[96] the process of transmission of such knowledge by way of Latin translations continued on into the thirteenth century, especially in the court of Frederick II.[97]

At Paris, considerable attention appears to have been given to Ptolemy's *Almagest,* as noted above. The Latin translation of this work was utilized along with the writings of such Moslem astronomers as Alfraganus and Albategni by John of Sacrobosco in the composition of his *Sphaera mundi,* a work which was itself to become the chief astromical textbook and subject of commentaries or lectures in the thirteenth and succeeding centuries.[98] John of Sacrobosco, it might also be noted, composed in France his treatises on the calendar (*Computus*), on the astrolabe, and possibly also that on the *Quadrant* attributed to him.[99]

Several other university scholars at Paris concerned themselves with astronomy, and those of whom mention might be made utilized Ptolemy's *Almagest* along with works of Moslem astronomers. This was true, for example, of William of Auvergne, Bishop of Paris (1228-1248). In his *De universo* especially, he exhibited his acquaintance with the above authors. However, following Alpetragius, as Duhem noted, William of Auvergne challenged and opposed a number of Ptolemy's doctrines, and specifically that of the hypothesis

93. C. H. HASKINS, *Studies in the History of Mediaeval Science*, Cambridge, Mass., Harvard University Press, 1927, p. 53 seq., 103-110, 157-165; P. DUHEM, *Le système du monde*, Paris, reprint edition by Hermann, 1958, III, 216 et seq. For further manuscripts and editions, see THORNDIKE and KIBRE, *Catalogue of Incipits*, 1963, Index, col. 179-180, 263, (comm.) 348, 479, 818, 1035-6, 1082, 1245, 1359, 1421.

94. HASKINS, *Studies in Mediaeval Science*, p. 369.

95. P. DUHEM, *Le système du monde*, III, chap. V et seq.

96. HASKINS, *Studies in Mediaeval Science*, chap. II; L. THORNDIKE, *History of Magic and Experimental Science*, 1923, II, chap. XXXVI. For a large number of astronomical manuscripts dating from the thirteenth century, see L. DELISLE, *Bibliothèque de l'École des Chartes*, 1871, p. 47 et seq., p. 463-65.

97. HASKINS, *Studies in Mediaeval Science,* p. 245 et seq.

98. L. THORNDIKE, *The Sphere of Sacrobosco and its Commentators*, Chicago, University of Chicago Press, 1949.

99. *Ibid.*, p. 3-4.

of epicycles and excentrics.[100] Moreover, both Albert Magnus and St. Thomas Aquinas are credited with having made an abbreviated version of the *Almagest.*[101] Albertus Magnus further wrote a tract or commentary on the sphere of the stars,[102] and perhaps also composed the *Speculum astronomiae,* which appears under his name.[103] St. Thomas, too, may have composed other tracts on astronomy. Among those attributed to him are the *De iudiciis astrorum*[104] and *De motoribus corporum celestium.*[105] Similarly, Robert Grosseteste, Bishop of Lincoln, who like John of Sacrobosco, spent the greater part of his teaching career in Paris, made use of the works of Ptolemy, together with those of Moslem authors, for his astronomical writings, particularly on the *Sphere* and on the calendar (*De arte computi*).[106] And his disciple, Roger Bacon, utilized, in addition to the works of Ptolemy, those of Albategni, Thebit, Arzachel, and Alfraganus.[107]

Moreover, Bacon like Robert Grosseteste, well known for his interest in astronomical studies, in his discussion of astronomy in the *Opus maius,* differentiated between what he termed theoretical astrology or astronomy, and practical astrology. Theoretical astrology or astronomy, he asserted, considers the heights, size, number or quantities of all celestial bodies and of celestial phenomena reduced to quantity, discontinuous as well as continuous. He noted the information provided by Ptolemy, Alfraganus and the other astronomers on the number of the heavens and of the stars, their size, shape, and magnitude, and their distances from the earth, insofar as this could be ascertained by means of instruments. He considered also their accounts of the rising and setting of the signs of the stars, and the numbers and varieties of eclipses. However, according to Bacon, theoretical astronomy is not limited to the celestial orbs alone, it deals also with such matters as the size and shape of the habitable earth, the great divisions which are called climes and the differences in the horizons and in the days and nights in varying climes.[108] Bacon went on next to consider practical astrology. The latter, he explained, enables us to know the aspects, actions, and all the changes that take place in the heavenly bodies. It considers comets, rainbows, and all the other changing phenomena in the air, and provides data on their positions, altitudes, magnitudes and forms. And the astronomer can obtain this information, Bacon asserted, by using suitable instruments, by tables and by

100. DUHEM, *Le système du monde*, III, p. 249 et seq., 252 et seq.; THORNDIKE and KIBRE, *Catalogue of Incipits*, 1963, cols. 1067, 1401.

101. *Ibid.*, col. 1006.

102. *Histoire littéraire*, XVI, 118; THORNDIKE and KIBRE, *Catalogue of Incipits*, 1963, col. 1602.

103. *Ibid.*, col. 975, for MSS and editions.

104. *Ibid.*, col. 154, 536, 1227.

105. *Ibid.*, col. 1201.

106. ROBERT GROSSETESTE, *De sphaera*, ed. BAUR, *BGPMA*, IX, 10 ff.; also BAUR, *ibid.*, XVIII, p. 26. For other manuscripts and editions, see THORNDIKE and KIBRE, *Catalogue of Incipits*, 1963, cols. 289, 761-763, and for his other works relating to astronony, *ibid.*, Index, col. 1813.

107. BAUR, XVIII, 46; on Roger Bacon's work at Paris, see DUHEM, III, p. 260 et seq., and especially 265 et seq.; and see *Opus maius*, Pt. IV, BRIDGES ed., I, 224 et sq., BURKE trans., I, 246 et seq. For astronomical works under his name, see further THORNDIKE and KIBRE, *Catalogue of Incipits*, 1963, col. 504, 1281, 1547, and Index cols. 1755-56, for other of his works.

108. *Opus maius*, Pt. IV, BRIDGES ed., I, p. 109, 224 et seq.; 376 et seq.; BURKE trans., I, p. 128; 246 et seq.; 391 et seq.

canons or specific rules formulated for such verification. Bacon went on then to note the practical application of the knowledge derived from such observations and studies in human affairs here on earth, in the making of judgments regarding the present, the past, and the future.[109] Bacon thus accepted in astrology the efficacy of general predictions. These were based upon the principle, he maintained, that the human body was in fact affected by some exterior causes and was subject to celestial influences. Bacon went on further to explain that the soul could be stimulated or directed toward certain actions which could not necessarily be determined, yet could be foreseen or foretold.[110]

Of the usefulness of astronomy and of its importance to other sciences as well as to men in all walks of life, both Robert Grosseteste and Roger Bacon appear to have had no doubt. Grosseteste held that astronomy assists other sciences such as alchemy, medicine, botany and gardening, that is, the growing of plants and vegetables. He noted that it is also necessary for naval science or navigation.[111] Furthermore, according to Roger Bacon, astronomy is as necessary to rulers of both church and state as it is to the navigator, farmer, alchemist and physician, especially for the election of favorable times.[112]

Moreover, Robert Grosseteste, Roger Bacon and other scholars in the French *studium* concerned themselves with other astronomical and closely allied mathematical matters in addition to those already named. They wrote on refraction, perspective, and on the calendar. On the last named, there appears to have been a considerable interest particulary in the University of Paris. Both Roger Bacon and Robert Grosseteste were concerned with the reform of the calendar while Alexander of Villedieu and John of Sacrobosco composed general tracts on the *Computus* or church calendar.[113] And the recognition of the importance of adequate and more precise measurement was reflected in further treatises on astronomical instruments, of which the work done at Paris by Franco de Polonia on the construction of the astronomical instrument called *Torquetus* is the most worthy of note.[114]

Similarly in Oxford, in the second half of the thirteenth century, astronomy was an important subject of study in the newly established Merton College. Although Walter of Merton had formulated statutes for a college expressly for the training of secular clerks, the College became prominent especially as a school for astronomy, on the foundations laid down, as Professor Crombie has

109. *Ibid.*, Pt. IV, BRIDGES ed., I, p. 109-110; 376 et seq.; BURKE trans., I, p. 128; 392 et seq.; *Histoire littéraire*, XVI, p. 118.

110. *Opus maius*, BRIDGES ed., I, 276 et seq.; 376 et seq.; BURKE trans., I, 291 et seq.; 392 et seq.

111. GROSSETESTE, *De artibus liberalibus*, ed. BAUR, p. 4-7; BAUR, *BGPMA*, XVIII, p. 22-23; ROGER BACON, *Opus minus*, ed. BREWER, p. 313 et seq., 375-89; ROGER BACON, *Communia naturalia*, I, 1, Dist. 1, chap. 2 (*Opera hactenus inedita Rogeri Baconi*, fasc. III).

112. *Opus tertium*, ed. A. G. LITTLE, 1912, p. 12-14; also in his introduction to the *Secretum secretorum*, p. 8.

113. THORNDIKE and KIBRE, *Catalogue of Incipits*, 1963, col. 167, 643, 826-27, 1557, and for the various commentaries on them, see *ibid.*, Index, col. 1729; also the *Computus ecclesiasticus*, *ibid.*, col. 1165.

114. *Ibid.*, col. 383, 1463, 1476; *Histoire littéraire*, XVI, p. 118.

shown, by Robert Grosseteste and Roger Bacon, both of whom may actually not have been members of the Merton school.[115]

In conclusion, it might be asserted on the basis of the foregoing study, especially of the University of Paris, that the mathematical or quadrivial arts, although no longer in their traditional framework, did continue into the thirteenth century to constitute an integral part of the university arts curriculum. That is, they were now one part of one of the three philosophies making up the arts curriculum. Attention to this fact was drawn by the anonymous master of arts, who in about 1230 or 1240, composed a manual in the form of questions for candidates preparing for the examination for the baccalaureate and for the license to teach. According to the anonymous master of arts, the mathematical arts were one of the three divisions making up natural philosophy, the other two being metaphysics, which he had precede the mathematical arts, and physics, which he had follow. St. Thomas Aquinas, too, had pointed up the new organization of the arts curriculum. He corroborated the fact that the mathematical arts were only one of the subdivisions of one of the three philosophies. But he placed them as one of the three subdivisions of speculative philosophy, the other two divisions being rational (grammar, rhetoric, and logic), which, according to St. Thomas, should precede mathematics; and *physica* or natural science, which should follow. That is, St. Thomas along with other of his contemporaries, namely Robert Grosseteste and Roger Bacon, held the view that mathematics provided the gateway for natural science or physics.

Of the other sources providing evidence on the mathematical arts in the university teaching and which have been only lightly tapped for this study, mention has been made of the biographies and of the works of scholars who were members of the university at Paris as well as at Oxford, also of extant manuscripts containing works on mathematical subjects belonging to the thirteenth century at Paris, as well as of thirteenth century collections of *Quodlibeta* and *Questiones disputatae.* All these attest the concern with the mathematical arts at Paris. To what extent similar evidence can be compiled for the other universities of the thirteenth century is still a matter of conjecture. Until such evidence is found and studied, the actual status of the mathematical arts or the traditional *Quadrivium* in the other thirteenth century universities remains an open question.

115. GUNTHER, *Early Science at Oxford*, II, p. 31 et *passim*. See also on the Oxford school, A. C. CROMBIE, *Grosseteste and Experimental Science*, Oxford, Clarendon Press, 1953, p. 187-188, and notes.

II

THE BOETHIAN *DE INSTITUTIONE ARITHMETICA* AND THE *QUADRIVIUM* IN THE THIRTEENTH CENTURY UNIVERSITY MILIEU AT PARIS

Although the Boethian *Arithmetica* has already received attention from scholars concerned with Boethius' place in the cultural history of western Europe in the middle ages,[1] the specific role that this work played in the framework of the *quadrivium* in the thirteenth century French university milieu has so far not been set forth. It is this lacuna that the present study would endeavor to fill. Before turning to this task, however, a brief review or account of the nature of the work and of its history in the west before the close of the twelfth century may be in order. The so-called Boethian *Arithmetica* is the Latin translation or paraphrase by Anicius Manlius Boethius of the Greek text of the *De Institutione Arithmetica* of Nicomachus of Gerasa, who flourished about 100 A.D., and was a popularizer of neo-Pythagorean doctrines.[2] Like the Pythagoreans he stressed the importance of the theory or philosophy of numbers

1 The most comprehensive work on Boethius in the Middle Ages is that of H.R. Patch, *The Tradition of Boethius: A Study of His Importance in Medieval Culture* (New York: Oxford University Press, 1935). Professor Patch has incorporated the information of the chief writers on the subject who wrote before him on Boethius. Although Professor Patch brought his account up through the fifteenth century his focus was general and literary in nature and he did not relate the work specifically to the thirteenth century university milieu. For recent estimates of Boethius, see the article by Lorenzo Minio-Paluello in the *Dictionary of Scientific Biography*; also, William H. Stahl, *Roman Science* (Madison: The University of Wisconsin Press, 1962), pp. 198 ff. and Gillian R. Evans, articles, especially Introductions to Boethius's „Arithmetica" of the 10th to the 14th century in *History of Science*, 16 (1978), 22-41.

2 See especially Nicomachus of Gerasa, *Introduction to Arithmetic*, trans. by M.L. D'Ooge, with studies in Greek arithmetic by F.E. Robbins and L.C. Karpinski (*University of Michigan Studies*, Humanistic Series, XVI; New York: Macmillan, 1926); David Eugene Smith, *History of Mathematics* (2 vols., New York: Ginn and Co., 1951-53), I, pp. 127-29, 178-79; also Sir Thomas Heath, *A History of Greek Mathematics* (2 vols., Oxford: Clarendon Press, 1921), I, pp. 10 ff. A critical edition of Boethius' *De Institutione Arithmetica* by G. Friedlein (Leipzig, 1867; reprinted: Minerva G.M.B.H., Frankfurt a.M., 1966), pp. 3-173, was made on the basis of eight MSS from Bamberg and Munich of the 10th through the 12th century. The text is also included among Boethius' *Opera omnia* in Migne's *Patrologia latina* (1860), LXIII, col. 1079-1168. A new edition of the *Arithmetica* has been announced by Professor Jean Schilling of Nancy as forthcoming in 1970, but so far has not appeared. MSS of the work are fairly numerous. In addition to the eight MSS utilized by Friedlein, and those listed by L. Thorndike and P. Kibre, in *A Catalogue of Incipits of Mediaeval Scientific Writings in Latin* (Cambridge, Mass.: Mediaeval Academy of America, new and revised edition, 1962, henceforth designated as TK), col. 465, 768, 959, 991; as well as those noted by Menso Folkerts, in his edition of *„Boetius" Geometrie II* (Wiesbaden: Franz Steiner Verlag GMBH, 1970), the following MSS have been noted: London, British Library (henceforth designated as BL) Arundel 339, 13th cent., ff. 1r-31r; Harleian 549, 10th cent.; 1737, only a part of the *Arithmetica*; 2510, 13th cent., ff. 136-167r; 3595, 10th cent., ff. 1r-48v; Lansdowne 842 B., 15th cent., ff. 1r-50v; New York, Columbia Univ. Plimpton MS c. 1294, indicated by D.E. Smith, I, 180; Paris, Bibliothèque Nationale (henceforth indicated as BN) 6401, 9th cent., ff. 15-138v; 6639, 10th cent., ff. 73-151; 7039, 10th cent., f. 95, incomplete; 7185, 9th cent., ff. 1-40v, Gloss, 12th cent., ff. 41r-47r; 7189, 12th cent., ff. 1-50; 13020, 9th cent.; 14064, 9th cent.; 14065, 13th cent.; 16201, 13th cent., ff. 6v-34; 17858, 10th cent., ff. 3ra-36ra; and it was also included in the library of Richard de Fournival 39, c. 1250 (Delisle, *Le Cabinet des MSS*, Paris, 1874, II, p. 526; Folkerts, p. 38).

under the Pythagorean principle that „all things that can be known have number" and „all things are numbers."[3] Under this aegis arithmetic was taken out of the realm of practical utility or commercial transactions and was raised to the level of speculative thought.

In preparing the *De Institutione Arithmetica* for Latin users, Boethius asserted that he had not made a literal translation of the Greek text but had rather given a free interpretation. He had condensed where Nicomachus was diffuse and expanded where further explanatory information seemed essential, adding formulas and demonstrations familiar to Latin scholars.[4] However, Boethius adhered to the general Pythagorean or neo-Pythagorean character of the Nicomachean text. That is he retained the philosophical rather than the mathematical side of arithmetic. In general, the work therefore had less appeal or application to mathematicians and those concerned with numerical calculation or simple reckoning than to philosophers and philosophy. The *De Institutione Arithmetica* in its Greek form had earlier drawn the attention of the second century Platonist, Apuleius of Madaura, who is credited with having translated it into Latin, although no trace of this version has as yet been found; also among others, of the fourth and fifth century neo-Platonists, Iamblichus and Proclus, both of whom commented on it, as well as of Martianus Capella, who cited the work possibly secondhand.[5] Moreover, in the Boethian translation or paraphrase, the Nicomachean *De Institutione Arithmetica* came to provide the basic text in western Europe for the study of arithmetic in its philosophical or theoretical rather than practical aspects. By its content Latin scholars were introduced to the divisions of numbers and their nature and properties, and were provided with a vocabulary and descriptive account of mathematical forms and terms. These comprised, among others, even and odd numbers, numbers separate and unified, absolute and relative, prime, deficient or defective numbers, perfect, abundant or redundant or overperfect numbers, linear numbers, rectalinear, polygonal, triangular, quadratic, pentagonal, hexagonal, heptagonal numbers, also solids, cubic, pyramidal, and circular or spherical numbers, as well as the ratios or proportions and proportionalities of numbers. In addition there were descriptions of the relation between arithmetic and geometry, or arithmetical geometry, and of harmonic proportion in the sense of Pythagoras and Plato.[6]

Boethius' translation of the *De Institutione Arithmetica* may well have been part of his general plan to make available in Latin the Greek writings essential for the study and mastery of the seven liberal arts as a prelude to the quest for wisdom or philosophic truth. In the schema canonized in the medieval schools, the four mathematical arts, arithmetic, music, geometry, and astronomy, or the *quadrivium*, generally followed the first three of the arts,

The Arithmetica was first printed separately at Augsburg, Ratdolt, 1488 (Arnold C. Klebs, *Incunabula Scientifica et Medica*, Bruges: The Saint Catherine Press, 1938, henceforth cited as Klebs, 191.1); and with the *Opera* (Venice: Gregoriis, 1491, 1492, Klebs 192.1; and Venice: Gregoriis, 1497, 1499, Klebs 192.2). An *Epitome in duos libros arithmeticos Boethii* by Jacques Lefevre d'Etaples, was printed with Jordanus Nemorarius, *Arithmetica*, at Paris: Higman and Hopyl, 1496 (Klebs 563.1). The commentary on Boethius' *Arithmetica* by Jean de Muris was printed in 1515 (Cf. TK 959).

3 Heath, p. 67.

4 *De arith.*, Praef.: „... paululum liberius evagatus alieno itineri, non vestigiis, insisto. Nam et ea, quae de numeris a Nicomacho diffusius disputata sunt, moderata brevitate collegi et quae transcursa velocius angustiorem intellegentiae praestabant aditum, mediocri adiectione reseravi, ut aliquando ad evidentiam rerum nostris etiam formulis ac descriptionibus uteremur." Friedlein, pp. 4-5: 29-4.

5 Heath, pp. 10 ff., 66 ff., 98-99; William H. Stahl, Richard Johnson, and E.L. Burge, *Martianus Capella and the Seven Liberal Arts*: Volume I: *The Quadrivium of Martianus Capella* (Records of Civilization: Sources and Studies, LXXXIV; New York and London: Columbia University Press, 1971), p. 156.

6 *Boetii de Institutione Arith.*, Libri duo ed. G. Friedlein, 1966, pp. 3-173. For the definitions of the mathematical terms, see Heath, pp. 74 ff., 91-112; and D.E. Smith, *History of Math.*, II, 1953, pp. 16 ff.

designated as the *trivium* at a later time, comprising grammar, rhetoric, and dialectics. Although Boethius is believed to have coined the term *quadruvium* or *quadrivium*, the actual grouping of the four branches went back to Plato, as well as to Archytas, in the fourth century before Christ.[7] Plato, as Professor Merlan has noted, represented the two aspects of the four mathematical arts, namely their elementary character (in the *Laws*) as grammar school subjects taught for practical purposes only, without any claim to being philosophical in nature or intent, and their position in the *Republic*, as preparation for philosophy or wisdom, the highest form of knowledge.[8]

In the differing interpretations of the role of the subjects of the quadrivium, Professor Merlan has drawn attention to the fact that the transition from the belief that they were elementary branches of learning to the view that they were philosophical in intent was made smoothly for arithmetic, geometry, and astronomy. But for the fourth branch, music, this was not so easy, since music as performed, or as produced in composition, or as enjoyed esthetically and so on, had little necessarily to do with music as the philosophy of sound or of acoustics.[9] Boethius, following Nicomachus, had adhered to the concept of not only the philosophic importance of the four branches of the quadrivium but also of their close interrelationship since as *mathematica* their common subject was quantity. And this quantity was either discontinuous or continuous, that is discontinuous either per se as in arithmetic, or in relation to another, as in music or harmony; and continuous either without motion as in geometry, or in motion as in astronomy. Thus the quadripartition was specifically that of quantity.[10]

In addition to this quadripartition, the *mathematica* or *quadriviales* were also encompassed within the Aristotelian concept of the tripartition of theoretical knowledge, corresponding to the tripartition of being, into physical, mathematical and theological, or the three states or spheres of being, namely of ideas (theological), mathematical, and physical. As Professor Merlan has noted, this theory of the tripartition of being into theological, mathematical and physical, persisted through the Middle Ages and was clearly set forth in the thirteenth century by St. Thomas Aquinas. It was also in evidence in the tripartite character of the curriculum of the Faculty of Arts at Paris, in the three divisions of natural philosophy into *physica, mathematica,* and *metaphysica* (the divine science).[11]

As set forth by Boethius and before him by Nicomachus and Plato, the four branches of *mathematica*, whose common constituent was quantity, were intimately connected in the quadrivium. They were said to constitute the fourfold or fourpronged road toward philosophical truth. Without knowledge of all four of them the seeker for truth would find it impossible

7 Heath, I, pp. 10 ff., citing Plato's *Republic* (VII.522C, 525A, 526B); and F.S. Benjamin Jr., and G.J. Toomer, editors and translators of *Campanus of Novara and Medieval Planetary Theory: Theorica Planetarum* (Madison, Milwaukee, and London: The University of Wisconsin Press, 1971), p. 372. On Boethius and the quadrivium, see also Etienne Gilson, *La Philosophie au Moyen Age: Les Origines Patristiques à la Fin du XIVe Siècle* (2nd ed., Paris: Payot, 1947), pp. 140-41.

8 P. Merlan, *From Platonism to Neoplatonism* (2nd ed., The Hague, 1960), pp. 88 ff., citing the *Protagoras* (318E), the *Laws* (817E), and the *Republic* (VII 530 D). In regard to the Platonic curriculum and the quadrivium, see the appendices to the *Republic*, Book VII, in *The Republic of Plato*, ed. by James Adams, 2nd ed. by D.A. Rees (Cambridge: University Press, 1969), pp. 164 ff.

9 Merlan, pp. 94-95.

10 *Ibid.*, pp. 89 ff., 94-95. *Boetii Inst. Arith.*, I. 1: „Horum ergo illam multitudinem, quae per se est, arithmetica speculatur integritas, illam vero quae ad aliquid, musici modulaminis temperamenta pernoscunt, immobilis vero magnitudinis geometria notitiam pollicetur, mobilis vero scientiam astronomicae disciplinae peritia vendicat...." Friedlein, 1966, p. 9: 1-6.

11 Merlan, p. 224; and see below.

to reach his destination or achieve his goal.[12] Yet, despite this emphasis upon the interrelationship of the four branches, it is impossible to determine with any degree of certainty, in the present state of our knowledge, whether the four were in fact studied with equal attention and devotion either in the earlier schools or in the universities of the thirteenth century. For purposes therefore of this study we shall concentrate on one of the four branches, namely on arithmetic, which, in the opinion of Boethius, was the one that should be studied first,[13] since all the other branches are dependent upon it and it alone was independent of the others. Boethius in placing arithmetic first, was, it might be recalled, following the Nicomachean progression of arithmetic, music, geometry, and astronomy, rather than that of the Varronean arrangement of geometry, arithmetic, astronomy, and music.[14]

The adoption of the *De Institutione Arithmetica* as the basic textbook on the theory of numbers in areas and times far removed from Ostrogothic Italy of the early sixth century provides an interesting illustration of the propagation of texts derived from the Greek. Beginning with the utilization of the work by Cassiodorus for his *Institutiones* or *Introduction to Divine and Human Readings*, the work was looked upon as the principal source from which knowledge of the art or theory of numbers might be derived. It thus accompanied the more practical abacus arithmetics and other texts on calculation. As Professor Patch and others before him have shown, the work was incorporated into the teaching of the cloister and cathedral of St. Gall, Reichenau, Laon, Hildesheim, Rheims, Chartres, Paris, and so on, or wherever the curriculum was organized on the plan of the seven liberal arts. Moreover, such prominent early scholars as Bede, Alcuin, Rabanus Maurus, Gerbert, Helperic, Hroswitha and many others had culled pertinent information from the *De Institutione Arithmetica.*[15] In the twelfth century, Boethius and arithmetic appeared in the allegory, attributed to Honorius of Autun, of the return of the soul from its exile of ignorance to its true homeland by means of the ten arts depicted as cities through which the soul must pass on its way to its true homeland. Arithmetic, the fourth city, was portrayed with Boethius teaching the art of even and odd numbers.[16]

12 *Boetii Inst. Arith.* I.1: „...haud quemquam in philosophiae disciplinis ad cumulum perfectionis evadere, nisi cui talis prudentiae nobilitas quodam quasi quadruvio vestigatur...." (ed. Friedlein, 1966, p. 7: 23-26); and *ibid.* „Quibus quatuor partibus si careat inquisitor, verum invenire non possit, ac sine hac quidem speculatione veritatis nulli recte sapiendum est. Est enim sapientia earum rerum, quae vere sunt, cognitio et integra comprehensio.... Constat igitur, quisquis haec praetermiserit, omnem philosophiae perdidisse doctrinam. Hoc igitur illud quadruvium est, quo his viandum sit.... (ed. Friedlein, 1966, p. 9: 6-10, 26-29).

13 *Boetii Inst. Arith.*, Praef.: „Cum igitur quattuor matheseos disciplinarum de arithmetica, quae est prima, perscriberem..." (ed. Friedlein, 1966, p. 5: 6-7).

14 See my article, „The *Quadrivium* in the Thirteenth Century Universities (with special reference to Paris)," in *Actes du Quatrième Congrès International de Philosophie Médiévale: Arts Libéraux et Philosophie au Moyen Âge* (Montreal: Institut d'Etudes Médiévales, and Paris: Librairie Philosophieque J. Vrin, 1969, henceforth to be cited as *Actes*, 1969), p. 181; also W.H. Stahl, *Martianus Capella and the Seven Liberal Arts,* 1971, pp. 154-55, note 35. See above I 181.

15 Patch, pp. 36 ff., citing the earlier literature on the subject. See also H.L. Heiberg, *Geschichte der Mathematik und Naturwissenschaften in Altertum* (Munich, 1925), pp. 49ff.; and the brief historical survey of the quadrivium, and of arithmetic in particular, in W.H. Stahl, *Martianus Capella and the Seven Liberal Arts*, 1971, pp. 154 ff.

16 *Ibid.*, Patch, pp. 36 ff. and the „De animae exsilio et patria, alias, De Artibus," attributed to Honorius of Autun, in which the exile is ignorance and the fatherland, wisdom. Migne, *Patrologia*, CLXXII, col. 1243-1246: 1244, „cap. v. Quarta civitas arithmetica.... In hac, Boetio docente, par et impar numerus..." See also Eva Matthews Sanford, „Honorius, presbyter and scholasticus," *Speculum*, 23 (July, 1948), p. 419.

Furthermore, Professor Patch drew attention to the indebtedness to Boethius of such prominent thirteenth century scholars as Alexander Neckam, Albertus Magnus, Thomas Aquinas, Michael Scot, Roger Bacon, and Robert Grosseteste, all of them associated at one time or another with the University of Paris.[17] However, he made no attempt to single out for specific study the use of the *De Institutione Arithmetica* by these authors, nor the continued presence of the work as a textbook for the study of arthmetic among the quadrivial arts in the university curriculum.[18] This then is the twofold task toward which this study is directed, with particular emphasis upon the Parisian university milieu.

Although there were in the thirteenth century several other French as well as non-French university centers, none of these could be considered as representative of the era as Paris. The University at Paris was a truly international association and was acknowledged as the intellectual center of Europe in the thirteenth century. It drew scholars not only from all parts of the French kingdom but also from the British Isles and continental Europe as well.[19] And insofar as the scholars whose works are to be considered were at one time or another in Paris, their writings may be examined for our purpose without regard to whether they were of English, German, Hungarian, Italian, Spanish, Scandinavian or of any other origin.

In general, as suggested earlier, little attention until recently had been drawn to the fate of either the Boethian *Arithmetica* or the quadrivial arts in the University of Paris in the thirteenth century. As noted in my previous study on the quadrivium in the thirteenth century University of Paris,[20] this neglect may be accounted for in part by the paucity of information on the subject in the thirteenth century university documents. However, as also suggested earlier, there are other available sources that may be tapped. The latter comprise student manuals or guides and the writings of either professors or scholars known to have been associated with the university as well as others in the immediate vicinity whose direct connection cannot be ascertained but who in all likelihood came in close contact with the community of scholars in the rather restricted geographical confines of the city of Paris. In addition, there is the evidence provided by extant manuscripts of texts either of earlier vintage or by contemporary authors who were regent or teaching masters in the university.[21] A sampling of only a portion of such resources has been possible for this study. But these few have reinforced the views earlier expressed. The mathematical or quadrivial arts were being taught within the larger and more comprehensive framework of the three philosophies, rational, natural, and moral, that made up the Faculty of Arts, which at Paris as elsewhere had taken over the task of providing the basic groundwork of the university educational program. As noted earlier, the quadrivial arts constituted one of the three divisions of natural philosophy, under the heading of *mathematica*, the other two being *physica* and *metaphysica.*[22]

17 Patch, pp. 39 ff.

18 For recent suggestions in this regard, see my earlier study in *Actes*, 1969, pp. 175 ff.; also the brief summary on the quadrivium by Mgr. Glorieux, *La Faculté des Arts*, (Paris: J. Vrin, 1971), pp. 33-34.

19 See my *Nations in the Mediaeval Universities* (Cambridge, Mass.: Mediaeval Academy of America, 1948), pp. 14 ff. and the references there noted.

20 *Actes*, 1969, pp. 175-91; also, Philippe Delhaye, „Arts libéraux et Programmes scolaire au XIIIe siècle," *Actes*, 1969, pp. 162-73; and Glorieux, *La Faculté des Arts*, 1971, pp. 33-38. See above I 175-191.

21 *Actes*, 1969, p. 176, and n. 8. See above I 176 and n. 8.

22 *Actes*, 1969, pp. 180-81; and St. Thomas Aquinas, *The Division and Methods of the Sciences: Questions V and VI of his Commentary on the De Trinitate of Boethius*, translated with introduction and notes by Armand Maurer (3rd rev. ed., Toronto: The Pontifical Institute of Mediaeval Studies, 1963), pp. xiv-xv. As indicated in my article named above, St. Thomas had asserted that the old divisions into trivium and quadrivium were no longer adequate to comprise the whole of speculative philosophy. And in the tripartite division into mathematical, natural, and divine or metaphysics, he had held that the mathematical

Moreover, for the teaching of the first of the quadrivial arts, arithmetic, the Boethian *De Institutione Arithmetica* appears to have maintained its position as a basic text, and this was the case despite the fact that there were available for the study of arithmetic in the thirteenth century, in its various practical as well as other aspects, a wealth of materials both old and new. To the many tracts on calculation, abacus arithmetic, mathematical games, and simple reckoning, of earlier vintage, there had been added the treatises on algorisms where Hindu-Arabic numerals made an early appearance, as well as other practical treatises and pedagogical instruments, as Guy Beaujouan has shown in his account of elementary texts for the teaching of arithmetic in the universities.[23] However, despite this abundance of practical materials, the Nicomachean *Arithmetica* in the translation or paraphrase by Boethius was named as the text in arithmetic by the anonymous Paris master in the examination manual dated between 1230 and 1240 prepared for students coming up for examinations for degrees or for the license in arts at Paris.[24] The Boethian *Arithmetica* had similarly been named together with Euclid, that is apparently the sections on numbers of the *Elements*, in an earlier list of textbooks prepared probably by Alexander Neckam at the close of the twelfth century while he was teaching the quadrivial arts at Paris.[25]

Furthermore, the tendency to relate or combine the Boethian *Arithmetica* with the new Hindu-Arabic mathematics[26] is illustrated in the *Algorismus Vulgaris* of John Halifax or Sacrobosco.[27] Although the name of John of Sacrobosco, an English scholar who taught at

arts should precede studies in natural philosophy or physics. In his opinion, the mathematical arts among which he placed arithmetic first, would prepare the mind, or open the way for the apprehension and understanding of the other physical or natural sciences. For a slightly different division of the three philosophies, see Father James A. Weisheipl, „The Place of the Liberal Arts in the University Curriculum during the XIVth and XVth Centuries," *Actes*, 1969, p. 210. See also above for the tripartition of theoretical knowledge.

23 For the place and importance of arithmetic in the university curriculum, see my previous study in *Actes*, 1969, pp. 181 ff.; also Guy Beaujouan, „L'enseignement de l'arithmétique élémentaire à l'Université de Paris aux XIIIe et XIVe siècles. De l'abaque à l'algorisme," in *Homenaje à Millas-Vallicrosa* (Barcelona: Consejo superior de investigaciones cientificas, 1954), I, pp. 93-124. Beaujouan's recent study, „L'enseignement du Quadrivium," Estratto da Settimane du Studio del Centro italiano di studi sull'alto medievo, XIX, *La Scuola nell'occidente Latino dell'alto medioevo* (Spoleto, 1972), pp. 639-723, relates in large part to music and to treatises other than those of the *Arithmetica*. For another indication of the variety and amount of mathematical literature available to the student in the later thirteenth century, see the introduction to Roger Bacon, *Communia mathematica*, ed. by Robert Steele in *Opera hactenus inedita* (Oxford: Clarendon Press, [1909-42]), fasc. 16, pp. viii-ix.

24 „Huius vero scientie auctor est Nicomachus, Boetius vero translator:" Barcelona Archivio de la Corona de Aragon Ripoll 109, f. 134v. This MS was discovered by Mgr. Martin Grabmann, „Eine für Examinazwecke abgefasste Quästionensammlung der Pariser Artistenfakultät aus der ersten Hälfte des 13. Jahrhunderts," in *Mittelalterliches Geistesleben: Abhandlungen zur Geschichte der Scholastik und Mystik*, II(1936), 189; and my article in *Actes*, 1969, p. 181 and note 40; also Delhaye, *loc. cit.*, p. 166.

25 „Institutis arismetice informandus, arismeticam Boecii et Euclidis legat:" Charles Homer Haskins, *Studies in the History of Mediaeval Science* (2nd ed. Cambridge, Mass.: Harvard University Press, 1927), p. 374; also Mgr Glorieux, *La Faculté des Arts*, p. 33.
For the combination in the teaching of arithmetic of the Nicomachan arithmetic with the section on numbers from Euclid's *Elements*, book VII, see W.H. Stahl, *Martianus Capella and the Seven Liberal Arts*, pp. 156-157; also Father J.A. Weisheipl, „Curriculum of the Faculty of Arts at Oxford in the early Forteenth Century," *Mediaeval Studies*, XXVI(1964), p. 170.

26 See my article in *Actes*, 1969, p. 182. See above I 182.

27 *Ibid.*, p. 183 and n. 53. For 13th century MSS of the *Algorismus*, see TK 991. To the 13th cent. MSS there listed might be added: London BM Harley 3353, 13th cent., ff. 76r-86v. The work was printed with the title: *Tractatus de arte numerandi*, together with an English translation, by J.O. Halliwell, *Rara mathematica* (2nd. ed., London: Maynard, 1841), pp. 1-26.

Paris, nowhere appears in the university documents of the thirteenth century, his presence is attested by another master, Bartholomew of Parma, who commented on Sacrobosco's *Sphere.*[28] The prose tract on the *Algorisms* as well as Sacrobosco's tract on the *Sphere*, both of which became basic textbooks for the teaching of two of the quadrivial arts, that is arithmetic and astronomy, are extant in thirteenth century manuscripts.[29] The *Algorismus*, a comparatively short tract which treated of various arithmetical operations and included the new Hindu-Arabic numerals from zero through nine was composed between 1220 and 1245 and constituted one of the major textbooks popularizing the new Arabic arithmetic. Yet it opened with the well known phrase from the second chapter of the first book of the Boethian *Arithmetica*: „All things that proceed from the first origin of things are formed in numerical ratio," and followed this with the definition of number as multitude composed of collected units and materially as a collection of units added one to another.[30] The *Algorismus* deals with the nine operations of the art of numeration, namely: addition, subtraction, halving, doubling, multiplying, dividing, progression, and extraction of cubic and square roots.[31] John of Sacrobosco also drew from Boethius his discussion of the extraction of roots and the explanation for the correspondence of numbers to geometric figures, and he summarized what Boethius had said of linear numbers.[32]

In addition to John of Sacrobosco's own citations and borrowing from the Boethian *Arithmetica* in his *Algorismus*, there were citations to the *Arithmetica* by the commentators on Sacrobosco's other popular university textbook, the *Sphere*. In one of these commentaries dated 1271, the author, Robertus Anglicus, a professor at Montpellier and also probably at Paris,[33] in his discussion of the number and position of the elements, recalled both the doctrine of Plato on means and proportion and the assertion of Boethius that „All things which proceed from the primeval origin of things are formed in numerical ratio."[34] And in another commentary, which is anonymous, the author drew from Boethius in the introduction to his translation of Nicomachus, the statement that: „Among all the sciences the quadriviales are the most suited for bringing one to wisdom" and the assertion, from the first chapter of Boethius' *Arithmetica*, that if anyone should neglect the four sciences that make up the quadrivium he would be unable to discover the truth. And further, that no one ignorant of these

28 As noted in the introduction to *The Sphere of Sacrobosco and its Commentators*, edited and translated with introduction by Lynn Thorndike (Chicago: University of Chicago Press, 1948), p. 2, n. 4.

29 For 13th cent. mss of the Algorismus, see note 27 above and for the *Commentary* by Petrus Philomenus de Dacia, found in 13th and 14th century mss, TK 681. Even more numerous are the 13th cent. mss of the *Sphere*, as indicated in TK 1524, 1577. The *Sphere* was also printed frequently by incunabula presses. See Klebs, 874, 1-30; and in Portugese 875.1.

30 „Omnia quecumque a primeva rerum origine etc." as in *Arith*. I.2, ed. with slight editions, Friedlein, p. 12: 14-15. „Omnia quaecumque a primaeva rerum natura constructa sunt, numerorum videntur ratione formata." And for the definition of number: „Numerus est unitatum collectio, vel quantitatis acervus ex unitatibus profusus..." *Ibid.*, p. 13; *Arith*. I-3: 10-12.

31 See Halliwell, pp. 1-26, for the text of the *Algorismus* or „Art of Numeration."

32 *Ibid.*, also Beaujouan, in *Homenaje à Millas-Vallicrosa*, 1954, p. 16. Cf. Boethius, *Arith*. ed. Friedlein, pp. 86 ff; 90 ff.

33 Thorndike, *The Sphere of Sacrobosco*, especially pp. 1-2; also P. Duhem, *Le Système du monde* (Paris: Hermanns, 1958), III, pp. 291-298 and for MSS, TK 337, 1596. The *Commentary* in both Latin and English translation is printed by Thorndike, pp. 143-98, 199-246.

34 „Lectio II," *Ibid.*, pp. 149-150; and p. 204: „... sicut dicit Boetius, Omnia que a primeva rerum origine processerunt ratione numeri sunt formata." Cf. *Arith.* I,2. ed. Friedlein, p. 12: 14-17: „Omnia quaecumque a primaeva rerum natura constructa sunt, numerorum videntur ratione formata. Hoc enim fuit principale in animo conditioris exemplar."

four sciences is suited to philosophizing.[35] The author then, probably to prove that he was not wanting in this regard, went on to repeat from Boethius the assertion that mathematical science relates to quantity which is dual in nature, that is either discontinuous or continuous. The discontinuous comprises number considered in itself, which is arithmetic, and number in relation to another which is music; and quantity that is continuous and unmoved which is geometry or quantity that is continuous and moved which is astronomy.[36]

Moreover, the Boethian *Arithmetica* provided the basis for another thirteenth century work on arithmetic, that of Jordanus Nemorarius, who may possibly be the same as the Jordanus of Saxony, who was a master of arts at Paris, a member of the Dominican Order, and the author of a number of mathematical tracts.[37] Although his *Arithmetica* was based on the Boethian work, Jordanus had expanded the two books of that text into ten books, of which the first treated the common attributes of numbers, their parts and composition; the second, proportions and common attributions of proportionalities; third, of the first composition of numbers and proportions; fourth, of proportionality; fifth, of addition, subtraction, and parts of proportion; sixth, of numbers squared and cubed; seventh, of odd and even or equal and unequal numbers; eighth, of the forms of numbers; ninth, of equality and inequality; and tenth, of the median or arithmetical music. However, the *Arithmetica* of Jordanus differed from that of Boethius since it made use of letters instead of concrete numbers. Jordanus had also incorporated a number of additional demonstrations and examples into his work, a procedure for which he was criticized by his contemporary, Roger Bacon.[38]

In all probability the continued use of the Boethian *Arithmetica* in the thirteenth century was due to its philosophical tenor and the degree to which the work lent itself to the speculative aspects of mathematical and scientific exposition. In the thirteenth century the work was cited by several theologians. One of these, Robert Grosseteste, bishop of Lincoln (d. 1253), primarily an Oxford scholar, had nevertheless spent some time in Paris.[39] He is moreover

35 Anon. Comm. on John of Sacrobosco's *Sphere*: Thorndike, *The Sphere of Sacrobosco*, Appendix II, p. 451: „Nota quod inter omnes scientias quadriviales maxime sunt appetenda que maxime faciunt ad sapientiam, quod patet per Boetium primo arismetrice sue ubi dicit quod sunt quatuor partes exponentes se, id est, quadrivium, quia si quis caret verum inveniri non potest et sine quorum speculatione aliquis non potest habere speculationem veritatis. Et etiam dicit alibi, Hiis quatuor ignoratis nullum dico aptum ad philosophandum." Cf. Boethius' *Arithmetica*, ed. by Friedlein, 1966, p. 9: 5-8: „Quibus quattuor partibus si careat inquisitor, verum invenire non possit, ac sine hac quidem speculatione veritatis nulli recte sapiendum est...." (*Ibid.*, p. 9: 10-13) Quod haec qui spernit id est has semitas sapientiae ei denuntio non recte esse philosophandum, siquidem philosophia est amor sapientiae, quam in his spernendis ante contempserit."

36 „Modo ille scientie quadriviales sunt mathematice que diversificantur, quia mathematica scientia est de quantitate. Modo duplex est quantitas, discreta et continua. Discreta que est de numeris est duplex. Vel numerus consideratur in se ut unus duo est, vel in alio ut duplum triplum. Sic quantitas continua est duplex, quedam est immota et de illa est geometria, quia est de magnitudinibus etc. que sunt absoluta ab omni motu et materia saltem secundum rationem. Quedam est quantitas que est continua mota et de illa est astronomia...." Lynn Thorndike, ed., *The Sphere of Sacrobosco*, Appendix II, pp. 451-52. Cf. Boethius' *Arithmetica*, ed. by Friedlein, 1966, p. 9: 1-6, cited above n. 10.

37 For Jordanus Nemorarius, see my article in *Actes*, 1969, pp. 182-83, and notes; also. E.A. Moody and Marshall Clagett, *The Medieval Science of Weights* (Madison: The University of Wisconsin Press, 1960), pp. 3-4. For his many mathematical works, see the index to TK under Jordanus Nemorarius, and especially for the *Arithmetica*, ibid., 1600. Another 13th century MS of the *Arithmetica Jordani (de Nemoraria)* is at Paris: BN 16644, 13th cent., ff. 2r ff. This MS was deeded to the Sorbonne by Gerard of Abbetsville. Jordanus also has an *Algorismus*: TK 237, 431. See above I 182-183.

38 Paul Abelson, *The Seven Liberal Arts* (New York, 1939; reprinted New York: Russell and Russell Inc., 1965), p. 105, and my article in *Actes*, 1969, p. 183; for Roger Bacon's criticism, see below. See I 183.

39 For his Paris sojourn see Ludwig Baur, „Die Philosophie des Robert Grosseteste Bischofs von Lincoln (d. 1253)," *Beiträge z. Geschichte d. Philosophie des Mittelalters*, Münster, XVIII, Heft 4 (1917), 4-5, n. 1.

associated specifically by Professor A.C. Crombie with the development of a new scientific procedure, through the utilization of mathematics. Without this discipline, upon which the investigation of natural phenomena is dependent, according to Grosseteste, man cannot achieve a scientific understanding of nature. Mathematics, in his view, provides the means to throw light on nature and natural phenomena.[40] However, although Grosseteste cited the Boethian *Arithmetica* in his tract on „Lines, angles, and figures,“[41] he relied more heavily on geometry than on the *Arithmetica* for his demonstrations.[42] He also gave considerable attention to the other two mathematical arts, that is to music and astronomy.[43]

On the other hand much more extensive use was made of the Boethian *Arithmetica* by Roger Bacon, Grosseteste's disciple. Bacon, a member of the Franciscan Order, as well as a master of arts, probably in the University of Paris, appears in any case to have spent a goodly part of his academic career in Paris.[44] Although generally outspoken in his criticism of contemporary mathematicians, Bacon expressed agreement with the views set forth in the Boethian *Arithmetica* and cited it frequently. He placed Boethius first among authorities on the subject and cited him for the statement that if the seeker after truth should lack knowledge of the four branches of *mathematica* (the quadrivium) he would be unable to achieve his goal; and for the further assertion that „without this speculative knowledge nothing of the truth could rightly be known.“[45] Bacon had explained that the *mathematica* comprise the four sciences of geometry, arithmetic, music, and astrology, placing under the latter both the judicial and operative aspects of the science.[46] And he repeated the statement from Cassiodorus that these four sharpen our perception and are instructive for all other sciences which indeed cannot be taught without mathematics, as Boethius had suggested in the prologue to the *De Arithmetica.*[47] Bacon also repeated the phrases from the *Arithmetica* that among all

40 For Robert Grosseteste, see especially A.C. Crombie, *Robert Grosseteste and the Origins of Experimental Science*, 1100-1700 (Oxford, Clarendon Press, 1953), pp. 44 ff., with references to earlier bibliography in note 1; also *ibid.*, p. 50; my article in *Actes*, 1969, p. 185; and Ludwig Baur, „Die philosophischen Werke des Robert Grosseteste, Bischofs von Lincoln (d. 1253),“ *Beiträge zur Geschichte der Philosophie des Mittelalters*, Münster, IX (1912), 59-60: „Utilitas considerationis linearum angulorum et figurarum est maxima, quoniam impossibile est sciri naturalem philosophiam sine illis.“

41 „De lineis, angulis et figuris,“ ed. Baur, *Beiträge z. Gesch. d. Philosophie*, IX (1912), p. 61: „Item, linea recta habet aequalitatem sine angulo; sed melius est aequale quam inequali, ut dicit Boethius in arismetica sua.“ (Boethius, *Arith.* I,32; II,1; Friedlein, pp. 66, 77.)

42 Crombie, pp. 32 ff., 50, 59; „De Natura locorum,“ ed. Baur, *Beiträge z. Gesch. d. Philosophie*, IX (1912), pp. 65-66: „His igitur regulis et fundamentis datis ex potestate geometriae diligens inspector in rebus naturalibus potest dare causas omnium effectuum naturalium per hanc viam.“ See also *Actes*, 1969, p. 185.

43 *Ibid.*, pp. 186, 189. See „De Artibus liberalibus,“ ed. Baur, *Beiträge* IX (1912), 1-5, for music; p. 5 for astronomy; and p. 4 for arithmetic and geometry.

44 *Ibid.*, p. 177; also Lynn Thorndike, *A History of Magic and Experimental Science* (New York, 1923), II, chap. LXI.

45 Roger Bacon, „Communia mathematica,“ in *Opera hactenus inedita*, ed. by Robert Steele (1909-42), fasc. 16 (1940), p. 7: „Incipio a Boetio. Dicit enim in prologo Arismetrice secundo mathematice ,Quatuor partibus si careat inquisitor, verum minime invenire potesta sine hac quidem speculatione veritatis nulli recte sapiendum est.' “ Cf. Friedlein, p. 9: 6-8; *Arith.* I. 1. For the lines quoted, see n. 12 above.

46 Bacon here follows the Varronean order, transmitted by Martianus Capella, which differed from the Nicomachean order of arithmetic, music, geometry (or in the variant, geometry, music), and astronomy. L. Baur, „Die Philosophie des Robert Grosseteste Bischofs von Lincoln (d. 1253),“ *Beiträge z. Gesch. d. Philosophie des Mittelalters*, XVIII, Heft. 4 (1917), pp. 17-18. Grosseteste followed the unusual order of music, arithmetic, geometry and astronomy. *Ibid.*, 1917, p. 18.

47 Roger Bacon, *Opera hactenus inedita*, ed. by Robert Steele (Oxford: Clarendon Press), fasc. V, pp. 2-3; „... et dicitur hec mathematica dicitur doctrinalis vel disciplinalis quia omnes alie sciencie per hanc docentur et sine illa non possunt doceri. Quod etiam Boethius in prologo Arithmetice...“ Boethius, *Arith.*

those of ancient authority who under the leadership of Pythagoras sought to attain the pinnacle of perfection in the disciplines of philosophy none could do so without the knowledge of the four mathematical sciences.[48]

Roger Bacon furthermore gave preference in the *Communia mathematica* to the Boethian work over that of his contemporary, Jordanus Nemorarius, whose *Arithmetic* in ten books, as previously noted, was largely based on that of Boethius. As between Jordanus and Boethius, Bacon asserted, the latter's *Arithmetica* is the better of the two and more useful. Jordanus, in Bacon's opinion, had included a superabundance of demonstrations, a failing that Bacon asserted, wasted too much time.[49] So many demonstrations were superfluous and unnecessary, he insisted, and if it were not for them and the difficulties they create, one could within a year know as much as anyone would learn in the course of twenty years, as experience has clearly shown.[50] Bacon further cited, on the subject of proportionality, Boethius and Jordanus as well as Adelard (Alardum) of Bath in the commentary on five of the *Elements* of Euclid that he had translated.[51]

Roger Bacon's agreement with the views expressed in the Boethian *Arithmetica* was further exemplified in several other instances. Although he had not followed Boethius' lead by placing geometric progression before that of arithmetic, Bacon made clear his adherence to the view expressed in the Boethian *Arithmetica* that without the speculation engendered by arithmetic, which teaches the species of numbers and the reasons for their operations, attainment of wisdom would be impossible.[52] Moreover, in his *Questiones altere supra libros prime philosophie Aristotelis (Metaphysica* I-IV), Bacon referred to Boethius' *Arithmetica*, in the course of a discussion of the question whether numbers are the foundations of things as the Pythagoreans and Platonists had asserted. He agreed that they were, ,,since Boethius has written in the *Arithmetica*, ,whatever is has proceeded from the primeval origin of things, therefore numbers are the beginnings of things...' "[53] He similarly acquiesced in the application of the term wisdom or philosophy to mathematics since ,,as is written in the *Arithmetica*, ,Wisdom is made up of those things that are true.' "[54] In sum, Bacon was articulate in his conviction, expressed at great length in the *Communia mathematica*, and the *Opus maius*, part four, as well as in other of his works, that the Boethian *Arithmetica* was of great importance

I, 1; Friedlein, pp. 7 ff. See also Bacon, *Opus maius*, ed. by J.H. Bridges (reprinted Frankfurt/Main: Minerva G.M.B.H., 1964), I, pp. 103 ff.

48 ,,Inter omnes prisce auctoritatis viros qui Pictagora duce... haud quemquam in philosophie disciplinis ad cumulum perfectionis evadera nisi cui talis prudentie nobilitas quasi quadrivio vestigatur..." *Opera hactenus inedita*, ed. by Robert Steele, fasc. XVI (1940), p. 7; Boeth. *Arith.* I.1, ed. by Friedlein, p. 7: 21-25.

49 ,,Communia mathematica," *Opera hactenus inedita*, ed. by Robert Steele, fasc. XVI, p. 47; ,,Jordani ex fontibus Boetii oriuntur. Unde optimus liber est *Arismetica* Boetii et utilior quam liber Jordani, quia pauca de numeris demonstranda sunt..."

50 For Bacon's criticisms of the mathematical teaching of his day, see *ibid.*, pp. xi, 117-18.

51 *Ibid.*, p. 83: ,,hec tres proportionalitates sunt medietates et secundum Boetium et Jordanum in Arismetica et secundum Alardum Batoniensem in expositione quinti Elementorum Euclidis quam tradidit..." and again *ibid.*, p. 86, ,,Sed continua proportionalitas potest esse in Arismetica medietate et in musica sicut in geometrica ut patet in exemplis et Boetius hoc edocet in Arismetica." Adelard of Bath made his translation of Euclid in the twelfth century. See *ibid.*, introd., p. ix.

52 See above note 45.

53 Ed. Robert Steele with the collaboration of F.M. Delorme, O.P., *Opera hactenus inedita* (Oxford: Clarendon Press, 1932), fasc. XI, p. 81. Cf. *Arith.* I.2, as cited in note 29 above.

54 *Ibid.*, p. 111: ,,Mathematica dicitur sapientia vel philosophia videtur; scribitur in Arismetica ,Sapientia est eorum que vere sunt." Cf. *Arith.* I.1: ,,Est enim sapientia earum rerum quae vere sunt..." Friedlein, p. 9: 8-9.

and also that mathematics was necessary and useful in every science including the divine science.[55]

The Boethian *Arithmetica* was also utilized by another member of the Franciscan Order, Saint Bonaventura (d. 1274), who taught in the University of Paris between 1248 and 1255.[56] Bonaventura has been shown to have been very much interested in the significance of numbers. The recent editor and translator of his „Collations on the Six Days" asserts that „In almost every one of his works and frequently in the present one, there are elaborate references to the numbers 3, 6, 7, 12, 144, 666, and 1000, in which he sees logical links with the realities of heaven and earth."[57] It is not surprising therefore that Bonaventura found much of interest to him in the Boethian *Arithmetica*. For example, in the „Third Collation" of the „Six Days of Creation," which he used as a literary and symbolic framework, Bonaventura referred to the Boethian *De Arithmetica* among other authorities for his expressed views „on oneness." „Indeed if oneness were able to know the sum total of its potencies, it would know all the lines passing through the center. Oneness, however, is more a principle than the mathematical point, for oneness is an essential part of number, while the point is a principle but not a part."[58] Furthermore, he utilized the Boethian *Arithmetica* among other works in the „Fourth Collation" in referring to mathematics. „Now these sciences prepare for the understanding of Scripture, as is clear in the case of perfect numbers, and of the decreased and increasing number, as it appears with the perfection of the number six which is perfect of itself... Likewise, concerning the two first cubic numbers, 8 and 27: twice two times two equals 8, and three times three times three equal 27, and they can be related through no other numbers than 12 and 18, for 12 is to 18 as 18 is to 27, in the proportion of one and a half, which contains the whole and its intermediate."[59]

Finally, Bonaventura utilized Boethius' *Arithmetica* in the „Eleventh Collation" on the vision of God's Trinity. „According to Boethius, inequalities have their origin from equality. Likewise if something essentially different is produced by God, by necessity there must be produced first something substantially the same, for before the extrinsic there is in the intrinsic, as is evident."[60]

Boethius' *Arithmetica* was similarly utilized by another contemporary of Roger Bacon, the learned and sainted Albertus Magnus, of the Order of Preaching Friars, whose intellectual activities are closely associated with Paris although his native home was in the Germanies. Albertus, too, like Bacon, expounded mathematics at considerable length in several of his writings, and is the author of a commentary on Euclid as well as of other mathematical writings.[61] He is credited further by the *Histoire Littèraire* with a commentary on the *Arithmetica Boetii*.[62] However, diligent search focused at the Bibliothèque Nationale in Paris has not so far led to success in locating such a work. Nevertheless Albertus has in his own writings exemplified both his interest in the quadrivial or mathematical arts and his use of the Boethian *Arithmetica*.

55 *Opus maius*, ed. J.H. Bridges (reprinted, 1964), I, pp. 97 ff.; 175 ff.

56 Etienne Gilson, *La Philosophie au Moyen Âge: Des Origines Patristiques à la Fin du XIVe Siècle* (2nd ed., Paris: Payot, 1947), pp. 439 ff.

57 „V. Collations on the Six Days," *The Works of Bonaventura, Cardinal, Seraphic Doctor, and Saint*, trans. form the Latin by José de Vinck (Paterson, New Jersey: Anthony Guild Press, 1970), introduction.

58 *Ibid.*, pp. 43-44; cf. *Arith.* I.7. Ed. Friedlein, p. 16.

59 *The Works of Bonaventura*, 1970, pp. 66-67. Cf. *Arith.* I. 20, ed. Friedlein p. 41 ff.

60 *The Works of Bonaventura*, 1970, p. 162. Cf. *Arith.* I. 32, Friedlein, p. 66.

61 B. Geyer, „Die mathematischen Schriften des Albertus Magnus," *Angelicum*, XXV (1958), 159-175, including the text of the Commentary on Euclid at pp. 170-175.

62 *Histoire littèraire de la France*, Paris, 1824, XVI, 113. The statement is also repeated by Mgr. P. Glorieux in *La Faculté des Arts et ses Maitres au XIII*e *siècle*, 1971, p. 76.

In addition to citing the *Arithmetica* specifically on the subject of the science of numbers, in his *Commentary on the Sentences,*[63] Albertus Magnus drew attention to the quadrivium and to the four mathematical disciplines in his work on *Metaphysics.*[64] He there took care to make clear the liberal and speculative rather than utilitarian character of the mathematical sciences of the quadrivium, that is of arithmetic, music, geometry, and astrology (*sic*). They are called liberal, he held, when they are exercised not for any utilitarian purpose but for themselves alone, since in the same way as man is free, that science is termed free or liberal that has no other utility than that of the science itself.[65] Similarly, the mathematical sciences are speculative, he continued, when they are pursued wholly for knowledge or for the science itself. Albertus had already affirmed the principle that the aim of all speculation is to know the truth, whereas the aim of practice is the work itself.[66] He also went on to assert that the speculative character of the mathematical sciences is not based on opinion but entails the speculative intellect. They are thus designated as true sciences and are distinguished as *doctrinales* and *disciplines*. They do not require experience and are taught simply by the master's demonstration. Hence inexperienced youth could greatly excell in them. This differentiates them from the physical sciences where experience is necessary. For unlike the *physicales* which are concerned with matter and hence are subject to motion, change, or both in time, the *mathematicales* which are not constituents of physical matter have their definitive form through demonstration.[67]

Furthermore, in his discussion of the Pythagorean doctrine that numbers are the beginnings of things, Albertus quoted the passage from the Pythagorean *Arithmetica* to the effect that unity is that by which each thing is one.[68] He went on then to assert that unity is in no way joined to number and to draw attention to the fact that Boethius, in transferring the substance of the words of Pythagoras into his discussion of the substance of number in the second chapter of the *Arithmetica*, had asserted that „Everything that proceeds from the primeval nature of things has been formed in numerical ratio" for this was the principal exemplar in the mind of the Creator.[69] But as Albertus explained in his *Summa Theologia*, the number which attended the divine ratio is not the number of forms; it is the number of proportion where the two extremes, as Boethius says, are connected by arithmetical means.

63 Albertus Magnus, *Commentarius in Sententias*, ed. A. Borgnet (Paris, 1890), XXVII, 15 (II Sent. Dist. 1, Art. 5): 2. Item Boetius in prohemio primi Arithmeticorum dicit sic: Numerorum scientiam ille hujus humane molis conditor Deus primam (*sic*) suae habuit rationis exemplar, et ad hanc conjuncta constituit quaecumque fabricante ratione, per numeros assignati ordinis invenire concordiam."

64 Albertus, *Metaphysicorum Libri XIII*, ed. A. Borgnet, Paris, 1890, VI, 1 ff., 32.

65 *Ibid.*, VI, 31-32 (Metaph. I.II.6-7): Scientie methematicae formas stantes habentes quae principium liberorum sunt sciendi in ipsis...hoc modo enim liberalis dicitur quae non alterius utilitatis causa quaeritur. Et hec modo sunt liberales illae quae dicuntur esse de quadrivio scilicet arithmetica, musica, geometria, et astrologia..."

66 *Ibid.*, VI, 31: „Finis autem omnis speculationis est scire et veritas: et praxis omnis finis est opus: ergo scientiae sunt speculativae: hi ergo prosecuti sunt scientiam propter notitiam simpliciter: non causa alicuius utilitatis...."

67 *Ibid.*, VI, pp. 1-2 (Metaph. I, 1, 1).

68 *Ibid.*, VI, p. 62 (Metaph. I.IV.2): „Pythagoras in Arithmetica, unitas est quaelibet res una est...." Cf. *Arith.* I. 7, ed. Friedlein, p. 16.

69 *Ibid.*, VI, 64 (Metaph. I.IV.2): „Et hoc quod dixit Boetius substantiam verborum Pythagorae transferens, et de substantia numeri in principio *Arithmeticae* loquens: ‚Omnia quae a primaeva rerum natura constructa sunt, numerorum videntur ratione formata: hoc enim fuit principale in animo conditoris exemplar...' " Cf. *Arith.* I. 2, ed. Friedlein, p. 12. See note 34 above, for the citation.

He noted too that Boethius had similarly asserted that this number cannot be understood as mathematical number but rather as ideal number.[70]

The views expressed by Albertus Magnus regarding the mathematical or quadrivial arts were similarly expounded by his disciple, St. Thomas Aquinas. St. Thomas asserted that arithmetic formed the principal part of mathematics and should precede geometry as well as astronomy or astrology, and music.[71] He had also in the *Commentary on the Ethics* outlined the order of learning or teaching as logic first, since it taught the method of all philosophy; and next the mathematicales or quadriviales, arithmetic, music, geometry, and astronomy, since as indicated by Albertus, they require no experience; thirdly, natural philosophy; fourthly, moral philosophy; and finally, divine philosophy or metaphysics.[72]

For another order of learning, it may be of interest to note that in a work entitled *Liber de Apprehensione* attributed to Albertus Magnus that is probably not by him, but is printed with his other works by Borgnet,[73] the recommendation to students is that they first study *physicis* (natural philosophy) then *mathematica* (the arts of the quadrivium), and finally complete their studies in the divine science or metaphysics. The reason given for this order is that it corresponds to the order of nature in which sense apprehension is first, then the intellect receives the *mathematica* abstracted from sensible matter.[74]

This same order of study is also found in the section on the mathematical sciences by Vincent of Beauvais, the learned Dominican friar who was closely associated with the French monarch Louis IX as royal chaplain, librarian, and tutor to the royal children, for whom he composed an educational tract.[75] Although Vincent of Beauvais cannot be directly associated with the University of Paris, his three or four part *Speculum* indicated that he was apparently in close rapport with the intellectual and scholarly community in Paris.[76] He devoted one entire book (Liber XVI) to *mathematica* in the second part of the *Speculum*, that is the *Speculum Doctrinale.*[77] And he there asserted that mathematics should be read or studied after natural philosophy or natural science because the latter considers form as it is in matter, whereas the former or mathematics is abstracted by the intellect. And since sense apprehension is prior to intellectual apprehension it should come first.[78]

70 Borgnet VI, 61 (Metaph. I.IV.2); also *Summa Theologiae* II, tract. I, Q. 4, m. 2, ad 3, ed. Borgnet XXXII, 76: „Numerus quem attendit ratio divina in constituendo res, non est numerus formarum, sed est numerus proportionis...." See also Albertus, In II Sentent. Dist. 1, A. Art. V, Borgnet XXVII, 15: „Boetius in prohemio primi Arithmeticorum...constat autem quod de numero mathematico istud non potest intelligi: ergo necesse est, quod intelligatur de numero ideali qui praecessit omnia ideata."

71 St. Thomas Aquinas, „In XII libros Metaphysicorum," *Opera Omnia*, Paris, 1875, XXIV, 468b. (Metaph. IV, lect. 1).

72 St. Thomas Aquinas, „In X libros Ethicorum ad Nicomachum," *Opera Omnia*, 1875, XXV, 503-504 (Ethica VI, lect. 7).

73 Borgnet, V, 556 ff. „Liber de Apprehensione a quibusdam adscriptus." Preceding the above text which is in the form of a dialogue, is the statement that the work is ascribed by some to Albertus, but is rejected as not authentic by others, among them J. Quetif and J. Echard, *Scriptores ord. Praed.* (2 vol., Paris, 1719-21; new ed., I-VI, Paris, 1910-1913).

74 Borgnet, V, 607: Liber de apprehensione Pars VI.5: „Ideoque bene studentes primo in physicis, postea ad mathematica venerunt, et tandem in divinis finiunt vitam in ipsis felicitati cupientes...."

75 L. Thorndike, *History of Magic and Experimental Science*, II, 458.

76 Vincentius Bellovacensis (Vincent de Beauvais), *Speculum quadruplex sive Speculum maius naturale/ Doctrinale/ Morale/ Historiale*. Photocopy of the edition of 1624: Ex officina typographica Baltozaris Belieri, Duac. Photocopy made in Graz, Austria, 1965. For incunabula editions, see Klebs 1036.1-3, 1037.1-3.

77 „Tomus secundus: *Speculum Doctrinale*. Liber Decimus sextus. De mathematica."

78 *Ibid.*, end of cap. 1, 1504: „Haec scientia [id est mathematica] post naturalem legenda est, quia naturalis

Vincent of Beauvais described mathematics as the discipline which considers abstract quantity and deals with invisible forms of visible things just as *physica* deals with the visible causes of visible things. He then went on to explain in the fashion of the Boethian *Arithmetica* the fourfold aspect of quantity as either separate and permanent, that is arithmetic or number; or successive, that is music, the number of sounds; or quantity continuously mobile, that is astronomy; or immobile, as geometry.[79] The authority to whom Vincent of Beauvais turned after Boethius was Michael Scot, the noted scholar, translator, and astrologer, whom Professor Lynn Thorndike characterized as „the leading intellectual in Western Europe during the first third of the thirteenth century."[80] Boethius' *Arithmetica*, Book One, was cited not only for the above fourfold aspect of quantity but also for the statement that no one can attain the pinnacle of perfection in the disciplines of philosophy unless he is possessed of the nobility of intellect achieved through the comprehension of truth. And without knowledge of the four parts of the *mathematica* as noted above, the seeker for truth would be unable to find it.[81]

Vincent of Beauvais further cited Boethius on the primacy of arithmetic, among the mathematical arts, and he repeated the statement that arithmetic is the discipline of numbers, about which the first Greek to write was Pythagoras. And he was followed by Nicomachus, whose work was translated into Latin first by Apuleius and then by Boethius.[82] He reported from Boethius the well known phrase „All things which were constituted from the primeval origin of things seem to have been formed from the ratio of numbers"[83] and cited him on several other occasions as well.

With this encyclopedia we may bring to a close our brief foray into some of the evidence reflecting and exemplifying the continuity of interest in, and utilization of, the Boethian *Arithmetica* and the quadrivium in the university milieu at Paris. The survival of interest in these relics of Greek antiquity particularly among philosophers and theologians is an interesting demonstration of the persistence of the Greek elements in western intellectual history and the extent to which they were adapted and molded to the new interests of medieval scholars.

considerat formam prout est in materia: haec autem prout est abstracta, scilicet intellectu, apprehensio enim sensus prior est, quam apprehensio intellectus."

79 *Ibid.*, cap. 1, 1503; *Arith.* I.1, ed. Friedlein, pp. 8-9.

80 *Ibid.*, cap. 1, 1503. For Michael Scot, see Lynn Thorndike; *Michael Scot*, (London: Thomas Nelson and Sons Ltd., 1965), and especially pp. 54 ff. for his interest in numbers.

81 Vincent de Beauvais, *Spec. doct.* cap. II, 1504; *Arith.* I.1, ed. Friedlein, p. 9. See n. 12 above for the quotation.

82 Vincent de Beauvais, Spec. Doct., cap. V, 1506: „*Jsid. in lib. 3 Etymo*. Arithmetica est disciplina numerorum. Graeci namque numerum a *Rythmom* dicunt. Hanc apud Graecos primum conscripsisse Pithagoram autumant, et postmodum a Nicomacho diffusius esse dispositam, quam apud Latinos primus Apuleius, deinde Boetius transtulerunt."

83 Vincent de Beauvais, *Spec. doct.*, cap. VI, 1507: „Boetius ubi supra. Omnia quaecumque a primaeva rerum natura constituta sunt, numerorum videntur ratione esse formata..."; also *ibid.*, cap. vii, 1507, et passim. For the citation from Boethius, *Arith.* I, 2, see n. 30 above.

III

ALBERTUS MAGNUS ON ALCHEMY

Albert's interest in alchemy,[1] the art, in his words, that best imitates nature,[2] is revealed in the references to the subject in his authentic writings, particularly the *Book of Minerals* (*Liber mineralium*), his *Commentary on Aristotle's Meteorology*, and other tracts. He had investigated and made a careful study of the subject in the course of his inquiry into the nature of metals, for guidance in which he had sought in vain for the treatise by Aristotle.[3] Without that guide, he was, as he reported, obliged to follow his own devices and to set down what he had learned from philosophers or from his own observations. He had thus at one time become a wanderer, journeying to mining districts to "learn by observation the nature of metals." "And," he stated, "for the same reason I have inquired into the transmutations of metals in alchemy, so as to learn from this, too, something of their nature and accidental properties."[4] Among the

---

[1] For previous accounts of this subject see especially J. R. Partington, "Albertus Magnus," *Ambix* 1 (1937), 3-20; Lynn Thorndike, *History of Magic and Experimental Science* (New York, 1923) 2: 569-573; also my "Alchemical Writings Ascribed to Albertus Magnus," *Speculum* 17 (1942), 499-518; and Albertus Magnus, *Book of Minerals* translated into English by Dorothy Wyckoff (Oxford: Clarendon Press, 1967; henceforth indicated as Wyckoff), introduction pp. xxx-xxxii. See below VII.

[2] Albertus Magnus, *Liber mineralium* (*Opera omnia*, ed. A. Borgnet, Paris 1890, vol. 5, p. 61; henceforth indicated as *Min.* with number of book, tractate, and chapter): *Min.* III.1,2; Wyckoff, p. 158.

[3] *Min.* I.1,1; III.1.1; Wyckoff, pp. 9, 153, 263, item 14; and 267, item 8.

[4] *Min.* III.1,1; Wyckoff, p. 153; Partington, p. 11.

names of the philosophers to whom Albert had turned were some of the principal authorities on alchemy, current in the twelfth and thirteenth centuries in Latin translation from the Arabic, comprising chiefly Hermes, Callisthenes (that is Khālid ibn Yazīd), Democritus, Gigil, and Avicenna.[5] Of these Albert relied principally upon Avicenna (Abū ʻAlī ibn Sīnā, 980-1037), utilizing both the apocryphal and authentic tracts appearing under his name. Albert thus cited a section of the supposititious Avicenna tract *On the Soul in the Art of Alchemy* (*De anima in arte alchemiae*), one of the most influential of the alchemical tracts upholding the possibility of the transmutation of metals.[6] Naming the work, "The Physical [Stone]," Albert referred only to the final section, the "Exposition of the physical stone by Avicenna to his son Aboali (Abū ʻAlī)," which circulated as a separate tract.[7] In addition, Albert utilized the so-called "Letter of Avicenna to King Hasen (or Hazen), the philosopher," in which is set forth the view commonly held in the thirteenth century, that quicksilver (mercury or *argentum vivum*) and sulphur are the materials of all metals and hence basic to the alchemical process.[8] This so-called newer theory of the components of metals, Albert contrasted with the older view expressed by Aristotle, that metals are formed from a subtle fatty moisture (*humidum unctuosum subtile*) combined with a subtle earthy tincture.[9]

In addition, in his search for "immediate efficient causes existing in the material and transmuting it,"[10] Albert continued his critical

---

[5] For Hermes and the others named, see below.

[6] *Min.* III.1,4 and 9; Wyckoff, pp. 161 and 177; also 283-284. Ascribed to Avicenna, the work is printed in J. J. Manget, *Bibliotheca chemica curiosa* (Geneva, 1702) 1: 633-636, especially p. 634. Although the tract purported to have been prepared in 1012, it was probably written in Spain about 1140 and appears to have been translated into Latin from the Arabic in 1235 (Partington p. 3).

[7] *Min.* III.1,4; Wyckoff, pp. 161 n.1, 284; Dorothy Waley Singer, *Catalogue of Latin and Vernacular Alchemical Manuscripts in Great Britain*, 3 vols. (Brussels, 1928-1931) 1: 117.

[8] *Min.* III.1,4,9; Wyckoff, pp. 161, 177-178, 284. *The Letter of King Hasen* is printed in L. Zetzner, *Theatrum chemicum*, 6 vols. (Strasbourg, 1659-1661) 4: 863-874. For manuscripts see L. Thorndike and P. Kibre, *A Catalogue of Incipits of Mediaeval Scientific Writings in Latin*, new and augmented edition (Cambridge, Mass., 1963; henceforth indicated as TK with column number), 1036. The authenticity of this tract as by Avicenna has not generally been accepted although Stapleton (H. E. Stapleton, R. F. Azo, M. Hidayat Husain, and G. L. Lewis, "Two alchemical treatises attributed to Avicenna," *Ambix* 10 (1962), 41-83) who discovered an Arabic manuscript of this text suggested it was an early work of Avicenna written before he "abandoned his belief in transmutation": Wyckoff, p. 284.

[9] *Min.* III.1,2; Wyckoff, pp. 155-159; Partington p. 10.

[10] *Min.* I.1,4; Wyckoff, p. 19.

evaluation of so-called authorities and the operations of alchemy. He characterized as erroneous the opinions of Hermes, Empedocles, Democritus, "and some of those in our own time who are practitioners of alchemy," and who are concerned with the generation of stones. These authorities mistakenly suggested, he reported, that all stones are produced by accident without a specific cause for their production,[11] whereas the true or productive cause, Albert asserted, is a "mineralizing power."[12] The making of stones, he concluded, by the operations of the alchemists is even more difficult than the making of metals.[13] Albert had earlier noted that just as metals are formed from water congealed by intense cold and dryness,[14] just so is the work of the alchemists performed, that is by separating and sublimating the humidity of iron.[15] Moreover, in the operations of alchemy, he noted that mercury (*argentum vivum* or quicksilver) that is dried by much burning and mixture with sulphur will be coagulated by heating in a furnace with green wood.[16]

Albert next went on to draw attention to the discussions unfavorable to the transmutation of metals which he attributed also to Avicenna, wrongly citing the "Letter to King Hasen" as the source rather than Avicenna's tract on minerals, *De congelatione et conglutinatione lapidum*.[17] In this treatise which has been shown to be an excerpt from the authentic book *Book of the Healing of the Soul* (Kitāb al-shifā'),[18] Avicenna disparaged the "claims of the alchemists" whose "power to bring about any true change of metallic species," he denied with the words, "Let practitioners of alchemy know that they cannot transmute one form of metal into another, but only make something similar. . . .As to the rest, that is that specific differ-

---

[11] *Min.* I.1,4; Wyckoff, pp. 18-20.

[12] *Min.* I.1,5; Wyckoff, p. 22.

[13] *Min.* I.1,5; Wyckoff, p. 23.

[14] *Min.* III.1,7; *Meteor.* III.5 unicum (Borgnet 4: 701).

[15] *Meteor.* IV.2.9 (Borgnet 4: 761a).

[16] *Meteor.* IV.3,2 (Borgnet 4: 775); Partington p. 10.

[17] The *De congelatione* was translated into Latin ca. 1200 by Alfred of Sareshel. Frequently cited by Latin authors, it was often attributed to Aristotle as Albert noted. *Min.* III.I,9; Wyckoff, pp. 177, 178; Partington p. 4. It was cited with an English translation by E. J. Holmyard and Mandeville, *De congelatione et conglutinatione lapidum* (Paris, 1927), pp. 45-54. For MSS and earlier printed editions, see TK 1565; and Wyckoff, pp. 283-284; also A. C. Crombie, "Avicenna's Influence on the Medieval Scientific Tradition," in *Avicenna: Scientist and Philosopher. A millenary symposium*, ed. G. M. Wickens (London: Luzac and Co., 1952), 87-88; and bibliography in n. 14.

[18] Holmyard and Mandeville, p. 41.

ences between metals may be removed by some clever method, I [Avicenna] do not believe. . .possible."[19] Albert went on also to paraphrase Avicenna's further statement (in the "Letter to King Hasen on Alchemy") that he had examined the books of those upholding "the art of transmutation" and had found them devoid of the reasoning that belongs to every art. He had found most of their content nonsensical. Moreover, an examination of the books of those who opposed the art of transmutation revealed that their arguments and reasoning were too feeble and trivial to destroy belief in the art.[20] Hence it appeared prudent to add that "specific forms are not transmuted, unless perhaps they are first reduced to prime matter (*materia prima*) . . . and then, with the help of art, developed into the specific form of the metal" desired.[21] Albert then added to Avicenna's stricture his own criticism of the alchemical literature: "I have examined many alchemical books, and I have found them lacking in [evidence] and proof." They merely rely "on authorities," and conceal "their meaning in metaphorical language, which has never been the custom in philosophy. Avicenna is the only one who seems to approach a rational [attempt], though a meagre one, towards the solution of the above question, enlightening us a little."[22]

Albert, moreover, was critical of opinions expressed by alchemists which did not coincide with those of Aristotle or Avicenna. He cited the undeniable but nonspecific statement that metals are made up of all the elements, expounded in the *Book of Alchemy*, by Hermes, the mythical or legendary founder of alchemy, who was probably of Greek origin but was known to the west through Latin translations from the Arabic.[23] Albert also characterized as "the strangest and most ridiculous of all opinions, the one that held that '*calx* (quicklime) and *lixivium* (lye) are the material of all metals'," an opinion he attributed to Democritus. Albert asserted that this statement about

---

[19] Text in Holmyard, p. 54; *Min.* III.1,9; Wyckoff, p. 177; Partington, p. 3.

[20] *Min.* III.1,9; Wyckoff, p. 177 n.2.

[21] *Min.* III.1,9; Wyckoff, p. 178. The quotation is from the *De congelatione*, Holmyard and Mandeville, p. 55.

[22] *Min.* III.1,7; Wyckoff, p. 172.

[23] *Min.* III.1,4; Wyckoff, p. 162; also pp. 282-283. Hermes' work referred to here may have been the *Emerald Table* (*Tabula smaragdena*) included in the Pseudo-Aristotle, *Secret of Secrets*, translated from the Arabic into Latin by Plato of Tivoli (fl. 1134-1135). Hermes is credited with the ascription of the names of the planets to the names of the metals. *Min.* III.I,6: Wyckoff, pp. 168-169. He is also credited with the quotation from the *Emerald Table* that "earth is the mother of metals and heaven their father": Wyckoff, p. 169.

the material of metals does not fit the fact, and is incorrect.[24] He further referred to the opinion "that alchemy is the science that confers upon inferior metals the nobility of the superior ones," expressed by Callisthenes;[25] and to the attempt "to prove that fused ash is the material of metals," reported in the book of *Secrets* by "Gigil of Moorish Seville," which Albert noted, "has now been returned to the Spaniards."[26] Albert went on to characterize Gigil's arguments in defense of his assertion as "unconvincing and stupid," and "Gigil himself" as "a mechanic and not a philosopher" who relied too greatly upon "the mechanical operations of alchemy" and was guilty of making incorrect assertions regarding natural science.[27]

Albert next drew attention to the procedures and objectives of the alchemists. "The experience of the alchemists," he asserted, "confronts us with two grave doubts. For they seem to say that the specific form of gold is the sole form of metals and that every other metal is incomplete — that is, it is on the way toward the specific form of gold, just as anything incomplete is on the way toward perfection." Thus metals lacking the form of gold in their material "must be diseased." Hence to cure or remove these diseases the alchemists endeavor "to find a medicine which they call the *elixir*, by means of which they may remove the diseases of metals. . ." and bring "out the specific form of gold."[28] Continuing further with the use of the *elixir* and the transmutation of metals, Albert asserted that since "it is found by experience that by means of the *elixir* copper turns to silver, and lead to gold, and iron likewise to silver," the alchemists erroneously conclude "that the specific form of all metals is one and the same, but the diseases of the material are many," an opinion with

---

[24] *Min.* III.1,4; Wyckoff, p. 162. See also *Min.* I.1,4; Wyckoff, p. 20 n. 8, and p. 281; Partington p. 10. Albert, as Professor Wyckoff suggests, may have thought he was citing Democritus of Abdera (fifth cent. BC), one of the founders of the atomist philosophy, known only through Aristotle who was a severe critic of Democritus' theories. More likely, however, as Professor Wyckoff suggests, Albert may have seen a reference to a Democritus in the *Turba philosophorum* (*The Conference of Philosophers*), edited by J. Ruska (Berlin, 1931) and by Plessner (1954). Albert, however, would have thought them to be one and the same person.

[25] *Min.* III.1,7; Wyckoff, pp. 171-173, 283. Callisthenes, apparently for Khālid ibn Yazīd ibn Mu'āwiya, author of the *Book of the Three Words* (*Liber trium verborum*). The work is printed in J. J. Manget (1702) 2: 189-191.

[26] Gigil (Abū Dā'ud ibn Juljul) a physician of Spain in the tenth century. Wyckoff, p. 163; *Min.* III.1,4; Wyckoff, pp. 161-164, 284. As Professor Wyckoff indicates, the Christians reconquered Seville in 1248.

[27] *Min.* III.1,4; Wyckoff, p. 163.

[28] *Min.* III.1,7; Wyckoff, p. 171. On the *elixir* as a medicine, see *Min.* I.1,1; Wyckoff, p. 10.

which Albert would not concur. He went on rather to discuss the means, that is the use by the alchemists of "calcination, sublimation, distillation, and other operations," to induce the *elixir* to penetrate into the material of metals, and hence possibly "to destroy the specific forms of metals that originally were in the material. The material that remains can then with the help of the alchemical art be reduced to another specific form, just as seeds are helped by ploughing and sowing or [as] nature is helped by the efforts of the physician."[29] This explanation, Albert noted, was not acceptable to "Hermes and Gigil, and Empedocles and almost all that group of alchemists," who appeared to defend the "stranger" principle "that in any metal whatever there are several specific forms and natures, including one that is occult and one that is manifest."[30] Albert himself had earlier expressed his opinion that in the case of the "experiments which the alchemists bring forward," to establish the validity of their conclusions, they do not offer enough proof.[31]

Albert then went on further to compare the procedure of the skillful alchemists with that of the skillful physicians, and also to enlarge upon his theory of nature's role. The skillful physicians, he asserted, "by means of cleansing remedies clear out the corrupt or easily corruptible matter that is preventing good health — the end which physicians have in mind. In doing so, they strengthen and aid the power of nature, directing it to bringing about natural health. [Good] health will [thus] be produced by nature, as the efficient cause; and also by art as the means and instrument." The skillful alchemists also proceed similarly in transmuting metals. They first cleanse thoroughly the mercury or quicksilver and sulphur, the constituents of metals; then, when this is done, "they strengthen the elemental and celestial powers in the material, according to the proportions of the mixture in the metal that they intend to produce." Thus "nature itself performs the work, and not art, except as the instrument, aiding and hastening the process."[32] "The alchemists appear, in this manner, to produce and make real gold and real silver, since the elemental and celestial powers can produce in artificial vessels, if they are formed like those in nature, whatever they produce in natural vessels. Hence "whatever nature produces by the heat of the sun and stars, art also

---

[29] *Min.* III.1,7; Wyckoff, pp. 173-174.

[30] *Min.* III.1,8; Wyckoff, pp. 174-175.

[31] *Min.* III.1,7; Wyckoff, p. 173.

[32] *Min.* III.1,9; Wyckoff, p. 178.

produces by the heat of fire, provided the fire is tempered so as not to be stronger than the self-moving formative power in the metals."[33] The inclusion of the "stars" as an agency influencing chemical operations is further exemplified in Albert's assertion in his *De causis elementorum* that "when skilled alchemists work during the waxing of the moon, they produce purer metals and stones." Albert also referred to the introduction by Hermes of the association of the seven planets with the seven metals so that the substitution of the names of the planets for the metals, such as *sol* for gold, *luna* for silver, and so on, became common practice.[34] In general, Albert noted, "of all the operations of alchemy, the best is that which begins in the same way as nature," that is "with the cleansing of sulphur by boiling and sublimation, and the cleansing of quicksilver, and the thorough mixing of these with the material of metal; for in these by their powers, the specific form of every metal is induced." Moreover, the alchemist proceeds by destroying "one substance by removing its specific form, and with the help of what is in the material producing the specific form of another [substance]."[35]

Although Albert recognized in the above directions the theoretical validity of the alchemical process he was obliged to admit that he had never seen it successfully carried to completion. He thus stated that "we have rarely or never found an alchemist, as we have said, who [could] perform the whole [process]." It is true that "One of them may indeed produce with the yellow *elixir* the color of gold," and with "the white *elixir*, a color similar to silver"; and "may endeavor to make the color remain fast when it is placed in the fire and has penetrated the entire metal just as a spiritual substance is put into the material of a medicine." He may by this operation induce a yellow color, while at the same time "leaving the substance of the metal unchanged."[36] Such operators Albert denounced as "deceivers." Without doubt they are deceivers. . .since they do not make real gold and real silver." And yet most alchemists follow this practice in whole or in part. "For this reason I have had tests made on some alchemical gold, and likewise silver, that came into my possession, and it endured six or seven firings, but then, all at once, on fur-

---

33 *Min.* III.1,7; Wyckoff, p. 178.

34 *De causis elementorum* I.2,7 (Borgnet 9: 615); *Min.* III.1,6: Wyckoff, pp. 168-169.

35 *Min.* III.1,9; Wyckoff, p. 179.

36 *Min.* III.1,8; Wyckoff, p. 176.

ther firing, it was consumed and lost and reduced to a sort of dross."[37]

In accord, moreover, with his view that the aim of a natural scientist is not merely to accept the statements of others, but rather to make an effort to observe the phenomena at first hand, Albert supplemented the knowledge of alchemy that he had derived from past authorities in his reading of books on medicine and alchemy, with the results of his own observations and experiences. From his visits to mining districts, metal workshops, and alchemical laboratories, he had acquired a practical acquaintance with the nature of metals by a direct observation of processes in nature. "I have learned," he explained, "by what I have seen with my own eyes, that a vein flowing from a single source was in one part pure gold, and in another silver. . . ." And "[from what] miners and smeltermen have told me. . .[that] what artisans have learned by experience is also the practice of alchemists who, if they work with nature, transform the specific form of one metal into another."[38] Furthermore, from visits to laboratories, in all probability in Cologne and Paris, Albert reported on the results of his inquiries into "the transmutation of metals in the art called alchemy" which he had directed to contemporary workers in the field, that is the "alchemists of our time," whose names he does not reveal.[39] He referred to alchemical experiments which showed that watery moisture is easily converted into vapour, and to the use of the alembic.[40] He noted that minerals that seem to be intermediate between stones and metals are important reagents in alchemy since they may be influenced by laboratory treatment. And he added, "On these substances depends most of the science of those who endeavor to convert one [metal] into another."[41] He had further reported on operations similar to those of the alchemists, such as drying of mercury by frequent burning and mixture with sulphur or when placed in a hot furnace with green wood,"[42] or of the forming of metals "from water congealed by intense coldness and dryness."[43] And he also went on to note in his exposition of the alchemical art, which as earlier noted he had

---

[37] *Min.* III.1,9; Wyckoff, p. 179.

[38] *Min.* III.2,6; Wyckoff, pp. 200-201; also *Min.* III.1,1; Wyckoff, pp. 153-154.

[39] Partington, pp. 9-11; *Min.* I.1,4; also III.1,1; Wyckoff, pp. 20, 153-154.

[40] *Min.* III.1,3; Wyckoff, p. 156.

[41] *Min.* V.1; Wyckoff, pp. 239-240, 241 ff.

[42] Partington, p. 10, citing *Meteor.* IV.3,2 (Borgnet 4: 775).

[43] See the preceding note.

termed the best imitator of nature, that of the two major constituents, sulphur is known as the father and quicksilver as the mother, "as the writers on alchemy metaphorically" suggest.[44] Moreover, he drew attention to the fact that since in alchemy there is no better way of proceeding than with the yellow *elixir* made with sulphur, the alchemists have observed that there is an unctuousness in sulphur so intensely active in burning that it burns all metals, and in burning blackens everything on which it is cast. Hence, the alchemists recommend that the sulphur be washed in acid solutions and that it be cooked until no more yellow liquid comes forth. These solutions may then be sublimed until all the unctuousness capable of burning has been removed, and there remains only as much subtle unctuousness as can endure the fire without being reduced to ash. This is, Albert added, "expressly stated by the authorities, Avicenna, Hermes and many others, who are men of great experience in the nature of metals." Albert had also noted unskilled alchemists at work in the digestion or boiling by moist heat of the earthiness in the moisture in metals.[45]

The foregoing details regarding Albert's concern with alchemy provide convincing evidence of his interest in the subject. They also demonstrate Albert's belief in the possibility of the transmutation of metals, although he judged the process to be very difficult and beset with the errors and imitations of imposters. "For [as quoted by Partington] alchemical gold does not gladden the heart like the real gold, and is more [easily] consumed by fire, yet transformation may really be produced by exspoliation of properties by alchemical operations, as Avicenna teaches."[46] Albert's desire to explore the entire matter of the possible transmutation of metals as thoroughly as possible is further exemplified by his study of the principal authorities and direct observation of alchemical procedures in laboratories as well as by association with contemporary alchemists whose names he does not provide. However, there appears to be a dearth of contemporary evidence to attest that Albert himself was considered an adept alchemist or that he engaged in or performed the alchemical processes he describes. He appears rather to have been an acute observer, an onlooker, but not an active participant in the laboratory experiments.

---

[44] *Min.* IV,1; Wyckoff, p. 204.

[45] *Min.* III.1,2; Wyckoff, p. 158.

[46] Partington, p. 13, citing Albertus Magnus, *Sententiae* II.vii, F. 8 (Borgnet 27: 154 f.)

Despite the lack of contemporary and specific evidence of Albert's direct participation in alchemical laboratory procedures, his fame and repute as a skilled alchemist became manifest not long after his death. By the mid-fourteenth century he is mentioned in catalogues as author of an alchemical tract[47] and is credited with having had as a disciple in this art, Roger Bacon, the English schoolman.[48] Nor did this repute diminish in the fifteenth and sixteenth centuries. In a collection of Stowe manuscripts, Hugh of England named Albert as one of the several authorities in the field.[49] This fame, whether deserved or not, appears to have motivated the attachment to Albert's name of some twenty-eight or more tracts on alchemy.[50] They appear in manuscripts dating from the close of the thirteenth century with the major number in the late fourteenth or fifteenth century. How much of this literary output can be attributed to the common practice in the Middle Ages of attaching to such treatises the names of prominent churchmen in order to give them respectability and insure their acceptance cannot be determined. Nor does the explanation that Albert was confused with a chemist who lived at Cologne, provided by Naudé in his "Apology for all Great Personages Who Have Been Falsely Suspected of Magic,"[51] seem adequate. What does appear clear is the fact that for the most part the alchemical tracts bearing Albert's name as author reflect, in keeping with Albert's authentic writings, an active interest in not only the philosophical bases of the alchemical art but also in its practical and experimental aspects.

The individual alchemical treatises that appeared under Albert's name have elsewhere been enumerated and analyzed briefly together with the manuscripts and printed editions in which they are found.[52]

---

[47] See my "Alchemical Writings Ascribed to Albertus Magnus," *Speculum* 17 (1942), 499; also "The *Alkimia Minor* ascribed to Albertus Magnus," *Isis* 32 (1940 [1949]), 267-268 n. 5, for the MS 4 Qq A 10, formerly in the possession of the Speciale family and now in the Communal Library of Palermo. See below VII 499, IV 267-268 n. 5.

[48] Kibre, "Alchemical Writings Ascribed to Albertus Magnus," p. 499, and the references there cited; also Paris, Arsenal MS 2872, 14th cent., f. 46, "et le dit Roger estoit disciple de frère Albert. . . ." See below VII 499.

[49] London, British Library MS Stowe 1070, 15th cent., ff. 32-37: Hugh of England, *Secreta secretorum artis philosophorum*, inc. "After the mynde of Hermes, Plato, Morien, Geber, Aristotill, Virgill, Albert, Avicen etc. . . ." See also Partington, p. 17, for other citations.

[50] See my "Alchemical Writings Ascribed to Albertus Magnus," pp. 499-518; also my "Further Manuscripts Containing Alchemical Tracts Attributed to Albertus Magnus," *Speculum* 34 (1959), 238-247. See below VII 499-518 and IX 238-247.

[51] Kibre, "Alchemical Writings," p. 499; and G. Naudé, *Apologie pour tous les grands personnages qui ont esté faussement soupçonnes de magie* (Paris, 1625) chap. xviii. See below VII 499.

[52] See the references in note 50 above.

Hence it will perhaps suffice here merely to draw attention first to some general characteristics of the tracts and second, to choose some examples for more specific comparison with the information contained in Albert's authentic works. In general the treatises are free from the mystifying and allegorical features upon which Albert himself in the *Book of Minerals* had cast aspersion as characteristic of alchemical tracts. In this respect the imprint of Albert's didactic method, noteworthy for clarity of expression and systematic arrangement, was strong enough to influence those who professed to write under his name. As in Albert's exposition to his confreres of the Aristotelian scientific corpus, the professed purpose of the authors of the alchemical tracts, in the majority of cases, was to explain to their readers in as simplified a fashion as was necessary for their understanding, the art of alchemy, its theory and practice.

The above features are exemplified specifically in the *Little Book of Alchemy* (*Libellus de alchimia* or *Semita recta*), the tract most consistently attributed to Albert and extant in manuscripts dating from the close of the thirteenth century.[53] The clear, concise, and well ordered account of alchemy contained in this tract resembles Albert's treatment of other topics of natural science in his authentic works. It also provides an excellent introduction to the alchemical art of the late thirteenth and fourteenth centuries. The author is particularly concerned with making known to his confreres, the aims, accoutrements and processes of alchemists and the alchemical art. His instructions are detailed and even repetitious in character. They are, moreover, together with the frequent cautions and admonitions, largely practical in nature. Yet, true to the professed author's ecclesiastical calling, the work opens with the phrase from Ecclesiasticus: "All wisdom is from the Lord God." However, despite the fact that the suggestions contained in the tract are largely practical in nature and might perhaps have emanated from Albert, the author's style, beginning with the introduction, differs pointedly from that of Albert in his authentic works. For example, the introductory phrases con-

[53] See my "Alchemical Writings," pp. 500, 511-515; and "Further Manuscripts," pp. 238-244, for example Vatican MS Palatine 978, late 13th or beginning 14th cent., ff. 33r-46v; also British Library Additional MS 41486, end of 13th cent., ff. 7-8, containing selections of the work. This manuscript was brought to my attention by T. C. Skeat, then Deputy Keeper of the Manuscripts at the British Museum. See also *Libellus de alchimia ascribed to Albertus Magnus*, translated [into English] from the Borgnet Latin edition by Sister Virginia Heines, S.C.N. (Berkeley: University of California Press, 1958; henceforth cited as *Libellus de alchimia* [1958]), p. 75. See below VII 500, 511-515 and IX 238-244.

tain the author's stated conviction that he has found what he was seeking; not, however, (in his words) "by my own knowledge, but by the grace of the Holy Spirit. Therefore, since I discerned and understood what was *beyond nature*, I began to watch more diligently in decoctions and sublimations, in solutions and distillations, in cerations and calcinations and coagulations of alchemy and in many other labors until I found possible the transmutation into gold and silver, which is better than the natural [metal] in every testing and malleation."[54] This does not coincide with Albert's view in the *Book of Minerals*. There he had expressed his belief that while the transmutation of baser metals into gold was theoretically possible, it had not so far been accomplished by the alchemists; also that while the alchemists were able to produce a metal similar to gold, their product was inferior to natural gold or silver and did not stand the accepted test for gold.[55] Moreover, while the author of the *Little Book of Alchemy* looked "beyond nature," Albert had repeatedly stipulated that the observation of nature and natural processes provided the best guide.[56]

Yet despite these essential differences it appears evident that the author of the *Little Book of Alchemy* was acquainted with Albert's work, or at least utilized similar sources. He repeated from Avicenna's *Congelatio* the phrase which he mistakenly attributed to Aristotle, "Let the masters of alchemy know that the species of things cannot be changed," and the accompanying statement, here also attributed to Aristotle, "I do not believe that metals can be transmuted unless they are reduced to prime matter, that is purified of their own corruption by roasting in the fire." Only then is transmutation possible.[57]

The treatise itself also has some interesting features. Among these are the enumeration of possible errors and the list of specific precepts to guide those undertaking the enterprise. For example, attention is drawn to the fact that some were incapable of carrying out certain sublimations "because they failed to grasp the fundamentals"; "others because they used porous vessels." Also, in the precepts, the first provided that "the worker in this art must be silent and secretive

[54] *Libellus de alchimia* (1958), pp. 2-3.

[55] See above, and *Min.* III.1,9; Wyckoff, pp. 178-179.

[56] See above, also *Min.* III.2,6; Wyckoff, pp. 199-201.

[57] *Libellus de alchimia* (1958), pp. 9 and 10; and see above; also *Min.* III.1,4; Wyckoff, pp. 161-162.

and reveal his secret to no one";[58] and the eighth "that no one should begin operations without plenty of funds. . .for if he should. . .lack funds for expenses then he will lose the material and everything."[59] Contributing further to the practical nature of the tract are the descriptions of the various utensils, furnaces, ovens, and flasks; then the spirits: quicksilver, sulphur, orpiment, and sal ammoniac; and finally the *elixir* or *fermentum*, the medicine or philosophers' stone capable of transmuting baser metals into gold and silver.[60]

Another even more practical tract, the *Alkimia minor*, is attributed in the manuscripts to "Brother Albert of Cologne of the Order of Preaching Friars."[61] Best described, perhaps, as a laboratory manual, it has directions for the preparation of chemical substances, for the dyeing of metals red or white, that is the transmutation into gold or silver, and for the preparation of the *elixir* or medicine, the transmuting agent. Like the *Little Book of Alchemy* or *Semita recta*, of which it seems to include abstracts, the *Alkimia minor* appears to have been in circulation by the mid-fourteenth century, although no manuscripts of the text earlier than the fifteenth century have been located so far. However, the tract is listed with the same opening words among the books contained in a collection of alchemical treatises of the early fourteenth century.[62] The text itself gives no indication of the date of composition, although the chemical knowledge coincides with that of similar writings of the thirteenth and fourteenth centuries. The tract provides details of laboratory procedure and of apparatus and utensils. The directions are simple and straightforward with no attempt to mystify. Yet, the work does conform to the common practice of assigning names of planets to the minerals, and it also makes use of the term medicine as a synonym for *elixir*, the transmuting agent. Similarly, the use of "to redden" (*ad rubeum*) or "to whiten" (*ad album*) for the gold or silver making recipes can be found. An explanation for the use of these terms is given in the *Book of Minerals*.[63] Many of the chemical substances utilized were already described in such works as the *Book of Minerals* and the *Little Book*

---

[58] *Libellus de alchimia* (1958), pp. 3-4, and 12.

[59] Ibid., p. 14.

[60] Ibid., pp. 12-19.

[61] For the edition and analysis of the text, see Kibre "The *Alkimia Minor* Ascribed to Albertus Magnus," *Isis*, 32 (1940 [1949]), 268-300. See below IV 268-300.

[62] Ibid., p. 268 n 5.

[63] "*Alkimia Minor*," p. 270; *Min.* IV.7; Wyckoff, p. 231. See below IV 270.

of Alchemy. In general, the *Alkimia minor* is characterized by a total lack of attention to theory; the emphasis is on actual procedure and practice. Many of the processes listed, such as sublimation and distillation, for example, are common to pharmacy as well;[64] and there is great variety in the laboratory apparatus.[65] Included were furnaces, the baker's oven (*furnus panis*), and the furnace of reverberation, the dung bath, marble slab, alembics, aludel, recipient (*ampulla*), and various kinds of jars, flasks, and vessels; earthen, copper, and glass, closed or open; a descensory, that is a vessel or retort used in distillation by descent, and pestles of iron or wood, as well as a mallet or hammer.

A further tract attributed to Albertus Magnus for which there are no fourteenth-century manuscripts extant but which is named in the same fourteenth-century alchemical miscellany as the *Alkimia minor*,[66] is that entitled "On the hidden things of Nature" (*De occultis naturae*).[67] This treatise provides a survey of the various alchemical doctrines set forth by alchemical authorities chiefly of Arabic origin. The work bears only a slight resemblance to the other alchemical tracts ascribed to Albertus Magnus. It professes to have been written in response to a request by a reverend father,[68] addressed in the course of the work. Unlike either the *Semita recta* or the *Alkimia minor*, with which it is frequently found in the manuscripts, the *De occultis naturae* relates more to the theoretical side of alchemy than to the practical although both aspects are covered. The author has utilized a large number of writers with the intention, he informs us, of making it unnecessary for the reader to consult them further since their principal doctrines will have been transferred in briefer form to the present compendium. In general the treatise appears to resemble more the alchemical writings of the fourteenth rather than those of the thirteenth century in its predilection for alchemical jargon, allegorical devices, and mystical phraseology.[69]

---

[64] "*Alkimia Minor*," pp. 271-272. See below IV 271-272.

[65] Ibid., pp. 272-273.

[66] "Manuale d'alchimia miscellanea membranceo del secolo XIV," Palermo, MS 4 Qq A 10. See "*Alkimia minor*," p. 268 n. 5; also P. Kibre, "The *De Occultis Naturae* attributed to Albertus Magnus," *Osiris*, 11 (1954), 24 n. 7. See below V 24 n. 7.

[67] Ibid. pp. 23-39; also "Albertus Magnus, *De Occultis Nature*" *Osiris*, 13 (1958), 157-183, for an edition of the text. See below VI.

[68] Kibre, "*The De Occultis Naturae*," (1954), pp. 24-25. See below VI 24-25.

[69] Ibid., pp. 34-35.

Of the remaining alchemical treatises appearing under Albert's name, it may suffice to note here two further examples. The tract *On Alchemy* (*De alchimia*)[70] which appears not to have been available before the fifteenth century, bears a close relationship with the *Book of Minerals* in several of the arguments presented and in the discussion regarding alchemy. It is distinguishable from the *Little Book on Alchemy* (*Libellus de alchimia* or *Semita recta*) by the opening words: "Callisthenes one of the earlier founders of our art after Hermes. . . ." In addition to Callisthenes, the author names other authorities similar to those included in Albert's discussion in the *Book of Minerals*, such as Hermes, and Avicenna. In addition he names Geber Hispanus[71] instead of Gigil and attributes to him the statement with some verbal changes, that Albert expresses as his own, in the *Book of Minerals*, namely that he has examined certain alchemical books and has found them to be without distinction and with their intention hidden under the guise of allegory. The author here also follows the current practice of using the names of the seven planets as synonyms for the metals, a practice that Albert attributed to Hermes. But he fails to repeat here the references to the influence of the heavens in the alchemical process found in the *Book of Minerals*. On the other hand he follows Albert's emphasis upon the principle that alchemy imitates nature and hence that it is necessary to observe carefully and closely natural processes.[72]

The other tract attributed to Albert that we would note here, namely the *Compound of Compounds* (*Compositum de compositis*) attracted attention in the fifteenth to seventeenth centuries when it was translated into French and English. However, the text in the late manuscripts resembles closely that found without Albert's name as author in a fourteenth-century manuscript at Edinburgh. In that text the work is said to have been collected and promulgated by masters at Paris in the year 1331. However, in the later manuscripts at Paris and the Vatican it is clearly attributed to Albertus Magnus.[73] In the course of the work reference is made to "our *Book on Minerals*" which is suggestive of Albert. There are included in the tract discus-

---

70 P. Kibre, "An Alchemical Tract Attributed to Albertus Magnus," *Isis*, 35 (1944), 303-316.
See below VIII 303-316.

71 Ibid., p. 303.

72 Ibid., pp. 303-304.

73 P. Kibre, "Alchemical Writings Ascribed to Albertus Magnus," p. 506, item 8.
See below VII 506.

sions on the theory of alchemy along with practical recipes for the preparation of vermillion and of white sublimate.[74]

Of the remaining alchemical treatises appearing under Albert's name, none, with the exception of those that are also ascribed to other authors as well, appeared before the fifteenth century. Although the relation of these alchemical texts to Albert is tenuous to say the least, they do attest to his repute as an adept alchemist in the decades and centuries following his death.

---

[74] Partington, pp. 17, 19-20. A copy in French translation is contained in a manuscript at the Beinecke Library (Yale University, New Haven, Conn.), MS Mellon 19, 15th cent., ff. 28v-32r: "Incipit tractatus Alberti qui intitulatus Compositum de compositis." I am preparing an edition of this text.

IV

THE *ALKIMIA MINOR* ASCRIBED TO ALBERTUS MAGNUS

In the category of the more practical treatises in alchemy may be placed the hitherto unedited *Alkimia minor* attributed in the manuscripts to Brother ALBERT OF COLOGNE of the order of preaching friars, that is to the well known Dominican scholar, ALBERTUS MAGNUS (1193-1280 A.D.), whom Dr. THORNDIKE named " the dominant figure in Latin learning and natural science of the thirteenth century " (1). The work may well be characterized as a laboratory manual with its straightforward and concise directions for the preparation of chemical substances, the dyeing of metals, red or white, symbolical for the transmutation into gold or silver, and the preparation of the elixir or medicine, that is the transmuting agent. Parts of the work (2) were apparently abstracts from or supplementary to the more extensive *Semita recta* or *De alkimia* which, of all the alchemical compositions parading under his name, seems most likely to have been the work of ALBERTUS MAGNUS (3).

Both the *Semita recta* and the *Alkimia minor* appear to have been in circulation by the middle of the fourteenth century. Manuscripts of the former (4) testify to that fact, while in the case of the latter, although no manuscripts from before the fifteenth century have thus far been located, the listing of such a tract, with the same opening words, among the books contained in an

(1) LYNN THORNDIKE, *History of Magic and Experimental Science during the first Thirteen Centuries of Our Era*, New York, 1923, II, 521.

(2) See below.

(3) Ed. as *Libellus de alchimia*, in D. ALBERTI MAGNI Opera omnia, A. et. Æ. BORGNET, Paris, 1898, XXXVII, 545-573. See also L. THORNDIKE, *op. cit.*, II, 571-73; J. R. PARTINGTON, " ALBERTUS MAGNUS on Alchemy," in *Ambix*, 1937, I, 9-13; and my survey of the " Alchemical Writings ascribed to ALBERTUS MAGNUS," in *Speculum*, 1942, XVII, 499-518. See below VII.

(4) A list of the manuscripts of the *Semita recta* is contained in the survey of ALBERT's alchemical writings noted above.

alchemical collection of the early fourteenth century (5), may serve to place it before the fifteenth century. The inclusion of ALBERT's name as author of the *Alkimia minor* is found in all four of the extant manuscripts. But this provides no justifiable reason for accepting the authenticity of the ascription. The practice by medieval writers on alchemy, in order to give their works greater authority, of sending them forth under the names of personages prominent in the ecclesiastical world is well-known and is responsible for the ascription of many such treatises not only to ALBERTUS MAGNUS, but also to RAYMOND LULL, THOMAS AQUINAS, and to a host of others. Yet in the case of ALBERTUS MAGNUS, one is strongly tempted to believe that there is some basis for accepting the ascription of some of the several alchemical works bearing his name. Thus in the *De mineralibus*, the authenticity of which has nowhere been doubted, ALBERT demonstrates his interest and probable belief in the transmutation of metals and reveals his acquaintance with many of the processes, apparatus, utensils, and aims of the practical chemistry of his epoch. He mentions the alchemists of his time and has apparently visited their laboratories (6). On the other hand, the absence of manuscripts earlier than the fourteenth century and the failure of his immediate biographers to assign any such works to him, throw doubt upon the veracity of the ascriptions.

The present treatise itself provides little means either for dating it or for ascertaining its authorship. If it is identical with the work in the fourteenth century alchemical collection it was

---

(5) See item 30 : Item tractatus fratris Alberti qui incipit dilecto in christo fratri N. ordinis predicatorum, in " Exemplum librorum alchimicorum quos habet reverendus frater dominicus monacus monasterii sancti Proculi de bononia," no. 46, in *Manuale d'alchimia miscellaneo membranceo del secolo XIV*, Palermo, MS. 4 Qq A 10, formerly in the possession of the Speciale family and now in the Communal library of Palermo. I have transcribed the item from a film copy of DI MARZIO's reprint made in 1872 of CARINI's description. The photostat was loaned to me by the kindness of Dr. W. J. WILSON, of the Department of Manuscripts at the Library of Congress.

(6) Cf. P. KIBRE, " An Alchemical Tract attributed to Albertus Magnus," in *Isis*, 1944 (1945), XXXV, 303-316; *Opera omnia*, BORGNET, Paris, 1890, V, 1-103. See also THORNDIKE, *History of Magic and Experimental Science*, 1923, II, 567-69; PARTINGTON, in *Ambix*, 1937, I, 9-13; M. BERTHELOT, *La chimie au moyen âge*, Paris, 1893, I, pp. 290-92; BERTHELOT, *Introduction à l'étude de la chimie*, 1889, pp. 260-61. See below VIII.

composed not later than the middle of the fourteenth century. The chemical knowledge portrayed is also closely related to that of other similar writings of the thirteenth and fourteenth centuries (7). No authors or alchemical writers are cited in the work although there is mention made of the *Dicta philosophorum* (8).

Despite this failure either to date the treatise more exactly or to fix with certainty its authorship, the *Alkimia minor* is of interest for the history of scientific thought and for the general history of alchemy and technology. It may be said further to illustrate BERTHELOT's dictum that this science, reputed to be purely chimerical and cited occasionally as one of the aberrations of the human intellect, belongs in the field of positive history (9). The treatise provides details regarding the status of chemical knowledge in the late thirteenth and early fourteenth centuries. It describes actual laboratory procedure common at the time, and gives the names of the various apparatus and utensils in use. The directions are simple, there is no attempt to mystify nor to resort to the allegorical form of exposition found in some alchemical writings (10), and there is a lack of the magical and occult features frequent in these treatises. Occasionally, however, in common with the majority of such works and in accord with the generally accepted astrological doctrine that each planet

(7) See especially VINCENT OF BEAUVAIS, *Speculum naturale*, Vol. I, Lib. VI-IX; (I have used the incunabulum edition, at the Union Theological Seminary in New York City, of [Nurembergae, ANTH. KOBURGER, 1485], Vol. I); also the *Speculum doctrinale*, Lib. XII, caps. 105-133; edition of Argentinae, [sine nota] JOANNES MENTELIN [1473], Vol. II, at the Union Theological Seminary. The information from VINCENT OF BEAUVAIS is summarized in BERTHELOT, *La chimie au moyen âge*, 1893, I, pp. 280-289. Cf. ROBERT STEELE, " Practical Chemistry in the Twelfth Century : Rasis de aluminibus et salibus," *Isis*, 1929, XII, pp. 10-46. Much the same information is found in the alchemical manuscript analyzed by Dr. W. J. WILSON, " An Alchemical Manuscript by ARNALDUS DE BRUXELLA," *Osiris*, 1936, II, pp. 220-405.

(8) This term is applied to various recensions of an alchemical compilation. See D. W. SINGER, *A Catalogue of Latin and Vernacular Alchemical Manuscripts in Great Britain and Ireland dating from before the XVIth Century*, Brussels, 1928-1931, items 12, 18, 19, 20, 24; corr. 11 A, 16 A, 24 B.

(9) M. BERTHELOT, *Introduction à l'étude de la chimie des anciens et du moyen âge*, Paris, 1889, preface p. v. It is significant that in the *Speculum doctrinale* attributed to VINCENT OF BEAUVAIS, alchemy is listed among the mechanical arts : De artibus mechanicis, Lib. XII.

(10) In this regard see L. THORNDIKE, *History of Magic and Experimental Science*, 1934, III, 75 *et seq.*

governed some mineral, namely the Sun, gold, the Moon, silver, Venus, copper, Mars, iron, Saturn, lead, Jupiter, tin, and Mercury, quicksilver, the names of the planets are substituted for the corresponding metals. Thus *sol* appears for gold, *luna* for silver, and *mars* for iron. The use of such a term as medicine as a synonym for elixir or the transmuting agent, though mystifying to the modern reader, was in accord with the prevalent theories of the thirteenth and fourteenth centuries. Similarly the use of "ad rubeum" or "ad album" for the gold or silver-making recipes frequently appears in such compositions (11). An interesting explanation of the use of these terms is provided by ALBERTUS MAGNUS in the fourth book of the *Liber mineralium :*

> The fact, however, must not be ignored, that gold which is found as yellow or saffron-colored becomes by decoction red, because the absorption of the whiteness of the material element is greater than of the redness of the formal element. Hence the alchemists wishing to make gold strive for the *elixir* to redden. This they call medicine. It is the object of their desire that it embody four characteristics, namely that of color, penetration, imperishability in fire, and consolidation, and they call this redness of the sun (rubeum solis). Likewise the *elixir* that they seek for silver-making should display the color of whiteness, should be penetrative, and should not evaporate in fire. Also it should have subtlety. And this they call whiteness of the moon (album lunae). Hence Hermes says that this is the root on which all such philosophers are sustained, that the red of the sun is the medicine, likewise the white of the moon (12).

Although most of the chemical substances utilized in the present treatise were already described in such works as ALBERT's *De mineralibus* and the *Semita recta* or *Libellus de alchimia*, as it is entitled in BORGNET's edition, the distinguishing features of the present tract are the total disregard for theory and the emphasis

(11) Caps. 16, 17, 24, 32, below; *Lib. de alchimia*, ¶ 12 : De generibus medicinarum et nominibus earum; ¶ 47, Borgnet XXXVII, 552, 568. See also W. J. WILSON, in *Osiris*, II, 292.

(12) *Lib. mineral.* IV, cap. 7, BORGNET V, 93 : Non autem ignorandum est, quod aurum quasi citrinum et croceum invenitur, quod tamen per decoctionem rubescit propter materialis principii quod album magis quam formalis quod est rubeum, consumptionem : propter quod alchimici volentes aurum facere, student ad elixir rubeum, quod medicinam vocant : et studium eorum est quod quatuor in se habeat, colorationem videlicet, et penetrationem, et immortalitatem in igne, et consolidationem : et hoc vocant *rubeum solis*. Elixir autem ad argentum student habere colorationem albedinis, et quod sit penetrativum, et non evaporet ab igne, et habeat subtilitatem : et hoc vocant *album lunae :* propter quod dicit Hermes, qui est radix super quam omnes Philosophi sui sustentati sunt, quod rubeum solis medicina est, album vero lunae.

upon actual procedure and practice. Each recipe opens with a brief statement as to the necessity or importance of the particular mineral in the present operation and then at once goes on to the steps to be taken for its preparation. Two examples from the text will illustrate this :

Rubification and solution of the atrament. Chapter one.

Atrament is necessary for this work. It is a black earth having the odor of sulphur. Take it therefore and grind it up very finely and enclose it carefully in a clean jar and put it on a slow fire for two hours. Afterward you may increase the fire until the jar becomes red hot, and you may leave it at such heat for the night. In the morning upon opening [it] you will find in the jar a very red substance which is called flower of atrament (flos atramenti). Then take this red substance and grind it up with sal ammoniac and sublimate from it the sal ammoniac and do this three times. After that put it on a marble [slab] in the cellar or in a damp place and it will be resolved into a very red liquid (aquam), which you should preserve carefully in a glass jar. For it is the noble fixed water with which the spirit and bodies are imbued with a red color that they never lose and it is one of the bonds of the spirits.

. . . .

On tartar and its preparation. Chapter seven.

Tartar is a very noble thing and relates to this science. Take it therefore and you will calcine it in a strong fire for three days. After it has been placed on a marble [slab] in a damp place it may be dissolved. Afterward it may be congealed again and once again dissolved in clear water. And this can be repeated four times. Then you will have a very noble oil of tartar with which the spirits are formed as well as dissolved, and [with which] they enter. Keep [it] therefore by itself apart.

Among the various processes, many of them common to pharmacy as well as to chemistry and the industrial arts (13), which are referred to in this treatise, are sublimation, that is the vaporization of a solid or liquid by application of heat and its recondensation (14), and distillation both through the alembic with the application of heat and through the filter (15). Use is also

---

(13) Reference has been made to the very useful glossary index of terms given by R. Steele, " Practical Chemistry in the Twelfth Century," *Isis*, 1929, XII, pp. 42-46; and by W. J. Wilson, " An Alchemical Manuscript by Arnaldus de Bruxella," *Osiris*, 1936, II, 383-401. The indices at the close of the various volumes on the history of alchemy by Berthelot are also valuable in this regard.

(14) Caps. 1, 6, 7, 9-12, 14, 17, 18, 25, 29. See also *Libellus de alchimia*, ¶ 30, Borgnet XXXVII, 559; W. J. Wilson, *loc. cit.*, II, 311.

(15) Caps. 5, 8, 20, 21, 22, 23, 28-31; *Lib. de alchimia*, ¶ 35, ¶ 48, ¶ 49, Borgnet XXXVII, 561, 568-69; W. J. Wilson, *loc. cit.*, II, 306-307, 309; Berthelot, *La chimie au moyen âge*, Paris, 1893, I, 161.

made of calcination, pulverization and grinding (16); of assaying, boiling or cooking (17); and of cementation (18), dissolution and resolution or liquefaction (19). Coagulation is named synonymously with congelation, that is solidification and crystallization (20). There is frequent mention of fixation or solidification either of a liquid or gaseous substance (21). Other processes included are ceration or the reduction to the consistency of wax (22), purging or purifying usually by washing (23), melting (24), deadening (mortificare) (25), and alchemical coloring, that is rubification or gold making and whitening or silver making (26).

The laboratory apparatus and utensils are also those usually described as part of the equipment of the alchemist, practical chemist or pharmacist of the period. Included are the furnaces, the baker's oven (furnus panis), and the furnace of reverberation (27); the dung bath (28), marble slab (29), alembics, aludel, recipient (ampulla), and various kinds of jars, flasks, and vessels, earthen, copper, and glass, closed or open (30); also a glazed

---

(16) Caps. 1, 2, 4, 7, 9, 10, 11, 13, 14, 15, 16, 17, 18, 25, 26, 27, 32; *Lib. de alchimia*, ¶ 31, ¶ 51, ¶ 53, BORGNET XXXVII, 559, 569, 570; W. J. WILSON, *Osiris*, 1936, II, 311.

(17) Caps. 9, 25; 8, 21, 27, 28.

(18) Caps. 27, 32. See also *Lib. de mineralibus*, I, tract II, cap. 7, BORGNET V, 20-21; BERTHELOT, *Introduction à l'étude de la chimie des anciens et du moyen âge*, 1889, p. 15; W. J. WILSON, in *Osiris*, II, 314.

(19) Caps. 1-7, 14, 16, 31; *Lib. de alchim.*, ¶ 34, ¶ 46, BORGNET XXXVII, 560-61, 567; W. J. WILSON, in *Osiris*, II, 324.

(20) Caps. 4, 5, 6, 7, 16, 17, 20, 22, 25, 30-32; *Lib. de alchimia*, ¶ 32, ¶ 50, BORGNET XXXVII, 560, 569; BERTHELOT, *Introduction à l'étude de la chimie*, 1889, p. 210; W. J. WILSON, in *Osiris*, II, 322.

(21) Caps. 7, 9, 10, 11, 12, 13; *Lib. de alchim.*, ¶ 33, ¶ 43, BORGNET XXXVII, 560, 565; W. J. WILSON, in *Osiris* II, 321; BERTHELOT, *La chimie au moyen âge*, Paris, 1893, I, 155, 157.

(22) Cap. 5; *Lib. de alchim.* ¶ 36, BORGNET XXXVII, 561; W. J. WILSON, in *Osiris*, II, 330.

(23) Cap. 4, 6, 9, 16, 17; W. J. WILSON, in *Osiris*, II, 306.

(24) Cap. 30, 32.

(25) Cap. 9.

(26) Caps. 10, 13, 15, 24, etc.

(27) Caps. 9, 26, 27; cf. *Lib. de alchim.* ¶ 4-8, Quod furni sunt necessarii; BORGNET XXXVII, 550-51.

(28) Caps. 16, 18, 22, 23, 25, 32.

(29) Caps. 1, 7, 9, 17.

(30) Caps 16, 23, 24, 29, 31 (alembic); caps. 9, 10 (aludel); caps. 13, 18, 29, 32 (ampulla); and various other vessels, caps. 1, 5, 8-9, 11-12, 18, 20, 22, 28, 29, 32.

parapsis (31), glass cucurbite (32); stoppers of glass or of cloth (33), a descensory, that is the vessel or retort used in distillation by descent (34); and pestles of iron or wood, as well as a mallet or hammer (35).

The *Alchimia minor* is reproduced below from a photostat of the manuscript at Venice, Biblioteca San Marco VI.214 (Valentinelli XVI, 3), 1472 A.D., fols. 180r-189v (A); with variant readings in the footnotes from three Paris manuscripts (36) at the Bibliothèque nationale : 6749B, 1481 A.D., fols. 48r-52r (B); 7162, 15th cent., fols. 80v-85r (C), except for slight variations identical with the preceding; and Nouvelle acquisition 1293, 15th-16th cent., fols. 59-61v (D). The last named, containing only the first sixteen chapters, has a greater number of variations than the others, and is more carelessly written. Headings to the chapters have only been added later in the margins. The other two Paris manuscripts are practically identical although there are some minor differences, which suggest that one has been copied from the other. The text in the Venice manuscript is the most complete, also it is the most legible and the most systematically arranged of all. The omissions which occur in the Paris manuscripts, indicating that these texts may have been copied from an earlier text similar to that in the Venice manuscript, are often due to the copyist carelessly dropping a line or two where the same word has been repeated within the space of a few lines. Examples of this may easily be detected in the transcription of the text (37). The Venice manuscript is the only one in which the headings have been numbered. In the transcription from the Venice manuscript no general attempt has been made to emend the text; the spellings of this manuscript have for the most part

(31) Cap. 5; W. J. WILSON, *Osiris* II, 323.

(32) Caps. 29, 31, 32; *Lib. de alchim.* ¶ 52, BORGNET XXXVII, 570.

(33) Caps. 29, 32.

(34) Cap. 23, *descensorium*.

(35) Cap. 26, 13.

(36) Photostatic copies of the text in the four MSS. were obtained for me through the good offices of Dr. W. J. WILSON of the Library of Congress, Mr. DONALD GOODCHILD, Corresponding Secretary of the American Council of Learned Societies, and The Mediaeval Academy of America, from the revolving fund of the Modern Language Association in the manuscript division of the Library of Congress.

(37) See for example notes 110, 116, 148, 337, 369, 382, 409.

been retained, with the exception of the substitution of *j* or *v* for consonantal *i* or *u* where these would make the reading more easily comprehensible. Differences in word order or spelling in the other manuscripts are not noted, except where these are especially marked (38).

Before proceeding to the Latin transcription of the text it will perhaps prove useful to provide a brief summary of its contents. This work like several of ALBERT's authentic writings is addressed to a brother of his order and has as its stated purpose the exposition of that science called "alchemy," in which the author claims to be adept. Its plan as set forth in the introductory paragraph is to describe first certain essential preparations and then the elixirs or the compositions of medicines that change substances into red and white, or gold and silver. There are 32 divisions or very short chapters each of which is numbered in the Venice manuscript. The first eight divisions describe the preparation or rubification and dissolution of the atrament (39) (cap. 1), the calcination and solution of alum of Yemen (40) (cap. 2), the dissolution of the greenness of copper (41) (cap. 3), the preparations of sal communis or common salt (42) (cap. 4), of sal alkali from clavellated ashes of the calcined dregs of wine (43) (cap. 5), and of sal ammoniac (44)

---

(38) Since this transcription was made I have noted an additional MS text at the Vatican, Palatine 1330, 15th cent., fols. 60v-72r, where it is placed between parts of the *Semita recta*. This text follows closely that of the Venice MS. What further appears as an abbreviated version of the *Alkimia minor* is found in a Florence, Riccardian MS : 1243 (s. III, 18), 15th cent., fols. 17r-48v. See *Speculum*, 1942, XVII, 502, 511, item 23. See below VII.

(39) *Lib. de alchim.* ¶ 22; *De mineral.* V, 3, BORGNET XXXVII, 556; V, 99.

(40) Alum belongs to the early Greek tradition and is also found in DIOSCORIDES, PLINY, etc. BERTHELOT, *Introduction à l'étude de la chimie*, Paris, 1889, p. 236. Alum from Yemen is said to have been preferred as the best : STEELE, "Practical Chemistry in the Twelfth Century," *Isis*, 1929, XII, 42; *Lib. de alchim.* ¶ 21, ¶ 20 additio, ¶ 22, additio; *De mineral.* V, 4, BORGNET XXXVII, 555-56; V, 100.

(41) Viride eris, *Lib. de alchim.* ¶ 24, BORGNET XXXVII, 556-57.

(42) *Lib. de alchim.* ¶ 18; *De mineral.* V, 2, BORGNET XXXVII, 554; V, 98.

(43) Salt prepared from the clavellated ashes of dried and calcined lees of wine. Cf. DU CANGE II, 1937, p. 333 : "cineres clavati qui ex fece vini siccata et combusta conficiuntur," (1332 A.D.). See also *Lib. de alchim.* ¶ 20, BORGNET XXXVII, 555.

(44) For various changes in the meaning of the term see BERTHELOT, *Introduction à l'étude de la chimie*, 1889, p. 45, n. 2, pp. 237-38. *Lib. de alchimia*, ¶ 17, ¶ 41, BORGNET XXXVII, 553-54, 564. See also W. J. WILSON, in *Osiris*, II, 302.

(cap. 6), also the preparation of tartar (45) (cap. 7), and of urine of boys (46) (cap. 8).

The second part of the work relates chiefly to the processes of sublimation and fixation : the sublimation of mercury (47) (cap. 9), of sulphur (48) (cap. 10), and of arsenic (49) (cap. 11). Two methods of fixation are described, that is by subjection to heat (cap. 12), and through the application of oil of tartar (cap. 13).

Then follow, in part three, directions for the preparing of the waters of metals necessary in all elixirs for making gold or silver (50) (cap. 14), for the coloring of the spirits (51), which must be done before the medicines are prepared (cap. 15), and for the preparing of the medicines for making gold (ad rubeum) (52) (cap. 16), and for making silver (ad album) (cap. 17), and also directions for the preparing of various fixed or solidified oils : oil of gold for gold making (cap. 18), oil of mars for iron oxide (crocus martis) (cap. 19), and oil of Roman vitriol (cap. 20). Next are given directions for preparing the non-fixed or volatile oils : oil of sulphur (cap. 21), oil of the greater stone, prepared from human blood (cap. 22), and oil of the ferment (cap. 23). A résumé of the method of composing the medicine, that is the transmuting agent or elixir (cap. 24), follows. The remaining sections contain recipes for treating the golden stone, or gold marcasite (53) which is

---

(45) Cf. *Lib. de alchimia*, ¶ 23, BORGNET XXXVII, 556.

(46) Cf. R. STEELE, *Isis*, 1929, XII, 46; *Lib. de mineral.* V, 2, BORGNET V, 99.

(47) Cf. *Lib. de alchimia*, ¶ 13, ¶ 30, ¶ 37, BORGNET XXXVII, 552-3. 559, 562-63.

(48) *Lib. de mineralibus*, IV, I; *Lib. de alchim.* ¶ 14, ¶ 38, BORGNET V, 83-84; XXXVII, 553, 563.

(49) *Lib. de mineralibus*, V, 5; *Lib. de alchim.* ¶ 16, ¶ 39, BORGNET, V, 100; XXXVII, 553, 563; ¶ 40, p. 564; BERTHELOT, *Introd. à l'étude de la chimie des anciens...*, p. 238, quoting from DIOSCORIDES, PLINY, and VINCENT DE BEAUVAIS.

(50) *Lib. de alchim.* ¶ 10-11, BORGNET XXXVII, 552; W. J. WILSON, *Osiris*, II, 296-301.

(51) *Lib. de alchim.* ¶ 10, ¶ 47, BORGNET XXXVII, 552, 568; W. J. WILSON, *Osiris*, II, 266.

(52) *Lib. de alchim.* ¶ 12, De generibus medicinarum et nominibus earum, BORGNET, XXXVII, 552; W. J. WILSON, *Osiris*, II, 292.

(53) R. STEELE, "Practical Chemistry in the Twelfth Century," *Isis*, 1929, XII, 45, describes marcasites as "a variety of pyrites, either gold, silver, copper, or iron." Cf. *Lib. de mineral.* V, 6, BORGNET V, 101 : In alchimicis etiam iste lapis principalis cibus est, cum quo cibatur argentum vivum ad elixir album ex argentea marchasita, ad elixir rubeum ex aurea.

said to produce the perfected body or gold (corpus perfectum s. sol) (cap. 25), for the preparation of crocus ferri (54), that is iron oxide (cap. 26), also for the making of stone or lime (calculum or calcutium) (cap. 27) from the filings of old copper, and of vitriol (55) (cap. 28). A second recipe for crocus ferri follows (cap. 29). Then come further directions for preparing lime (calcutium) and vitriol (cap. 30); for the distillation of mercury which is afterward congealed to the elixir for the great gold (cap. 31); and finally for the combination of all the foregoing to form the perfect medicine (cap. 32).

Incipit trac[ta]tus alkimie fratris ALBERTI DE COLONIA (1).

Dilecto (2) in Christo patri (3) N. ordinis predicatorum (4) ALBERTUS eiusdem ordinis salutem in domino. Ex cunctis nostre scientie libris et secretorum (5) abditis diligenti indagatione prehibita relictis causarum divinis (6) et divinarum causis attestantibus quidem (7) vel negantibus quam alkimialiter (8) appellamus scientiam iuxta petitionem vestram, huiusmodi non (9) ignora ea que experti sumus, tria vobis in scriptis redigimus ex omnibus fallaciarum discreta (10) contestibus. Primum enim quasdam

---

(54) Crocus ferri or Crocus martis, the iron or black oxide was a popular medicinal remedy in the Middle Ages as well as in the sixteenth and seventeenth centuries.

(55) Although frequently said to have been first used by ALBERTUS MAGNUS, vitriol dates back to the 8th century and is used in the *Compositiones ad tingenda*, BERTHELOT, *La chimie au moyen âge*, 1893, I, 14.

. . . .

(1) B, C : Incipit alkimia minor Alberti magni episcopi ratisponensis ordinis fratrum predicatorum. D begins without title, " Item dillectissimo..."

(2) Dilectissimo, B, C, D.

(3) Fratri, B, C, D.

(4) A. fol. 180r.

(5) secretis, B, C.

(6) differentiis et differentiarum causis attestantibus (attemptantibus, C), B, C; differentiis et differentiarum vel differentiarum, D.

(7) quidem, omitted, B, C.

(8) alkimialem, B, alkymealem, C; alquimialem, D.

(9) Huiusmodi non ingrato ea que experta sumus, B; non negato ea que experta, C; petitionem vestram non ignoro eam, D.

(10) descripta, C; descripta conceptibus, D.

preparationes (11) huic operi necessarias brevi sermone monstravimus demum vero elixiria i. medicinarum compositiones (12) in album vel rubeum corpora permutantes (13) consequenter insinuabimus.

Rubificatio et solutio attramenti capitulum primum (14).

Attramentum est huic operi necessarium. Terra quidem (15) nigra est odorem habens sulfureum. Accipe ergo ipsum (16) et minutissime conteras et in ollam novam (17) diligenter concludas et ignem per duas horas lentum subicias (18). Postea vero ignem augeas donec olla rubescat (19) et in tali calore per noctem dimittas. Mane quidem aperiens (20) rubicundissimam in olla invenies qui flos attramenti dicitur. Accipe ergo hoc (21) rubeum et contere cum sale armoniacho et sublima ab eo salem armoniacum (22) et hoc tertio (23) fac. Postea pone super marmorem in cellario vel in loco humido et resolvetur in aquam rubicundissimam etiam (24) diligenter in vitreo vase conserva (25). Est enim aqua nobilis fixa cum qua (26) spiritus et corpora rubeo [fol. 180v] colore quem numquam dimittent (27) informantur et est unum de retinaculis spirituum.

---

(11) Primum est quasdam preparationes. Secundo (secundum est, D) sublimationes ac (et, C) fixationes huic operi necessarias, B, C, D.

(12) medicinas componendas, D.

(13) permutantia et sequenter, B, C; mutantes, D.

(14) B, De attramento preparatio sequitur; C, De atramento ad idem folio 40 [i.e. 69r, new numbering, to section on the same subject in the *Semita recta*, cf. BORGNET XXXVII, 556]; D, omits heading and begins : Item hatramentum huic...

(15) omitted, B, C; in D the four words after *necessarium* are omitted, and the reading is : " necessarium est. Hodorem..."

(16) omitted, B, C, D.

(17) olla nova, B, C.

(18) D, fol. 59v.

(19) rubificat, C.

(20) aperias rubicundissimum, B, C; aperias et invenies cum rubicundissimo qui flos atramentum dicitur, D.

(21) omitted B, C, D.

(22) omitted, B, C; sale armoniaco, D.

(23) fac et pone super, B, C; et hoc fac ter postea ponas, D.

(24) quam, B. C, D.

(25) serva, B.

(26) written " cum aqua," A; nobilis fixa cum qua, B, C; nobilis cum qua, D

(27) dimittunt, B, C; dimitit informata, D.

Calcinatio et solutio aluminis iameni capitulum secundum (28).

Alumen iameni etiam huic operi est necessarium. Accipiatur (29) ergo in olla nova (30) et diligenter argilletur. Et in calore ignis (31) ut attramentum pernoctare et quod mane in olla repertum fuerit nive albius ut superius de attramento dictum est. In albissimam aquam resoluatur cum aqua (32) spiritus et corpora albificantur colore albo (33) quem numquam dimittent.

De viride eris eodem modo capitulum tertium (34).

Viride quidem eris operi (35) necessarium est ut per omnia de attramento dictum est in aquam rubeam soluitur (36). In qua sunt multa secreta nam unum (37) de retinaculis spirituum est.

De preparatione salis communis capitulum quartum (38).

Sal (39) communis multum spectat ad hanc artem (40) et scientiam quoniam ipse aperit et claudit et corrodit infirmitates et superfluitates spirituum et (41) corporum cuius talis est preparatio. Accipias (42) ergo et calcinetur et in aqua calida (43) dissoluatur et iterum conjeletur (44) et hoc quater faciendum est ut eius

---

(28) B, De alumine iameni; C, De alumine iameni ad idem folio 40 [i.e. 69r new numbering]; heading omitted in D but in margin is : De alumine iameni preparatione.

(29) accipe, B, C.

(30) in olla nova concludatur et fortiter lutetur, D.

(31) ignis per noctem dimittatur et quod mane repertum fuerit, B, C; ignis ut atramentum per noctare dimitte et cum mane repertum fuerit nivem, D.

(32) cum qua, B, C, D.

(33) albo qui numquam dimittetur, B, C; colore quam numquam dimitetur, D.

(34) B, De viride eris; C, De viride eris ad idem folio 41 [69v, new numbering], D omits heading but has in margin : De viride tamen preparatione.

(35) nostro operi, B, C, D.

(36) soluatur, B; soluatur in hac autem aqua, C; resoluitur, D.

(37) omitted, B, C; nam unum, omitted, D.

(38) B, De sale communi; C, De sale communi ad idem fol. 40 [i.e. 39v, or 68v, new numbering]. D gives heading in margin.

(39) C, fol. 81r.

(40) artem et, omitted, B, C, D.

(41) B, fol. 48v; et corpora, B, C.

(42) accipiatur, B, C; accipe, D.

(43) aquam calidam dissoluetur, B, C.

(44) written con*i*eletur throughout in A; congeletur, B, C; coaguletur, D. This use of consonantal *i* to represent soft *g* is not uncommon, especially in middle English MSS.

terreitas et superfluitas (45) qui alios purgare debet absoluatur et deponatur (46).

De preparatione salis alkali capitulum quintum (47).

Sal alkali nobilissimus quidem (48) sal est nostro operi valde (49) necessarius cuius (50) pre [fol. 181r] paratio talis est. Accipiatur cinis (51) clavellatus parte una calcis vive tantumdem et (52) vasi in panno lineo et spisso. Supponatur (53) aqua fervens ut inferius distilletur et in tantum (54) perfundatur donec nulla acuitas in cineribus relinquatur. Postea quod (55) distillatum est per filtrum distilletur et in vase ereo bulliatur donec nichil aque apparens in fundo vasis (56) lapis durissimus conjeletur quod sal alkali dicitur. Ponatur (57) ergo in olla nova et subiciatur ignis lentus donec tanquam cera fundatur et currat. Postea ignis augeatur quousque rubescat et in aliam ollam subito (58) perfundatur et in loco sicco custodiatur quia statim solueretur (59) in aquam. Accipe ergo et in aquam claram (60) dissoluas (61) postea evanescente aqua (62) ad ignem conjeles et sic tertio fiat (63). Demum vero (64) in resolutionis fovea (65) marmori superpositus dissoluatur.

---

(45) superfluitas (removetur, C) quia (et, C), B, C.

(46) ponatur, D.

(47) B, Salis alkali; C, De sale alkali primo (?) ad idem fol. 40 [i.e. 39v, or 68v, new numbering] et fol. 26; D has heading in margin, Sal alkali.

(48) qui, B, C.

(49) omitted, B, C, D.

(50) eius, B.

(51) cineris clavellati pars calcis, B, C; cineris clavellati pars una, D.

(52) tantumdem vasi, B, C; rasi (?), D.

(53) supponatur et desuper ponatur aqua, B, C.

(54) tantumdem, C.

(55) omitted D.

(56) donec in fundo vasis in aquis durissimis congeletur qui, B, C; donec in fundo vasis nichil de aqua apareat et in aquis durissimis coaguletur qui sal, D.

(57) D, fol. 60r.

(58) omitted, B, C.

(59) resolueretur, D.

(60) aqua clara, B, C.

(61) dissoluatur, D.

(62) Written aqua et ignem in A; aquam ad ignem congelas (coagules, D), B, D.

(63) fac, B, D.

(64) omitted, D.

(65) fovea marmori suppositus dissoluatur, B; resolutionem fovea marmoris, C; foveam marmoris superponatur et dissoluitur, D.

De sale armoniaco et eius preparatione capitulum sextum (66).

Sal armoniacus operi nostro est necessarius. Est per eum enim (67) non transmutantur corpora in album vel rubeum set per eum reducuntur (68) spiritus in corpora planetarum. Precedit enim spiritus et parat ingressum et purgat (69) omnia corpora a sua nigredine et relinquit sibi (70) spiritus fixos (71) coniunctos perseverantes et recedit. Accipiatur (72) ergo et per se sublimetur et in aqua clara (73) postea dissoluatur et iterum evanescente aqua (74) conjeletur (75) et hoc tertio fiat et sic est optime preparatus in omni opere necessarius. [fol. 181v.]

De tartaro et eius preparatione capitulum septimum (76).

Tartarum nobilissima res est et spectat ad hanc scientiam (77). Accipe (78) ergo ipsum et in igne (79) vehementi per triduum calcinabis postea in loco humido marmori superpositum (80) dissoluatur. Postea (81) conjeletur et iterum in aqua clara dissoluatur et hoc 4° iteretur et (82) habebis oleum tartari nobilissimum cum quo finguntur (83) spiritus et soluuntur (84) et ingrediuntur. Custodi ergo ad partem per se.

De urina et eius preparatione capitulum octavum (85).

---

(66) B, De sale armoniaco; C, De sale armoniaco ad idem folio 39 [68r, new numbering]; D, has heading in margin.

(67) tamen, B, D; per eum spiritus tamen non transmutat, C.

(68) introducuntur, B, D; introducuntur spiritus et parat ingressum et purgat spiritus confixos coniunctos, C.

(69) purgat enim, D.

(70) ibi, B, D.

(71) confixos, B, C.

(72) Accipe, D.

(73) aquam claram, with postea omitted, D.

(74) omitted, D.

(75) congeletur et optime preparatus est et in omni opere, B; coaguletur (congeletur, C) et sic optime preparatus est, C, D.

(76) B, De tartaro; C, De tartaro ad idem folio 40 [fol. 69v, new numbering]; D has heading in margin.

(77) artem, B, C.

(78) Accipias, B, C; Accipiatur, D.

(79) ignem vehementem, D.

(80) suppositum, B, C; supradictum, C; marmoreum suppositum, D.

(81) This and the following words to " et hoc " are omitted, B, C, D.

(82) et hoc quater cum quo fixetur spiritus, D.

(83) fixantur, B, C.

(84) sublimentur, D.

(85) B, Urina pueri; C, De urina puerorum ad idem folio 8 [i.e. fol. 37r, new numbering]; D has heading in margin.

Urina puerorum 12. annorum etiam (86) huic operi necessaria preparanda est (87). Accipiatur ergo urina puerorum bonum vinum bibentium quia melior est et acutior et (88) de ebdomada in ebdomadam eius residentia subtrahatur et (89) per 7. ebdomadas postea per filtrum distilletur in vase vitreo usque ad tertie partis consumptionem (90) bulliatur demum in urinali superposito alembicho distilletur (91) operi necessaria preparata.

Secunda pars de sublimatione mercurii capitulum nonum (92).

Postquam diversarum rerum huic operi necessarias preparationes attulimus consequens est ut (93) de sublimationibus et fixationibus (94) plenius disseramus et primo de sublimatione mercurii postea de singulis ut ordo postulat (95) narrabimus. Accipe ergo unam libram mercurii et unam libram calcis corticum ovorum sive marmoris albi sive viridis (96) eris et aliquantulum salis armoniaci (97) et super marmorem cum aceto fortissimo rorabis (98) et for [fol. 182r] titer incorporabis donec de mercurio nichil appareat. Postea per noctem in furno panis desiccetur. Hoc facto temptabis (99) si ex hoc nummus fricatus albescit (100) et si albescit nondum (101) bene mortificatus est et iterum cum aceto rorabis (102) et incorpores (103) et assabis et totiens (104)

---

(86) qui est nostro opere, D.

(87) est preparanda sic. Accipe, D.

(88) C, fol. 81v; bona viva bibentium quia melior et acutior et de edomadam [*sic*] in edomadam eius residentiam, D.

(89) et hoc, B, C, D.

(90) ad tertiam partem consumationem bullietur (bulliantur, D), C, D.

(91) distilletur est operi necessario preparata, C; alambicho distillatur operi nostro preparato, D.

(92) B, De sublimatione mercurii; C, De sublimatione mercurii ad idem fol. 42 [i.e. fol. 72v, new numbering]; D has heading in margin.

(93) nunc, D.

(94) omitted, C.

(95) B, fol. 49r.

(96) viride eris, B, C.

(97) armoniaci et tritere super [fol. 60v] marmorem, D.

(98) fortissimo roborabis et fortiter incorporabis donec de mercurio nichil, B, C; fortissimo et incorporabis bene usque nichil de mercurio, D.

(99) temperabis, B; temptabis si ex hoc minus, D.

(100) words between here and *nondum* omitted by B, C.

(101) nundum, B, C.

(102) cerabis et totiens quod nichil de ipso adhereat, D.

(103) omitted, B, C.

(104) et totius, B.

quod de ipso mercurio (105) nichil nummo adhereat et tunc bene mortificatus est. Accipe ergo et contere (106) et in vase aludel constituas (107) et ignem lentum per medium diem subicias aperto foramene (108) vasis tunc laminam foramini superponas (109) et si aliquid humiditatis (110) adhereat ad hunc ignem lentum continues (111) donec nichil (112) humiditate appareat tunc foramen claudas et ignem fortifices usque ad vesperas. Postea magis fortem (113) adhibeas per duas horas et dimitte infrigidari (114). Mane aperies quod vivum (115) superiacet pulverizatum ut nix, abstolatur et reconde et quod vivum est iterum sublima et sic reitera donec totum pulverizatum habeas. Postea accipe hoc pulverizatum et cum tantumdem salis communis preparati conteras et in aludel sublima et quod sublimatum est (116) reserva et iterum feces sublima donec totum sublimatum habeas (117) et iterum cum novo sale (118) quater sublima et sic est (119) optime purgatus (120).

De sublimatione sulphuris capitulum decimum (121).

---

(105) mercurio, omitted, B, C, D.

(106) cooperias, B, C; conteras ipsum, D.

(107) conservans ad ignem, B, C; constituas et in ignem, D.

(108) written foramen, A; constituas tunc laminam foramen vassis, D.

(109) supponas, C.

(110) written humiditates. C, has in aliquid humiditatis adhereat tunc foramen claudas et ignem, with intervening words omitted; D, aliquis humiditas.

(111) continuas, B, D.

(112) nil humiditatis adhereat, B; nichil humiditas. Tunc foramen claudas, D.

(113) fortem ignem, B, C.

(114) infrigidare et, D.

(115) vivum sublimatum est fecibus reddas et conteras ut prius. Quod vero fecibus subiacet pulverisatum ut nix abstollatur et reconde et iterum quod vivum est sublima et hoc totum donec pulverisatum habeas. Postea accipe, B, C; vivum sublimatum est fecibus redeas et conteras ut prius quod non super fecibus pulverizatum ut nix abstolatur et reconde et iterum quod vivum est sublimetur. Reytera donec totum habeas pulverizatum cum tantumdem salis communis preparati conteras, D.

(116) est, omitted, B. C omits words following aludel sublima and ends, et hoc est optime purgatus et preparatus ad fixandum.

(117) totum sublimetur et iterum, D.

(118) totum, B.

(119) erit, D.

(120) optime purgatum et preparatum ad fixandum, B, C, D.

(121) D has heading in margin : De sulfuris preparatione sublimatione et dealbatione.

Sulfur operi (122) necessarium sic sublimatur et dealbatur. Recipe (123) ergo sulfur et in aceto per biduum lente (124) bulliatur et despumetur (125). Postea cum tantumdem de fuligine (126) ferri conteratur et in aludel per (127) diem sublimetur cum magis lento igne quam mercurius et [fol. 182v] hoc tertio (128) conteratur et sublimetur cum eisdem fecibus postea cum tantumdem salis communis quater sublimetur et erit album precellens nivem (129). Reconde ergo preparatum fixationi (130).

De sublimatione arsenici (131) capitulum undecimum.

Arsenicum vero nature sulfuree (132) est subtilioris vero substantie et ipsum non est necesse (133) decoquere. Inbibatur ergo cum aceto (134) quater et desiccetur. Postea cum tantumdem de fuligine ferri contere (135) et per omnia ut superius (136) de sulfure dictum est sublimetur et erit albissimum aptum (137) ad fixandum.

De primo modo fixationis capitulum duodecimum (138).

Accipe (139) de quocumque horum trium (140) sublimatorum

---

(122) Sulfur enim sublimatum et dealbatum operi nostro erit necessario, D.

(123) Accipe ergo et in aceto, B, C, D.

(124) lento igne, C; bene, D.

(125) here spelled dispumetur; cum spumetur, B, C; despumentur, D.

(126) ferrigine, with, vel fulligine, in the lower margin, B; tantumdem vel fulligine ferrugine ferri, C; cum tantum de fulliginis ferri conteratur, D.

(127) C, fol. 82r.

(128) secundo, D; tertio conteratur et sublimetur cum magis lento igne quam mercurius cum eisdem, B.

(129) with variations in word order in, B, C, and D.

(130) fixationem, D.

(131) D has heading in margin : De arsenici preparatione fixatione et sublimatione.

(132) sulphuris, B, C; Arsenicum natura sulphuris est subtillioris vero substantie ipsum non est necesse dequoqui [*sic*]. Inbibatur, D.

(133) necessare, B, C.

(134) aceto forti, B, C, D.

(135) conteratur. B, C, D.

(136) omitted, D. There is considerable variation in word order in both B and C.

(137) preparatum, D; paratum, B, C.

(138) B, C, De primo modo fixationis spirituum; D, fol. 61r, heading in margin.

(139) Accipe ergo, B, C; Recipe de unoquoque, D.

(140) omitted, B, C, D; sublimatorum quod, D.

volueris et pone (141) in vase terreo vitreato sine foraminibus (142) in cineribus callidis (143) et ignem competentem subicias donec quod inferius (144) est sublimetur. Postea revoluatur vas ut subiaceat quod superius emanebat et sic totiens iteretur (145) donec nichil ascendat et figatur quod intus est forsitan in decem diebus fiet vel undecim.

De secundo modo fixationis capitulum tertium decimum (146).

Secundus quidem (147) modus fixationis est qui fit per imbibitionem cum oleo tartari. Imbibas et conteras et in ampulla vitrea reponas (148) cineribus condas ignem lentum subiciens desiccetur vel ponas ipsum in scudella vitrea et cum martello trita fortiter satis ut reducatur in pulverem tegu [fol. 183r] lam cum carbonibus desuper pone tempore veris, in estate pone ad solem ut desiccetur et sic facias ut fixetur et currat super laminam. Postea frange ampullam tuam et iterum cum oleo conteras (149) et inbibas et desicces et hoc septies fac et habebis spiritus fixos (150) et ingredientes ad album et ad rubeum preparatos.

Tertia pars de aquis metallorum. Capitulum 14^m^ (151).

In omnibus (152) elixiriis ad album vel (153) rubeum componendis necessarie sunt aque metallorum. Recipe (154) ergo lunam sive solem et subtillissime (155) limabis et (156) cum aceto fortissimo per novem dies dimittas. Postea cum armoniaco (157)

(141) impone, B, C, with in vase, repeated in B.

(142) foramine, et, D.

(143) callidis ponatur, D.

(144) perfectus est sublimatum, D. In B and C, the paragraph ends here : inferius (est, C) sublimetur et erit albissimum paratum ad fixandum.

(145) omitted, D, and the paragraph ends with quod intus est.

(146) De secundo modo fixationis spirituum, B, C.

(147) omitted, C, D.

(148) reponens (reponas in, D) cineribus calidis. Condas ignem lentum. Subicias donec desiccetur. Postea frange, B, C, D.

(149) conteratur et imbibas, B, C.

(150) fixos ad ignem ducentes ad album, D.

(151) B, C, De solutione corporum; D has heading in margin.

(152) In omnibus enim, B.

(153) et ad rubeum componendi, D.

(154) Accipe ergo, B, C; Recipe lunam vel solem, D.

(155) B, fol. 49v.

(156) in aceto, B, C, D.

(157) cum sale armoniaco, B, C, D.

conteras et sublima et hoc tertio fac postea in fovea resolutionis marmori (158) superponatur (159) et soluatur (160).

De coloratione spirituum. Capitulum quintumdecimum (161).

Colorationes (162) enim spiritus secundum hunc modum ante medicinarum compositiones faciende sunt. Accipiatur ergo spiritus quem colorare volueris et cum aqua attramenti sive viridis eris ad rubeum ad album vero cum aqua aluminis iameni septies inbibatur conteratur et desiccetur.

De medicina ad rubeum (163). Capitulum sextumdecimum.

Accipe (164) ergo in nomine domini unam partem mercurii facti rubei cum aqua attramenti et fixi et pone super laminam ferream in loco humido et (165) dissoluetur in aquam rubeam in qua (166) tantumdem sulfuris rubificati et pulverizati mittas et dimit [fol. 183v] te donec in eos (167) dissoluatur. Postea accipe (168) unam partem aque sive calcis auri et istum (169) admisceas ut dissoluantur et uniantur. Demum vero (170) in urinali superposito alembicho in aquam callidam (171) distilletur et habebis spiritus puros claros et sine (172) nebula. Pone ergo

---

(158) marmoris, B, C; fovea solutionis marmoris subponatur et resoluetur, D.

(159) supponatur, C, D.

(160) soluetur, B, C; resoluetur, D.

(161) B, De bona coloratione medicine; C, De bona coloratione medicine, quere in folio 48 [i.e. fol. 77r, new numbering, in the text of the *Semita recta*]. The text on the folios indicated has been checked. But I do not have on hand photostats with which to make a careful collation.

(162) colorationes enim spirituum, B; colorationes enim secundum vel hunc modum ante medicinarum compositiones faciendi sunt. Accipiatur ergo quod colorare, D.

(163) B, De elixire rubeo. The text in C is found on fol. 48 [fol. 77v, new numbering]. Cf. note (161) above.

(164) Recipe ergo partem unam mercurii rubificati cum aqua, D.

(165) et, omitted, D.

(166) in qua quedam aqua tantumdem sulphuris bene sicati et pulveris sicati, B; in qua quedam aquam tantumdem sulphur rubificati et pulverizati, D.

(167) in eos, omitted, B; mittas donec dissoluatur, D.

(168) accipe, omitted, D.

(169) in istis commisceas ut, B, D.

(170) vero, omitted, B, D.

(171) callidam in caldario (caldariam, D) distilletur, B, D; et habebis spiritus, omitted, D.

(172) sine nebula vel nebulla, D.

hanc aquam in topicam (173) cecam et lento igne conjela. Postea quod conjelatum est sub fimo dissoluas et dissolutum conjela et habebis tincturam fixam coniunctivam et perseverativam (174). Pone ergo de hoc rubeo partem unam super 100 partem cuiuslibet metalli purgati et calcinati et est superbonum (175) in omni examinatione et malleatione. Probatio huius medicine (176) hec est quia conjelatur in laminam rubeam transparentem. Accipiatur enim (177) modicum huius et superponatur lamine candenti. Et si fluit (178) nec fumigat perfecta est. Sin (179) autem reiteretur super eam conjelatio et distillatio in fimo donec quod dictum est eveniat.

De medicina ad album capitulum decimum septimum (180).

Accipe unam partem mercurii albi et unam partem arsenici albi et tertiam (181) aque sive argenti calcinati et super marmorem fortissime conteras et (182) tantumdem salis armoniaci et sublima ab eis salem armoniacum (183) et hoc quater fiat et in loco humido dissoluatur et per omnia ut superius dictum est fiat et conjelabitur in laminam albam cristallinam transparentem. Proice de hoc albo partem unam super 100 partem (184) cuiuslibet

(173) copidam terream in lento, D. I have failed to find a definition in dictionaries for the term *topica, copica*, or *copida*, which is here intended to indicate a vessel without any opening.

(174) perseverantem... super centum partes cuiuslibet, B, D.

(175) et erit bonum [D, fol. 61v] semper et in omni examinationem et malationem, D; erit bonum semper, B, C.

(176) Probatio enim huius medicine est quod congelatur, B; Probatio enim huius medicine est in laminam rubeam transparentem, D.

(177) Accipe ergo, D; Accipiatur ergo modicum de hoc, B.

(178) si fluit nec incipit fumigare perfecta est, B; si fluit vel fluit ne fumiget perfecta est, D.

(179) sin autem reiteratur super eam dissolutio et congelatio donec, B; si non faciat parvam predictam reiteretur super eam disolutio et congelatio donec quod, D.

(180) B, De elixire albo. In C, the text is on fol. 48 [77r, new numbering]. D diverges from this point and after three paragraphs beginning respectively, Item aqua sal armoniaci necessaria est vini facere ut ita...; Item calcinatio sulphuris ante fixationem; and Item vassa de terra oportet hanc primo..., it ends. The treatise of Paulus de Ursinis follows.

(181) The word, argenti, which follows in A is marked for deletion. B has, lune et super marmorem, with the intervening words omitted.

(182) cum, B.

(183) omitted, B.

(184) omitted, B.

metalli purgati et calcinati et est (185) semper bonum in omni malleatione et examinatio [fol. 184r] ne. Consulo tamen quod nunquam tingas (186) aliquod metallum nisi purgatum et calcinatum sit quia spiritus (187) ingredi non possunt nisi sint (188) purgati et si ingredirentur post primam vel tertiam examinationem evanescerent et tinctura separaretur ab eis (189). Et nota quod sal nitrum in pastatum cum vitello ovi et calce cuiuscumque corporis reducit ipsam calcem ad corpus.

De oleo auri ad opus solis capitulum octavum decimum (190).

Ad opus solis primo partem (191) ipsius solis puri (192) cum odore saturni pulverizati (193) vel ipsum quo vis modo calcina. Et habeas aquam tertiam ex sale nitro ex sale armoniaco et vitriolo ana de quolibet cum media parte alterius predictorum cinabrii distillata (194) quam aquam saltim quatuor (195) vicibus ex pulvere solis (196) distilla. Quo facto ponderetur pulvis et si sit una pars habeant (197) e due parte salis armoniaci bis sublimati et sex vicibus a predicto sole sublima (198) semper adiungendo de novo sale armoniaco sublimato s. per sublimationem minuatur. Quo facto pone solem alteratum in vase nitido (199) cohoperto sub fimo equino per 5 dies (200). Et si adhuc non sit solutum ponatur per unam noctem ad (201) aerem ita tamen quot ab alio (202) non tangatur et iterum ponatur in callido fimo ut prius

---

(185) erit, B.
(186) tangatis, B.
(187) calcinatum quia spiritus corpus, B.
(188) omitted, B.
(189) The paragraphs ends here in B.
(190) B, De oleo auri; in C, the text is on fol. 48 [fol. 77v, new numbering].
(191) omitted, B.
(192) puri pariter, B.
(193) pulverisa et, B.
(194) distillati, B.
(195) decem, B.
(196) solum, B.
(197) habeas duas partes, B.
(198) predicto pulvere salis semper sublima, B.
(199) B, fol. 50r.
(200) tres dies, B.
(201) in aere, B.
(202) aliquo, B.

dictum est per 5 (203) dies et dissoluetur in substantiam olei quod serva per se in amppulla clausa.

De oleo martis capitulum decimum nonum (204).

Quod autem dictum est de sole fiat in croco martis excepto quod tres sublimationes salis [fol. 184v] anima (205) in ipso sufficiunt quod serva per se.

De oleo vitrioli romani capitulum 20^{m} (206).

Ad tertium capitulum sic procede. Recipe (207) vitriolum romanum viride et tere subtiliter et tritum et pone in aceto forti. Et dissoluetur et erit valde viride quod distilla per filtrum. Demum distillatum supra lentum ignem conjela et conjelatum pone in vase terreo clauso luto sapientie et vas stet in igne reverberationis per diem unum. Deinde extrahatur et aperiatur vas et vitriolum valde rubeum invenietur quod iterum ut prius dictum est, dissolue, distilla et conjela a quo conjelatio salem armoniacum bis (208) sublimatum. Tere, sublima et postea procede in (209) dissolutione sicut dictum est de sole. Ista tria olea sunt fixa et perfecte tingentia.

De oleo sulfuris capitulum 21 (210).

Nunc procedendum est ad olea (211) non fixa volatilia et primo in sulfure procedamus. Accipiatur sulfur quamvis (212) et tere minutissime cum quarta sui salis nitri et ponatur ad bulliendum per diem unum in capitello forti semper colligendo nebulam super natantem quousque non videatur plus ascendere. Et si (213)

---

(203) sex dies, B.

(204) B, De oleo martis; in C, the text is on fol. 48 [fol. 77v, new numbering].

(205) salis armoniaci, B.

(206) B, De oleo vitrioli sequitur operatio bona; in C the text is on fol. 48 [fol. 77v-78r, new numbering].

(207) Vis, B.

(208) bis vel ter, with, sublimatum, omitted, B.

(209) ad dissolutionem, B.

(210) B, De oleo sulphuris, B; in C, the text is on fol. 48 [fol. 78r, new numbering].

(211) written, olia; non fixa sed, B.

(212) quantumvis, B.

(213) sint sicut, B.

sint due uncie (214) salis nitri et aluminis plumosi ana imbibatur ex ipsis primis duobus quibus bene simul incorporatus (215) ut salsa ponantur (216) ad distillandum super lentum ignem quousque oleum exeat citrinum. Deinde ut sanguis rubeum quod profacto [fol. 185r] proprio reservetur.

De oleo lapidis maioris capitulum 22^{m} (217).

Sic in aqua et oleo rubeo procedetur. Recipe (218) sanguinem humanum hominis rubei quantum placet et conjeletur ad ignem ita quod maior pars aque recedat. Pars remanens in loco (219) ponatur in vitro clauso sub fimo equino per 15 dies. Deinde ponatur ad distillandum cuius aqua totaliter per se colligatur (220). Demum oleum citrinum cum igne (221) rubeo simul reponatur. In vase vitreo clauso per dies 10. sub fimo equino callido collocetur et iterum distilletur de qua di̦stillatione solus ignis rubeus rese̦rvetur.

De oleo fermenti capitulum 23 (222).

Accipiatur pasta ex frumento bene fermentato (223) et modicum decoquatur (224) in fimo equino per 30 dies ita quod panis sit bene putrefactus. Deinde piscetur (225) optime et ponatur in vase descensorii de terra forti vitreato (226) et ita aptetur quod nichil de eo (227) possit descendere preter (228) oleum. Et hoc fieri potest cum lamina ferrea minutim perforata. Et super

---

(214) salis mixta est ex sulfure et quarta salis nitri, alie due oz. salis nitri et aluminis, B.

(215) incorporatis, B.

(216) ponatur, B.

(217) B, De oleo lapidis marmoris; in C the text is on fol. 49 [fol. 78r, new numbering].

(218) Accipe, B.

(219) Marked for deletion in A.

(220) colligetur, B.

(221) igneo, B.

(222) B, De oleo fermenti panis; in C, the text is on fol. 49 [fol. 78r, new numbering].

(223) fermentata, B.

(224) decoquatur et postea ponatur in fimo equino, B.

(225) piscetur per optimum, B.

(226) written vitriato.

(227) omitted, B.

(228) nisi, B.

descensorium fiat ignis fortissimus quousque (229) per ignem fortissimum nichil amplius descendat et quod descensum est per alembichum distilla et rubeum serva.

De modo compositionis medicine capitulum 24m (230).

Sic in dei nomine procedas ad compositionem de omnibus sex oleis supradictis pone (231) partes equales in alembicho ceco et ille (232) alembichus aptetur in caldario [fol. 185v] aqua pleno ita quod non tangat fundum caldarii et aqua ascendat (233) olea predicta extra alembich in caldario per 4 digitos (234) et semper ferveat (235) aqua in quantum potest et in eadem custodiatur quantitate donec de oleis nichil penitus (236) plus ascendat. Set in fundo convertantur (237) in pulverem rubicundum et tunc completa (238) sunt Dicta philosophorum dicentium, si sciveris facere fixum volatile et volatile fixum artis perfectionem invenisti. Et alterius qui dicit (239), si sciveris spiritus (240) et corpora summe depurata coniungere per minima perfectionis opera tibi indubitanter complebuntur (241) de predicta medicina una super 50 album in rubeum mutat mutatione perfecta.

De lapide aureo i. marchasita aurea capitulum 25m (242).

Accipe marchasitam auream (243) et contere et cribra (244)

---

(229) usque nil amplius descendat, with, per ignem fortissimum, omitted, B.

(230) B, De modo compositionis; C, De modo compositionis oleorum supradictorum, the text occurring on fol. 49v [78v, new numbering]. At the close of this section the text resumes on fol. 53v [82v, new numbering].

(231) B, ponas [fol. 50v] partes equales.

(232) iste, B.

(233) ascendat supra, supra olea predicta extra alembicum..., B.

(234) written digites, A; digitos, B.

(235) serveat, B.

(236) omitted, B.

(237) convertatur, B.

(238) impleta, B.

(239) dixit, B.

(240) spiritus et, omitted, B.

(241) compatebunt de medicina supradicta primus una supra quinquaginta albi in rubeum, B.

(242) C, fol. 82v, the text resumes again here. The intervening text between caps. 15 and 25 is found on fols. indicated above. Heading, B, C, De lapide aureo.

(243) auream et est aurum finum in limatura s. in laminibus mirabiliter, C.

(244) omitted, C.

postea commisce (245) cum tantumdem mercurii (246) et sublima et sublimationem fecibus redde et hoc septies fiat (247). In septima vice remanebit mercurius in fundo solubilis (248) quem pone in parapsidem vitreatam (249) in fimo callidissimo et desuper pone catinum (250) unum et cohoperi eum (251) cum fimo et in tertia die invenies solutum (252). Tunc accipe tantumdem solis (253) calcinati et pone in aqua predicta super lentum ignem et dissoluetur (254) totum. Postea lento igne conjela et pone in fimo predicto et die tertia invenies solutum (255) tunc habeas calcinatum (256) lune lb. ii (257). Et aque predicte lib. I. et inbibe et assa et reduc et erit corpus perfectum (258) s. sol.

De croco ferri capitulum 26^{m} (259).

[fol. 186r] Accipe (260) de limatura acuum que sint de bono calibe et lava ipsam in scutella vitreata cum aqua clara molendo cum (261) pistello ligneo vel ferreo et colando aquam turbidam (262) et adendo aquam claram et totiens hoc iterabis (263) donec aqua exeat clara postea limaturam sic lotam (264) pone in scudella predicta ad desiccandum (265) super ignem lentum (266) quousque

---

(245) misce, B, C.
(246) mercurii sublimati, et sublimati iterum sublimationem, C.
(247) fiet, B, C.
(248) solutibilis, B.
(249) written, parasidem vitriatam, A; parapside vitreata, B, C.
(250) coopertorium, B, C.
(251) omitted, B, C.
(252) dissolutum, B, C.
(253) salis, B; salis communis et, C.
(254) dissoluitur, B, C.
(255) dissolutum, B, C.
(256) calcem, B, C.
(257) libram unam, B, C.
(258) id est, B; id est sol, followed by Ista recepta est tu. (?) bene secretum spiritus, C.
(259) B, C, De croco ferri.
(260) Recipe (Accipe, C) limaturam acuum de bono calibe, B, C.
(261) eam, C.
(262) turpidam, B.
(263) iterando, B, C.
(264) lavatam, B, C.
(265) siccandum, B, C.
(266) levem, B, C.

aquositas evanescat. Postea (267) cum dicta (268) limatura siccata (269) misce tertiam partem sui de sulfure et (270) vitriolo et simul iterum tere subtiliter (271) super porfidum. Et postquam optime insimul trita fuerint in pasta ipsa in dicta scudella vitreata cum aceto et cum spatula ducendo (272) et incorporando fortiter donec sint ut (273) pasta mollis non tamen ut superemineat (274) aqua. Postea dimitte quiescere quousque videris (275) ipsam pastam facere bullas (276) et quasi velle calefieri. Tunc iterum revolve cum spatula et misce bene et plana et dimitte stare aliquantulum et videbis (277) ipsam misturam (278) fumare et tumescere et crepare quod (279) non tangas sed permitte (280) stare et post paululum videbis ipsam inflammari (281) et exinde flammam sulfuris accensi exire per ipsas crepaturas. Et sic permitte (282) per noctem stare donec totus fumus et calor (283) evanescat. Et invenies ipsam limaturam rubeam ut sinopidem (284). Tunc habeas catinam (285) ferream magnam et grossam seu scudellam vitreatam et pone in ea dictam limaturam rubificatam. Et accende super eam (286) et circa eam carbones ita quot igneatur cacia [? capsa] vel scudella et limatura. Et super (287) ipsam [fol. 186v] limaturam agita cum pistello ferreo seu spatula in ipsa cacia (288) ut perfecte (289) pulverizetur et

---

(267) Postea misce, B, C.
(268) predicta, B.
(269) written, siccatum, A; exsiccata, B, C.
(270) in vitriolo, B, C.
(271) subtilissime in porfiritico, B, C.
(272) deducendo, B, C.
(273) in pasta, B, C.
(274) supraemineat, B, C.
(275) videas, B; videns, C.
(276) bullias, B, C.
(277) vides, B; videris, C.
(278) mixturam incipere fumare, B, C.
(279) quam, B, C.
(280) permittas, B, C.
(281) inflammari et ascendi et, B, C.
(282) dimitte, B. C.
(283) C, fol. 83r.
(284) sinopide, B, C.
(285) craterem, B, C. Catina (a crucible); the feminine form seems unusual.
(286) Et accende super eam carbones ita ut igniatur cacia seu scutella, B, C.
(287) per, B, C.
(288) capcia, B.
(289) ipse, B, C.

calcinetur et sulfur totum evanescat quod potest evanescere in furnum (290) et relinquatur ipsa limatura rubicundissima et subtilis (291) et tunc (292) calcina ipsam per se solam in furno reverberationis per diem et noctem et si plus melius valebit et tunc habebis optimum crocum ferri (293).

Quomodo fit calculum [capitulum] 27^{m} (294).

Accipe (295) libras quattuor laminarum caldariarum (296) eris veteris et igneas et extinguas (297) in aceto in quo bullierit (298) tartarum et sal et lava et frica optime ut perfecte mundentur (299) ab omni sorde. Postea cementa eas cum libris 3. vitrioli romani vel ciprini vel cuperosse (300) in olla terrea faciendo primo stratum (301) de vitrioli pulverizato et postea ex dictis laminibus et sic (302) alternatim facies (303) usque ad summam (304) olle et dictam ollam pone in furno reverberationis et des (305) ignem per tres dies et noctes et si plus melius vel pone in 3° solario superiori ubi coquuntur lapides. Tunc desiste ab igne (306) et infrigiditate frange ollam predictam et invenies dictas laminas conbustas (307) que trite erunt rubicundus (308) pulvis et hoc est optimum (309) calcarium quod pone ad partem (310) et serva.

---

(290) fumum, B.
(291) subtillissima, B, C.
(292) B, fol. 51r; tunc calcina ipsam limaturam rubicundissimam, C.
(293) ferri quem pone (pones, C) ad partem, B, C.
(294) De calcutio eris, B, C.
(295) Postea recipe, B, C.
(296) caldarie, B, C.
(297) extingue, B, C.
(298) bulietur, B, C.
(299) mundetur, C.
(300) vel cipri vel coperose, B, C.
(301) letum (omitted, C) in dicta olla de dicto vitriolo pulverizato et postea, B, C.
(302) omitted, C.
(303) faciendo, B, C.
(304) summum, B, C.
(305) da, C.
(306) et dimitte refrigescere et, B, C.
(307) predictas combustas, B, C.
(308) rubicundi pulveris, C.
(309) optimum calcinatum, B, C.
(310) et serva, omitted, B, C.

Preparatio vitrioli (311) capitulum 28^m.

Postea recipe vitriolum (312) rubificatum quod remanet tibi in fundo vasis in sublimatione mercurii ad album et tere ipsum et pone in aqua callida et [fol. 187r] bullita ita (313) ut dissoluatur in ea sal quod fuerat (314) sibi admixtum et (315) dissoluetur cum sale (316), aliud de vitriolo de quo non cures et tunc dimitte pausare et distilla ab eo aquam per filtrum et iterum superpone aquam callidam ut siquid de sale remanserit dissoluatur (317). Postea distilla per filtrum aquam et residebit vitreolum (318) in fundo privatum sale rubeum quod postea (319) exsicca in scudella vitreata ad solem vel super lentum ignem et habebis vitriolum optime rubificatum quod tere et pone ad partem (320).

De preparatione croci ferri capitulum 29 (321).

Nunc omnibus predictis preparatis. Recipe supradicti (322) croci ferri partem 1. et salis armoniaci citrini partem aliam et misce (323) et subtilissime super lapidem et ita pone in ampulla vitri rotunda et pone super lapidum fornacis (324) primo ignem lentum ore ampulle aperto (325) quousque humiditas evanescat postea ore ampulle clauso cum petia linea (326) fortifica ignem quousque ascenderat (327) salis pars que ascendere potest. Et forte (328) in hac prima vice invenies tangendo cum baculo ipsa (329) fixa in fundo vasis. Cave tamen ne sal armoniacus

---

(311) B, C, De vitriolo rubeo.
(312) vitriolum rubeum seu rubificatum, C.
(313) omitted, B, C.
(314) fuit, B, C.
(315) C, fol. 83v.
(316) cum sale adde de, B, C.
(317) dissoluetur, B, C.
(318) rubeum privatum sale quod, C; inserted in the margin of B.
(319) reposita in scutella, B.
(320) et serva, B, C.
(321) B, C, without heading.
(322) predicti, B, C.
(323) misce et tere, B, C.
(324) super fornacem et subice primo, B, C.
(325) apertum, A; aperto, B, C.
(326) linita fortiffica fortifica [*sic*], B; linita fortifica ignem, C.
(327) written ascerat, A; ascenderit salis armoniaci, B, C.
(328) forte hoc prima vice invenitur, B, C.
(329) opera fixa, C.

qui sublimatur obturet (330) os ampulle quia inpetu (331) vaporis subfacti (332) frangeretur ampulla et perderetur opus totum (333). Tunc dimitte infrigidari et frange ampullam et tere (334) subtilissime iterum super lapidem salem armoniacum quem invenies sublimatum (335) cum eo quod remansit in fundo. Et iterum [fol. 187v] pone in alia ampulla et pone supra (336) cineres in fornace. Et da ignem per omnia faciendo ut supra quousque fundatur (337) in fundo vasis et currat hoc reitera septies vel pluries donec fundatur quod in fundo est ad lumen candele et habebis crocum ferri fusum et ceratum. Postea tere ipsum subtilissime et dissolue ipsum in duplo sui vel pluries (338) aceti distillati per alembichum callidi et dimitte quiescere et distilla quod ex eo distillatum (339) est cum aceto (340) per filtrum. Et iterum adde de aceto callido et misce ut residuum quod (341) ibi erat de subtili dissoluatur et remanebit (342) terreitas quam abiecte (343). Postea hoc totum dissolutum et distillatum iterum distilla ut (344) sit clarum. Postea pone totum (345) acetum (346) distillatum cum croco ferri soluto in urinalibus in cineribus supra fornacem locatis (347) usque ad os. Provideas tamen (348) ne dictum acetum inpleat nisi (349) tertiam partem urinalis aut parum plus et superpone (350) urina-

---

(330) obturetur, B, C.
(331) impetus, A; impetu, B, C.
(332) suffocati frangetur, C; suffocati, B.
(333) tuum, B, C.
(334) optime et subtilissime, B, C.
(335) sublimatum in ampula cum eo, B, C.
(336) cum cineribus, B, C.
(337) fundatur quod in fundo est ad lumen, intervening words omitted, B, C.
(338) pluris, B; plures, C.
(339) dissolutum, B, C.
(340) cum aceto, omitted, B, C.
(341) quod remanet desubtili, B; quod maneat, C.
(342) et remaneat terreitas in fundo, B.
(343) abice, B, C.
(344) B, fol. 51v.
(345) dictum, B, C.
(346) C, fol. 84r.
(347) Written locati (?), in A; super fornacem locatem, with in cineribus, omitted, B, C.
(348) Et provideas ne, with tamen omitted, B, C.
(349) plusquam, B.
(350) suppone, C.

libus alembichum (351) cum receptaculis suis et subicies ignem lentum (352) quousque (353) acetum distilletur. Et quod solutum fuerit ex dicto croco ferri (354) remaneat in spissatum in fundo cucurbite ad modum mellis solidi. Tunc extrahe de dictis cineribus et pone totum in una ampulla magna ita quod excedat totum tertiam partem ampulle. Et pone ipsam ampullam in cineribus usque ad collum [su]per fornacem ut scis et subice levem ignem quousque [per os] (355) ampulle tota aquositas evanuerit. Tunc aperi aliquantulum cineres ita (356) ut videas discopertam ampullam a cineribus fere tertiam partem (357) corporis ampulle et [fol. 188r] claude os ampulle cum uno stupone (358) petiarum lini et augumenta ignem quousque fundatur ut (359) videas in vase fusum et liquidum ut oleum. Tunc subtrahe ignem et dimitte infrigidari et postea extrahe ampullam tuam et frange ipsam super loco mundo et invenies crocum tuum optimum (360) preparatum conversum in lapidem rubeum ut sanguis qui statim soluitur in (361) manus vel loco humido quem (362) pone ad partem ut humorem non sentiat ne soluatur quia incontinenti solueretur (363) et iterum vade ut supra.

De preparatione calcutii et vitrioli (364) capitulum 30.

Eodem modo facias de predicto calcutio et de predicto vitriolo rubificato s. de unoquoque per se (365) terendo partem cuiuslibet eorum cum totidem (366) salis armoniaci et fundendo et soluendo in aceto et distillando per filtrum et conjelando (367) et fundendo

---

(351) alembic, B.
(352) levem, B; et subicias ignem levem, C.
(353) usque totum acetum, B, C.
(354) omitted, B, C.
(355) per os, omitted from A, is found in B, C.
(356) ita, omitted, B, C.
(357) tertia parte, B.
(358) stopone, B; stapone, C.
(359) et, B, C.
(360) optime, B, C.
(361) inter, B, C.
(362) quod, B, C.
(363) paragraph ends here, C.
(364) B, C, De calcutio soluto.
(365) scilicet de unaquamque, with per se omitted, B, C.
(366) tamendum, B, C.
(367) coagulando, B, C.

per omnia (368) sicut fecisti de croco ferri et habebis calcutium conversum in lapidem rubeum solubilem (369) et preparatum. Et attramentum conversum in lapidem rubeum solubilem et facibilem et preparatum pone ergo quodlibet (370) per se ad partem in loco humido (371) in quo humorem non sentiat.

De preparatione mercurii ad soluendum (372) capitulum 31.

Accipe postea libras duas (373) vitrioli romani vel de cipro vel cuperosse (374) et libram sensim salis nitri. Et oz. 4 viridis eris et tere bene simul (375) et pone in cucurbita cum alembicho (376) ad distillandum ut (377) sis et de hac aqua (378) facias magnam quantitatem. Postea recipe mercurii crudi partem 1. et pone ipsam in una cucurbita vitrea et superpone [fol. 188v] eius (379) triplum de aqua predicta distilla (380) et superpone (381) alembichum absque lutatione cum recipiente suo. Loca super fornacem in cineribus et subice ignem et dissoluetur dictus mercurius (382) in dicta aqua et postea continua ignem. Distilletur tota aqua et invenies mercurium tuum conjelatum in rubeum pulverem. Cui postquam infrigidatum fuerit redde iterum aquam ei s. suam (383). Et iterum distilla et sic reitera ter. Postea (384) redde sibi dictam aquam iterum et dissolue ipsum in ea et conjela

---

(368) per omnia faciendo, B, C.

(369) solutibile et fusibiliter et preparatum, B; solubilem et fusibilem et preparatum, C. The sentence following is omitted down to the second preparatum, in B, C.

(370) quodlibet illorum per se, B, C.

(371) humido, omitted, B, C.

(372) B, C, De mercurio rubificato soluto.

(373) Postea recipe libram unam vitrioli, B; C [fol. 84v] Recipe libram vitrioli Romani.

(374) vel cupiose, B; vel cuperose, C.

(375) insimul, B, C.

(376) alembic, B.

(377) scis, B, C.

(378) aqua, omitted, B, C.

(379) ei triplum sue, B; suppone ei triplum sui de aqua predicta, C.

(380) distillata, B, C.

(381) suppone, C.

(382) mercurius, omitted, B; also the words following aqua up to Et invenies, omitted, B, C.

(383) aquam suam et iterum distilla et sic reitera ter, B, C.

(384) Postea iterum redde, B, C.

ipsum solum (385) usque ad mellis spissitudinem et habebis mercurium tuum rubificatum et preparatum ad soluendum (386) pro rubeo (387) vel melius. Quando dicitur quod inbibatur cum dicta aqua usque ad spissitudinem mellis non est verum set debet accipi ipse mercurius ter solutus et conjelatus in dicta aqua et bene fixus et rubeus et fundi ut de calcutio et croco ferri et vitriolo diximus cum sale armoniaco ter et postea solui in aceto distillato. Et distillari per filtrum et coniungi cum dictis equa portione et predictis addatur pars una vel plus solis calcinati et soluti. Et fiant totum una aqua que postea coaguletur et habebis elixirium ad solem magnum.

De compositione omnium predictorum (388) ad medicinam perfectam capitulum 32m.

In nomine domini (389) accipe predictorum croci ferri preparati (390) et vitrioli preparati ana partem I. et tere quodlibet per se postea misce insimul et tere (391) subtilissime super lapidem et pone in ampulam ro [fol. 189r] tundam et (392) grossam et pone in cineribus supra fornacem prout scis et subice (393) ignem ut liquidissime fundatur ut oleum tunc subtrahe ignem et dimitte frigidari (394) et frange vas et invenies lapidem unum rubeum seu nigrum quem frange et invenies fractionem similem fractioni margarite rubee foliate quam (395) iterum tere (396) et dissolue in aceto distillato et coagula in cucurbita. Et recipe acetum (397) et sic fac ter vel quater ut optime subtilientur (398) et incorporentur ultimo coagula in predictis cucurbitis (399) ad spissitudinem

(385) solum, omitted, B, C.

(386) dissoluendum, B, C.

(387) Both B and C omit the remainder of this chapter and continue immediately with the section headed, De compositione totius elixir.

(388) B, C, De compositione totius elixir.

(389) Postea in nomine domini, B.

(390) et calcutii preparati et, B; et calcutii et, C.

(391) tere iterum, B, C.

(392) ampulla rotunda et grossa in cineribus, B, C, with et pone omitted.

(393) subice(sse, C) ignem quousque liquidissime, B, C.

(394) infrigidari (et) Frange ampulam, B, C.

(395) quod, B, C.

(396) B, fol. 52r.

(397) acetum per alembicum et iterum redde sibi acetum et sic, B, C.

(398) sublimetur et incorporetur, B, C.

(399) concurbitis, C.

mellis sollidi et pone in ampulla grossa (400) quam pone (401) in cineribus supra (402) fornacem et subice (403) ignem levem ut substantia (404) aquositatis evaporet aceti deinde (405) obtura os (406) ampulle et fortifica ignem ut fundatur in oleum (407) et permitte frigescere et tunc frange ampullam tuam et invenies lapidem rubicundissimum quem statim tere subtilissime et pone in ampulla plani fundi et obtura os cum pasta (408) et cum petiis vel gipso vel calce viva cum flore istorum duorum in pastatis cum albumine ovi vel quomodocumque s. argilla vel stuppino vitreo ut non respiret. Et tunc loca in fimo calido et humido mutando fimum semper de ebdomado [*sic*] in ebdomadam ita ut semper sit callidus et humidus et hoc facias quousque quod (409) in ampulla est soluatur in aquam claram rubicundissimam ut sanguis et absque turbulentia quod sit si scies bene preparare fimum in 40 diebus quod si non fuerit tunc tene in fimo quousque [fol. 189v] sic contingat. Eodem modo dictum mercurium (410) rubificatum et solutum in dicta aqua (411) vitrioli et sal nitri et viridi eris ultima vice conjelatum usque ad mellis spissitudinem et preparatum ut dictum est locabis in ampulla plani fundi et obturabis os eius et pones in fimo ad soluendum (412) per omnia ut de croco (413) et de aliis dictum est donec soluatur in aquam claram. Postea recipe (414) aque predictorum trium s. croci ferri calcutii et vitrioli solutorum in fimo (415) ut dictum est partem 1. et misce

---

(400) ampullam grossam, C.

(401) quam pone, omitted, B, C.

(402) super, B.

(403) subicesse, C.

(404) ut sola aceti aquositas, B; ut folia aceti aquositas evaporet, C.

(405) demum, B, C.

(406) C, fol. 85r.

(407) ut oleum, B, C.

(408) cum pasta vel gipso vel calcem inmisceas cum albumine ovi vel cum peciis vel quocumque modo ne respiret (respiretur, C). Et tunc lota, B, C.

(409) quod (quousque, C) fiet. Scies (Scias, C) bene preparare fimum in 40 diebus, with the intervening words omitted, B, C.

(410) mercurium omitted, B, C.

(411) aqua mercurii et sal(salis) nitri, B, C.

(412) soluendum faciendo per omnia, B, C.

(413) ut de croco dictum est aliis (ante, C), B, C.

(414) Accipe aquam, B, C.

(415) in fimo omitted, C.

insimul dictas aquas et iterum pone sub fimo (416) predicto ut optime soluatur (417) et incorporentur et fiant unum et cum clarificata fuerint pone ea ad conjelandum (418) in vase longo in cineribus lentissimo igne per octo dies vel plures quousque coagulentur (419) lento igne in laminam rubeam transparentem. Et si fortem ignem dederis fundetur (420) ut oleum cuius partem unam proice super 70 lune (421) preparate cum sale communi calcinate et reducte (422) ter vel quater ita quod ter (423) in cimento vel mercurio conjelati (424) in lunam et habebis solem optimum ad omnia iudicia. Et si de (425) dicta aqua composita ex dictis quatuor quando ponis eam ad conjelandum poneris (426) quintam sui partem solis laminati subtiliter (427) et postea coangulaveris ut dictum (428) est meliorem habebit ingressum et melius valebit quod si postquam coagulatus (429) iterum solueris et coagulaveris cadet (430) una supra 100 et cetera. Finis. Explicit liber secundus fratris Alberti de ordine predicatorum.

---

(416) modo predicto, B, C.
(417) optime dissoluantur, B; dissoluentur, C.
(418) coagulandum, B, C.
(419) coagulantur, C.
(420) fundatur, C.
(421) written lunam, A; lune, B, C.
(422) reduce, B, C.
(423) stet, B, C.
(424) mercurii coagulanti, C; mercurii congelati, B.
(425) Et si dicta aqua composita fuerit ex dictis (predictis, C), B, C.
(426) posueris suam, B, C.
(427) omitted, B, C.
(428) tamendum est, C.
(429) coagulantur, B, C.
(430) B ends : unam supra centum 100 et sic est finis. Ego frater Albertus ordinis predicatorum ista opera experta et probata inveni. Explicit alkimia minor fratris Alberti. C ends : unam partem supra centum et hoc est finis. Ego frater Albertus ordinis predicatorum ista opera experta et probata inveni. Explicit alkimia minor fratris Alberti. Deo gratias.

V

THE *DE OCCULTIS NATURAE* ATTRIBUTED TO ALBERTUS MAGNUS

Among the several alchemical treatises attributed to the now sainted thirteenth century Dominican scholar, Albertus Magnus (1), is one which in a fifteenth century manuscript at the British Museum bears the intriguing title, " On the hidden things of nature," or " De occultis naturae " (2). Of particular interest because it provides a survey of alchemical doctrines as set forth by various alchemical authorities, chiefly of Arabic origin, this text, is, however, as yet unedited and unpublished. The work is also found in another fifteenth century manuscript now at the Vatican library in the Palatine collection (3). It there follows after the *Semita recta* (4) and the *Alkimia minor* (5), and is designated

---

(1) See the survey of such works in my article, " Alchemical writings ascribed to Albertus Magnus," *Speculum*, 1942, *17:* 499-518. See below VII.

(2) For convenience in citation, a list of the abbreviations utilized and their equivalents, has been given in Appendix I.

BMar 164, 1422 A.D., fols. 127r-131r. On fol. 127r, in the upper margin is the titulus : " Albertus Magnus, De occultis naturae," followed by a recipe and then the opening words of the text : " In mutuo allocutionis tractatu rogasti me ut veritatem," followed by another recipe in the same hand. Two other recipes in different hands fill the page. The text itself begins again on fol. 127v, with a repetition of the incipit as given above. Frequent marginal notations occur throughout the manuscript.

(3) VAp 1330, 1463 A.D., fols. 92r (old numbering, 85r)-101v. At the top of fol. 92r is the heading indicated in the text, then lower down : " Hic incipit alius liber fratris Alberti de Colonia ordinis predicatorum. In mutuo allocutionis tractatu rogasti me ut veritatem in magisterio (veritatem magisterii, in BMar 164) scientie alchimie sub compendio designarem ..." I am now preparing an edition of the text.

(4) For manuscripts and editions of this work, see *Speculum*, 1942, *17:* 511 ff., item 25. See below VII 511ff.

(5) See my edition of this work in *Isis*, 1949, *32:* 267-306. In VAp 1330, ol. 60v, the tract is designated as " Liber secundus." See above IV.

as " Liber tertius " in the upper margin of the manuscript, and as " Alius liber " in the rubric preceding the body of the work (6). No earlier manuscripts of the work have thus far been located. But it was apparently already in circulation in the fourteenth century, since a work with the same opening words was listed among the books in an alchemical collection at one time owned by a monk of the Benedictine monastery of San Procolo at Bologna (7).

The two fifteenth century manuscript copies of the text were apparently made from variants of an earlier exemplar since there are wide verbal differences between them. On the whole the earlier of the two manuscripts, that at the British Museum, is more concise than the other, frequently omitting qualifying phrases and other matter found in the Vatican Palatine manuscript. However, the former contains additional matter covering some two leaves after the close of the text in the latter (8).

Although it is not possible to determine with any degree of certainty the authenticity of the ascription to Albertus Magnus, it is of interest to note that the " De occultis naturae," the title by which, for convenience, we shall designate the work, bears only a slight resemblence to other alchemical treatises ascribed to Albertus Magnus. It professes to have been written in response to a request by a reverend father, addressed in the course of the

---

(6) See note 3 above.

(7) " Exemplum librorum alchimicorum quos habet reverendus frater dominicus monacus monasterii sancti Proculi de bononia." For a description of this collection, now in the Communal library at Palermo : MS 4 Qq A. 10, formerly in possession of the Speciale family, see *Isis*, 1949, *32:* 268, note 5; and W. J. WILSON, in *Osiris*, 1936, *2:* 236. Item 46, no. 27, of this collection reads : " Item liber fratris Alberti qui incipit In mutuo allocutionis..." See above IV 268, note 5.

(8) The text in VAp 1330, ends at fol. 101v : " ... dimittit corpus animam que sibi sic introducitur etc. Finis liber Alberti Magni philosophi 16 Novembris per Henricum Valpod Familiarem Reverendissimi domini Caroli Sancti Petri qui fuit de Almanica nacione de Valle Cusa apud Teneri. Hic est finis libri Alberti." This ending does not appear in BMar 164, fol. 129v, which continues for two more leaves and ends at fol. 131r : " ... ut quidam dixerunt sapientes, et nos quandoque experti sumus. Qui sine sale operatur nihil operatur sicut qui cum arcu sine corda saggittaret. Deo gratias. Scriptum anno domini nostri Iesus Christi 1422° 21ª martii tunc sabbato (corr. above the line : die veneris) ante lectare (sic), etatis mee anno 34°, magistratus vero 3°, contrariantibus michi astris..."

work, who had asked that the author prepare a compendium setting forth the truth of the teaching of the science of alchemy (9). Unlike the *Semita recta* and the *Alkimia minor*, with which the " De occultis naturae " stands in close juxtaposition, particularly in the Vatican manuscript, the latter is more concerned with theory than with the practical side of the alchemical process. However, both theory and practice are represented. The author of the " De occultis naturae " enumerates at some length the various theories on transmutation and on the philosophers' stone held by prominent authorities in the field. He has for this purpose utilized a large number of writings, the names and authors of which, in so far as he knows them, are carefully reported in the course of the work. It is his hope, our author states, that his treatise will make it unnecessary further to consult many of these tracts since their principal doctrines will have been transferred in briefer form to the present compendium. And one may then, " like a vagabond abandon all the volumes of philosophy for this one beautiful and more concise volume" (10).

Included as one of the authorities is the curious Geber. He is cited frequently for the alchemical doctrines upon which the " De occultis naturae," along with many similar treatises, reputed to be of the thirteenth and fourteenth century, lean heavily (11). In the present work there is also utilized without indication of authorship the " Book of the Perfect Mastery," which frequently appeared in the manuscripts under Geber's name (12). Another

---

(9) See note 3 above; also BMar 164, fol. 127v; VAp 1330, fol. 92r, " Attendite inquam Reverende pater (ad) ea que sum vobis quasi memoralia traditurus..."

(10) BMar 164, fol. 128r; VAp 1330, fol. 94r : " Nunc autem (ne) universa philosophie volumina tanquam vagabundus aberres (oberres) uno pulchro et breviori volumine nunc facere nitor..."

(11) BMar 164, fol. 128r; VAp 1330, fol. 94r : " Dico autem ut Geber quod in argento vivo (et) sulfure..."; also BMar 164, fol. 128v; VAp 1330, fol. 96r : " Geber testatur dicens intentio nostra in opere maiori est sumi..." See also VAp 1330, fols. 96v, 98v, 99r; and BMar 164, fols. 129r, 129v, 130r, etc.

(12) VAp 1330, fol. 94r; BMar 164, fol. 128r : " Unde in libro perfecte administrationis traditur quodcumque corporum vel spirituum..."; also in VAp 1330, fols. 96r-v; 98r-v; 100v ; BMar 164, fols. 129r; 130r : " requiras in libro perfecti magisterii..." Cf. J. RUSKA in *Quellen*, 1935, *4*, Heft *3:* 7, " Liber perfecti magisterii sive administrationis." For manuscripts and editions of the work see TK, col. 723; CORBETT I, 22, 35, 38, 74 : II, 75, 112, 128, 132; W. J. WILSON, in *Osiris*, 1936, *2:* 237, 360.

well known author, prominent also as an alchemical authority, and referred to frequently by our author, is Rasis (13). There are a number of references too, without naming their author, to the "Light of lights" (14), and to the work on "Alums and Salts" (15), both of which are elsewhere often ascribed to Rasis. Several alchemical texts attributed to Avicenna and to Hermes were also utilized. Among those assigned to Avicenna (16), frequent reference is made to the " Epistle to King Hasem " (17). There are a number of tracts under Hermes' name, including probably the " Emerald Table " (18), as well as other works. A " Liber Hermetis," appears among the " experimental books " (19), cited as authorities for producing color changes in metals, along with such elusive titles as " Liber mercurialis "; and " Liber de transmutationibus". Included also in this group are a " Liber Archelai," presumably the Archelaus to whom a number of alchemical tracts are attributed (20); the " Liber Mappa Claviculae," which is in all probability the work of that title that was translated into

---

(13) VAp 1330, fol. 93v; BMar 164, fol. 128r : " Bubachar maiorem, Bubachari (Bubacarda) duodecim capitulorum librum artis..." Bubacar apparently is Rasis. See Appendix II.

(14) BMar 164, fol. 127v; VAp 1330, fol. 92v : " in lumine luminum," also BMar 164, fols. 128r-v; 129r-v; 130r-v; VAp 1330, fol. 94r-v; 96r; 99v; and 100v.

(15) " In libro aluminum et salium..." BMar 164, fols. 127v; 129v; 130r; VAp 1330, fols. 92v; 93r; 98v; 99v.

(16) BMar 164, fol. 128r; VAp 1330, fol. 94r : " In libro maioris Alboali Avicenne..." The same " Liber maior " with Avicenna's name is cited again several times : BMar 164, fols. 128v, 129v, 130r; VAp 1330, fols. 95r, 99v. It is possible that this may refer to the alchemical *De anima* attributed to Avicenna. See references in the Appendix (II).

(17) BMar 164, fol. 128r; VAp 1330, fol. 93v : " Ergo dixit Alboali id est Avicenna in Epistola transmissa ad regem Assem (Ascinde)..."

(18) BMar 164, fol. 130v : " De quo dicit Hermes in suo thelesio quod incipit : Verum sine mendacio..." This incipit identifies the work with the *Tabula smaragdina*. See Appendix (II).

(19) VAp 1330, fol. 93r; BMar 164, fol. 128r : " Liber (de) bobotie Hermetis (Hermete); and for the " Libri experimentales," BMar 164, fol. 128r; VAp 1330, fol. 93r : " multos libros experimentales invenies (hoc) ut est maxime liber ille qui dicitur Mercurialis, Liber mappa claviculae. (Iamdem) liber de transmutationibus, liber de bobotie Hermetis, et liber Archilai et multi alii tam antiquorum quam modernorum de quibus esset longum narrare..."

(20) " Liber Archelai," VAp 1330, fol. 93r; BMar 164, fol. 128r.

Latin by Robert of Chester in the twelfth century(21); and "many others both ancient as well as modern of which it would take too long to report" (22).

The author of the present treatise furthermore made use of a considerable number of alchemical collections, or compilations, such as the "Book of the seventy precepts," or *Liber septuaginta;* the "Book of the thirty precepts"; and the "Book of the twelve waters" (23). However, he cites most frequently the *Turba philosophorum* (24) as well as the "Allegories". The latter appear similar to the "Philosophical allegories of Hermes," or, as elsewhere indicated, the "Allegories of the wise men on the book of the Turba" (25). Several of the philosophers of the Turba, namely, Zenon, Bonellus, and Mundus, are also cited (26). Still other authors and works of alchemical repute named in the course of the work include King Kalid (27); Maria the prophetess (28); Senior (29); Morigenes or Morienus (30); the "Epistle to Euthe-

---

(21) "Liber mappa clavicule," *Idem.*

(22) See the end of the quotation in note 19 above.

(23) BMar 164, fol. 128r; VAp 1330, fol. 94r: "Si autem diversos modos actionis et compositionis affectas queras (quere) libros LXX preceptorum, XXX idem preceptorum, duodecim aquarum..." For other citations of the Liber septuaginata, see VAp 1330, fol. 92v; BMar 164, fol. 127v: "Respuo iuxta quod traditur in LXX"; VAp 1330, fol. 95v, "Quorum opinio aliter opinionem libri qui dicitur LXX fefellit..." or in BMar 164, fol. 128v: "Quorum opiniones liber qui..."

(24) "Sed verius dixit Turba animalia et plante..." VAp 1330, fol. 92v; BMar 164, fol. 127v; and other citations: VAp 1330, fol. 94r-v; 95v; 96r; 97r; 98v; 100v; 101r; BMar 164, fol. 128r-v; 129r-v; 130v; 131r.

(25) VAp 1330, fol. 97r; BMar 164, fol. 129r: "Et hoc probat allegoria dicens 'Si camelus...' Other citations are in VAp 1330, 96v; 99v; BMar 164, fol. 130v: "Allegoria sapientum..."; also at fol. 131r. *Ibid.*, fol. 128r; VAp 1330, fol. 94v, has: "In composito (commento) Geberis super eodem Allegoria sapientum..."

(26) VAp 1330, fol. 101v, "Hoc ayt Zynon..." Cf. Turba [Sermo XXVI], "Inquit Cinon..."; VAp 1330, fol. 101v, "Item Bonellus et in suo..." Cf. Turba [Sermo XXXVII]; VAp 1330, fol. 101v, "Hoc ayt Mundus philosophus." Cf. Corbett II, 141. The above section is omitted from BMar 164.

(27) VAp 1330, fol. 93v; BMar 164, fol. 128r: "in libro regis Calith..." The work is also cited in VAp 1330, fol. 101r; BMar 164, fol. 130v.

(28) VAp 1330, fol. 95r; BMar 164, fol. 128v: "Et hoc probat Maria..."; also VAp 1330, fol. 96r; BMar 164, fol. 128v-129r: "Et Maria clarius dixit..."

(29) VAp 1330, fol. 94v; BMar 164, fol. 128v: "De quo Senior ex siccitate...'

(30) VAp 1330, fol. 94r; BMar 164, fol. 128r: "Hoc idem Morigenes ait..." Other citations at VAp 1330, fol. 96r, 100r; BMar 164, fol. 129r, 130r.

sia " (31); the " Book of the furnace," which may be the thirty-second book of the *Septuaginta*, or the work of that title ascribed to Geber (32); the " Flores ethymologiarum " (33), and the " Lily torn from the thorns " (34).

Although most of the above works are believed to be of Arabic origin, they had, in large part, already become known in western Europe in Latin translations or paraphrases by the beginning of the fourteenth century, and possibly earlier. But they appear to have been seldom cited in such profusion before the middle of the fourteenth century (35). Hence their inclusion in the present treatise provides no definitive clues for determining either the latest date at which the work could have been prepared, or the authenticity of the ascription to the thirteenth century Albertus Magnus. The latter point appears, however, particularly dubious since few of the authors here named are included in the authentic writings of the Dominican scholar. Despite this fact the work which appears to stem from the fourteenth century is of interest because of the enumeration of such a considerable body of alchemical writings chiefly of Arabic origin. Their inclusion does emphasize the author's particular concern for Arabic writings on alchemy. This interest in Arabic which is also exhibited in the use of such terms as Azoc (36) for quicksilver, is further exemplified by the statement that one of the works utilized was either translated directly by the author himself, or at his request, from Arabic into Latin. Unfortunately no identifiable details regarding

---

(31) VAp 1330, fol. 94r; BMar 164, fol. 128r: " Et Euthesia qui pacientiam non habet..." Other citations at VAp 1330, fol. 100v; BMar 164, fol. 130v.

(32) BMar 164, fol. 128r; VAp 1330, fol. 93v, " Liber fornacis." See Appendix II.

(33) VAp 1330, fol. 92v; BMar 164, fol. 127r: " in floribus ethymologiarum..." and again, VAp 1330, fol. 96v; BMar 164, fol. 129r, " ...florum ethimologiarum..."

(34) VAp 1330, fol. 94r; BMar 164, fol. 128r: " In libro aureo qui dicitur Lilium velud ex spinis evulsum (emissum); " also VAp 1330, fol. 96r; BMar 164, fol. 129r, " ut traditur in Lilio..."

(35) Thorndike III, 41 ff.

(36) VAp 1330, fol. 95r, " sed Azoc est suum argumentum... decoquitur azoc ipsum ... postea loton id est sulfur vertit super eum scilicet azoc et reddit album et rubeum..." According to Ruska (*Quellen*, 1937, *6:* 37), Azoc, also written azoch, or azoth, is from the Arabic *az-zawriq* and is the equivalent of quicksilver.

the tract are provided since the name of the author of the translated work was not known (37).

Our present author obligingly sets forth for the consideration of his reader, in addition to the names and titles of previous alchemical authorities, a review and examination of their various theories on the alchemical processes and particularly on the means of producing the alchemical stone. Some, he asserted, held that the alchemical stone was to be found in minerals alone; some that it was in plants; others that it was in animal substances; and still others that it was produced by the aid of alums, dyes, and salts (38). But even within each of these groups, he continued, there was no agreement among the philosophers as to whether the stone was simple, or whether it was a composite mixture within one group of substances or a combination from several of them. Furthermore those who asserted that the stone was to be found in minerals alone differed among themselves on the question of whether it was to be found in the volatile spirits alone or in the bodies of the metals; or whether it was the result of a combination of these (39). Our author concluded that the foregoing were in part correct and in part incorrect (40). However, he insisted that those who stated that the alchemical stone was to be found either in the spirits alone or in the bodies alone might be said to have strayed from the path of truth (41). For the spirits which include quicksilver, sulphur, arsenic, and ammonium salt (sal armoniacus) and all the minerals which flee from fire, could persevere and resist the onslaught of fire only when they had been reinforced or joined with the metallic bodies (42). His view, which coincided

---

(37) BMar 164, fol. 129r; VAp 1330, fol. 96v: " utar stilo cuiusdam operis quod ego feci transferre (transferri, in VAp) de arabico in latinum cuius autorem ignoro in quo declaratur breviter et aperte quidquid in alchimia fuerat occultum..."

(38) BMar 164, fol. 127v; VAp 1330, fol. 92r.

(39) VAp 1330, fol. 92r; BMar 164, fol. 127r.

(40) *Idem:* " Dico quod predicti partim dixerunt bene et partim mali..."

(41) *Idem:* " Qui enim in spiritibus tamen (tantum) aut in corporibus dixerunt a veritatis tramite demarunt (deviarunt)."

(42) VAp 1330, fol. 92r-v; BMar 164, fol. 127r: " Spiritus enim tantum sunt argentum vivum sulfur et arsenicum sal armoniacum et ceteri lapides qui ab igne fugiunt dicuntur. Spiritus angelimi fugitive sue partes (cum per se) in igne non perseverant nisi cum corporibus fuerint sociati." For other instances of this union of spirit and body in the alchemical process see Thorndike, III, 91, 97,

with that of other late thirteenth and fourteenth century alchemical writers, was that the philosophers' stone resulted from the alchemical marriage, or conjugal union of two parents, sulphur and quicksilver (43). The alchemical stone was thus the offspring of the union of the spirit and the body, in which the spirits might be said to have refined the bodies, and the bodies to have bound down the spirit. This one would find, our author asserts, set forth in the *Lumen luminum*, and in the *De floribus etymologiarum* (44).

The author of the " De occultis naturae " further reviews and rejects as fatuous and puerile the theories and practical directions relating to transmutations which resulted merely in changes of the color of the metals to white or yellow, without a resultant and corresponding change in species. He describes and names the chief writings, " the experimental books," in which the methods of bringing about changes in color are set forth (45). He insists that the true art can be distinguished from these mere changes in color by virtue of the fact that the true art is accomplished with the aid of the Elixir or notable medicine. For it is the function of this medicine or Elixir to enter into the bodies of the minerals and to propel from them in projection all corruption at the same time that it brings about a complementary change in species (46). By this means alone the sought for result could be attained and there could be produced the single substance coordinated from many, a substance which had been fixed or set, and which when placed over fire would not be consumed, but would liquefy. The Elixir or medicine by which this result could be produced was

---

etc.; and cf. Albertus Magnus, " Lib. mineralium," *Opera omnia*, ed. A. Borgnet, (Paris, 1890-1899), V, 2.

(43) VAp 1330, fol. 92v; BMar 164, fol. 127v. On alchemical marriage, see Sherwood Taylor, *The alchemists*, 1949, pp. 148 ff.

(44) *Idem:* " Spiritus subtiliant corpora et corpora ligant spiritus." For the two works named see, above, notes 14, and 33.

(45) See note 19, above. Cf. Thorndike, III, 33; and the similar views presented in another alchemical tract attributed to Albertus Magnus : *Isis*, 1944 (1945), *35:* 304, col. 2.

(46) BMar 164, fol. 128r; VAp 1330, fol. 93v : " Est autem tertii ordinis quedam medicina nobilis quam appello omnem preparationem que quoniam corporibus diminitis advenit omnem corruptionem ab eis in sua proiectione propellit et cum eis perficit differentias complementi..."

further described as the antidote and condiment of all bodies, a view which the author of the " De occultis naturae " found supported by the " Book of King Kalid," and by Avicenna in the " Epistle transmitted to King Hasem " (47).

While our author held with Geber that the work of transmutation and the alchemical stone could best be produced by the union of quicksilver and sulphur (48), he was willing to point out that those who were interested in other methods for producing the interaction and composition of these elements would find such diverse means set forth in the books "Of the seventy precepts," " Of the thirty precepts," and " Of the twelve waters," as well as in the books " On alums and salts," in the works of Rasis, and of Avicenna, in the book " Of the furnace," and " in so many others that it would take too long to enumerate them " (49).

On the more practical side the present treatise gives some consideration to the preparation of the minerals that are most important for the production of the philosophers' stone, namely of sulphur, and silver, as well as of alums, salts, and of *atramenta* (50). In the section on the preparation of sulphur which precedes that on quicksilver, the reader is cautioned to be mindful of the fact that sulphur alone, since it is only a part of the process,

---

(47) BMar 164, fol. 128r; VAp 1330, fol. 93v : " Dixit Alboali (id est) Avicenna in Epistola transmissa ad Ascinde (Assem regem). Nos querimus inquit substantiam unam facere tamen ex pluribus aggregatam coadunatam fixamque super ignem posita in quam ignis non exprimit (imprimat) et liquatis permisceatur et liquefacit..."

Just preceding the last statement is : " Ista enim est medicina que Elixir a philosophis (est) nuncupata scilicet antidotum et condimentum omnium corporum diminutorum ad curandum et transformandum in solificum et lunificium verum."

For the " Epistle to king Hasem," see note 17 above; and for " Book of king Kalid", note 27, above. See also Appendix II.

(48) BMar 164, fol. 128r; VAp 1330, fol. 94r : " Dico autem ut Geber quod in argento vivo et sulfure propinquius opus queritur et facilius elicitur. Si autem diversos modos actionis et compositionis affectas quere libros LXX preceptorum, XXX idem preceptorum, duodecim aquarum, (idem preceptorum trium), aluminum et salium, bubachar maiorem bubacarda duodecim capitulorum librum artis, librum fornacis et quam plures alios quos longum esset narrare." See notes 23, 15, 32, above; and cf. *Isis*, 1944 (1945), *35:* 304-305. For other references to Bubacar (Rasis), see Thorndike, III, 651, 653 and Appendix II.

(49) See preceding note, end of the quotation.

(50) For *atramenta*, which W. J. Wilson defines as inks or vitriols, (*Osiris*, 1936, *2:* 343), see VAp 1330, fol. 98v; BMar 164, fol. 129v.

cannot accomplish the result sought after. This desired objective, it is reasserted, can be attained only with the aid of the Elixir which alone produces the redness or whiteness that cannot be overcome by fire. In support of this view is cited the authority of the Turba (51). Furthermore it is stated, other philosophers like Geber and Maria, the prophetess, would insist that a third ingredient the feces or ash, or copper should be added (52). Considerable stress is laid in this section upon the important processes of cleansing and coagulation.

Following the discussion on sulphur attention is given to the preparation and principal ingredients of silver, which is declared to be the best principle after gold and the nearest neighbor to gold (53). This account is succeeded by the consideration of the atraments, alums, and salts. Salt is declared " according to the wise men, to be the silver of the people since all men need it and it is the condiment of all." The salts particularly favored in the discussion are " sal nitrum," and " sal Iabar (Iabarbar) " of which the last named is said to be the noblest and best of all the salts (54). In the preparation of the salts are recommended the processes of ablution, calcination, sublimation, dissolution, distillation, congelation, and cerration (55).

There follows too a detailed description of the copper vessel (vase eneo) in which the commingling of minerals with the aid of fire takes place. Reference is made in this section to the " Book of the Perfect Mastery," the " Epistle to Euthesia," the " Book of king Kalid "; and to the philosophers of the Turba (56). The

---

(51) VAp 1330, fol. 95v; BMar 164, fol. 128v.

(52) VAp 1330, fol. 96r; BMar 164, fol. 128v-129r.

(53) VAp 1330, fol. 98r; BMar 164, fol. 129v.

(54) VAp 1330, fol. 98v; BMar 164, fol. 129v; the discussion on salts begins at fol. 99r (VAp 1330); and BMar 164, fol. 129v. " ... Vocaverunt ipsum sapientes argentum populi eo quod omnes gentes indigent ipso et est condimentum populi totius..." " ... Sal Iabarbar est nobilius et melius omnibus salibus." For the use in the *Alkimia minor* of sal nitrum, saltpeter, see *Isis*, 1949, *32:* 287; also W. J. WILSON, in *Osiris*, 1936, *2:* 289, 302, 256; and for a reference to Sal Iabar or Geber's salt in a fourteenth century treatise (*Icocedron*), see Thorndike III, 134.

(55) VAp 1330, fols. 99r-100r; BMar 164, fols. 129v-130r. See above IV 287.

(56) VAp 1330, fol. 100r; BMar 164, fol. 130r (heading is omitted) : " De vase eneo. Fiat itaque vas eneum spissum ad modum olle..." See below in Appendix II, for the works named.

additional matter in the Arundel manuscript also continues the discussion on procedures introducing considerable allegorical material. There are frequent citations too of such previous authorities as Tullius, probably Tullius Grecus (57), Hermes, Geber, the " Allegories of the Turba " or of " the Wise Men "; the Turba itself; and of the individual philosophers of the Turba, namely Bonellus, Zenon, and Mundus (58).

As indicated earlier the authors and works named in the course of the " De occultis naturae " provide little or no assistance in determining the *terminus ad quem* of the composition of the work, a fact which is paralleled by the theories of alchemy with which these authors are associated. In similarity to other alchemical treatises attributed to Albertus Magnus, the author of the present work asserted that he was guided not only by past authorities but also by his own experience (59). He emphasized in this regard the assistance afforded by a close observation of nature since the alchemical art imitates nature more closely than other sciences (60). He stressed patience as one of the most important virtues for the alchemical worker, since the operation and its results may be long delayed. Support for this assertion which may also be found in the *Semita recta*, he found in the " Epistle to Euthesia," which stated that he who lacks patience should withdraw from the work; and also in the Turba where it is indicated that the three important necessities for those who would engage in the alchemical art are patience, a lapse of time, and skill in the handling of the instruments needed in the process (61).

However, unlike the *Alkimia minor*, and other alchemical tracts attributed to Albertus Magnus, which were characterized particularly by their straightforward directions and concise exposition

---

(57) For two alchemical treatises ascribed to this author see Thorndike, III, 96, note 57.

(58) For these authors and philosophers see Appendix II.

(59) " Ego vero experientia didici..." VAp 1330, fol. 98r; also 98v; BMar 164, fol. 129v; 131r : " Quia experientia didici..."

(60) BMar 164, fol. 128v; VAp 1330, fol. 94v : " Ut fiat opus ex hiis ex quibus natura procedit..." " ...(in) alchimia que naturam pre aliis (scientiis) imitatur..."

(61) VAp 1330, fol. 94r; BMar 164, fol. 128r : " Et Euthesia qui pacientiam non habet ab opere manum suspendat..." " Dixit Turba : tria sunt necessaria (scilicet) patientia, mora, et instrumentorum aptatio..."

of laboratory procedures (62), the present treatise abounds in allegory and obscure devices and phraseology. Like the " Flower of the Lily " attributed to Arnald of Villanova, the " De occultis naturae " contains a " turgid mixture of mystical phraseology and practical instructions." It has in common with other fourteenth century tracts the same allegorical representation of the union of mercury and sulphur, in the marriage of man and woman, the merging of the body and the spirit, for the production or procreation of the alchemical stone or of the son who will not be assimilated by his parents (63). It discusses the analogies between the multiplication of species in the animal kingdom and the production of mineral substances; the relation of the camel and the bird; and whether the birds can produce fish(64). It further draws analogies between the production of the alchemical stone and the sowing of grain, the planting and fructifying of trees, the joining of brother and sister, the ferment of the grain and of that of gold (65), and finally of the bird's egg and of the philosophers' egg (66). In short the " De occultis naturae " contains a very large proportion of the curious alchemical devices and phrases characteristically found in alchemical treatises of the fourteenth century.

In conclusion therefore it may be pointed out that the author has achieved his purpose in so far as he proposed to prepare a compendium of the alchemical doctrines of his own time. That these were, however, not of the thirteenth but of the fourteenth century appears most likely. For while the author of the " De occultis naturae " leaned toward the thirteenth century sulphur-mercury theory of the production of the alchemical stone, his predilection for the alchemical jargon, allegorical devices, and

---

(62) See my editions of two of these tracts in *Isis*, 1944 (1945), *35:* 303 ff.; and *Isis*, 1949, *32:* 267 ff. See above IV and below VIII.

(63) See for examples of stock alchemical phraseology, Thorndike, III, 62-63; 75 ff.; and W. J. WILSON, *Osiris*, 1936, *2:* 289 ff.; and for the present treatise, VAp 1330, fol. 94v.

(64) VAp 1330, fol. 97r-v.

(65) VAp 1330, fol. 97v.

(66) VAp 1330, fol. 97v-98r. One whole leaf relating to this subject of the philosophers' egg which is found in the Vatican Palatine manuscript is omitted from the Arundel manuscript, where the discussion is limited to fol. 129v.

mystical phraseology, characteristic of fourteenth and fifteenth century alchemical tracts, distinguishes and differentiates him sharply from the thirteenth century Dominican scholar, Albertus Magnus. Nevertheless the treatise can be said to have an intrinsic interest as an example of the alchemical literature of the fourteenth century of which it is a particularly representative specimen.

APPENDIX I

The following is a list of the abbreviations utilized.

BMar : London, British Museum, Arundel Manuscripts.

Corbett I, II : JAMES CORBETT, *Catalogue des manuscrits alchimiques latins.* I : *Manuscrits des bibliothèques publiques de Paris* (Brussels, 1939); II : *Manuscrits des bibliothèques publiques des départements français* (Brussels, 1951). Reference is to pages in the volume.

DWS : DOROTHY WALEY SINGER, *Catalogue of Latin and vernacular alchemical manuscripts in Great Britain and Ireland*, Vols. I-III. (Brussels, 1928-1931). Reference is to item numbers.

Quellen : *Quellen und Studien zur Geschichte der Naturwissenschaften und der Medizin.*

Thorndike : LYNN THORNDIKE, *History of magic and experimental science*, Vols. I-II (New York, 1923); Vols. III-IV (New York, 1934).

TK : LYNN THORNDIKE and PEARL KIBRE, *A catalogue of incipits of mediaeval scientific writings in Latin* (Cambridge : Mediaeval Academy of America, 1937).

VAp : Bibliotheca apostolica Vaticana, Latin manuscripts, Palatine collection.

APPENDIX II

Authors and Works cited in the " De occultis naturae ".

For convenience the Latin forms of the titles have been retained. References are made to the numbered notes, in order to assist in locating them in the article.

Allegoria; or Allegoria sapientum, 25, 58. For the incipit, " Si camellus..." see TK 667; and see also TK 8, and 354; Corbett II, 111.

Aluminibus, see Rasis, *Liber de aluminibus et salibus.*

Archelaus, see *Liber Archelai.*

Avicenna, 16, 49. The " Liber maioris Alboali Avicenne," may refer to the alchemical *De anima.* See J. RUSKA, " Die Alchemie des Avicenne," *Isis*, 1934, *21:* 23 ff. See also TK 208, 257, 324; Corbett I, 34; and W. J. WILSON, *Osiris*, 1936, *2:* 284.
Epistola transmissa ad Regem Hasem (*de re recte*), notes 17, 47. For this work see J. RUSKA, in *Quellen*, 1935, *4*, Heft 3 : 6-7, nos. 18 and 21; also *Isis*, 1934, *21:* 20-23, where the work is said to be false; and the various references in TK 484, 724; Corbett I, 51, 183.

Bonellus, 26, 58. See J. RUSKA, ed. Turba [Sermo XXXVII], *Quellen*, 1931, *1*, 1-2 : 25, 145, etc.

Bubacar, i.e. Rasis, q.v.

Bubachardus, i.e. Rasis, q.v.

Euthesia, " Epistola ad Euthesiam," 31, 56, 61. For the treatise, (Rosinus ad Euthesiam), see Thorndike III, 43, note 6, for a manuscript said to be of the thirteenth century. See also TK 353, 716.

Flores ethymologiarum, 33, 44. Cf. J. RUSKA and W. HARTNER, *Quellen*, 1939, 7, 2-3 : 143, " nona questio de libro Etymologiarum in quo de ethimologiis philosophorum super lapidem animali..." The work was partly ed. by. J. RUSKA, *Osiris*, 1939, *6:* 3-9.

Geber, 11, 32, 48, 52, 58. On Geber, see J. RUSKA and PAUL KRAUS, " Der Zusammenbruch der Dschābir-Legende," *Forschungs-Institut für Geschichte der Naturwissenschaften in Berlin*, 1930, 3 Jahresbericht : 42 pp.; W. J. WILSON, in *Osiris*, 1936, *2:* 264, note 54; 360. A brief summary of Geber's theories is included in the recent survey by F. SHERWOOD TAYLOR, *The alchemists*, (New York : Henry Schuman, 1949), pp. 78 ff.; 91-94. For citations of Geber in other alchemical tracts attributed to Albertus Magnus, see P. KIBRE, in *Isis*, 1944 (1945), *35:* 303; and in works of the fourteenth century, Thorndike, III, 41, and 97 ff.

Hasem, Epistola ad regem, see under Avicenna.

Hermes, 18, 19, 25, 58. The incipit " Verum sine mendacio..." is that of the *Tabula smaragdina*, TK 770. See also TK 384, 590, 770; Corbett I, 146, 292; and R. STEELE and D. W. SINGER, " The Emerald table," *Proceedings of the Royal Society of Medicine, Section of the History of Medicine*, (Nov. 2, 1927), pp. 485-501, with references to earlier studies by J. RUSKA and M. PLESSNER, on the same subject. For other alchemical works of Hermes see TK 331, 353, 633, etc.

Kalid, see Liber regis Kalid.

Liber : " Ille philosophus cuius liber incipit : Omnes illi qui habitant..." See 37. I have been unable to identiy this work.

Liber Archelai, 20. See the works listed under Archelaus in TK 81, 245, 344, 462, 517; and in Corbett, I, 29, 97, 109; II, 127.

Liber duodecim aquarum, 49. For manuscripts and other references relating to the *Liber duodecim aquarum*, see P. KIBRE, in *Speculum*, 1942, *17:* 504-505, item 3. The work was also frequently ascribed to Rasis, Aristotle, Avicenna, etc. See TK 51-52; J. RUSKA and W. HARTNER, *Quellen*, 1939, *7*, 2-3 : 140. See below VII 504-505.

Liber fornacis, 32, 39. Cf. " Liber fornacis (qui est XXXII[us] de LXX[ta])," in M. BERTHELOT, *Archéologie et histoire des sciences*, (Paris, 1906), 342. The work is also ascribed to Geber, TK 143, 263, 704.

Liber maior perfectionis, see Avicenna, *Liber maior*.

Liber Mappae Claviculae, 21. See the references in TK 548, 661, 677; Corbett I, 43; II, 162; and the edition in *Speculum*, 1935, *10:* 72-81.

Liber mercurialis, 20.

Liber perfecte administrationis, see Liber perfecti magisterii.

Liber perfecti magisterii, 12, 56. Cf. J. RUSKA, in *Quellen*, 1935, *4*, 3 : 7, " Liber perfecti magisterii sive administrationis." For manuscripts and editions of the work see TK 723; Corbett I, 22, 35, 38, 74; II, 75, 112, 128, 132; W. J. WILSON, in *Osiris*, 1936, *2:* 237, 360.

Liber Regis Kalid, 27, 47, 56. This may in all likelihood be identified with the " Interrogationes regis Kalid et responsiones Morieni de omnibus in quibus totum magisterium Hermetis consistit." Cf. Thorndike II, 214-217; III, 652, 654; W. J. WILSON, in *Osiris*, 1936, *2:* 372-373; TK 33, 210, 387, 388; Corbett I, 32; RUSKA, *Quellen*, 1935, *4*, 3 : 5, no. 6.

Liber septuaginta preceptorum, 23, 32, 48. For this work which is often ascribed to Geber, see M. BERTHELOT, *Archéologie et histoire des sciences*, (Paris, 1906), pp. 310-363; J. RUSKA, " Die Siebzig

Bücher des Gabir ibn Hajjan," *Festgabe für E. O. v. Lippmann*, (Berlin, 1927), pp. 38-47; TK, 383, " Liber Deitatis, *or*, Divinitatis qui est primus de LXX "; Thorndike III, 653; DWS I, pp. 70-94, no. 74; Corbett I, 98. Cf. RUSKA, in *Quellen*, 1935, *4*, 3 : 7, no. 23. See also TK 320, under Geber; and 357, Liber septuaginta verborum.

Liber Smaragdinus, see under Hermes.

Liber de transmutationibus, 20.

Liber triginta preceptorum, 23, 48. This may be the same work as the " Liber triginta verborum," of Thorndike III, 654. It is also variously ascribed to Argenteus, Geber, and Aristotle, TK, 309; 587, 771; W. J. WILSON, in *Osiris*, 1936, *2:* 365.

Liber trium preceptorum, 48. This may be the same as the " Liber trium verborum," which is variously ascribed to Kalid rex, Rasis, Rudianus, etc., TK 33, 295, 326, 382, 525.

Libri experimentales, 19.

Lilium velut ex spinis evulsum, 34. See TK 426; Thorndike III, 63, 64, notes 32, 43; also W. J. WILSON, *Osiris*, 1936, *2:* 374.

Lumen luminum, see Rasis.

Maria, 28, 52. For Mary the alchemist, see TK 6, 8, 121, 201, 238, 249; Corbett I, 228, 262; and W. J. WILSON, in *Osiris*, 1936, *2:* 260, note; 261; 302; 310-311, note 123.

Morigenes, 30. This is probably the same as Morienus, TK 270; Thorndike III, 70, 73, 626, 639.

Mundus, 26, 58; see RUSKA, ed. Turba, *Quellen*, 1931, *1:* 23, 25, etc.

Opus, (translated from Arabic into Latin), 37.

Rasis, 13, 49. For Rasis and alchemy see the recent work of SHERWOOD TAYLOR, *The alchemists*, (New York, 1949), pp. 86 ff.; G. HEYM, and J. R. PARTINGTON, in *Ambix*, 1937-1938, *1:* 184-191; 192-196; and the references cited in *Osiris*, 1936, *2:* 264, note 54.

Bubacar (Bubachar) Maior, 13, 48. See TK 162, 387; and J. RUSKA, *Ubersetzung und Bearbeitungen von al-Razi's Buch Geheimniss der Geheimnisse*, 1935.

Bubachardi duodecim capitulis liber artis, 13, 48. This may be the same as the " Questiones libri Viridarii Ebubachar," noted by J. RUSKA, *Quellen*, 1939, 7, 2-3 : 143; *Osiris*, *6:* 3-9.

Liber de aluminibus et salibus, 15, 49. See the work of that title, translated into Latin in the late twelfth century by Gerard of Cremona, edited by R. STEELE, *Isis*, 1929, *12:* 10-46; also W. J. WILSON, in *Osiris*, 1936, *2:* 237, and the references cited at 264, note 54; also

TK, col. 643, incipit, " Scias quod attramenti..."; Corbett I, 30. Cf. J. RUSKA, *Quellen*, 1935, *4*, 3 : 7, no. 34.

Lumen luminum, 14, 44. For the work of this title opening, " Cum (de) sublimiori..." or " Cum studii solertis...", see the references cited in TK 133, 160; Corbett I, 28, 72, 89, 168; II, 100; and J. RUSKA, *Quellen*, 1935, *4*, 3 : 7, " Liber florum qui lumen luminum dicitur ab Avicenna compositus." See also J. RUSKA, " Pseudepigraphe Rasis Schriften," *Osiris*, 1939, *6:* 26-35. This work is variously ascribed to Aristotle, Avicenna, and Albertus Magnus.

Senior, 29. See TK 8, 143, 215, 365, 421, 661, 701; Corbett II, 144; Thorndike III, 44, note 10; also J. RUSKA, " Studien zu Muhammad ibn Umail...", *Isis*, 1935-36, *24:* 310-342.

Tullius (Grecus), 57.

Turba philosophorum, 24, 25, 26, 51, 56, 58, 61. See Thorndike III, 41, *et passim*, for the use of this work by fourteenth century alchemical authors. For other manuscripts and the edition, see TK 56, 162, 377, 661; and J. RUSKA, " Turba philosophorum," *Quellen*, 1931, *1*, 368 pp.

Zenon, 26, 58. Cf. RUSKA, Turba [Sermo XXVI], " Inquit Cinon...", *Quellen*, 1931, *1:* 25, 135, etc.

VI

ALBERTUS MAGNUS, *DE OCCULTIS NATURAE:* LATIN TEXT

The following pages contain the text of the alchemical *De occultis nature*, an edition of which was promised in an earlier issue of *Osiris* (1). As there described, the contents of this work are of considerable interest because they reflect a fairly wide acquaintance, on the part of the author, with Arabic treatises on alchemy, either in their original Arabic, or in Latin translation (2). Foremost among the works or authors utilized are the *Turba philosophorum* (3), from which a number of statements are taken; with other standard writers on the subject, such as GEBER, HERMES, RASIS, AVICENNA, and others following in close proximity (4). Worthy of note, too, is the absence of the names of Latin authors, who were fellow workers in the field in the thirteenth and fourteenth centuries, the two centuries which the alchemical doctrines presented would appear to cover. As earlier shown, the internal evidence for the date of composition of the work is meagre. The works utilized had already in large part become known in western Europe in Latin translation by the end of thirteenth century, but they were seldom cited in such profusion before the first half of the fourteenth century. Similarly, while the alchemical doctrines and theories, especially that of the sulphur-mercury theory of the production of the alchemical stone, might point to the late thir-

---

(1) *Osiris*, XI (1954), 23-39; and see especially, p. 23, note 3.

(2) In this regard may be noted the author's reference to a work which he has either translated or had translated from the Arabic into Latin : *loc. cit.*, p. 29, note 37. For a good summary of Arabic alchemy and alchemists, see especially the long note by W. J. WILSON, 'An alchemical manuscript by Arnaldus de Bruxella,' *Osiris*, II (1936), 263-64, note 54.

(3) For the edition of this text see especially J. RUSKA, 'Turba philosophorum,' *Quellen und Studien zur Geschichte der Naturwissenschaften und der Medizin*, I (1931), henceforth to be referred to as *Quellen*. And for other references to this work see *Osiris*, XI, 39. See above V 39.

(4) An alphabetical list of the authors has been given in the earlier volume, *Osiris*, XI, 36-39. See above V 36-39.

teenth century, the predilection of the author for allegorical devices, and symbols, relates him more definitely to the fourteenth century (5).

For the foregoing reasons, one is more prone than otherwise to doubt the attribution, in the extant manuscripts, of the work to the thirteenth century Dominican scholar of natural science, ALBERTUS MAGNUS. And this scepticism persists despite the fact that the work follows that author's custom of addressing a reverend father, in response to whose request, the task of preparing a compendium setting forth the truth of the teaching regarding the science of alchemy has been undertaken (6). For here the similarity appears to end. And unlike both the authentic writings of ALBERTUS MAGNUS and others on alchemy of probably spurious origin, the present work, as demonstrated earlier (7), abounds in the use of obscure phraseology, analogy, and allegory more commonly found in fourteenth and fifteenth century texts (8). One is therefore led to conclude that, in all probability, this tract provides but another instance of ghost writing in the medieval sense.

Yet despite the uncertainty of the authorship, the work has an intrinsic interest for the reasons set forth earlier. And these would appear to justify the publication of the text in order to provide for it a wider currency than the existing manuscripts would otherwise afford. The earlier of these two manuscripts, that at the British Museum (B), Arundel 164, dated 1422, and covering folios 127 recto to 131 recto (9), has been utilized as the basis of the transcription. Variants found in the second of the manuscripts, that at the Vatican (V), Palatin 1330, dated 1463, and covering folios 92 recto to 101 verso, are noted in the footnotes. In general, however, such minor variations as order of words, or spelling except in a few instances, have not been taken into account.

---

(5) The work was apparently composed no later than the fourteenth century, since it was already in circulation in the fourteenth century, if, as already indicated, it can be identified, as seems likely, with one of the books owned by a monk of the Benedictine Monastary of San Procolo at Bologna. See *Osiris*, XI, p. 24. For a similar discussion, in a fifteenth century manuscript, of the opinions of various philosophers on the subject, see W. J. WILSON, *Osiris*, II, 342 ff.; and in addition to the references cited in *Osiris*, XI, 25 ff.; the examples of allegorizing cited by W. J. WILSON, *loc. cit.*, II, 327, 347 ff. See above V 24, 25ff.

(6) See *Osiris*, XI, 24 ff. See above 24ff.

(7) *Loc. cit.*, XI, 33 ff.

(8) See the references in note 5 above.

(9) For earlier notices of this and the following manuscript see *Osiris*, XI, 23-24. See above V 23-24.

On the other hand, the sharp divergence of the two texts in the closing sections of the work have necessitated reproducing both endings in their entirety, that of the Vatican manuscript in the notes; and that of the British Museum, in the text. Photostats of both manuscripts have been utilized to supplement the examination of the manuscripts made at the libraries named.

It may further be pointed out that an effort has been made to preserve the peculiar flavor of the documents by retaining, for the most part their medieval spelling, except in those few instances where greater clarity might be achieved by changing *y* to *i* or by the doubling of an *l*. In addition, some uniformity has been introduced in the spelling of proper names; and titles of books have been italicized. Finally, punctuation and paragraphing not found in the manuscripts have been introduced. Outside of these exceptions, the transcription has endeavored to follow faithfully the manuscript versions.

ALBERTUS MAGNUS, DE OCCULTIS NATURE[1]

In mutue allocutionis tractatu rogasti me ut veritatem magisterii[2] scientie alchimie sub compendio designarem. Cumque de glorioso et mundanorum rerum affectu me sit huiusmodi sicut[3] de ipsius naturali processu me non piget studiosum perorare. Cum enim fructus arbor non efficit ex sue dulcedinis amenitate quam plures ut huiusmodi delectationis designare ethimologia manum ad stilum impellit. Attendite inquam reverende pater[4] ea que sum vobis traditurus quasi memoralia. Et ab hiis vestre discretionis industria in aliqua devians non declinet. Philosophorum namque plures mirificum opus alchimicum solum in mineralibus statuerunt. Alii autem in plantis; alii[5] in animalibus statuerunt.[6] Qui de mineralibus dixerunt diversi sunt adinvicem. Nam alii de spiritibus solum; alii de corporibus tantum; alii de aluminibus vitris et salibus fieri voluerunt. Qui vero in vegetabilibus seu in animalibus fieri putaverunt similiter fuerunt[7] discordes. Nam aliqui ex hiis solum et singuli; alii ex ipsis ammixtis. Alii ex utrisque

1. This titulus is followed in B, at fol. 127r, by an alchemical recipe; the first few words of the text; and other alchemical recipes. Then on fol. 127v, the opening words are repeated and are there followed by the text as indicated. In V, the titulus, "Hic incipit alius liber fratris Alberti de Colonia ordinis predicatorum," is given since the work there follows the *Semita recta*.

2. In magisterio : V.

3. Cumque deo glorioso et precipuo mundanorum rerum cum affectus meus habunda (? for abundantia) : V.

4. Pater ad : V.

5. Alli vero : V.

6. Posuerunt : V. Marginal notes from here on : B.

7. Sunt : V.

tum singulis tum mineralibus mixtis opus rectum effici crediderunt. Quorum omnium rectior se censetur opinio que ad finem intentum congruum statuunt operantem. Salva tamen reverentia maiorum. Dico quod predicti partim dixerunt bene, partim et male. Qui enim in spiritibus tantum aut in corporibus dixerunt a veritatis tramite deviarunt.

Spiritus enim tantum sunt argentum vivum, sulfur, arsenicum, et sal armoniacum. Et ceteri lapides qui ab igne fugiunt dicuntur[8] spiritus angelini.[9] Fugitive sue partes in igne non perseverant nisi cum corporibus fuerint sociati. Corpora namque ut sunt metalla et lapides que pugnam ignis expectant non leviter ingrediuntur intra "corpora" cum sint grossa, nisi cum spiritibus fuerint aggregata. Sed cum alternatim[10] desponsantur spiritus subtiliant corpora et corpora ligant spiritus. Unde dicitur in *Floribus Ethymologiarum*:[11] Corpora namque spirituum coagula sunt et ut in *Lumine luminum*[12] non possunt gravia nisi levium adiunctione[12a] superius levigari levia gravium inferius consortio detrudi. Qui vero dixerunt in *Aluminibus*[13] *et salibus*[14] et similibus minus bene dixerunt. In eis namque solis non poterit reperiri quia ea solvendo, coagulando, et assando paucam utilitatem impendunt transmutationis. Aliique tamen possunt in eis alterationem invenire laboriosam valde. Et hoc melius novit qui fuerit experientie durus. Magisterii tamen in eis invenimus subsidium et nature propinquum. Quare ipsam ab omni opere non abicio vel contempno[15] ad extrema. Item in aliis crescentibus operatio magis laboriosa putatur. Sed quicumque in animalibus seu in vegetabilibus ponunt scientiam possible quidem dicunt.[16] Sed non est in eis quia prius deficiunt in labore quam perfici sit possibile super hiis que optarunt non tamen ista. Respuo iuxta quod traditur in *LXX*.[17] Ait enim de animalibus loquens Philosophus plus valent prima vice ista quam res minerales centies iterate. Sed verius dixit *Turba*[18] scilicet animalia et plante non sunt lapides nostri

8. V, fol. 92v.

9. agilini fugitive cum : V.

10. alternatim congrue : V.

11. For the *Flores etymologiarum*, see *Osiris*, XI, 36; where the reference to J. Ruska, *Osiris*, VI (1939), 3-9, should be omitted. See above V 36

12. This work is variously ascribed to Aristotle, Rasis, Avicenna, Albertus. See the references listed in *Osiris*, XI, 39; also *loc. cit.*, VII (1939), 54 ff.

12a. adiunctione, repeated : B.

13. Here written 'animalibus'; but it is aluminibus in V; and is hence, in all likelihood, to be identified with the *Liber de aluminibus et salibus*, ascribed to Rasis. See next note.

14. 'Rasis, Liber de aluminibus et salibus,' was edited by R. Steele, *Isis*, XII (1929), 10-46. See also the other references relating to this work listed above V 38: and earlier in *Osiris*, II (1936), 264, note 54; also VII (1939), 39.

15. contempno quia sunt media inter spiritus et corpora et sine medio ut dicunt non potest fieri transitus cum, ad extrema : V.

16. aliter dicunt : V.

17. For the *Liber septuaginta*, often ascribed to Geber, see Ruska, *Quellen*, III (1935), 7, no. 23; *Osiris*, VII, 40 ff., and the other references listed; Above V (1954), 37-38; especially M. Berthelot, *Archéologie et hist. des sciences*, Paris, 1906, pp. 310-363. For a passage similar to the above see, *loc. cit.*, p. 310.

18. See *Osiris*, XI, 39, for the *Turba philosophorum*; and the edition by J. Ruska,

sed sunt iuvamentia ⟨ad⟩ lapidem nostrum.[19] Et hoc cognovit similiter Experimentator bonus.[20] Sicut et dixit quam pluries in radice huius operationis fuerunt diverse et in compositionibus sic variarunt. Unde[21] omnibus eorum dictis medullicis perscrutatis reperimus procreandorum medicinarum triplices in genere gradus[22] in speciali modi fuerunt infiniti. Nam[23] omnes hii dixerunt ut putaverunt forte non ut experti fuerunt. Statuunt enim unius ordinis medicinas inter se compositiones diversas quas proiciunt super diminuta corpora et eis solum alterationem imponunt. Et[24] adducunt insufficiens[25] complementum. Quare contingit postmodum alternatim mutari atque corrumpi. Ut est in ere et ferro per solum arsenicum dealbati et in omni sublimatione dealbativa et in medicamine quod auget auri et argenti colorem. Hec enim mutant. Sed in ista mutatione minime perseverant.

Et secundi ordinis alia medicina in plures similiter partes divisa quam omnem preparationem appellam[26] illam scilicet que imperfecta corpora in differentiam aliquam alterat complementi relictis differentis aliquibus corruptione omnino sicut est calcinatio corporum maxime mollium eorum que reductio per quam omne fugitivum deletur ab eis et huiusmodi.[27] Similiter et gravis illa medicina citrinans et dealbans funditis aliquibus tamen corruptionis differentiis derelictis. Et ut est illa coagulatio argenti vivi que fit in igne cum marcasita ⟨et⟩[28] arsenico. Et ut quidam volunt aluminibus ⟨et⟩[29] salibus adiunctione[30] quibus omnibus[31] diligenter administratis propter affinitatem quam habent cum ipso argento vivo coagulantur. Non tamen in verum corpus reducitur ut cinericium vel cimentum expectet. Quod enim ipsa fugitiva et immunda fugitivum in rectum fugant fatuum existimo et credere puerile. Ex istis itaque duobus ⟨fol. 128r⟩ modis multos libros experimentales invenies[32] ut est maxime liber ille qui dicitur *Mercurialis*,[33] *Liber mappe clavicule*,[34] *Liber de transmutatio-*

Quellen, I (1939), 137 : [Sermo XXIX], probably relating to the passage : 'Scitote, omnes huius doctrinae investigatores, quod non exit ex homine nisi homo, nec ex brutis animalibus...'. See above V 39.

19. nostrum quod est maritus et uxor : V.

20. bonus amplius : V.

21. Unde in : V.

22. gradus hoc et horum : V.

23. V, fol. 93r.

24. Et non : V.

25. The 'in' is added as a correction : B. sufficiens : V.

26. appellam sicut est separatio : V; omit : illam scilicet : V.

27. huiusmodi id est consimiles medicine : V.

28. V, only.

29. V, only.

30. adiunctione cum : V.

31. et non : V.

32. 'Enumerat libros experimentales mendosos,' top margin : B.

33. I have not been able to identify this work. The term '*Mercurialis*' is referred to as one of the three herbs found by HORTULANUS. See THORNDIKE, *Hist. of Magic and Experimental Science*, 1934, III, 181, note 17.

34. See *Osiris*, II, 242; and XI, 37, for references to this work and the edition in *Speculum*, X (1935), 72-81. See above V 37.

nibus,[35] *Liber bobocre Hermetis*, et *Liber Archilai*[36] et multi alii tam antiquorum quam modernorum de quibus longum esset narrare. Quia[37] in hiis inveniuntur capitula veritate nudata sola et ⟨in⟩ simplici locutione placita et hoc modo in toto vel in parte hodie reperimus operantes. Preterea illud[38] aurum vel argentum[39] quod educunt ut dicunt[40] post plurimas fusiones vel cementi vel cinericii examinatione[41] evanescit. Qui enim per alba albificant ⟨et⟩[42] per citrina citrinant eadem metalla specie[43] remanente prorsus deceptiones sunt. Est autem tertii ordinis quedam medicina notabilis quam appello omnem preparationem que quando corporibus diminutis advenit omnem corruptionem ab eis in sua proiectione propellit et cum eo perficit differentias complementi. Et [44] quidam unita sola est licet in plures diffunditur[45] partes quia multis modis actionis et compositionis pervenitur ad eam quam quidem[46] noverunt sapientes philosophi calumpni[47] quos deus sua pietate voluit adipisci prout in *Libro Regis Calith*[48] apertius testatur.[49] Insipientes[50] vero in ea querenda decipiuntur. Et quasi abissi profunda et pelagi alta natantes[51] quasi fessi resiliunt natationes sicque pro nullo reputantes eadem ista via precelsa neglecta alicui duarum premissarum inherent.[52] Quare accidit illis sicut accidit[53] illi qui[54] in suam faciem protinus decidet dum propositis gradibus altum per abrupta fantastice querunt ascendere.[55] Ego autem dico cum illis qui veritatem concedunt quod per medicinam tertii ordinis ab omnibus premissis aliis excusamur. Ista enim medicina est[56] elixir a philosophis[57]

---

35. I have been unable to identify this and the following work. For Hermes, see the references listed in *Osiris*, XI, 37. See above V 37.

36. For the various works attributed to ARCHELAUS, see the index of THORNDIKE and KIBRE, *Catalogue of Incipits of Mediaeval Scientific Writings in Latin*, (Mediaeval Academy, 1937); and the other references in *Osiris*, XI, 37. See above V 37.

37. Omitted : V.

38. Omitted : V.

39. V, fol. 93v.

40. dicunt se tenere : V,

41. examinatione protinus : V.

42. Omitted : B.

43. spiritu eorum : V.

44. Et hoc quidam una vice sola : V.

45. dividitur : V.

46. quidem partes vel quarum modos : V.

47. alumpni : V.

48. For the *Liber Regis Kalid*, see the references in *Osiris*, XI, 37. See also *Osiris*, II, 372-373. See above V 37.

49. attestatur : V.

50. Insapientes : V.

51. Omit : quasi fessi resiliunt natationes : V.

52. adherent : V.

53. Omit : accidit : V.

54. qui que : V.

55. ascensum : V.

56. est que : V.

57. philosophis est : V.

nuncupata scilicet antidotum et condimentum omnium corporum diminutorum ad curandum et transformandum in solificium et lunificium verum. Propterea[58] dixit Habohaly[59] Avicenna in *Epistola transmissa ad Assen*[60] *Regem*. Nos querimus, inquit, substantiam unam facere tamen ex pluribus aggregatam coadunatam fixam, que super ignem posita in quam ignis si imprimat et liquatis permisceatur et liquefiat cum ipso quod est in eo de substantia[61] liquefactiva; ingrediatur cum eo quod est in eo de substantia ingressibili et permisceatur cum eo quod est in eo de substantia[62] permiscibili; consolidetur cum eo quod est in eo de substantia consolidativa et figatur cum eo quod est in eo de substantia fixativa.[63] Non conburetur ab hiis que non adurunt aurum scilicet[64] et argentum et afferat consolidationem et pondus. Cumque pervenimus[65] ad has res ut ait: Pervenit ad nos intentio, et hec quidem medicina elicitur de corporibus aut[66] spiritibus pluribus aut singulis preparatis. Unde in *Libro perfecte administrationis*,[67] traditur quodcumque corporum vel spiritum si recta preparatione fuerit preparatum erit album videlicet vel rubeum elixir per se solum ut autem intelligatur recte preparare[68] superflua demere[69] absentia suplere preparatio enim recta in demptione[70] superflui. Et absentis[71] adiunctione versatur. Dico autem, ut Yeber,[72] quod in argento vivo[73] puro[74] propinquius opus queritur et facilius elicitur. Si autem diversos modos actionis et compositionis affectas quere libros *70 preceptorum*,[75] *30* illud[76] idem preceptorum, *12* illud[77]

---

58. Ergo: V.

59. Albohali id est: V.

60. ad Ascinde: V; omit: regem: V. For the 'Epistola transmissa ad regem Hasen,' with which this no doubt coincides, see the references above V 36.

61. Omit: liquefactiva ingrediatur cum eo quod est in eo de substantia: V.

62. Omit: permiscibili—substantia: V.

63. Fixativa et: V.

64. Omit: scilicet: V.

65. V, fol. 94r.

66. aut de: V.

67. This work is probably identical with the *Liber perfecti magisterii sive administrationis*; for which see J. Ruska, *Quellen*, IV (1935), 7; *Osiris* VII, 45 ff. Other references noted above VII 37. See also *Osiris*, II, 237, 360, 365, under Geber.

68. preparare supple: V.

69. Omit: absentia suplere: V.

70. deprecatione corrumpentis: V.

71. absentis necessarii: V.

72. For Yeber, or Geber, see the references in *Osiris*, XI, 36; to which should be added Ernst Darmstaedter, *Die Alchemie des Geber übersetzt und erklärt*, Berlin, 1922; also above, note 67 and V 36.

73. vivo et sulfure propinquius: V.

74. Omit: puro: V.

75. For the *Liber septuaginta preceptorum*, or *Liber septuaginta verborum*, often ascribed to Geber, see the references in note 17 above.

76. Omit: illud: V. For the *Liber triginta preceptorum*, above V 38. This may be the same as the *Triginta verba* attributed to Geber, see *Osiris*, II, 365.

77. Very probably this may be related to the *Duodecim verba* [for precepta?] also attributed to Geber, *loc. cit.*, 365. See above V 38.

idem preceptorum *Trium*,[78] *12 aquarum*,[79] *Aluminum et salium*,[80] *Bubacar maiorem*,[81] *Bubacarda 12 capitulorum librum artis*,[82] *librum fornacis*[83] et quam plures alios quos longum esset enarrare.[84] In his autem manifestum invenies potestatem et sine omni palliatione datam veritatem huius magisterii.[85] Si vero affectas in theorica queras[86] *Librum ⟨perfecti⟩ magisterii*,[87] in *Libro lumen*,[88] in libro Yebri,[89] in *Libro Maiori* Habohaly Avicenne,[90] in *Libro Turbe philosophorum*,[91] in [92]composito Yebri super eodem *Allegoria sapientum*[93] et in libro aureo qui dicitur *Lilium velud ex spinis emissum*.[94] Nunc autem ne universa philosophie volumina tamquam vagabundus oberres uno pulchro et breviori[95] volumine nunc facere nitor pro viribus et nos deus[96] ad hoc complendum[97] sua benignitate fecundet.

---

78. Similarly for the *Liber trium preceptorum* or *verborum*, variously ascribed to Kalid Rex, Rasis, Rudianus, etc., see *Osiris*, XI, 38. See above V 38.

79. See also *loc. cit.*, XI, 37; and *Osiris*, II, 366; VII, 67 ff.; for the *Liber duodecim aquarum*, variously ascribed to Albertus, Aristotle, Avicenna, Rasis, etc.

80. See note 14 above for the *Liber de aluminibus et salibus*.

81. For Bubacar (Bubachar) Maior, or Rasis, see *Osiris*, XI, 38-39; and the following note. See above V 38-39.

82. The work here referred to may be one of several of the works of Rasis. See especially *Quellen*, VII, 2-3 (1939), 143; and *Osiris*, VII, 31 ff. A work with a similar title, 'Duodecim capitula,' in Catalan, is attributed to ARNALD OF VILLANOVA. See *Osiris*, II, 368-369.

83. This may be the same as the 'Liber fornacis,' (qui est XXXIIus de LXXta), noted by BERTHELOT, *Archéologie et histoire des sciences*, (Paris, 1906), 342. It is also ascribed to Geber. See for example, THORNDIKE and KIBRE, *Catalogue of Incipits of Mediaeval Scientific Writings in Latin*, (Mediaeval Academy of America, 1937), 143, 263, 704.

84. narrare : V.

85. magisterii quam est in theorica : V. Ennumerat libros theorice : right margin, B.

86. querans in libro : V.

87. For this work, see note 67, above.

88. Lumen luminum : V. For the *Liber Lumen luminum*, variously ascribed to ALBERTUS, ARISTOTLE, AVICENNA, and RASIS, see references to it, *Osiris*, XI, 39, under RASIS; and in note 12, above. Above V 39.

89. Jeberis : V. For GEBER, see note 17, above.

90. The 'Liber Maiori Haboaly Avicenne,' may refer, in all likelihood, to the alchemical *De anima* attributed to AVICENNA. In this regard, see the references in *Osiris*, XI, 36, under AVICENNA. See also *Osiris*, II, 284, note 85; and p. 359.

91. See note 18 above, for the *Turba philosophorum*. See above V 36.

92. in commento Jeberis : V.

93. Alcharia sapientum : V. For the 'Allegoria sapientum,' see especially RUSKA, *Quellen*, I (1931), 328 ff.; and the index of THORNDIKE and KIBRE, *Catalogue of Incipits*, (1937). See also *Osiris*, II, 371.

94. ex spinis evulsum : V. For this work usually entitled, *Lilium velut ex spinis evulsum*, see the references indicated in *Osiris*, XI, 38; and *Osiris*, II, 374-375. Above V 38.

95. brevimodi : V.

96. debemus : V.

97. complementum : V.

Non tamen tacemus; in brevi tempore intelligas ut paucis diebus vel horis possit prima vice constitui.[98] Si quia aliorum veridicorum virorum modernorum respectu etiam operis nature veritas hocmodo citius terminatur. Dum[99] dicunt philosophi cum medicis[100] cuius compositum longi operis spatium anticipavit. Et Yeber in composito[101] dicit patienter sustine et[102] forte moratur. Hoc idem Morienus addit et ait[103] festinantia ex parte diaboli est. Et Euthesia[104] qui pacientiam non habet ab opere manum suspendat quia impediet eum festina credulitas. Omnis enim actio naturalium[105] habet modum et tempus determinatum[106] in quo minori vel maiori spatio perficitur. Propterea[107] Turba dixit : Tria sunt necessaria[108] : patientia, mora,[109] instrumentorum aptatio de quibus deo volente suo loco dicemus recto[110] sermone completo.[111]

Primum[112] itaque tradentur res in quibus propinqua veritas reperitur. Dico autem quod propinqua veritas sic se habet sine mendatio videlicet ut fiat opus ex hiis ex quibus natura procedit. Principia[113] quidem sunt que actione sua fundat natura ⟨fol. 128v⟩ ut dixerunt sapientes.[114] Diutissime[115] sunt operationes. Et sunt spiritus fetens, calidus et siccus et aqua viva quam similiter siccam nuncupant.[116] Ex hiis diversis tum[117] eorum proportionibus metalla constituuntur et procreantur. Similiter dixit utique quod[118] alchimia que naturam pre aliis[119] imitatur in actionibus suis lapis ad ipsam alchimiam[120] procreandam esset. Unus in mundo toto et qui ab hoc[121] errat in precipitium abissi cadit. De quo Turba : Recto illo quod est omnia et omnium una perfectio sequitur deo volente

98. Sed quia illud : V.

99. Unde : V.

100. medicina cuius longi temporis spatium : V.

101. commento : V.

102. et quia forte : V.

103. Morigenes ait et dicit : Festinantia quidam : V. For Morienus, or Morigenes, see the index of Thorndike and Kibre, *Catalogue of Incipits*, (1937). See also Ruska, in *Quellen*, I (1931), 9; and *Osiris*, II, 372-373.

104. For Euthesia, see the references in *Osiris*, XI, 36. See above V 36.

105. naturalis suum habet modum : V.

106. V, fol. 94v.

107. Quod dixit Turba : V.

108. necessaria scilicet : V.

109. mora et : V.

110. recto et : V.

111. completo. Sequitur de rebus : V.

112. De rebus in quibus propinqua veritas est. Primum : V.

113. Et prima quidem super que actionem suam fundat : V.

114. philosophi : V.

115. Diutissime ac fortissime sunt compositiones. Et : V.

116. nuncupant et : V.

117. tamen : V.

118. quod in : V.

119. allis scientiis : V.

120. alchimiam veraciter procreandus est : V.

121. ab hoc vero errat : V.

quod queritur. Hoc autem quod dicunt unum[122], non est numero[123] sed spiritus sicut vir et mulier duo sunt. Numero[124] unius tamen speciei ad filium producendum propterea dixit de hiis que sunt ut vir et mulier. Unde subdit mulier virum soluit et ipse tingit eam. Et idem in eodem ex duobus[125] fit filius qui non assimilatur parentibus. Ego dico quod hii duo vulgariter nuncupantur argentum vivum et sulphur.[126] Qui enim sulphur argento vivo desponsabit nature[127] invenit archanum[128]. De quo Senior[129] ex[130] caliditate unius et frigiditate et alterius et humiditate unius et siccitate alterius misceantur donec bene conveniant. Et *Lumen luminum* philosophando dixit : Non potest calidum nisi frigidum nec humidum nisi sicco adiunctionis modo quolibet temperari. Et quia videbantur imperfecta deinde subdit non possunt gravia[131] nisi levium superius levigari[132] nec levia nisi gravium inferius[133] consortio detrudi. Et[134] ita dico[135] quod[136] si quis hunc lapidem, de duobus compositis corporibus, coniungere[137] novit ad maximum perveniet archanum[138].

Sulphur[139] enim non est de veritate artis sed pars eius qui autem[140] sulphur per se opus compleat alchimicum non est aliud credere nisi vanum quia ipsum figi non potest nisi prius calcinetur. Sed cum commixto[141] facilius calcinatur et preparatur. Qui ergo querit ex eo opus elicere per

---

122. unum. Unum : V.

123. matrimonio : V. On the use of 'the marriage metaphor,' see the references in *Osiris*, II, 327; XI, 30.

124. matrimonio : V.

125. duobus nascitur filius : V. For such analogies to generation in the alchemical process, see THORNDIKE, *Hist. of Magic and Experimental Science*, 1934, III, 90-92.

126. Nam qui ipsum sulphur et argentum vivum desponsabit : V.

127. nature et invenit : V.

128. Add here : Supra dixit fiat opus ex hiis ex quibus natura procedit id est coniungit in unum ut sunt vir et uxor in carne una et dicit natura : Oportet ergo quod sint simul ut in metallo nam illud est primum desponsatum nature : V.

129. For Senior, see the references in *Osiris*, XI, 39; and see RUSKA in *Quellen*, I (1931), 9, 344 *et passim*, consult index. See above V 39.

130. ex siccitate, caliditate unius frigiditatis et humiditate : V. Omit : unius et siccitate : V.

131. Omit : gravia : V.

132. Omit : levigari: V.

133. inferius levigari : V.

134. consortio et : V.

135. V, fol 95r.

136. Omit : quod : V.

137. coniungere et amicari : V.

138. archanum. Sequitur de sulfure et eius veritate. : V.

139. De sulfure et eius veritate. Sulfur : V.

140. Omit : autem : V.

141. Add here : Id est cum corpore in quo est hoc forte possible licet minus durum huiusmodi tamen dicere non debent trahi ex alio argento vivo argentum vivum et corpus vivum in quod sulfur neque nisi unum corpus in quo sint ista ergo cum commixto : V.

se preparandum[142] non eliciet sed cum commixto quia cum eo perficitur et sine illo usque ad aspernationem magisterii protelatur. Cum sulphure[143] enim et arsenico fit tinctura et dant pondus[144] completum uterque ex metallis et ipsum[145] feditate purgat et illustrat. Et hoc probat Maria[146] dicens : Nichil est quod possit a lotone suam umbram vel suum colorem aufere sed azoc[147] est suum tegumentum. In primis quoniam loton decoquitur nam[148] cum eo colorat et cum eo album reddit postea loton[149] vertit super eum scilicet azoc et reddit album et rubeum[150].

Amplius autem et[151] argentum vivum non perfectissimum in sua natura neque in natura ad quam producit ipsam minera.[152] Sed ad quod producit ipsum artificium nam sub magisterio nichil utilitatis perfecte prestat sed potius corrumpit licet et hoc ipsum[153] proficuum sit iuxta quod dicit Habohaly Avicenna in *Maiore* de argento vivo loquens : Si nichil aliud[154] aliquid operetur lapis noster nisi in subtiliando corpora et reducendo ea ad modum suum,[155] satis nobis esset. Et ideo dico ut eo ipso cum magisterio[156] quia ipsum est fleuma[157] purum.[158] Philosophi quandoque vocant eum sulphur[159] et metalicum accerrimum propter sue mirabilis[160] virtutis effectus ut enim quidam[161] voluerunt. Ex ipso creavit deus omnes gentes et eorum statuit originem. Est tamen argentum vivum sulphureum sed cum regum expectat operatur opera magna et alta miranda. Ipse enim solus est unus et deus. Unus[162] philosophorum nullus sibi potest equiparari nec aliquid possit operari quod per ispum operatur quia est elixir[163] ad

---

142. Separandum : V.

143. sulfure et suo compari : V.

144. pondus et : V.

145. ipsum metallum : V.

146. For Maria, or Mary the alchemist, see the references in *Osiris*, XI, 38; also RUSKA, *Quellen*, I (1931), *passim*; consult index.

147. Azoc, also written azoch, azoth, from the Arabic 'az-zāwūq,' is quicksilver. See RUSKA, *Quellen*, VI (1937), 37.

148. nam Azoc ipsum lotonem colorat : V.

149. loton, id est sulfur, vertit : V.

150. rubeum precedens et iam dictum capitulum est tamquam argumentum. Iam sequitur effectus argumenti scilicet de argento vivo et de perfectione eiusdem sequitur : V.

151. Omit : et : V.

152. minera, for mineral, see *Medieval Latin Word List*, p. 266.

153. ipsum corrumpere perficuum : V.

154. aliquid : V.

155. suum, id est in spiritum sicut ipsum est satis : V.

156. magisterio utaris : V.

157. For 'phlegma' (?) or phlegm.

158. purum quia transmutationem quia fixio in puro operis : V.

159. vocant ipsum : V.

160. V, fol. 95v.

161. quidam dicere : V.

162. Omit : unus : V.

163. Written Ysir : B. Isir, id est lavamentum : V. For the various forms of elixir, see RUSKA, *Quellen*, I (1931), 29 : 'Iksir, icsir, ixir, iesir, yesir.'

album et ad rubeum. Lar.[164] <id est ignis> non potest ipsum superare quia ipsum fugat. Sed si rogus[165a] debite administrare ipsum argentum vivum fixat.[165b] Est ergo panis quesitus a philosophis.[166] Non[167] sulphur solum cum eo[168] cum sit tinctura rubedinis et videtur[169] uzifur. Propterea Turba : Argentum vivum fumo sulphuris occupatum fit [170]papaver. Non tamen sunt commixti ut quidam fatui putaverunt. Quorum opiniones[171] liber qui *70* dicitur refellit et ideo qui ipsum invicem in preparatione commisceri et amicari novit sciet unum de maximis secretis nature et unam viam perfectionis de qua sola dicemus sermone claro et aperto suo determinato loco licet multe[172] vie sint[173] ad effectum unum et unum intentum. Nostra tamen via brevior cunctis existit. Et est radix et caput omnium aliarum in qua nichil erit occultum qui tam dicta quam dicenda diligenter attendit. Concludo ergo[174] ex premissis <quod> ex his duobus opus perfici quia se invicem alterant et alterantur se invicem perficiunt et perficiuntur.[175] Et ut dicit Turba se invicem corrigunt et emendant. Et[176] ut dicitur in *illo Thelesino* quod incipit : Omnes illi qui habitant in abisso maris etc.[177] Tunc velox choruscatio debet resurgere illa si benedicta creatura patris lumen. Set clarius dixit Turba ex duobus fit filius qui non assimilatur parentibus. Hic[178] tamen maxima altercatio inter philosophos fuit. Quidam enim dixerunt quod ista[179] sufficiant ut iam probatum est.

Alii dixerunt quod debet eis addi tertium. In hoc tamen[180] diversificaverunt nam alii putaverunt tertium fecem scilicet cinerem. Ipsorum duorum,[181] alii illud quod ex hiis duobus procedit tertium ascripserunt. Quedam non dixerunt vere tertium debere adiungi,[182] de quo Yeber testatur dicens : Intentio nostra in opere maiori est sumi duas res quibus

---

164. id est ignis : V.
165a. rogus sibi : V.
165b. fixatur, ut in rebis dicitur. Hic est : V.
166. philosophis, id est fixus sulfur : V.
167. Omit : Non : V.
168. eo tamen mixtum fit tinctura : V.
169. vocatur, id est cinnabarium.': V.
170. occupatum sicut : V.
171. Opinio aliter opinionem libri qui : V.
172. multis vie : V.
173. Omit : sint : V.
174. igitur ex predictis quod : V.
175. Add here : Scilicet sulfur termini scilicet tinctura albi et rubei per quod apparet pater noster et argentum vivum spiritus latens in materia scilicet illa creata que pater argentum vivum illuminat illis coloribus quibus totus mundus illuminatur scilicet albo et rubeo. : V.
176. Et de illo dicit ille philosophus cuius liber incipit : Omnes : V.
177. I have been unable to identify this work. Cf. below, note 403.
178. Inter hoc tamen : V.
179. Ista duo : V.
180. V, fol. 96r.
181. duorum esse : V.
182. Omit : de quo : V.

adiungitur tertia. Et Maria clarius dixit ⟨fol. 129r⟩[183] : Accipe placidum[184] et colericum et territe sanguineum cum eis donec sanguineum fiat relictum tingendum.[185] Istud autem tertium corpus nuncupant. Inde Turba: Tertium est corpus venas habens cordis per quod mundus intelligitur[186] et corpus mundum. De quo *Lumen luminum :* Letantur[187] enim spiritus in corpora munda equalis complexionis et proprietatis sicut viri iusti ab omni nephario scelere sunt[188] immunes. Quorum dictis assentio et priorum dicta recusso. Si enim addatur corpus metallicum quod nichil aliud est in sui origine ut iam dixi quam argentum vivum et sulphur propterea duorum numerus in essentia nec augetur. Iuvat tamen ut traditur in *Lilio*[189] ad opus brevius et citius peragendum. Sicut enim argentum vivum et sulphur spiritus fugitivi quibus addi debent et conadiungi flegma[190] et colerica fixa ad opus brevius terminandum. Et inde[191] *Lumen luminum* non possunt gravia nisi levium[192] etiam ut supra prodest etiam ut in principio ponatur. Corpus quod postmodum non indiget fermentatione que[193] quando potest fieri. Nam Morienus[194] ait quod quidam ponunt fermentum in principio quidam in medio post dealbationem scilicet[195] vel incinerationem et quidam in fine id est in operis complemento. Tu autem propter has causas ponis predictas in principio corpus mundum quod est corpus et fermentum. Non enim spiritus et corpora complexantur adinvicem ut dicitur in *Perfecto Magisterio* nisi fuerint ab omni sorde optime mundi. Sed cum sic[196] fuerint, fit ex eis corpus spirituale. In aliis etiam lapidibus fixis non localibus parum utilitatis elicies. Unde dicit Turba : Si corpus quod non liquefit spiritum coagulet ne penetret ne perforet prohibetur. Unde vermilio draganto[197] namque coagulatur quod liquefieri prohiberet. Cave tibi cum taliter propter hoc non recuses. Vitriolum multum[198] enim poterit conferre quandoque elicias itaque tibi[199] ex hiis optimum argentum[200], ex his[201] premissis ex quibus opus possit confici. Quia iam brevem

183. Dixit, repeated, B.
184. Fleumaticum : V.
185. Omit : Istud autem, V.
186. et per ipsas corpus : V.
187. Ligant : V.
188. Omit : sunt : V.
189. For the work entitled *Lilium*, see note 94 above.
190. et enim : V.
191. Unde Lumen : V.
192. levium superius : V.
193. Omit : que : V.
194. Morigenes : V.
195. Omit : scilicet : V.
196. Omit : sic : V.
197. For 'vermilio draganto', see *Medieval Latin Word list*, pp. 143 and 452. See also for 'dragantum', and red vitriol, RUSKA, *Quellen*, I (1931), 331.
198. V, fol. 96v.
199. Omit : tibi : V.
200. argentum vivum et sulfur ex : V.
201. Omit : his : V.

doctrinam dedimus in eo secundum intentionem Yebri,[202] Turbe, *Allegorie*, et *Florum ethymologarum*. Verum[203] quia in istis[204] et in omnibus aliis libris non invenitur aperte declaratum illud quod elixir perficit et quomodo perficitur. Illud vobis tradam in aliquam rem epilogando dicta prout sum divina gratia consecuutus[205] experientiam et potius doctrinam paternam in quo declarandam utar stilo cuiusdam operis quod ego feci transferre de arabico in latinum cuius autorem ignoro in quo declaratur breviter et aperte quidquid in alchimia fuerat occultum et ponitur ibi manifeste quidquid[206] Turba et alii dixerunt diminute. Parcat mihi deus quia intendo eorum secreta propalam denudare et nos iuvet ad celandum archanum. Attendite inquam res iuvantes et perficientes opus excelsum sunt considerande. Sed potissime sit consideratio[207] tua in electione[208] pure substantie argenti vivi et est illud quod ex ipso sumpsit originem et ex illo creata est. Non[209] autem est pura materia in sui natura nec in tota sui substantia sed fuit pars illius.

Quando[210] autem aliam formam habet et vulgariter appellatur sanguineus et fleumaticus. Purum enim aurum est lapis pretiosus[211] er nobilior existit quod a colerico ignito non corrumpitur vel minuitur sed melioratur eius namque compactio[212] sanguinea est equalis qualitatis et clara ideo sapientes complexionem sanguineam[213] multum exaltaverunt et ab eo habuerunt complexionem[214] maioris elixir. Illustrat enim et ab adustione conservat quod perfectionis significatio est quia est substantia equaliter durans et est fermentum elixir.[215] Non enim perficit opus nec emundatur sine fermento quia est capistrum patris proprii et nullus coagulat[216] argentum vivum ⟨in⟩ corpore[217] magnesie in qua unum est cremans, alterum autem[218] fugiens, et[219] ipsum ergo est[220] illorum tincturas[221] recipiens ⟨et⟩ est sanguineum ergo precise[222] metallorum.

---

202. Jeberis : V.
203. Verum est : V.
204. hiis libris : V.
205. consecutus et : V.
206. propalatio : V.
207. ratio : V.
208. electione sulfuris pure : V.
209. Non enim fuit sulfur in : V.
210. De auro et alchimie forma. Forma enim alchimie vulgariter : V.
211. pretiosior : V.
212. complexio : V.
213. sanguineam eius : V.
214. compositionem : V.
215. Written lxir : B; Ysir : V.
216. congelat : V.
217. vivum in : V.
218. vero : V.
219. nisi : V.
220. est enim : V.
221. *sic* : B.
222. pretiosius : V.

Qui[223] est tinctura rubens et[224] pater proprius, transformat omne corpus cum ipso.[225] Inde Turba : Nisi aurum in sanguineum pones nil habes[226] aurum ⟨et argentum⟩ vivum. Dicimus argentum vivum rubificatur et in *Visione Belini*[227] supra quem fluvium dixit enim sanguineus pater meus sol[228] dedit mihi mirabilem potestatem quia[229] mea virtute vivifico et[230] illumino lumine.[231] Qui novit me coniungere cum materia mea in mundo nil melius. Ego enim procreo similem mihi ex[232] quolibet enim aliquod sibi simile procedit. Et quodlibet individuum genus[233] multiplicat[234] sue speciei et alterius etc.[235] Et egō dico[236] quod aurum nil aliud est quam sulphur fixum[237] et argentum vivum fixum.[238] In essentia tamen utrumque clarum et subtile minerici quod patet quia argentum vivum defectum[239] suscipit illud per splendorem etiam et fulgorem radiantem ostenditur quod clarum utrumque fugit[240] et quod non fuit sulphur illud comburens patet quia omnem preparationem[241] colerici igniti expectat non inficiatur. Hoc nisi qui sensu caret visus. Et ideo cum ipso commiscentur reges[242] defacili hospitantur et maxime pater. Et hoc probat *Allegoria*[243] dicens : Si camelus caput et aures pota ipsum lacte soluto et gallina generabit pisces. Hoc tamen dico fieri diuturna operatione subtilique artificio. Est enim aurum optime coniunctionis et ipsum longo tempore natura produxit. Non ergo poterit brevi tempore taliter destrui quod inde sequatur effectus. Si calcinatur tantum[244] inde modica sequitur utilitas. Oportet enim ut corrumpatur et putrefiat cum

---

223. Et quia est tua : V.

224. rubedinis secum inventum et argentum vivum pater prius : V.

225. V, fol. 97r.

226. habens. Et hoc dicunt philsophi quia qui aurum in venum vertit ad propositam iam pervenit : V.

227. This work may coincide with the 'Dicta Belini,' or 'Visio Arislei', noted by RUSKA, *Quellen*, I (1931), 332-333.

228. Omit : sol : V.

229. quia, repeated, V.

230. Omit : et : V.

231. lumine meo : V.

232. in quodam enim : V.

233. Omit : genus : V.

234. multiplicat ergo : V.

235. non : V.

236. dico tibi : V.

237. vivum : V.

238. Omit : fixum : V.

239. defacili : V.

240. Omit : fugit et quod non : V.

241. operationem : V.

242. reges et : V.

243. Written 'Aligoria,' B. For the incipit, 'Si camellus . . .' see THORNDIKE and KIBRE, *Catalogue of Incipits of Mediaeval Scientific Writings in Latin*, (1937), 667, where the work is attributed to Hermes; also *ibid.*, 354. See also RUSKA, *Quellen*, I (1931), p. 330.

244. tamen aut soluitur : V.

aqua de qua dicemus et est[245] quam valde desideratis.[246] Iste emundatio[247] et in terra sua aqua illa fructificat iuxta quod legitur in Turba : Nisi ⟨fol. 129v⟩ granum frumenti cadens[248] in terram etc. Et *Allegoria :* Qui non tristatur nec letatur. Qui non corrumpitur non emundatur. Et hec aqua[249] qualiter fiat[250] pervenire non poterit ad artificem dure cervicis.[251]

---

245. est aqua : V.

246. desiderat : V.

247. Iste ibi emendatur et terram suam : V.

248. cadat : V.

249. a omnia : V.

250. fiant : V.

251. A long section follows here in V : Et dixerunt sapientes mundifica animam ex omni sordicie ut aurum fiat venenum. Nam sapientes declaraverunt nobis cum dixerunt attendite ad aratores qui seminant et qui metent ⟨fol. 97v⟩ secundum mirabile quod est quoniam poteris ut seminetis aliud quam aurum et metetis aurum. Nam propinquus invenietis mortem quam hoc attendite ergo vos omnes qui queritis hanc scientiam ad corpora in quibus incorporatum est aurum quemadmodum incorporatus est fructus qui comeditur in ramis qui plantantur ut fiant arbores. Deinde fructificantur; quilibet arbor secundum suam radicem propriam. Quoniam ergo sperantes extrahere aurum ex ovo vel auripigmento vel sulfure vel similibus, intellige quod dixi vobis quia non est necesse ut amplius dicam. Nam pone fermentum in auro et dic qualiter fermentatur cum auro. Nam sicut fermentum farine fermentatur farina ita similiter fermentatur aurum auro id est cum farina auri. Et oportet similiter ut faciat sapiens et habeat intellectum huius artis. Precipio ei ut accipiat elizir ex ovo non generato ex ave. Et si dissoluit hunc ovum caveat ne ardeat vel comburat illud quod si ipsum comburit vel ardet penetrabit nec dissoluitur sicut quodlibet ovum quod si non elizir est sicut sal in albedinem, et imponas in eo aurum, nichil fecisti. Nam sine dubio et vere ex fermento fermentatur elizir sicut fermentatur farina. Quod si volueris rubedinem indiges fermento argenti continua decoctione donec sit citrina et erit fermentum auri. Fermentum auri aurum est et fermentum argenti argentum est. Et si volueris tincturam argenti quod est fermentum auri. Deinde venenum in duas partes. Et cum desiccatur pone venenum secundum super residuum ut putrefiat et tingat et dimite ipsum per quadraginta dies vel quinquaginta. Nam quidam ex sapientibus nominaverit ipsum ovum et res ovi. Ut prepararet obscuritatem et liquitatem quod admodum evenit huiusmodi qui pervenit ad materia et posuit digitum suum auricularem in eo cogitans ascendere totam aquam maris. Et ego docebo vos querentes hanc scientiam quod istud ovum quod nominaverunt sapientes ovum non est ovum avis ⟨fol. 98r⟩ nec generatur ex gallina sed est ovum sapientum quod assimulaverunt ob albedinem suam albedini ovi. Quoniam in ovo sunt septem colores. Similiter et in ovo sapientum. Et assimulaverunt ovo nec ovum est sed sunt plura quia dum miscetur unum cum altero fit unicumque. Et nunquam declaravit sapiens hoc quando recoluit hanc scientiam ubi dixit quando fermentum non poterat nasci in spica donec dissoluatur ad solem et umbram per 60 dies. Nam sapientes posuerunt omnia in similitudinibus et assimulaverunt hoc unicuique rei que intentio sapientum quidam nominaverunt ovum eorum galline nam multa sunt nomina que posuerunt sapientes lapidi nostro. Nam nominaverunt eum secundum similitudines rerum nec ipsa nomina sunt nomina eius vera sed sunt nomina ficta et ideo nominaverunt eum

Post[252] aurum autem argentum purum optimum principatum obtinet.[253] Et ipsum est[254] ex colerico mundo albo fixo claro quod dedit super substantiam fleumaticam mundam fixam claram. Sed in quantitate non superat illud et ideo est corpus mundum minus tamen sanguineo diminutum magis quam aurum et excepto sanguineo nullum corpus cum eo melius existit. Et ipsum auro vicinius est. Itaque fleumaticum purum[255] corpus elixir[256] albi in minori apte quam est rubedinis tinctura firma. Qui[257] novit ipsum subtiliare et figere secum associat scilicet[258] cum eo manet in pugna quia sunt frater et soror ut dicitur in disceptatione quam fecit cum sanguineo et iuxit[259] dum dixit argentum vivum.[260] Qui iungere[261] me novit[262] cum fratre meo et sorore mea gaudebit quia si[263] mille homines haberet cotidie in mensa sua divitiis tamen opulentis existit vel habundat. Nec mirum quia sunt unius originalis nature cum qua[264] gaudet incorrupta facta. Inde Turba : Natura naturam vincit natura naturam superat natura naturam[265] letatur. Igitur ista[266] duo premissa corpora reliquis sunt[267] digniora. Moneo te tamen quod[268] artis naturam non negligas quia ferrum[269] iungitur auro et argento, quod si fuerint[270] separati;[271] immutat colorem commixti sed auget illud in quantitate nec separare[272] potest[273] aliud artis ingenium ut Yeber testatur

---

ovum. Hoc est propter colores qui sunt in eo ovo. Quoniam in eo ovo est avis volans et sic in ovo sapientum est fugiens et non fugiens et cum commiscentur et putrefiunt fient omnes spiritus et propterea nominaverunt eum ovum galline quia quia ⟨sic⟩ est vivus et non mortus quia dum ovum ponitur sub gallina deus extrahit ex ipso avem. Similiter est de ovo sapientum quia in eo est anima et corpus et spiritus et est in eo quod fugit et non fugit.

252. In V, the line reads : De argento et eius principatu. Et suum habet principatum.

253. Post aurum : V.

254. Omit : est : V.

255. purum est : V.

256. written *Ysyr* : V.

257. Et hoc dico qui novit spiritum sublimare et fixare cum argento puro associat : V.

258. Omit : scilicet : V.

259. iuxit eum : V.

260. purum : V.

261. coniungere : V.

262. V, fol. 98v. Me novit, (repeated) : V.

263. quia si, repeated V.

264. qua eius natura : V.

265. namque : V. Cf. Ruska, in *Quellen*, I (1931), p. 119 : Turba, [Sermo XI].

266. Omit : ista duo : V.

267. sunt nobiliora et : V.

268. Omit : quod : V.

269. ovum : V.

270. fuerit : V.

271. adiunctum non mutet : V.

272. separari : V.

273. potest per aliquid : V.

in ultimo suo volumine. Dicit tamen ipsum separandum quia lividum est parum rubeum[274] et albedine non[275] mortificat ipsius tamen rubedo. Ego vero experientia didici quod est tinctura rubedinis defacili maxime si fuerit eius materia pura ad album vero tinctura est difficilis. Alia consideratio est in rebus de quibus non[276] procedit[277] in sulphure et argento vivo de quorum[278] natura suprascripsi.

Tertia[279] vero consideratio versatur inter ea que sunt media et[280] predicta corpora et spiritus in unum coniunguntur que multa sunt ut in principio retulimus. In hoc tamen loco[281] que necessaria sunt denotamus ut sunt alumina et sales et atramenta de quorum naturis in proprietatibus[282] alumina talia diximus. Atramenta enim plurima sunt. Sed ciprinum[283] nobilius deprehendi Yeber filius Abiecti in *Libro de rebis*[284] exposito ait: Atramentum purum nimis habet originem ex alcatem[285] et in eo habentur sulphuries subtiles qui tingunt forsitan et una suarum prelationum est quod retinet omne fugitivum ne fugiat. Idcirco[286] aperi cor tuum quia non submergitur nisi cum aquila. Et ideo dico quod hoc utaris[287] ad rubeum preparatum[288] loco sulphuris preparati.

Ad album vero utaris alumine[289] quod dicitur plume quia est, ut dicunt quidam, argentum vivum in perfectione diminutum. In libro vero[290] *Aluminum et salium*[291] traditur quod illud est[292] unguentum quod coagulavit siccitas terre calidum et humidum a[293] natura. Alii dixerunt calidum et siccum sicut et[294] vitreolum, hic est retentor omnium volantium, et mundator corporum; mundat enim corpora mundatione famosa. Mundat et[295] splendidat et addit in eorum tinctura. Ipsum est duplator unius triplator[296] duorum quadruplator trium. Et dixerunt quod alumen est

---

274. rubori : V.
275. non puram mortificationem tamen ipsius videbo. : V.
276. natura : V.
277. procedit scilicet : V.
278. quorum ratione et : V.
279. De mediis coniungens corpora Tertia : V.
280. que : V.
281. vobis : V.
282. proprietatibus aliquantulum dixeramus. : V.
283. citrinum : V. Over the word in B, is 'vitriolum.'
284. I have not been able to identify this work.
285. In the margin of B is written : 'alias ex colcathar.'
286. Et idcirco : V.
287. Omit : utaris : V.
288. paratum utere suo loco. Sequitur de alumine ad quod utitur. : V.
289. The preceding is indicated as a heading in V.
290. Omit : vero : V.
291. Cf. R. Steele, 'Practical chemistry in the twelfth century: Rasis, De Aluminibus et salibus,' *Isis*, XII (1929), 15 : cap. 3, 'Modus aluminis.'
292. V, fol. 99r.
293. Humidum in, V.
294. Omit : et : V.
295. Tamen, V.
296. Omit : duorum quadruplator : V.

nobilius omnibus lapidibus quia est frigidum propter acerbitatem suam et est conveniens omnibus rebus ad condiendum cum arsenico et sulphure convenientius. Cave tamen tibi in hoc[297] opere de mixtione ipsius sulphuris vivi aut arsenici quia multum protelat opus. Cave etiam ne multum de ipso alumine ingrediatur opus quia licet multa bona conferat tamen denigrat album colorem sue nature et postea non mutatur in[298] album nec[299] in rubeum.[300]

Salia[301] autem multi sunt generis sed in omni genere natura[302] calida et sicca et eum siccavit[303] ignis. De proprietatibus vero salis est[304] quod soluit argentum et addit fortitudine ignis in argento albedinem et mutat ipsum a corporeitate ad spiritualitatem. Sic agit in auro et rubedinem in eo addit. Lavat corpora ab inquinatioribus eorum quia finit spurcicias cum eo calcinantur corpora et comburuntur. Vocaverunt ipsum sapientes argentum populi eo quod omnes gentes indigent ipso et est condimentum populi totius cum eo meliorantur creature, ut[305] Yeber nominatus testatur. Unde dico quod si studueris in eo invenies eius altitudinem et[306] totum absconditum eius est in eius solutione congregatione[307] et coagulatione. Ne ergo divites in hoc ut pro nostro opere[308] assumas quod levi eget compostione[309] magneque virtutis existit quod per se cum corporibus se artificio fixat si est quo per se et cum corporibus fugit ut est illud sal nitrum volatile.[310]

Sal[311] melius et nobilius est Yabar. Ipsum enim est mirabilis virtutis quoniam ipsum soluit argentum vivum in aquam et mutat fluentem quando cum eo fuerit exaltatum. Ipsum enim sal est unguentum siccitate ignis coagulatum ex natura calidum[312] et siccum subtile aperte in partem penetrativam[313] solum corpora et est copulator contradictoriarum et omnium spirituum cum[314] corporibus. Ipsum enim est[315] volans, lapis

297. hoc nostro opere, V.

298. Omit : in : V.

299. Omit : nec : V.

300. rubeum. Sequitur de salibus. : V.

301. De salibus. Salia multa sunt genera : V. 'Ex libro aluminibus et salibus, cap. 2°' : B, margin. On this subject see 'Rasis, De aluminibus et salibus,' in *Isis*, XII (1929), 15-16, 'De speciebus salium.'

302. naturaliter calidum et siccum et proprium : V.

303. siccavit caliditas : V.

304. et sua proprietas quod : V.

305. Hoc : V.

306. Omit : et : V.

307. Omit : congregatione : V.

308. opere id : V.

309. preparatione : V.

310. volatile. Sequitur de sale arsenico : V.

311. Sal Iabarbar est nobilius et melius omnibus salibus : V. The qualities here described as belonging to 'sal yabar' are similar to those attributed to 'sal armoniac'. Cf. 'Rasis, De aluminibus et salibus', in *Isis*, XII (1929), 18-19.

312. calida et sicca subtilis : V.

313. penetrat : V.

314. V, fol. 99v.

315. est spiritus : V.

generans ad elixir adiutor et nisi esse[316] cum eo, non solueretur, non ingrederetur, non compleretur elixir nec poneretur unum cum alio nec intraret unum[317] aliud volans est et existens una cum corporibus. Corpus autem[318] hoc Habohaly[319] in *Maiori :* Si posueris eum loco ignis acris vel sulphuris aut cuiuslibet non errabis in opere ad quamlibet enim se inclinat[320] Et *Lumen luminum* ⟨fol. 130r⟩ cum almizadir[321] omni[322] esse volo quare vero ad aquas ab omni pulvere receptas ad decoquendum et adiunxit ipsum tamquam valde necessarium estimat. Et subdit igitur ipsum a vilo abesse censeo. Et paulo post addit Almizadir solum tibi servat in libro *Aluminum et salium* videtur[323] quod si deus non creasset[324] ipsum non perficeretur elixir[325] et vanum esset studium alchimicum. Ego dico cum patre meo cuius anime deus misereatur quod philosophi multum commendaverunt salem et[326] non tamen dixerunt ubi opus erat et qualiter subministrat. Dixit[327] quod in eo esset occultum et[328] absconditum et monuit me dicens sapienti pauca sufficiant. Qui sine sale operatur nichil agit quia ut ait *Allegoria* : Corpora mortuorum in sepulcris attenuant propterea[329] dono veniam. Hoc tamen[330] tibi me dixisse sufficiant. Considerandum est in purgatione predictorum non enim congruit cum lapidibus non preparatis aliquid operari. Est enim lapis preparatus thesaurus rei et aspectum complementum ut gravioribus abiectis partibus opus cum purioribus facilius compleatur de quibus plenius traditur in *Libro maiori perfectionis*.[331] Et Habohaly[332] in *Maiori* dixit : Nisi prepares totum quod ponis in elixir erit aurum vel argentum[333] acre. Sed hanc preparationem necessariam philosophi multipliciter descripserunt ut[334] est ablutio calcinatio sublimatio solutio distillatio congelatio et inceratio[335] etc.,[336] de quibus esset longum narrare. Sed teneo ut traditur in libro *Lumen luminum* preparari dicitur quidquid ignem sumit, sive vegetabile sit vel animale aut potius de

316. Omit : cum eo : V.
317. unum in : V.
318. De : V.
319. Alboali : V.
320. inclinat materiam : V.
321. For 'Almizadir', or Mizadar, see RUSKA, *Quellen*, I (1931), p. 331.
322. omnia eoque non enim cum aquis variis quoniam ipsum : V; omit : esse — adiunxit : V.
323. Traditur : V.
324. creasset Almizadir sive Iabarbar. Non : V.
325. alchimia : V.
326. Omit : et : V.
327. Dixit salem in eo sale est : V.
328. Omit : et V.
329. propterea deo veniam imploro : V.
330. Omit : tibi me : V.
331. For this work, see above, note 67.
332. Albohali : V.
333. Luna : V.
334. Et : V.
335. Ceratio : V.
336. Omit : etc. V.

minera productum. Dico igitur quod in hoc opere preparatio subiungenda tibi sufficiat. Inquit[337] autem ipse[338] aurum et argentum sine calcinatione subtiliatur. Argentum vero[339] vivum abluitur. Vitriolum et ferrum calcinantur ut auferatur ab eis sulphur adurens et remaneant munda et eorum augeatur[340] siccitas. Sales autem in aqua dissoluimus coagulans et dessiccans ut purgentur a terrestritate et ut accidentalis humiditas protinus evanescat. In primis itaque te exerceas ut devenias ad alia. Et hec in[341] tua mente reconde ut dicit Morienus[342] in hiis que igne comburuntur quale proficuum utilitatis expectas. Est[343] et alia non inefficax consideratio de proportione spiritus a corpore et hoc philosophi celaverunt. Solus autem Yeber nos illuminavit dicens : Si summa volatilis superaverit summam fixi ingemueris addere de substantia fixi et econverso. Ego dico quod spiritus solo igne figi possunt diutius tamen protelatur opus. Quanta autem pars in nostro opere sufficit suo loco dicetur.[344] Et dico quod minima[345] pars sufficit corporis[346] ignis extrahatur proportionalis proportio in quo sepe contingit errare artificem rudem, qua propter considerandus est debitus vasorum modus.[347]

Fiat[348] itaque vas eneum spissum ad modum olle cuius altitudo sit palme unius[349] et dimidii et in orificio ipsius sit amplitudo unius palme et[350] modicum plus. In fundo vero sit amplitudo unius palme aliquantulum minus. In medio fundi sui habeat foramen unum ad capacitatem digiti pollicis. In[351] circuitu vero foraminis illius duos ordines foraminum equi distantium[352] per congrua spatia et sint numero ad minus duodecim[353] et sit quodlibet eorum capax principium digiti indicis. Similiter habeat duos similes foraminum ordines in circuitu[354] in mediate supra fundum scilicet in pariete[355] in quo quidem pariete supra fundum ad altitudinem palme[356] minuente fiat hostium quadratum per quod manus ingredi libere valeat. Et iuxta orificium ipsius vasis inferius per duos digitos habeat tria foramina equi distantia ad digiti minorum CX^{m}. Et totum os ipsius

---

337. In quo, V.
338. Opere, V.
339. Enim, V.
340. V, fol. 100r.
341. Omit : V.
342. Morigenes : V.
343. Iste : V.
344. Tradetur : V.
345. minima ceteris : V.
346. corporis si : V.
347. modus. Sequitur de vase eneo : V.
348. Preceded by heading : De vase eneo : V.
349. Omit : unius : V.
350. et quod : V.
351. Et in : V.
352. Duos ordines equi distantium foraminum : V.
353. Written *12* : B.
354. circuitu vasis : V.
355. pariete circumcirca : V.
356. Omit : palme : V.

vasis cohoperiatur lamina enea grossiori et[357] sit tribus magnis foraminibus perforata ut[358] per quodlibet ipsorum pugillum clausum valeat pertransire et stet bene sigillata cum vase inferiori quasi essent unum corpus et altitudo ipsius[359] lamine vas inferius per digitum excedat. In cuius circuitu supra laminam tamen vas eneum subtile ad modum medii pilii[360] expansi mobiliter collocetur. In latitudine tamen inferioris olle premisse[361] quasi ad altitudinem palme unius sint foramina duo aliis invicem opposita per que duo baculi quadrilateri deferro transeant et non moveantur super quos enea lamina rotunda collocetur que distat undique a lateribus olle per duos saltem digitos iunctos ut ignis in mediate percutiat laminam[362] et calor expansus inter laminam et latera vasis[363] transcendat superius ubi sint vasa vitrea superius vitreata.[364]

Postquam[365] prelocuti sumus de rebus[366] quibus scitur veritas propinqua et de[367] perficientibus ipsum opus et corpora proportione vasis. Restat modo etiam videre de ingenio quod possit per minima commisceri. Super quo philosophorum processit summa. Nam quidam dixerunt quod totalis adiunctio fiat cum solutione; quidam cum igne et solutione; quidam cum igne solo quorum omnium diversitates requiras in *Libro perfecti magisterii* quam propter in hiis non insisto. Sed in hoc opere teneo cum illis qui cum igne solum admiscendo procedunt. Moneo vos[368] attendere que diximus tamen abluta et munda et com⟨fol. 130v⟩miscens ea in unum fortiter et cum suo igne donec figantur. Itera donec fiat unum corpus homogeneum.[369] Suus autem ignis dicitur quod non prorsus rennuit fugitivus. De quo dictum fuit ad Euthesium[370] ipsa compositio nec ostendit modum[371] ignis. Ego autem teneo ut dicit *Lumen luminum* quia tam magnus ignis quam maximus superafficiunt[372] levis adhibendus erit; levem autem intelligo quantumcumque[373] patienter sustinet. Et propter hoc dicit Turba : Veneramini[374] reges habentes naturam in gratia[375] ministri iniu-

357. et lamina : V.
358. Omit : ut : V.
359. Omit : ipsius : V.
360. 'pilii', apparently for 'pillei (cap)'. See *Medieval Latin Word list*, p. 311. Fol. 100v follows : V.
361. premisse et : V.
362. Omit : et calor—laminas : V.
363. Repeat : et latera vasis : V.
364. vitreata. Sequitur de commixtione rerum etc. : V.
365. De commixtione rerum. Postquam : V.
366. rebus in : V.
367. Omit : de : V.
368. vos igitur : V.
369. homogeneum per totum. Suus : V. Nota digestio proprio seu iccui (?) : B, margin.
370. For 'Euthesia', see THORNDIKE and KIBRE, *Catalogue of Incipits*, (1937), 353, 716; and THORNDIKE, *Hist. of magic and exper. science*, III, 43, note 6.
371. Omit : modum : V.
372. efficiant super hoc : C.
373. quantumcumque spiritus : V.
374. Venerant : V. Cf. Turba, Sermo XXIX, *Quellen*, I (1931), 138.
375. gratia reges namque magnanimi sunt ministri : V.

riam non patientes. Nam si iniuriam eis feceris et ultra quam sustinere possint violentiam eis inferre cog:s te dimittunt proposito privatum et laborem perdes. Secundum quantam partem ignis levis quia sui levitate argentum vivum purum ingressum in corpus mundum ipsum corpus attenuat dum cum eo putrescit. Sed[376] ignis[377] aliquo vigore cum ⟨aqua⟩[378] viva modo subtiliat corpus citius. Et hoc Turba :[379] Introducite citrinum servi rubei filium sue odorifere uxori in balneum ut post ablutionem coeant quia communiter artem g'gnunt ad[380] quod similiter confert almizadir. Inde Calid :[381] Amizadir fuscorum eis[382] adiunge vel appone. Contritio manualis cum aqua calcanti similiter. Confert scilicet ad partium subtiliationem et fixionem. Inde Turba :[383] Terite ipsos donec coniungantur et fiant unum. Et Calid : Quidam in eo sunt adiuncti cum aquis aluminibus et salibus. Quidam vero non sunt adiuncti prodest etiam humiditas extranea quia illa[384] intentente et illa humiditas secum recessit que est in puro argento vivo illa scilicet intrinseca corruptibilis,[385] de[386] qua expellenda versatur intentio et hoc cum ignis levitate. Quia Turba : Nichil est quod ita extrahat humiditates fixantes sicut ignis levis et hoc dico quia fleumaticus multum habet de humiditate quam ab eo separare non est possible nisi[387] per ignis violentiam cum cautela de quo modo non est curandum ad presens aut per conservationem eius quod nunc querimus. Si vis autem dicitur ignis acer. Ut supra[389] dictum est in igne namque qui homogenea cumulat et etherogenea segregat argentum vivum purum et corpus se invicem alterant. Quandoque enim apparet nigra violacea; quandoque crocea et cinericia[390] et crocea ad modum iridis tendentia. Et hoc propter diversitatem ignis et vasis et tempus aspiciendi. Sed in fine fit rubeum propter incinerationem quia tunc agit sulphur et patet Azoc. Et qui agebat[391] primo[392] impatiens transfertur.[393] In liquefactione aut fit venenum croceum tingens et hoc ignis facit cuius officium est sibi similem sentire colorem. Et hoc potius dicunt de natura fermentantis esse et hanc administrationem ponit Turba dicens : Accipite

376. V, fol. 101r.
377. Omit : ignis : V.
378. aqua : V.
379. Cf. Turba, Sermo [XXIX] : 'Introducite citrinum cum sua uxore . . .,' *Quellen*, I (1931), p. 138.
380. Omit : ad : V.
381. For this author, usually written, 'Kalid', see note 48 above.
382. The reading is not entirely clear here.
383. Cf. Turba, Sermo [XXIX], as in notes, 374, and 379 above.
384. illa naturaliter : V.
385. corruptibilis sulfurietatibus argenti vivi : V.
386. Omit : de : V.
387. nisi aut : V.
388. eius in suo igne : V.
389. Omit : dictum est : V
390. Omit : et crocea—tendentia : V.
391. Omit : agebat : V.
392. primo congelat : V.
393. translatum est. Et in : V.

aquam lucentem que nulli miscetur[394] coinquinationi et suo commiscite compari et[395] coquite donec opus peragatur. Et iterum accipite aquam que est de frigoris natura seminate in ea aurum ibi enim putrescit. Oritur crescit et multiplicatur.[396]

De[397] medio autem quod ea coniungit figurative loquitur *Allegoria Sapientium :* Vidi hominem iam necatum et cupit scire quis eum interfecerit, et ecce apparuit mihi iuvenis bipennem manibus habens, prisco sanguine coinquinatam. Repetam igitur ut dicam quod tota hec est sublimationis intentio, scilicet ut remota terreitate illorum et abiecta similiter ex eis, furiosissimam et subtilissimam partem quam ignis fit caliditate que aliis adustionem aliis corruptionem tantum adducit. Remaneunt nobis quod in equali caliditate consistit, sine adustione vel fuga, et simplicem habet fixionem sine adustionis fuga, et hoc totum fuit per determinatam corporis amministrationem inrogo. Ideo dixit Turba :

---

394. Commiscere ignationi in suo miscetur compari, V.

395. Omit : et : V.

396. V diverges entirely at this point. It continues : Cum enim aqua hec sit ⟨fol. 101v⟩ de natura frigoris ut ibidem. Cavendum est ab igne. Ostendo natura huiusmodi qualiter corporeas vertit in spiritum. Ostendo quam admirabilis natura qualiter omnibus imminet ac omnia superat et est acetum acerrimum quod fecit aurum esse merum spiritum sine quo aceto nec albedo nec nigredo nec rubor nec rubigo fieri potest. Et scitote quod cum corpore commiscere et fit unum cum eo. Vertit ipsum spiritum spirituali vero igne tinctura invariabili que deleri non potest. Item BONELLUS (*) et in sua aqua congelate que aqua est venenum. Dicitur quod est quasi nativitas et vita eo quod est anima ex multis extracta rebus nam eius tinctura vita est hiis quibus introit detrementum et mors corporibus ex quibus extrahitur. Ut ait ZENON (**) : Item dicitur aqua permanens sine que nichil fit. Vis enim eius est spiritualis sanguinis. Contrita enim cum corpore illud in spiritum. Vertite sibi adinvicem mixta et in unum redacta se invicem vertunt. Corpus scilicet incorporat spiritum spiritus vero corpus in spiritum tinctum prout sanguis vertit. Nam omne quod spiritum habet et sanguinem habet. Ut ait MUNDUS (***) philosophus : Cum enim corpus penetrat venenum ipsum corpus in variabili colore colorat et nunquam dimittit, corpus animam que sibi sic introducitur etc. Finis libri Alberti Magni philosophi 16 Novembris per Henricum Valpod familiarem Reverendissimi domini cardinalis Sancti Petri (****) qui fuit de Almanica nacione de Valla Cusa apud Treveri. Hic est finis libri Alberti.

Following the above work there begins a tract attributed to Hermes at folio 102r. 'Hic incipit liber Hermetis summi philosophi . . .'

397. B, fol. 130v, continues without a break.

(*) For BONELLUS, one of the authors in the Turba, see especially Sermo [XXXVII], *Quellen,* I (1931), pp. 144-145; also pp. 25-26.

(**) ZENON, also written ZIMON, SIMON, CINON, is similarly one of the authors of the Turba. See *Quellen* I (1931), 25.

(***) MUNDUS, is another of the Turba authors, see *loc. cit.*, I, 23, *et passim.*

(****) The reference is to Cardinal NICHOLAS OF CUSA.

Rogorum scientiam minerale[398] munus est scientie, eritque reiteratio :[399] inbibitionis, assationis et conservationis in suo lari fit substantia una fixa que dicitur unum. Et hec *Allegoria* : Ista nigra primo fuit, postea rubea, et inde citrina, postremo vero est venenum tingens. Cavete vobis in liquefactione, quia nisi subito fortificaveritis ignem ut vitrifactoriam dat fusionem. Accidit quandoque non cito ingreditur propter errorem caliditatis. De quibus duobus erroribus non paveatis aqua emundabitur nam uterque sit sublimata : argentum vivum cum medietate sui salis armoniaci. Tere sublimatum cum duplo sui de argento mixto cum argento vivo locis equaliter et omnia in ampulla superponans per iii horas. Dimitte ut leviter fundatur; postmodum contritum in aere; sub divo pone. Aquam educit que erit ad incerandum melior cunctis. Si laborem cupis deponis in phiala; pone in alembico. Cum hac itaque aqua nobile tere confectionem in qua cerasti (?)[400] et assa et tere et assa et hoc reitera ad proportionem cironis (?).[401] Donec levi igne calcinatur tantum leviter fundatur quia nos querimus medicinam leviter ingredientem fusibilem ut aquam que metallis cito admisceatur per minera (?).[402] Similiter et argentum vivum purum ante eius fugam in lari. Et ideo nos posuimus in opere plus de fleumatico quia talem medicinam querimus de qua loguitur *Allegoria*. Dicit : Planta hanc arborem et edifica ei domum rotundam et pone ei hominem maxime etatis. Dico quod senex ille de fructu arboris illius comedere non cessabit in veram proportionem quam mire nature quod illius animam senis in iuvenile corpus transmutaverit, et pater filius factus est. Ego dico quod hic est filius benedictionis qui omnes subditos fulgida dignitate coronat. De quo dicit Hermes in suo *Thelisino* quod incipit : Verum sine mendacio[403] ille qui omnem rem subtilem vincit, omnemque rem solidam penetrabit, quia subtile dignius est grosso et rarie (?) spisso, quorum omnium causa brevioris intelligentis, brevius et verius subiungam. Exemplum. Recipe ergo in Dei nomine : auri puri et argenti uncia 1[404] ad minus ⟨fol. 131r⟩ argenti vivi uncie 4, salis arsenici uncia 1, salis nitri uncia 1; corpus cum spiritu malgama et super lapidem tere et lava cum aqua et sale. Ferveat leviter in oleo communi claro cum modico aluminis plume et iabar per diem unum, hoc fac per triduum oleum qualibet die renovando; separa eum de oleo cum aqua calida; tere cum aqua calida et sale; ut omnis nigredo recedat, terge, linteo, mundo, predictos sales admisce. Et tere tamdiu cum aqua aluminis de pluma vel vitriolo, et tunc pone in urinali apta in suo lari et sicca igne levi; extrahe in francum, tere sine liquore, reduc in similibus vasis ad ignem similem per diem naturalem ad minus per alium fortiorem ut saltem in motus fiat. Si quid vero ascenderit quandoque reduc eum ad

---

398. This reading is uncertain; but it is apparently 'minerale' for mineral. See *Medieval Latin Word list*, p. 266.

399. In the margin is written : 'His ponit exemplum de opere lapidis.'

400, 401, 402. These are uncertain readings.

403. For this work see THORNDIKE and KIBRE, *Catalogue of Incipits*, (1937), 770; and *Osiris*, II, 371-372. The incipit identifies the work as the *Tabula Smaragdina*. For the name *Thelisino* see above.

404. The sign for ounce ℥ is given here. Since the author's use of Arabic numbers is a characteristic feature of the text, they have been reproduced here.

feces, sed post tertium diem reduc ad ignem levem. Iterum extrahe in francum; tere cum aqua sua, et totum reitera et assidua cum contritione et assatione donec fiant unum homogeneum per totum quod accidit circa 22 reiterationes. Et hoc nota quod ignis utrobique in qualibet reiteratione gradatim debet augeri. Cumque videris eam fixam, gaude, postmodum vigorem ignem et lunam talem cum quo ultimo fixa sit per unum diem naturalem ad minus, tunc cum aqua simplici reduc ad eundem ignem parum plus fortiorem per alium diem, et illa sepius imbibendo et paulatim ignem augendo. Reitera ad minus noviens donec tibi calcinatum et pulverum aspectu appareat, et hoc fieri potest et melius in ampullis; et si plus feceris calcinationem melius erit. Ultimo vero fac ignem flamme subito per diem si non liquefit subito fusione bona errasti, quia fuit determinata privatam humiditate ut vitrificatoriam det fusionem aut ullam. Si vero leviter liquatur super laminam ignitam, recte opus extraxisti, quia erit tingens circa centennarium transcendens, de quo accipe partem, id est de puro argento vel auro partes 4, de iabar autem vice tincte uncia 1, tere totum et coque per similes gradus ignis et ita infra pauciores dies scilicet statues elixir priori potentius in effectu. Hoc enim modo roge secretum et lege quia non indigebis reiteratione totali, si prima vice recte peregeris. Si autem longius opus cupis, loco argenti vivi pone cinobrium, quia experientia didici quod ignis non poterit extrahere nigredinem nisi circa 48 dies et indigebis diutiori tritatione et sublimatione seu assatione. Item si addis vel alumina vel sulphur, addis ad laborem sicut in operatione quarundam operationum deprehendi. Tu autem ab hac via nostra non devies; habeas mentem fidelem; quia ut dicit Tulius in hac operatione, dato quod habeas elixir nisi in Deo mentem habeas adhuc. Nichil habes quia forte in crastinum morieris. Cela istud capitulum quia est de Turba scilicet secundum expositionem quam retulit in commento. Dicit Turba : Oportet ut corpus flamma ignis occupatum dirivetur et debile fiat cum aqua in qua illud est. Que verba Yeber exponens ait : Insipientes autem aquam haurientes in nobis aquam esse, qui si libros legisset, scivisset utique aquam esse permanentem; que quidem absque suo corpore commixta et facta sint unum permanens esse non potest; contrita enim cum corpore quod philosophi exposuerunt; nutu Dei corpus illud in spiritum versum. Contrita enim et sibi invicem mixta; se invicem tinctuerit. Corpus enim incorporat spiritum, spiritus vero corpus in spiritum tinctum ut sanguis vertit. Ergo dico cum *Allegoria* quod nisi spiritualia corporea feceritis nolite elixir blasphemare sed opus. Sed hoc totum diminutum subiicio ut quidam dixerunt sapientes; et nos quandoque experti sumus. Qui sine sale operatur nihil operatur sicut qui cum arcu sine corda sagittaret. Deo gratias.

Scriptum anno domini nostri Iesu Christi 1422° 21^{a} martii tunc sabbato ⟨corr super lin. : die veneris⟩ ante Letare, etatis mee anno 34°, magistratus vero 3°, contrariantibus michi astris, aut peccatis propriis, in tantum quod spire nec invidie, scelerata lues corrosit egenum; spurcicie soboles physis propellit alumpnum; sed patientiam habe quoniam pro iustitia patris. Et licet saturnalia cum martialibus inimicentur; arrident tamen iovialia cum veneraris. Inestimabili enim gaudio exultat cor meum, nesciens quid fortuna paret aut que sit causa gerendi tripudium tantum, quis motor in orbe creavit flagrantis convivi iubilum sibi nesciue instat. Quis furor, o superi; quis fervor tenet amantem. Anda soror soror anda, mee non inscia pene. Quidquid tamen fortuna disponat in omnibus intentionibus Dei sumus, qui est gloriosus et benedictus in secula. Amen.

VII

ALCHEMICAL WRITINGS ASCRIBED TO ALBERTUS MAGNUS

THAT Albertus Magnus, the distinguished Dominican scholar of the thirteenth century, was deeply interested in and quite probably a believer in the possibility of the transmutation of metals has already been demonstrated by the recent study of J. R. Partington from the various passages in Albert's authentic writings bearing on alchemy as well as by the earlier analysis of his interest in the subject by Lynn Thorndike.[1] Numerous references to alchemy in Albert's commentaries on Aristotle's *De caelo et mundo*, and the *Meteorology*, as well as in his own five books on minerals (*Mineralium libri v*), have been noted in support of Albert's favorable attitude toward the Hermetic art. He had acquired his theoretical knowledge of the subject largely from the Latin translations of Arabic works on alchemy, and his practical acquaintance with it through his visits to laboratories in Cologne and Paris. He was acquainted with contemporary workers in the field and makes references to the 'alchemists of our time.'[2] On the other hand Albert's interest in the subject appears not to have been noted by his contemporaries, although there is associated with his name a fairly large body of alchemical literature dating chiefly from the fourteenth and fifteenth centuries. How much of this can be attributed to the common medieval practice of attaching to such treatises names of prominent ecclesiastics in order to give them greater authority, it has so far been impossible to determine. One explanation for the currency of alchemical tracts under Albert's name is put forth by Naudé who in his 'Apology for all the Great Personages who have been falsely suspected of Magic,' states that Albert is confused with a chemist who lived at Cologne.[3] Hence the alchemists have used his name. Whether authentic or not there is without doubt a close relationship between the writings in alchemy circulated under Albert's name and his avowed interest in the art. Albert's reputation as a skilled alchemist appears to have been fairly widespread by the middle of the fourteenth century, when he is even credited with having had as a disciple in this art, Roger Bacon.[3a]

Although as has been indicated above there have been several accounts of the alchemical treatises in print under Albert's name, very little account has so far been taken of such tracts in manuscripts.[4] The present study is intended therefore

[1] J. R. Partington, 'Albertus Magnus on Alchemy,' *Ambix*, I (1937), pp. 9–13; Lynn Thorndike, *A History of Magic and Experimental Science* (New York: Macmillan, 1923), II, pp. 569–573. For earlier bibliography on this subject, see especially R. P. Laurent, O.P., and R. P. Congar, O.P., 'Essai de bibliographie Albertinienne,' *Revue Thomiste*, XIV, n.s., no. 65, p. 448.

[2] Partington, *loc. cit.*, pp. 9–10.

[3] G. Naudé, *Apologie pour tous les grands personnages qui ont esté faussement soupçonnes de magie* (Paris, 1625), Chap. XVIII.

[3a] Thorndike, *History of Magic and Experimental Science* (1923), II, p. 571; D.W. Singer, *Catalogue of Latin and Vernacular Alchemical Manuscripts in Great Britain and Ireland* (Brussels, 1928–1931, 3 vols.), I, No. 193. See also James Corbett, *Catalogue des manuscrits alchimiques Latins* (Union Académique Internationale, Brussels, 1939), p. 279.

[4] Professor Thorndike, *op. cit.*, II, pp. 569–571, has indicated several manuscripts containing alchemical writings under Albert's name. It was at his suggestion that the present study was begun.

to provide a preliminary survey of the manuscript literature, to indicate its relationship to the printed works, and to Albert's authentic compositions. The detailed analysis and evaluation of the individual treatises, is, however, reserved for a later more detailed account of their contents in relation to other contemporary tracts on the same subject. Before proceeding to the tabulation of the treatises it may be of some interest to note which of them were already in circulation before the close of the fourteenth century, the earliest date of their appearance, and which might therefore have the best claims to authenticity. Among these may be indicated the *Alkimia minor* (2)[1] which is listed under Albert's name in a fourteenth-century alchemical miscellany and is intended to serve as a laboratory manual. Several of its short concise recipes are also found in the *Semita recta* (25) which is likewise included in the same alchemical miscellany. The *Semita recta* is the best known of Albert's works on the Hermetic art and it appears in numerous manuscripts as well as in the printed collections of Albert's writings. Suggestions as to its probable authenticity are based on the fact that its clear, concise, and well ordered account of the subject resembles Albert's treatment of other topics of natural science in his authentic compositions. The manuscript texts of the *Semita recta* vary greatly among themselves. Some have been abridged, others have been added to, and the interpolations are frequently of a much later date than the original matter. Any final decision as to whether or not the work is genuine would need to await a careful examination and sifting of these manuscripts.

The *Semita recta* is followed in one manuscript by a third tract attributed to brother Albert in the aforesaid fourteenth-century alchemical miscellany. This Work which is entitled, *De occultis naturae* (15), in an Arundel manuscript purports to be a compendium of the truth in the mastery of the alchemical art. It reiterates much that is contained in the *Semita recta* and other works of like nature. Another treatise, the socalled *Compositum de compositis* (8), which is repeatedly attributed to Albertus in late manuscripts and in the printed alchemical collection of Zetzner is found anonymous in a fourteenth-century manuscript at the Advocates' Library in Edinburgh, Scotland.[2] The work is described at the close as a 'Composite of composites abstracted by philosophers and compiled by masters.' It is said to have been authorized and promulgated at Paris in the year 1331. In the body of the work the author speaks in the first person singular and refers to his previous treatise on minerals, which might be said to bear out the attribution to Albertus Magnus in the later manuscripts. The work also contains a systematic exposition of the alchemical art which is suggestive of the *Semita*

[1] The numbers in parentheses refer to numbered items in the list below. For the hitherto unedited Latin text and an analysis of its contents, see my article, 'The *Alkima minor* Attributed to Albertus Magnus,' above IV.

[2] An analysis of this text, without the identification is contained in L. Thorndike, *History of Magic and Experimental Science* (New York: Columbia Press, 1934), III, pp. 133–134. Professor Thorndike has kindly loaned me his photostat of the manuscript, which I have now compared with my notes of the same work in manuscripts at Paris, *BN 7147*, 1535 A.D., fols. 1^r–12^v, and at *Vatican 4092*, fifteenth century, fols 42^r–47^v, as well as with the printed text in Zetzner.

recta although the contents of the two works are not the same. However, in the Paris manuscript of the work which was copied by Oronce Finé in 1535, the tract is entitled, 'The Book of Alchemy which is called Semita recta.'[1] Although there is considerable verbal variation between the texts of the Latin manuscripts of the *Compositum* their general content is the same. In the Edinburgh text, however, the introductory section beginning, 'Talentum mihi . . .' which usually identifies the work is omitted. Also all three manuscript texts end differently. At the close of the Paris text there is added a long section not found in the other versions. The printed text as reproduced by Zetzner, on the other hand omits several lines found in the earlier sections of the Edinburgh text and after the first three sections deviates entirely from the manuscript versions.

A *Practica alchimiae* (18) under Albert's name is found in a late fourteenth- or early fifteenth-century manuscript. In it are considered the alchemical processes of sublimation, calcination, and the coloring or transmutation of the metals into gold (rubeum) or silver (album). The treatise also contains directions for the preparation of mineral waters essential to the art as well as for the preparation of the elixir, and is, as its title implies, chiefly a practical guide for use in the laboratory.

Of the other treatises on alchemy circulated under Albert's name no manuscripts earlier than the middle of the fifteenth century have so far turned up. Included among these tracts is a general work on the art which opens with the statement from Calixtenes (1), here named as one of the founders of alchemy, that alchemy is the science that imparts to inferior metallic bodies the nobility of the superior bodies. It is interesting to note that Albert quotes a similar statement from Calixtenes in his *De mineralibus*.[2] In 1468 this tract which begins with Calixtenes' statement was apparently one of a collection of books sold at Paris.[3] Another of these works is the *Libellus de alkimia* (13), in which the author calling himself, Albert, states that he will elucidate the secrets of the art for the service of all since so many are cut off from them through ignorance. Here again the plan and exposition are similar to the *Semita recta*. Still further tracts include a description of the composition of the elixir in fifteen operations (10); also a 'Concordance of the philosophers on the stone' (9) in which the author endeavors to demonstrate that although there is verbal disagreement among the philosophers they all are in general agreement in substance. Though they may describe the op-

[1] This fact has led Dr. Corbett into the error of confusing this work with the *Semita recta* or *De alchemia* printed in Borgnet's edition of the *Opera omnia* of Albertus Magnus (Paris, 1890–1899, 38 vols.), XXXVII, pp. 545–573: James Corbett, *Catalogue des manuscrits alchimiques Latins* (Brussels, 1939), p. 56.

[2] *Lib. mineral.* III, 1, 7, *Opera omnia*, Borgnet, V, 68: 'Callisthenes enim praecipuus in hac sententia, dicit alchimiam esse scientiam quae inferioribus metallis nobilitatem attribuit superiorum.' This is quoted in the course of a discussion as to the truth of the alchemists' theory that gold is the only perfect metal, and all other metals are imperfect and striving for perfection. On this moot question Albert claims to have examined the alchemical books which he reports, however, are without figures or proofs, 'hiding their intention by metaphors, which is not the habit of philosophy.' See my forthcoming account of this text in *Isis*.

[3] Corbett, *Catalogue des manuscrits alchimiques Latins* (Brussels, 1939), p. 293; 'Albert Magni Colistenus. . . . '

erations or processes under different terms or signs and designate the stone under various names they all tend toward one end. Unlike the bulk of the other tracts on the art attributed to Albertus Magnus this work emphasizes the importance of mercury alone as the material of the stone. The prime importance of mercury above the other minerals is further discussed in the 'Book of the Eight Chapters' (16), which appears to be extant only in the printed edition of Zetzner. Quicksilver or mercury is here stated to be the ferment and the elixir which produces gold or silver in the alchemical process. On the other hand the more generally accepted theory expounded in the other works attributed to Albert, namely that both mercury and sulphur are the essential material of the stone, is set forth in the *Compendium alchemiae* (7) on the origin and material of metals. In this tract, although the principal substance is said to be mercury, the productive spirit (spiritus foetens) is stated to be sulphur. All metals are said to be of the same basic substance or matter although they differ in form.

In addition to the foregoing the fifteenth-century manuscripts contain under Albert's name a work entitled, *Propositiones* (20), which contains short statements regarding the practical aspects of the alchemical art; also a tract revealing the 'Secret operations' (24). In this last named work the familar astrological doctrine of favorable and unfavorable times as applied to alchemical operations is introduced. There is further a *Secreta philosophorum* (23) which claims to have been extracted from the secrets of the philosophers. Its avowed intention is to confine itself to the proofs of operations without discussing their theories, causes, or deceptions, a procedure which is strongly suggestive of the *Alkimia minor*. In fact the general plan of its contents as stated in the opening paragraph further resembles the *Alkimia minor* since it is to describe first the essential preparations, secondly, the sublimations, and thirdly, the elixir for whitening or reddening, that is silver and gold-making. In the body of the work, however, this plan is not closely adhered to and its arrangement differs from that of the *Alkimia minor* although many of the same recipes are included. A separate treatise on the 'Regimen of the work on the stone' (22) is found in at least three fifteenth-century manuscripts under Albert's name. Another work on secrets, that is the *Secretum secretorum* or *Practica alkimiae* (19) is apparently also attributed to Albertus Magnus in a Sloane manuscript where it is immediately followed by the *Semita recta*.

Several works which belong to the general core of alchemical literature in the later middle ages are also found under Albert's name. Such for example are the various tracts on waters or liquids (3); the *Experimenta* (11), or reports of actual laboratory observations; the *Clavis sapientiae* (4), usually attributed to Ortulanus; the *Liber Perfecti magisterii* (17), which more generally appears under Rasis' name, as well as several 'Recipes' (21).

The frequency and character of the alchemical writings encountered in the manuscripts under the professed authorship of Albertus Magnus reflects an active interest in not only the philosophical basis of the art but also its practical and experimental aspects. In general these treatises are free from the mystifying and allegorical features upon which Albert himself in the *De mineralibus* cast aspersions as characteristic of alchemical books. In this respect at least the imprint of his didactic method, noteworthy for its clarity of expression, and systematic arrangement was sufficiently strong to influence those who professed to be his mouthpiece. As in the case of Albert's exposition to his confrères of the Aristotelian scientific corpus, the main purpose of the author in the great majority of these tracts was to explain to his brethren, in as simplified fashion as was necessary for its understanding, the art of alchemy, its theory and practice.

The following list of alchemical texts which appear under Albert's name has been arranged alphabetically so far as possible by the first important word of each title. Variant titles, however, of the same tract have been brought together under a common title, the choice of which may be somewhat arbitrary. Manuscript and other references follow directly after the titles, with opening and closing words where these would be useful for further identifications. For manuscripts before 1500 in the British Isles, reference is made to Mrs Dorothea Waley Singer's Catalogue where more complete descriptions of these codices may be found. For those from Paris, although this work was completed before the appearance of Dr James Corbett's Catalogue, reference by page is made to his work. Printed editions are also indicated. Where it has so far not been possible to consult the manuscript either directly or in photostat, an asterik (*) is placed before the manuscript. For economy and brevity of citation a system of abbreviations has been employed similar to that previously utilized in Thorndike and Kibre, *Catalogue of Incipits of Mediaeval Scientific Writings in Latin*, Mediaeval Academy, 1937.[1]

[1] BL Bodleian Library, Oxford
BM British Museum, London
BN Bibliothèque nationale, Paris
Borgnet Albertus Magnus, *Opera omnia*, edited by A. Borgnet (Paris, 1890–1899), 38 volumes.
BU University Library, Bologna
Cassel Landesbibliothek, Cassel
CLM Codex Latinus Monacensis (Bayerische Staats-Bibliothek), Munich
Copenhagen Bibliotheca regia Hafniensis, Copenhagen
Corbett James Corbett, *Catalogue des manuscrits alchimiques latins*, (Union académique internationale, Brussels, 1939). Reference is to page.
CU Cambridge University
CUL University Library, Cambridge
DWS Dorothea Waley Singer, *Catalogue of Latin and Vernacular Alchemical Manuscripts in Great Britain and Ireland* (Brussels, 1928–1931), 3 vols. Reference is to item number.
Ea Erfurt Stadtbücherei, Amplonian collection
FL Biblioteca Laurenziana, Florence
FN Biblioteca nazionale, Florence
FR Biblioteca Riccardiana, Florence
KlaB Bischöfliche Bibliothek, Klagenfurt
Lami Jo. Lami, *Catalogus codicum manuscriptorum qui in Bibliotheca Riccardiana Florentiae asservantur*, (Leghorn, 1756).
Manget J. J. Manget, *Bibliotheca chemica curiosa*, Geneva, 1702, 2 vols.
Na Biblioteca nazionale, Naples
Prag (Formerly Republic and University Library, Prag)
Thorndike Lynn Thorndike, *A History of Magic and Experimental Science*, I–II (New York, 1923); III–IV (New York, 1934).
VA Bibliotheca Apostolica Vaticana, Latin manuscripts
VE Bibliotheca Marciana, Venice (The shelf marks added in parentheses are those of Valentinelli's *Catalogue*)
VI (Formerly National-Bibliothek), Vienna
Wo Landesbibliothek, Wolfenbüttel
Zetzner L. Zetzner, *Theatrum chemicum* (Strassburg, 1659–1661), 6 vols.

1. Alchimia[1]

DWS 180: *BM Sloane 3457*, fifteenth century, fols 40–50v: Introd. 'Calistenus unus de antiquioribus post Hermetem artis nostre inventoribus . . . ' Text: 'Scias itaque quod omnis . . . / . . . evolat et humidum suum unctuosum fuerit compositum. Et est finis magni Alberti.'

BM Sloane 3120, seventeenth century, fols 174–192v: 'Incipit tractatus Alberti qui sic incipit. Calixtenus unus philosophus capitulum primum est hic obmissum . . . Principia immediata sunt . . . / . . . mercurio vivo communi. Finis.' Postscript: 'Calcinatio . . . / . . . funditur super siccum. Finis alchemie Alberti magni.'

BU 270(457), III, fifteenth to sixteenth century, pp. 77–97, apparently identical with *BM Sloane 3120*: 'Incipit tractatus Alberti, qui sic incipit Callixtenes unus philosophorum cuius capitulum primum est hic obmissum. Principia immediata sunt sulfur et mercurius . . . / . . . aliquid liquidum funditur super siccum. Finit alchimia Alberti Magni.'

2. Alkimia minor

*PALERMO *4 Qq.A.10*, fourteenth century, item 46, no. 30: 'Item tractatus fratris Alberti qui incipit Dilecto in Christo fratri N. ordinis predicatorum . . . '[2]

BN 6749B, 1481 A.D., fols 48r–52r, 'Incipit alkimia minor Alberti Magni episcopi ratisponensis ordinis fratrum predicatorum. Dilectissimo in Christo N. fratri ordinis predicatorum . . . / . . . soluveris et coagulaveris cadet unam supra centum 100 et sic est finis. Ego frater Albertus ordinis predicatorum ista opera experta et probata inveni. Explicit alkimia minor fratris Alberti.'

BN 7162, fifteenth century, fols 80v–85r, except for some verbal variations, is identical with the text in the preceding manuscript. The sections [15–24] are on fols 77r (old numbering, 48r)–78v.

BN nouv. acquis. 1293, fifteenth century, fols 59–61v: 'Item dillectissimo in Christo fratri N. hordenis predicatorum . . . / . . . dissolutio et congelatio donec quod dictum est eveniat.' The remaining sections of the work are missing.

VA Palat. 1330, fifteenth century, fols 60v–72v, in the midst of the Semita recta: 'Dilectissimo in Christo fratri N. ordinis predicatorum Albertus . . . / . . . (72r) Compositio omnium predictorum ad medicinam perfectam artis . . . (72v) Explicit liber secundus.'

VE VI.*214*(*XVI,3*), 1472 A.D., fols 180r–189v, 'Incipit trac(ta)tus alkimie fratris Alberti de Colonia. (D)ilecto in Christo patri N. ordinis . . . / . . . quod si postquam coagulatus iterum solueris et coagulaveris cadet una supra 100 etc. finis. Explicit liber secundus fratris Alberti de ordine predicatorum.'

3. Aquae, which also appear anonymous, or ascribed to Aristotle
Aquae duodecim.[3]

BN 6514, thirteenth to fourteenth century, fols 40v–41v, Anon. 'Incipit liber xii aquarum . . . Libelli huius series . . . Primum ergo de aqua rubea . . . De aqua rubicunda. Ovorum vitellos equaliter . . . / . . . et domos illuminat operi enim summe necessaria.'

BN 7156, thirteenth to fourteenth century, fols 145v–146r: 'Incipit liber xii aquarum.

[1] Thorndike, II, p. 570. My transcription of this text from the two Sloane MSS is forthcoming in *Isis*.

[2] This is one of 72 items contained in a catalogue of alchemical books in the Palermo Ms. I have transcribed the item from a photostat copy of the description (the Di Marzo reprint of Carini's description) loaned to me through the kindness of Dr W. J. Wilson. See also item 23 below, *Secreta philosophorum* which treats of the same general subject matter. Corbett, pp. 49, 111, 215.

[3] Thorndike, II, 569; DWS 1063; W. J. Wilson, *Osiris*, II (1936), p. 366; Corbett, pp. 20, 78, 88.

Ovorum vitella equaliter teres . . . / . . . auripigmenti crocei v. partes . . . Explicit liber de xii aquis.'

BN 7158, fifteenth century, fol. 112^{r-v}: 'Incipit liber xii aquarum. Ovorum vitella equaliter . . . / . . . et rubescet et colorem ac naturam auri suscipiet quam in perpetuum non amittet. Explicit liber de xii aquis.' This is much shorter than the preceding text.

BU 138(104), fifteenth century, fols 235^{v}–237^{r}, 'Incipit liber xii aquarum Alberti Magni. De prima aqua (aqua ovorum). Ovorum vitella equaliter teres ut in medulla . . . / . . . Explicit liber xii aquarum' followed by an 'Additio ad supradicta . . . et soluit omne corpus. Amen.'

BU 270(457), fifteenth to sixteenth century, pp. 108–111, is identical with the preceding.

FN Palat. 887, fifteenth to sixteenth century, fols 89^{r}–90^{v}: 'Incipit liber xii aquarum et primo de aqua rubicunda. Ovorum vitella . . . / . . . mollescat. Explicit liber xii aquarum;' fols 91–93^{r}, 'Incipit liber duodecim aquarum. Libelli huius series xii splendescat capitulis. Primum de aqua rubicunda . . . Primum ergo de aqua rubea quomodo et ex quibus componatur . . . ' fols 93^{r}–94^{v}, 'Item alius modus xii aquarum. Libelli huius series . . . / . . . in hoc libello ultimam hanc aquam describit et sic est finis. Explicit liber xii aquarum. Deo gratias.'

FN Palat. 981, fifteenth century, fols 70^{r}–71^{r}, 'Incipit liber xii aquarum Aristotelis. Libelli huius aquarum series . . . '

Geneva 82, sixteenth century, fols 146^{r}–157^{v}: 'De aquis. Aqua rubicunda sic fit. Recipe ovorum vitella . . . / . . . hoc toties donec tuam assequaris voluntatem.'

**Palermo 4 Qq.A.10*, fourteenth century, item 46, no. 36, 'Item liber xii aquarum qui incipit libelli huius . . . '

**Prag 1984(X.H.6)*, fourteenth century, fols 29^{v}–30^{v}

Aqua mercurius et oleum sulphuris.[1]

**CUL 220(Dd.IV.45)*, small 4to, sixteenth century, 2 paper leaves in an alchemical miscellany: Inc. 'Opus istud multis diebus abscondebatur. Circa quod primo principaliter est notandum quod mercurius . . . / . . . et ego Albertus dico quod sum expertus istas duas operationes et quod non est aliud opus perfectum (a) me . . . et scias quod omnia alia sunt vana et illusoria. Deo gratias.'

Aqua vitae.[2] See also Experimenta.

**VI 5315*, fifteenth century, fols 128–133: Albertus, De aqua vitae. 'Inter cetera domini Alberti Magni aquarum experimenta . . . '

VA 5377, fourteenth to fifteenth century, fols 137^{r}–138^{r}, 'Consequitur tractatus aquarum magistri Alberti de Alamania et primo de aqua vitae contra calidas et frigidas passiones. Aqua composita contra calidas et frigidas passiones est dupplex. Quedam frigidis . . . / . . . et hec de aqua composita contra frigidas passiones tam ab antiquis philosophis quam etiam a modernis comprobata fuit.'

4. Clavis sapientiae. This is the work of Ortulanus, De secretis naturae (DWS 32). It is ascribed to Albertus in **BL Ashmole 1448*, fifteenth century, fols 259–262 (DWS 32, xiii): 'Incipit tractatus libri qui vocatur Clavis sapientiae secundum Albertum. Laus (et) honor virtus et gloria . . . ' In *FN Palat. 887*, 15–16c, fols 17^{r}–23^{r}, it is ascribed to Ortulanus: 'Incipit Ortulanus de secretis naturae. Laus (et) honor . . . '; and also in *FR 1165* (L.111.34), fifteenth century, fols 47^{r}–49^{v}.

   Probably the same treatise is that in *Cambrai 924(823), fourteenth to fifteenth century, fols 168–175, 'Incipit liber qui vocatur Clavis sapientiae. Tu qui legis istum librum noveris quod in exemplari . . . '

5. Colors, various tracts on:

**CU Corpus Christi Coll. 243*, thirteenth to fourteenth century, fols 1–58^{v}, Incipit liber Alberti de coloribus et virtutibus lapidum.[3] This is the Ps. Albertus, *Lapidarium*,

[1] Thorndike, II, p. 570, note 4. [2] *Ibid.*, II, p. 798, note 5. [3] Thorndike, II, p. 567, note 2.

incipit: 'Habete celi silentium . . . ' It has little alchemical content. Other MSS of the work are *BN 7156, thirteenth to fourteenth century, fols 175–192, Anon. Tractatus de nominibus lapidum et eorum proprietatum (Corbett 80); *VA Regin. 1106, ff. 1–;

*Glasgow Hunterian 468 (v.6, 18), fourteenth to fifteenth century, also in part in *BN 7337, f. 121; and *VA 1043, fifteenth century, fols 397ʳ–402ʳ (A. Pelzer).

**Ea Q.189*, thirteenth to fourteenth century, fols 67–68, Notae de coloribus, fortasse Alberto Magno attrib. Inc.: 'Lazurium fit multis modis . . . '

Coll. Amplonius Ratynck, Bücher-Verzeichniss von 1412, Phil. nat. 5, De coloribus Alberti M.[1]

**Wo 672*, 1444 A.D., fols 37–60, Albertus, Liber de coloribus.

6. Commentary on Aristotle's *Secretum secretorum*

DWS 35: **BL Fairfax 22*, fourteenth century, fols 31–38ᵛ, Inc.: 'Artis sapientibus sermo comprobandus . . . / . . . descriptio galli . . . pedes rane vel bufonis. Explicit alchemica magistri Alberti'; **BM Harley 3528*, fifteenth century, fols 9ᵛ–10ᵛ, Anon. Inc.: 'Ars a sapientibus comprobanda . . . / . . . et est luna perfecta in omni examinatione etc.'

7. Compendium alchemiae.[2] See also De occultis naturae.

**Wo 676*(627 Helmst.), 1444 A.D., fols 1–24ᵛ.

**Wo 676*(627 Helmst.), 1444 A.D., fols 91–130, German free translation.

Printed in Zetzner II(1659), 123–126: 'Compendium Alberti Magni de ortu et metallorum materia supra quam spagyricus radicalia principia fundet. Materia vero principalis . . . / . . . putrefactionis si eius praeparationem nosti, felix Medicus eris, totis conatibus in eo votum tuum dirige, Vale.'

BN fonds français, nouv. acquis. 4114, seventeenth to eighteenth century, pp. 1–9: 'Abregé d'Albert le Grand de l'origine et naissance des métaux, sur laquelle les spargyristes fondent et tirent ses principes radicaux. La matière principale de tous . . . (Traduit par le Rᵈ P. A. tiré du *Theatre chim.* tom. 2, p. 123).'

**BM Sloane 976*, fifteenth century, fol. 32ᵛ, Compendium Alberti super artem alkimie. This is part of the *De mineralibus* (DWS 176, xiv).

8. Compositum de compositis[3]

Edinburgh, *Advocates' Lib. 20.8.1*, fourteenth century, fols 6–40ᵛ: Anon. 'Oportet itaque artificem naturam inspicere et procedere ex hiis ex quibus procedit natura. Natura autem prout cognonovimus . . . / . . . accendans. Postea de ipso proice unam supra 1000 et iterum de eo id est super alias 1000.1000. partes donec totius numerus compleatur. Explicit compositum de compositis abstractis a philosophis et compilatis a magistris Parisius divulgatum et auctorisatum anno 1331 mense Maii. Hec scripta anno eodem revoluto.'

VA 4091, fifteenth century, fols 42ʳ–47ᵛ, 'Tractatus domini fratris Alberti Episcopi Ratisponensis ordinis praedicatorum. Talentum mihi traditum negoti(ati)onis domini non abscondam ne maledictione . . . ' The second paragraph begins: 'Natura . . . ' The work closes, 'super mille et iterum de eo unam super mille alias partes totius numerus compleatur. Amen. Explicit. Amen.'

BN 7147 (Colbert 1639), sixteenth century, fols 1–12ᵛ, 'Alberti Magni Liber alkimie, qui Semita recta vocatur. Talentum mihi . . . / . . . sui similem exhibet colorem nec

[1] W. Schum, *Beschreibendes Verzeichniss der Amplonianischen Handschriften-Sammlung zu Erfurt.* (Berlin, 1887), p. 809.

[2] Partington, *Ambix*, I (1937), p. 17.

[3] Partington, *Ambix*, I (1937), pp. 17, 19; Corbett, p. 56, where the work is incorrectly identified with the *Semita recta.*

vires ignis pertimescit. Explicit liber de semita recta Alberti Magni in secretis nature operibus et alkimicis introducens. Orontius Scribebat Parisiis. 1535.'

**Na V.H.134*, fifteenth to sixteenth century, fols 8r–14v

**CUL 1255*, 6(Ff. IV, 12, 13), 1528–1529 A.D., fols 227–249r, 'Albertus In Compositum de composito.'

Printed in Zetzner, IV (1659), 825–841, Alberti Magni Compositum de compositis. Inc. 'Talentum mihi traditum negotiationis . . . ' This paragraph ends with the sentence: 'Oportet igitur naturam inspicere artificem et procedendum est ex quibus natura procedit.' The next paragraph (Cap. I) opens: 'Naturam autem prout cognovimus . . . ' This printed version, however, deviates from the MSS after the close of the third section (p. 830) where there begins: 'Nota. Natura seu materia lapidis philosophorum . . . '

**BM Sloane 276*, sixteenth century, fol. 3

English translations: **BM Sloane 3180*, 1582 A.D., fol. 12; **Sloane 3630*, seventeenth century, fols 70–74, 'Upon the work or science of alchimie named, "Compositum de compositis" ' (Ayscough, p. 477).

French translation: *BN fonds fr. nouv. acquis.* 4114, seventeenth to eighteenth century, pp. 13–63, 'Le composé des composez d'Albert le Grand . . . Traduit sur le traité d'Albert le Grand, qui se trouve dans le *Theatre Chymique*, p. 825, dans le 4 vol.'

9. Concordantia philosophorum in lapide[1]

Printed in Zetzner IV(1659), 809–824: Inc. 'Licet in ista materia videntur philosophi ad literam fore discordes tamen concordando . . . / . . . totum opus in perfectione cum operis instantia et continuatione, et ipsius reiteratione cum adjutorio altissimo sit completum, cuius nomen sit benedictum in secula seculorum. Amen. Finis.' It appears anonymously in Part I of H. Condeesyanus, *Harmoniae imperscrutabilis Chymico-Philosophicae* (Frankfurt, 1625), pp. 228–260; and as by Antonius in Part II, pp. 144–174.

BN fonds français 2012 (Colbert 4447), sixteenth century, fols 49r–70r, 'Le traicte de Albert le Grant de la Concordance des philosophes en la pierre. Je ssache que en ceste matierie les philosophes sonent bens discordans . . . / . . . Cy fine le livre de Albert de la Concordance des philosophes en la pierre.' (Corbett 233).

Duodecim aquae, see Aquae

10. Elixir[2]

**BM Sloane 3457*, fifteenth century, fols 109–113v, 'Compositio elixiris mineralis secundum Albertum Magnum Theutonicum summum philosophum.' Inc. 'Elixir ex mineralibus requirit xv operationes octo scilicet ex parte spirituum tres ex parte corporum perfectorum et tres ex parte imperfectorum et unam in proiectione elixiris . . . '

11. Experimenta

**BM Harley 79*, fifteenth century, fol. 46 (DWS 1001, vii), 'Experimentum de aqua ardenti quod fecit frater Albertus menciom in libro methaurorum ubi tractat de fulgore et tonitruo . . . '

BN nouv. acquis. 1293, fifteenth century, fols 118r–122v, 'Incipiunt quedam experimenta in scientia alchimie iuxta scientiam Alberti Magni. Quomodo fit aqua acuta. Recipe unam libram aluminis . . . (fol. 118v) Incipiunt alia sperimenta in scientia alchimie iuxta (scientiam) Alberti Magni quomodo fit aqua acuta vel acutissima . . .

[1] Partington, *Ambix*, I (1937), p. 17.

[2] DWS 181. I follow the corrected readings given by L. Thorndike, 'A Study of Complex Scientific Manuscripts,' *Isis*, XXIX (1938), pp. 389–390, n. 80.

(fol. 122v) . . . et habebis verum aurum ut dictum est de aliis. Explicit opus magistri Alberti Magni' (Corbett 218).

BU 270(457), fifteenth century, xv, 3, fols 1r–21v, 'Ex Floridis. In Christi nomine. Amen. Sciendum vero est quod iste sunt species cum quibus sublimari debet mercurium crudum idest vinum . . . / . . . in pulverem ossium arborum cum viscositate malve. Expliciunt experimenta omnium receptorum Alberti. Deo gratias.'

FL Ashburnham 1448, fifteenth century, fols 157r–158v, 'Incipiunt alique experimenta Alberti Magni et primo de aqua vite. Aqua vite ponitur loco balsami naturalis quoniam omnes virtutes . . . ' Then follow recipes for 'aqua aromatica,' and for 'aqua acuta metallum dealbans.' Other recipes include directions 'Ad faciendum lapides ardentes ut candela;' for 'Ignis grecus,' and 'Ignis tonitrus.' The work ends: ' . . . et semper movebis quousque sit factum rubeum. Expliciunt alique experimenta secundum Albertum Magnum.' Some of these recipes are also found at the end of the *De mirabilibus mundi* frequently attributed to Albertus Magnus: (Thorndike, II, 736–737).

VA Palat. 1144, fifteenth century, fols 74r–78v, Incipiunt experimenta Alberti Magni. 'Omnis scientia est de genere bonorum operativa . . . (fol. 76r) Sequitur de lapidibus et eorum virtutibus. Magnes ferrogineus inditus et teutonicus in provincia qui Francia . . . / . . . et hec sunt lecta fratris Alberti Coloniensis.' This is apparently excerpted from the *Liber Aggregationis* (DWS 1069; Thorndike II, 722 *et seq.*). But see also *De mineralibus*, Lib. II, Tract. II, cap. 9, Borgnet V, 40: 'Magnes sive magnetes lapis est ferruginei . . . Ego vidi invenire in partibus Teutoniae in ea provincia quae Francia orientalis vocatur . . . '

12. Fundamenta alchemiae: Listed by S. Ayscough[1] as in **BM Sloane 513*, fifteenth century (3), p. 154, is probably only an extract. See DWS 650, ii; and 177, vii.

13. Libellus (de alchymia). This bears a close resemblence to the *De occultis naturae*, and to the *Compositum de compositis*.

BU 139(105), fifteenth century, pp. 107–121, 'Incipit libellus ab Alberto compositus. Quoniam ignorantia mentis multi fuerant execati, igitur ego Albertus ad summam alkemiam volens provenire ad utilitatem omni hoc opusculum duxi componendum in quo opusculo secreta artis omnia elucidabo (p. 108). In primis igitur sciendum est quod materia metallorum omnium est ex argenti vivi substantia coagulata ex vapore sulphuris ut in libro de mineralibus decerniavimus(?) Ego igitur hoc ad oculum volens probare . . . / . . . dum regnat iupiter. Explicit libellus Alberti. Sit laus et gratia Christo. Amen.'

Notabilia Alberti Magni. See Semita recta (DWS 177, viii)

14. Mirror of Lights (Speculum luminum).

DWS 183: 'Part I. Inc. "In seeking out the sothenes of this craft that men call alchemy . . . " '; with the following fifteenth century manuscripts listed:
**CU Trinity Coll. 916*, pp. 121–142; *CUL Kk VI, 30; fols 1–35v;
**BM Sloane 513*, fols 155–168, which at the close has, 'Explicit Semita recta alkymye Alberti.'

15. De occultis naturae.[2]

DWS 182: **BM Arundel 164*, 1422 A.D., fols 127v–131. Inc. 'In mutue allocutionis tractatu rogasti me ut veritatem . . . / . . . vel operatur sicut qui cum arcu sine corda sagittat etc. Deo gratias.'

[1] S. Ayscough, *A Catalogue of the Manuscripts Preserved in the British Museum Hitherto Undescribed* (London, 1782), p. 477, under Albertus Magnus.

[2] Thorndike II, p. 570, citing the Arundel Ms.

VA Palat. 1330, 1463 A.D., fols 92^r (old numbering 85^r)-101^v, following the *Semita recta.* 'Hic incipit alius liber fratris Alberti de Colonia ordinis predicatorum. In mutuo allocutionis tractatu. Rogasti me ut veritatem in magisterio scientie alchimie sub compendio designarem. Cumque deo glorioso . . . / . . . Cum enim corpus penetrat venenum ipsum corpus in variabili colore coloratur et numquam dimittit corpus animam que sibi sic introducitur etc. Finis libri Alberti Magni philosophi 16 Novembris per Henricum Valpod familiarem seren. domini Carlis (Cardinalis?) Sancti Petri qui fuit de Alamania natione de Valla Cusa apud Trenti. Hic est finis libri Alberti.'

Palermo 4 Qq.A.10, fourteenth century, item 46, no. 27, 'Item liber fratris Alberti qui incipit in mutuo allocutionis . . . '

Apparently not the same is *FN Palat. 887,* fifteenth century, fols 83^r–85^r, Anon. De occultis naturae libellus perutilis incipit. Argenti vivi materia est humiditas . . . ' (Cf. DWS 176, XV). Rather it suggests the following.

16. Liber octo capitulorum.[1]

Printed in Zetzner, IV(1659), 841–862; Alberti Magni Liber octo capitulorum de lapide philosophorum. Librum autem istum dividam in octo capitula. Cap I, Inc.: 'Argentum vivum est frigidum et humidum et Deus creavit cum eo omnes mineras . . . ' The eighth chapter ends: ' . . . alteret in complemento lunifico vel solifico certo pretiosissimum super omne mundi pretium. Deo gratias qui creavit illud, qui est benedictus in secula seculorum. Amen. Explicit liber octo capitulorum Alberti Magni.'

The work is ascribed to Avicenna in *Artis auriferae,* I, 405–437; and in Manget I, 626.

17. Liber perfecti magisterii. This is the work usually attributed to Rasis. It appears under Albert's name in *BN 7161,* fifteenth century, fols 48^r–53^v, 'Incipit liber Alberti Perfecti magisterii. Quoniam studii solertis . . . '

18. Practica alkimiae

VA Palat. 1339, fourteenth to fifteenth century, fols 146^r–154^v, 'Iucipit practica alkimie magistri Alberti. Incipit liber practice in arte alkimie. Item accipe salis communis quantum vis et cum qua re notata in sequente libro . . . (fol. 146^v) Sublimatio salis armoniaci in rubea . . . (fol. 147^v) Sublimatio sulphuris . . . (fol. 148^r) De preparationibus corporum . . . (fol. 148^v) Calcinatio solis . . . (fol. 154^r) Elixir de auripigmento . . . Elixir de mercurio . . . ' The work appears to end on fol. 154^v, with the last recipe that for 'Aqua tartari acuta.'

19. Practica in alchimiam or Secretum secretorum.[2]

**BM Sloane 323,* fourteenth to fifteenth century, fols 2–61^v: 'Hic incipit practica fratris Alberti in alchimiam que ab eodem dicitur secretum secretorum.' Inc. 'Secretum quod apud sapientissimos valde . . . ' The work is followed on fol. 61^v by the

[1] Partington, *Ambix* I (1937), p. 17.

[2] DWS 179; Thorndike II, p. 570, citing the Sloane Ms, and fol. 84^v as the end of the *Practica.* The date and foliation here given have been verified for me by my sister, Dr Adele Kibre, who inclines toward the dating of the Ms as fifteenth century rather than fourteenth century. There are two systems of numbering in the manuscript, one at the top of the page the other at the bottom. The upper numbers are those followed here in accordance with the Catalogue of Sloane Mss. In this pagination the flyleaf is numbered as 1 and the first occupied leaf of the manuscript as 2. The lower pagination considers the first occupied leaf as 1.

This work is not the same as the *Secretorum tractatus* printed in the *Artis auriferae,* III (1610), pp. 121–130. Cf. Partington, *Ambix* I (1937), p. 17. See item 24 below.

rubric: 'Item hic incipit alius liber alkimie qui quantum ad eius practicam valet.' The opening words, 'Omnis sapientia a domino deo est . . . ' indicate the *Semita recta* which ends on fol. 84v.

A 'Practica fratris Alberti Commentatoris' contained in *VA 4425*, fols 277v–278r, is clearly medical and probably by a physician named Albert. It opens 'Incipit capitulum de curis passionum oculorum. Oculorum calidas passiones flebotomia egeret . . . '

19a. Processus alchymici. This is listed by S. Ayscough[1] under Albertus Minor as in German in *BM Sloane 830*, 1575.

20. Propositiones artis alchemiae

BN 14,006, fifteenth century, fols 52r–53r, 'Propositiones maxime in arte alchimie Alberti ordinis predicatorum. Omnis pura res et munda a lapidibus rebus extraneis abstracta de sua minera sine aliqua preparatione . . . / . . . Ex ista maxime habetur quod lapis philosophorum componitur ex oleo incombustibili et sale fusible. Deo gratias Amen.'

FR 923(L.III.28), fifteenth to sixteenth century, fols 127r (old numbering 124r)-131r: 'Propositiones seu maximae artis alchimiae excellentissimi Alberti Magni ordinis philosophorum intelligentium secretum et primo propositio prima. Propositio prima. Omne purum et mundum extractum a sua minera a lapidibus cum rebus extraneis . . . / . . . Ex hoc maxime elicitur quod lapis physicus componitur ex oleo incombustibili et sale fusibili. Deo gratias. Amen. Expliciunt propositiones pulcherrime et perutiles Alberti Magni super arte alkimica. Laus deo.'

VA Barberini 273, fol. 210r in the bibliography of alchemical writings: 'Propositiones seu maxime artis alchemie. Propositio prima, omne purum et mundum . . . / . . . ex oleo incombustibili et sale fusibili!'

Probably a French translation is the following: **Chantilly 419(919)*, 4to, paper, sixteenth century, fols 19v–20v, 'La propositione over, masime de l'arte de l'alchimia di Alberto Magno de l'ordine de phy. che intendono il secreto.'

21. Recipes

DWS 28, iv: Receptum Alberti, in **CU Trinity 1363*, fifteenth century, fols 192v–196v, 'Hec est ars tota sed stultis valde remota. Hunc de scorpione . . . ' This corresponds to the chapter, De scorpione, found in several versions of the *Semita recta*.[2] English version anon. in *Oxford, Corpus Christi Coll. 226, fifteenth century, fols 94r–94v (DWS 28, ix).

DWS 495, De vase philocophico, paragraph 2, 'Lutum sapiencie sic fit secundum Albertum'; Mss **BM Sloane 976*, fifteenth century, fols 82v–83v; **BL Ashmole* 1450, fifteenth century, I, fol. 2r–v.

DWS 1094 A [Panacea]: 'Oleum preciosissimum contra omnia contraria huic nature secundum fratrem Albertum theotonicum.' Ms. **BM Sloane* 416, fifteenth century, fols 160r–160v.

VA 4092, fifteenth century, fol. 124v, col. 2: Oleum mercurii secundum magistrum Albertum

BN 7161, fifteenth century, fol. 109: 'Albertus ad solem' (Corbett, 105)

BN 14,005, fourteenth to fifteenth century, fols 123v–124: 'Opus magistri Alberti Ratisponensis episcopi quod reliquerat cuidam aurifabro dicto vulgariter Hammis von Haws . . . ' This is among the recipes for gold collected by Leonard de Maurperg in 1394[3] (Corbett, 174).

[1] S. Ayscough, *Catalogue of Manuscripts Preserved in the British Museum Hitherto Undescribed* (London, 1782), p. 477.

[2] Cf. DWS 177, paragraph 3; and item 25 below.

[3] J. Corbett, 'L'alchimiste Léonard de Maurperg (XIVe S.), sa collection de recettes et ses voyages,' *Bibliothèque de l'Ecole des Chartes* (1936), 131–141.

22. Regimen operis in lapide.

**FR L.III.XIII*: Albertus, Regimen operis ('In ora libri adnotatum est manu recentiori: "Adverte, Lector, quod iste Albertus non est Albertus Magnus," 'Lami, p. 13)

FN Palat. 887, fifteenth to sixteenth century, item XXII, fols 115r–128r: 'Incipit tractatus qui dicitur regimen operis secundum Albertum et adverte quod non est Albertus Magnus. Nota quod est lapis humidus phisicus qui effunditur de duobus montibus s. calido et sicco et calido et humido.[1] Accipe eum et pone in vase vitreo bene clauso et colloca sub fimo equorum per tres . . . / . . . tunc assa ipsum ut supra dictum est in piscidem (pixidem?) luteam donec fiat citrinus. Et sic est finis.' This text, except for some verbal differences, is the same as the following:

VE VI.214(XVI,3), 1472 A.D., fols 39r–52v: 'Incipit tractatus qui dicitur regnum secundum Albertum de separatione et preparatione elementorum. Nota quod lapis humidus philosophicus qui effunditur de duobus montibus est calidus et siccus et calidus et humidus . . . / . . . tunc assa ipsum ut supradictum est in piscidem luteam donec fiet citrinus et sic est finis. Explicit tractatus qui appellatur regnum secundum Albertum de separatione et preparatione elementorum deo gratias. Amen.'

23. Secreta philosophorum

FR 1243(S.III.18), fifteenth century, fols 17r–48v (old numbering, 1r–40v): Albertus Magnus, Secreta philosophorum (according to the table of contents at the beginning of the volume). 'Ihesus Christus. Liber fuerit Alberti ordinis predicatorum extractus de secretis philosophorum in quo obmisit omnes doctrinas et causas et solum probata posuit et fallacias reliquerat. Tria nobis scribens: Primo quasdam preparationes necessarias; Secundo sublimationes; Tertio elixiria ad album et rubeum. Hic obmisi prohemium propter brevitatem. Preparatio croci ferri . . . ' This is apparently an abbreviated version of the *Alkimia minor*,[2] since many of the same recipes are included although in a different order from the *Alkimia minor*.

FL Ashburnham 1448, fifteenth century, fols 87v–88v: 'Incipiunt secreta fratris Alberti de Colonia super materia quarundam herbarum lapidum et animalium . . . ' This is a part of the *Liber aggregationis*.[3]

VA Palat. 1248, fifteenth century, fols 114v–123r: 'Secreta de lapidibus. De lapide magnetis de obtalmio . . . ' This is also a part of the *Liber aggregationis*. The part on herbs with the usual incipit, 'Sicut dicit philosophus in pluribus . . . ' occurs at fol. 112r.

24. Secretorum tractatus[4]

**VE VI.215(XVI, 4)*, 1475 A.D., fols 19–26; Inc. 'Et ut intelligere possis artem maiorem veram . . . '

Printed in *Artis auriferae*, III (1610), 121–130. Inc. 'Et ut intelligere possis artem maiorem veram scilicet intentionem nostram, volumus ostendere in qua hora et in quo die debet esse inceptio huius nostri operis . . . / . . . erit sicut lac incerans, liquescens, penetrans ad modum aquae fixae super ignem pugnando, et tunc opus erit completum, et lauda Deum. Explicit Alberti Magni secretorum tractatio.'

25. Semita recta[5]

Printed in Borgnet XXXVII, 545–573, 'D. Alberti Magni, Libellus de Alchimia. Praef.: Omnis sapientia a Domino Deo est . . . (Chap. I) De diversis erroribus. Nunc autem

[1] Cf. DWS 28, Liber rebis.

[2] See item 2 above. Thus roughly the first 7 sections correspond to the last 7 chapters of the *Alkimia minor*, etc.

[3] See Thorndike II, 722 *et seq.*; DWS 1069.

[4] Cf. item 19 above.

[5] Thorndike II, pp. 570–573; Partington, *Ambix*, I (1937), pp. 18–19; DWS 177–178. Dr W. J. Wilson reports on a text of the 'Semita recta in alchimia' in 'An Alchemical Manuscript by Arnaldus

qualiter ad tanti operis . . . ' Then follow 57 chapters or short sections, the last, 'Qualiter ex supradictis omnibus perficitur Sol et Luna? Recipe unam partem mercurii . . . / . . . ne tingas cum illo aliquod metallum non purgatum, quia tinctura evanesceret post duas vel tres examinationes.' Next come 'Additiones. In libro Aristotelis de Perfecto magisterio . . . / . . . aquam solam, fiet Luna: si conjunxeris ignem, rubefaciet, Domino concedente.' The earlier editions with Albert's *Opera*, 1651, vol. XXI, pp. 1–17, and in Zetzner, II (1659), 423–456 are identical with that in Borgnet.

There are, however, variations in the manuscript texts as the following manuscript items will indicate:

BN 7162, fifteenth century, fols 62ʳ–76ʳ, 'Incipit prologus sequentis operis per magistrum Albertum philosophum. Omnis sapientia a domino deo est et cum illo fuit . . . ' (Corbett 110). This text follows closely that found in *FR 921*, fols 119ʳ–(134ʳ), and *VE fondo antico 323*, fols 241ʳ–272ᵛ. It closes: ' . . . fit tinctura qui vocatur elixir quod transmutat omnia metalla et non perogata (?) in solem et lunam quod melior est omni naturali. Sed ego volo ponere doctrinam nisi de uno tamen s. de scorpione. Explicit.'

BU 138(104), 1476 A.D., fols 171–182ᵛ: 'Incipit Semita recta fratris Alberti Magni de ordine fratrum predicatorum. Omnis sapientia a domino deo est et cum illo fuit semper. Quicumque igitur diligit sapientiam . . . ' The last chapter, 'De tinctura optima ad lunam faciendam,' ends: ' . . . aliquid metallum non purgatum quia evanescitur post secundam examinationem et tinctura fugetur. Explicit semita recta Alberti.'

BU 139(105), fifteenth century, fols 3–55, 'Incipit liber qui dicitur Semita recta. Omnis sapientia a domino deo est et cum illo fuit semper . . . ' This text is similar though somewhat fuller than that in *BU 138*, fols 171–182ᵛ. After the closing section given above (which here occurs at fol. 49ʳ, ' . . . et post 2 vel 3 examinationes et tincture fugeret'), the text continues for several folios and closes with the chapter, 'De praeparatione lapidis philosophorum qui dicitur rebis (Cf. DWS 177) Nunc ergo ex lapide ubique reperto qui vocatur rebis . . . / . . . et hoc est yxir(elixir?) quod transmutat omnia metalla in solem et lunam in una hora. Explicit Semita recta.' Then follow 'Notabilia. De distillatione aquae mercurii. Sume limature plumbi . . . / . . . Rubificatio mercurii. Explicit Semita recta et notabilia supradicta.'

CLM 12026, fifteenth century, fols 32ʳ–45ᵛ; 'Incipit prologus artis alchimie magistri Alberti de Colonia qui est flos florum et verus illuminator totius artis alchimie. Vidi quamplures libros de ista arte qui propter nimiam vanitatem et maxime incredulitatem acceptare non valebant. Vidi alios qui cum omnia diligentia faciebant . . . ' This corresponds roughly to the second paragraph of the first chapter in Borgnet, XXXVII, 546 (De diversibus erroribus). The chapter headings correspond to similar sections in the Borgnet text although they vary greatly in arrangement and there are fewer headings in the manuscript. The last chapter, 'Quomodo fiat tinctura,' ends ' . . . uncie faciunt libram. Explicit alchimia magistri Alberti de Colonia vir expertissimi in hac arte. Sequitur tractatus alius de alchimia valde notabilis.'

**Copenhagen Gl kgl. S. 236*, fol. chart., fifteenth century, fols 154–162, 'Liber magistri Alberti qui dicitur Semita directa. Omnis sapientia a Domino deo est . . . / . . . re[illegible] cum vasis collocentur.'

**FN Magliabech. cl. XVI.2(II.IV.230)*, item 3, 'Alberto Magno dell'ordine Pred. Libe[illegible] semita recta.'

**FN Magliabech. cl. XVI. cod. 15*, item 1

---

de Bruxella,' *Osiris*, II (1936), pp. 221, 364. This text Dr Wilson states, 'stands in a recension very different from all the printed editions and probably much superior.'

**FN Magliabech. cl.* XVI. *cod. 24*

**FN Magliabech. cl.* XVI. *cod. 37,* item 3, fourteenth century, Magister Albert, Semita recta.

**BL Ashmole 1448,* fifteenth century, pp. 47–73; (DWS 177, ix)

**BL Canon. Lat. Script. Eccles. 53,* fifteenth century, fols 49–75v (DWS 177, xii).

**BL Canon. Misc. 81,* fifteenth century, fols. 25–85v (DWS 178: Semita recta different from 177) 'Semita recta fratris Alberti ordinis predicatorum de arte alchimie feliciter incipit. In nomine Domine dei Patris omnipotentis incipiam scribere secreta secretorum . . . ' Opus Inc.: 'Alchimia est ars artium scientia scientiarum domina . . . '

**BM Sloane 323,* fourteenth century, fols 61v–84v (DWS 177, ii)

**CU Trinity Coll. 1363,* fifteenth century, fols 57–83 (DWS 177, iv)

**CUL Ff.* VI. *50,* fifteenth century, fols 111–140 (DWS 177, v)

FN Palat. 981, fifteenth century, fols 203r–264r, Albertus, Liber semita recta. Inc.: 'Totam nostram scientiam quem ex libris . . . ' This is the work or *Summa* usually ascribed to Geber as the opening words indicate.

*FR L.*III.XIII (Lami, p. 13): Semita recta.

*FR L.*III.XIII bis (Lami, p. 122): Liber Alberti Magni qui dicitur Semita recta.

*FR L.*III.XXXIII (Lami, p. 13): Liber Alberti Magni.

*FR 390(N.*III.XI*),* fifteenth century, fols 76r–108r, Semita recta Alberti Magni fratris Coloniensis. Omnis sapientia a domino deo est et cum illo fuerit semper . . . / . . . habebis effectus ad quos nos producat quoniam est benedictus in secula seculorum. Amen. Explicit alkimie Semita recta Alberti Magni fratris Coloniensis.' On fol. 85r–v are figures of the 'furnus philosophicus,' and 'furnus sublimatoris.'

*FR 921(L.*III.*16),* fifteenth century, fols 119r–(134r), 'Incipit alchimia fratris Alberti de ordine fratrum predicatorum. Omnis sapientia a domino deo est et cum illo fuit semper . . . / . . . (last chapter, 'Summa de lapide nostro ubique reperto qui vocatur rebis et nascitur in duobus montibus) omnia corpora in hora in solem et lunam. Explicit semita directa fratris Alberti Theutonici.'

*FR 923(L.*III.*28),* sixteenth century, fols 299r–311r, 'Epistola fratris Alberti super alchimia quae vocatur Semita recta. Omnis sapientia a domino deo est . . . / . . . et colorem et naturam auri in eternum non emittat. Finis.'

*FR 1165(L.*III.*34),* fourteenth century, fols 124r–132r, 'Incipit quidam tractatus de operatione seu preparatione rerum que operantur in arte ipsius alchimie feliciter. Ars alchimie inventa est ab alchimio philosopho qui chimia grece latine massa dicitur . . . ' (Cf. Borgnet, XXXVII, 547, cap. 2). The work ends as in Borgnet p. 572.

**Glasgow Univ. Hunterian 110,* fourteenth century, fols 27–35v (old nos. 25–33v): DWS 177, i.

*Oxford, *Corpus Christi Coll. 185,* fifteenth century, fols 48–70, without title; fols 70v–71v, Anon. and without title; fols 80–117 (DWS 177, XIII–XV).

*Oxford, *Corpus Christi Coll. 226,* fifteenth century, fols 59–69 (DWS 177, xvi)

**Palermo 4 Qq.A.10,* fourteenth century, item[1] 35, 'Incipit summa artis alkimie edita a domino Alberto episcopo que dicitur semita recta' (in the index, Alberti de Alamania). Rubrics: 'Explicit prologus, nunc videndum est quid sit alkimia . . . De fundamento huius scientie quod positum est videamus qualiter edificemus . . . De octo preceptis que in arte sunt servanda . . . ' According to the headings there is a general correspondence with the Borgnet text although there is considerable variation in arrangement. In addition like the list of rubrics at the opening of the text

[1] Transcribed from the film copy of Carini's description in the reprint by Di Marzo, which was loaned to me by the kindness of Dr W. J. Wilson. See also Julius Ruska, 'Uebersetzung und Bearbeitungen von al-Razis Buch Gehemnis der Geheimnisse,' *Quellen und Studien zur Geschichte der Naturwissenschaften und der Medizin* (1935), IV, n. 3, 5, 8.

in VE fondo antico 323, fol. 241r, there are two further headings at the end: De tribus lapidibus pretiosis principalibus, and De lapide scorpionis (Cf. DWS 177). These last two headings are not included in Borgnet. Item 36 of this same Palermo manuscript description continues: 'Expositio illius capituli quod incipit summe de lapide ubicumque reperto . . . ' (with notations) 'et vocatur ab Alberto in libro Semite lapis scorpionis.'

**Palermo 4 Qq.A.10*, fourteenth century, item 46, no. 29: 'Item semita recta fratris Alberti.'

**Prag 1765*(IX.E.9), fourteenth to fifteenth century, fols 58v–63v, Semita recta. Inc. 'Omnis sapientia a domino deo est . . . / . . . et tinctura evanesceret.' (Borgnet, XXXVII, p. 572, col. 2).

VA 4092, fifteenth century, fols 1r–8r, 'Semita recta Alberti. Omnis sapientia a domino deo est et cum ipso . . . / . . . (incomplete, ends at the close of the eight precepts) et in expensis deficerit tunc res et opus amittit et cum labore in damno. Iam satis dictum est de preceptis serva et custodi' (Borgnet, XXXVII, p. 550).

VA Palat. 1330, fifteenth century, fols 56r–60v, 73r–91v: 'Hic incipit liber fratris Alberti Almania de Colonia ordinis predicatorum super alkimia qui vocatur semita iustice. Prohemium in nomine patris dei omnipotentis. Incipiam scribere secreta secretorum (Cf. DWS 178) . . . ' The text continues as in VE fondo antico 323, fol. 242v. With paragraph 2 begins. 'Omnis sapientia a domino deo est et cum illo fuit . . . ' (corresponding to *VA 4092*, fol. 1r, although this text is somewhat fuller than the other). On fol. 60v, there intervenes the text of the *Alkimia minor* which occupies fols. 60v–72v, after which the text of the *Semita recta* resumes, the eight precepts occurring on fol. 74v. The last chapter, 'Sunt tres lapides principales in arte ista scilicet aliene rei . . . ' ends, 'et nota quod rebis debet esse acrius volatilis et non adustus ut dicit autor. Nota dicta magistri et domini Alberti Archiepiscopi Coloniensis semita directa nuncupata. Cui similis in hac scientia temporibus suis non caret (?). Et explicit iste liber hic et alius de eadem scientia incipit. Finis huius libelli.' It is followed by the tract beginning 'In mutuo . . . '

VE fondo antico 323, fifteenth century, fols 241r–272v, 'Incipit liber fratris Alberti de Colonia de ordine predicatorum super alchimia. Tabula totius libri secundum rubricas capitulorum ut videatur que et quot sunt . . . / . . . Expliciunt rubrice magistri Alberti de Colonia.' The rubrics number from 1 to 73, the last two: 'Item de tribus lapidibus (cap. 72);' and 'De lapide scorpionis idemque locorum reperte (cap. 73),' do not appear in the text, which closes with the chapter headed, 'Item de tinctura alia (cap. 71)' which corresponds roughly to chapter 57 of Borgnet's text.

The work opens (fol. 242v) 'Prohemium libri huius. In nomine dei patris omnipotentis incipiam scribere secreta secretorum multis incognita (Cf. DWS 178). Varia et completa capitula et meliores operationes de secreta arte alchimie . . . Prologus libri huius cap. secundum. Incipit prologus. Iste liber vocatur semita recta. Cum (fol. 243r) ergo ego frater Albertus de ordine predicatorum dilexeram scientiam . . / . . . sed tincturam procedens. Explicit semita recta edita a magistro Alberto de Colonia in alchimia preintegrato et approbato scriptus in Swodiutz (?) anno 1482 (LXXXII?).'

**Vienna 5489*, fifteenth century, fols 1r–48v; *5477*, fifteenth century, fols 1r–16v, Albertus Magnus, 'Semita recta alchimiae.'

**Wo 676* (627 Helmst.), 1444 A.D., fols 25–34, 'Declaratio magistri magistrorum super semitam rectam Alberti Magni.'

**Wo 3721*, 1468 A.D., fols 221–252v, Semita Alberti. Inc. 'Omnis sapientia a domino deo est . . . '

Excerpts of the Semita recta are found in the following:

**BL Ashmole 1451*, fifteenth century, II, fols 47v–48, 60 (DWS 177, x–xi)

**BM Harley 3542*, fols 17–25v (DWS 177, vi)

**BM Sloane 513,* fols 168v–178 (DWS 177, vii)
**BM Sloane 2135,* fols 20–21; 2170, fols 18–30; 3180, sixteenth century, Excerpta.
**BM Sloane 3744,* fols 117v–124 (DWS 177, viii): Notabilia Alberti Magni?
**BN fonds franç. 14797,* sixteenth century, pp. 157–177: Corbett, 251: 'Sequitur Practica magistri Alberti philosophi in suo libello continenti nuncupato semita recta.' Inc. 'Recipe in nomine domini unam partem aque mercurii albi . . . '
BN 7161, fifteenth century, fols 68r–(69r?): Nota de lapide philosophorum et preparatione eius. Albertus in Semita recta. Inc. 'Lapis philosophorum quem omnes querunt . . . ' This is probably Winandus de Rupheo Clipeo, Gloria mundi: Corbett, 100, Thorndike, III, 68, n. 57.

In the inventory of the library of Francesco Gonzaga (1407)[1] the following is probably also a part of the *Semita recta*: 'Albertus, Liber alchimiae,' Inc. 'Si hec ars est quomodo est . . . '[2]

English translations: **BM Sloane 316,* sixteenth century, item 3 (Ayscough, p. 477); fols 8–54;
**BM Sloane 317,* seventeenth century, fols 88–91v, 99
**BM Sloane 513,* fifteenth century, fols 155–168 (See item 14 above)
**BM Sloane 2128,* fifteenth century, fols 1–13v, Extracts in Latin and English. Inc. 'Many a regyon and contre . . . ' DWS 177, xviii.
**CUL Ee.I.13,* fifteenth century, fols 141–148v (DWS 177, xvii)
**CU Trinity Coll. 915(II),* fifteenth century, fols 15v–17 (DWS 177, xx)
**Oxford, BL Ashmole* 1490, sixteenth century (?), (pp. 26–33), fol. 93, 98–100v.
*Oxford, *Corpus Christi Coll. 185,* fifteenth century, fols 158v–160 (DWS 177, xix).
German translations: **BM Sloane 830,* 1575 A.D., fols 1–43v
Greek translation under the name Petrus Theotonicos:[3]
* *BN Greek 2419,* in fol., transcribed about 1460 by Georges Midiates, fols 279–287v
Italian translations: **FN Palat. 955,* fifteenth century, fols 31v–44r, 'Comincia "Semita retta" della archimia d'Alberto Magno.' Inc. 'Ogni sapientia da dio procede et con esso sempre fu . . . / . . . allora rectira l'aqua distilata sopra le sua fècie, et distilla; et cosi fa' tre volte. Finito el libro della archimia d'Alberto Magno, chiamato Semita recta.'
**VE Nani Cod. volg. 27,* fourteenth century: 'Il libro di frate Alberto arcivescovo di Cologna della magna sopra all'alchimia lo quale si chiama, La semita.' Inc. 'Nota che ogni scientia e sapientia viene dallo omnipotente Iddio . . . '
De separatione et praeparatione elementorum, see Regimen operis

6. Speculum secretorum[4]

This is the work usually ascribed to Roger Bacon.[5] It appears under Albert's name in the following manuscripts:
BU 138(104), fifteenth century, fols 233r–235r, 'Incipit speculum secretorum philosophorum Alberti Magni de secretis nature et sunt novem capitula. In nomine domini nostri Jhesu Christi. Ad instructionem multorum circha hanc artem studere volentium quibus deficit copia librorum hic libellus addatur qui titulus est et speculum secretorum videtur et illud ideo quia quasi ut in speculo . . . / . . . sub tali compendio propter penuriam librorum. Laudas igitur deum et ei gratias age qui vivit et regnat benedictus et gloriosus et pius per infinita secula seculorum. Amen.'

[1] Pia Girolla, 'La biblioteca di Francesco Gonzaga secondo l'inventario del 1407,' *Atti e Memorie, eale Accademia Virgiliana di Mantova,* Nuova Ser. XIV–XVI (1923), p. 67.
[2] Cf. Borgnet, XXXVII, 546; Praefatio, paragraph 4: 'Si haec res est quomodo est? et si non est . . . '
[3] Berthelot in 1889 stated that he had determined the general conformity of the Greek text with e Latin *Semita recta* by comparing them line for line: M. Berthelot, *L'Introduction à l'étude de la imie* (1889), p. 205 et seq.
[4] Thorndike II, p. 569. [5] DWS 197; A. G. Little, *Roger Bacon Essays* (1914), p. 413.

BU 270(457), fifteenth to sixteenth century, x, 2, pp. 99–107; 'Incipit Speculum secretorum philosophorum Alberti Magni de secretis naturae.' This is identical with the text in the preceding manuscript.

27. Transmutatio metallorum secundum Albertum Magnum et Geber

**KLaB XXIX.d.24*, 1421–1423 A.D., fols 22ʳ–95ʳ: Inc. 'Antiquorum toto nisi a me visa et perlecta de transmutatione metallorum . . . / . . . resultat bonitatis alternantis multiplicatio ut ex me(dici)nis quaedam suum duplum, quaedam triplum, quaedam centuplum. Explicit in Vallerendena.'[1]

28. Trifolium

**Lyons 317(253)*, sixteenth century, fols 2–9ᵛ: 'Nota de secretis alchimie artis. Scire te facio quod duo modi sunt corporum combustionis . . . / . . . Explicit Trifolium Alberti Magni. Finis. Amen.'

29. De vinis (It is not certain that the following are of chemical or alchemical significance).

**Bern 556*, fifteenth century, fols 110ᵛ–121ᵛ, 'Tractatus Alberti Magni de vino. De vino et eius proprietatibus tractare . . . '

*Esslingen, Kloster der Augustinereremiten, Inventory of 1488:[2] 'Item tractatus de proprietatibus vini et notabilibus multis bonis magistri et domini Alberti Magni episcopi Ratisponensis.'

*Karthause Salvatorberg, fifteenth century Catalogue: 'Albertus Magnus de preparacione vini, conservacione et reformacione et similiter fructuum, et multa alia bona ibi continentur. Quomodo conficiantur diversa vina ex diversis rebus pro diversis remediis eiusdem Alberti.[3]

**O.S. Aug.*: Item tractatus de proprietatibus vini et notabilibus multis bonis magistri et domini Alberti M. episcopi Ratisponensis.[4]

**Prag 2056(XI.E.9)*, fourteenth to fifteenth century, fols 135ʳ–142ᵛ, 'De reformatione vinorum et eorum conservatione.' Inc. 'De vino et eius proprietatibus . . . / . . . et sic successive in cibum sumantur.'

*Wiblingen, Benediktinerkloster, Book lists for the year 1432: 'Expliciunt notabilia de proprietatibus vini Alberti Magni, per Joannem Troycker de Ladenburg.'[5]

30. Unidentified and miscellaneous works:

*Amplonius Ratinck, Catalogue at Erfurt, 1410–1412: 'Alchimia,[6] "Liber Alberti Magni de hac re usque in finem voluminis de variis huius artis ingeniis et intencionibus, et est volumen valde bonum." '

**BL Ashmole 1490*, sixteenth century: 'Quedam ex Alberto Magno'

*Cassel, Landesbibliothek Chem. Folio *XIII.33*: Albertus Ratispon. Episc. In expositionem totius artis alchemice metrica compendiosa.

**FR L.III.XIII.bis* (Lami, p. 122): Alchimia Alberti Magni

*Karthause Salvatorberg, fifteenth century catalogue: 'Albertus Magnus, De alchemia.'[7]

[1] Cf. *De mineralibus*, Lib. III, cap. 9: Borgnet v, p. 70.

[2] P. Lehmann, *Mittelalterliche Bibliothekskataloge Deutschlands und der Schweiz*, (Munich, 1918), 37. [3] *Ibid.*, 1928, II, 438.

[4] D. Planzer, O.P., 'Albertus-Magnus Handschriften in mittelalterlichen Bibliothekskatalogen des deutschen Sprachgebietes,' *Albertus-Magnus Festschrift* (Freiburg, 1932), pp. 246–276.

[5] P. Lehmann, *Mittelalterliche Bibliothekskataloge Deutschlands und der Schweiz* (Munich, 1918), 435. [6] *Ibid.*, 1928, II, 41.

[7] *Ibid.*, II, 557; Schum, *Beschreibendes Verzeichniss der Amplonianischen Handschriften-Sammlung zu Erfurt* (Berlin, 1887), p. 817: 'Sequitur de alchimia que subalternatur philosophie naturali.'

**Prag 1984(X.H.6)*, fourteenth century, fol. 24r–v: 'Ista est operatio Mag. Alberti.'
**Turin 1488(K².IV.6)*, fifteenth century, fol. 198: 'Albertus Magnus, Alchemia.'
**Vienna 5509*, fifteenth century, fols 249r–251v: 'Notabilia alchymica ex Alberti Magni, Avicennae, Democriti aliorumque operibus.'

INDEX OF MANUSCRIPTS

(References are to numbered items)

Bern 556, fols 110v–121v 29

Bologna, University Library
- 138(104), fols 171–182v 25
- 138(104), fols 233r–235r 26
- 138(104), fols 235v–237r 3
- 139(105), pp. 3–55 25
- 139(105), pp. 107–121 13
- 270(457), fols 1r–21v 11
- 270(457), pp. 77–97 1
- 270(457), pp. 99–107 26
- 270(457), pp. 108–111 3

Cambrai 924(823), fols 168–175 4

Cambridge University Library
- Dd.IV.45 3
- Ee.I.13, fols 141–148v 25
- Ff.IV.12, 13, fols 227–249r 8
- Ff.VI.50, fols 111–140 25
- Kk.VI.30, fols 1–35v 14

Cambridge Colleges
- Corpus Christi 243, fols 1–58v 5
- Trinity 915 (II), fols 15v–17 25
- Trinity 916, pp. 121–142 14
- Trinity 1363, fols 192v–196v 21
- Trinity 1363, fols 57–83 25

Cassel Chem. Fol. XIII.33 30
Chantilly 419(919), fols 19v–20v 20
Copenhagen Gl kgl. S. 236, fols 154–162 25
Edinburgh, Advocates' Library 20.8.1, fols 6–40v 8

Erfurt, Amplonian
- Q.189, fols 67–68 5
- Catalogue of 1412, Phil. nat. 5 5
- Catalogue of 1412, Alchimia 30

Esslingen Kloster 29

Florence, Bibl. nazionale
- Magliab. cl. XVI. 2, item 3 25
- Magliab. cl. XVI. cod. 15, item 1 25
- Magliab. cl. XVI. cod. 24 25
- Magliab. cl. XVI. cod. 37 25
- Palat. 887, fols 17r–23r 4
- Palat. 887, fols 83r–85r 15
- Palat. 887, fols 89r–94v 3
- Palat. 887, fols 115r–128r 22
- Palat. 955, fols 31v–44r 25
- Palat. 981, fols 70r–71r 3
- Palat. 981, fols 203r–264r 25

Florence, Laurenziana, Ashburnham 1448, fols 87v–88v 23
- Laurenziana, Ashburnham 1448, fols 157r–158v 11

Florence, Riccardian
- L.III.XIII 22,25,30
- L.III.XXXIII 25
- 390 (N.III.XI), fols 76r–108r 25
- 921 (L.III.16), fols 119r–(134r) 25
- 923 (L. III.28), fols 127r–131r 20
- 923 (L.III.28), fols 299r–311r 25
- 1165 (L.III.34), fols 124r–132r 25
- 1165 (L.III.34), fols 47r–49v 4
- 1243 (S.III.18), fols 17r–48v 23

Geneva 82, fols 146r–157v 3

Glasgow Univ. Hunterian 110, fols 27–35v 25
- Hunterian 468 5

Karthause Salvatorberg 29, 30

Klagenfurt Bischöfl. Bibliothek
- XXIX.d.24, fols 22r–95r 27

London, British Museum
- Arundel 164, fols 127v–131 15
- Harley 79, fol. 46 11
- Harley 3528, fols 9v–10v 6
- Harley 3542, fols 17–25v 25
- Sloane 276, fol. 3 8
- Sloane 316, fols 8–54 25
- Sloane 317, fols 88–91v, 99 25
- Sloane 323, fols 2–61v 19
- Sloane 323, fols 61v–84v 25
- Sloane 416, fo.s 160r–160v 21
- Sloane 513, (3), p. 154 12
- Sloane 513, fols 155–168 14
- Sloane 513, fols 168v–178 25
- Sloane 830 .... 19a

Sloane 830, fols 1–43^{v} 25
Sloane 976, fol. 32^{v} 7
Sloane 976, fols 82^{v}–83 21
Sloane 2135, fols 20–21 25
Sloane 2170, fols 18–30 25
Sloane 2128, fols 1–13^{v} 25
Sloane 3120, fols 174–192^{v} 1
Sloane 3180, fol. 12 . . . . . 8, 25
Sloane 3457, fols 40–50^{v} 1
Sloane 3457, fols 109–113^{v} 10
Sloane 3630, fols 70–74 8
Sloane 3744, fols 117^{v}–124 25

Lyons 317 (253), fols 2–9^{v} 28
Munich CLM 12026, fols 32^{r}–45^{v} 25
Naples V.H.134, fols 8^{r}–14^{v} 8

Oxford, Bodleian
Ashmole 1448, pp. 47–73 25
Ashmole 1448, fols 259–262 4
Ashmole 1450, fols 2^{r}–2^{v} 21
Ashmole 1451, fols 47^{v}–48, 60 25
Ashmole 1490 30
Canon. Misc. 81, fols 25–85^{v} 25
Canon. Lat. Script. Eccles. 53, fols. 49–75^{v} 25
Fairfax 22, fols 31–38^{v} 6

Oxford, Corpus Christi College
185, fols 48–70; 70^{v}–71^{v}; 80–117 25
185, fols 158^{v}–160 25
226, fol. 94^{r-v} 21
226, fols 59–69 25

Palermo 4 Qq.A.10
no. 27 15
no. 29 25
no. 30 2
no. 35 25
no. 36 3

Paris, Bibliothèque nationale
Latin 6514, fols 40^{v}–41^{v} 3
Latin, 6749B, fols 48^{r}–52^{r} 2
Latin 7147, fols 1–12^{v} 8
Latin 7156, fols 145^{v}–146^{r} 3
Latin 7156, fols 175–192 5
Latin 7158, fol. 112^{r-v} 3
Latin 7161, fols 48^{r}–53^{v} 17
Latin 7161, fols 68^{r}–(69^{r}?) 25
Latin 7161, fol. 109 21
Latin 7162, fols 62^{r}–76^{r} 25
Latin 7162, fols 80^{v}–85^{r} 2
Latin 7337, fol. 121 5
Latin 14005, fols 123^{v}–124 21
Latin 14006, fols 52^{r}–53^{r} 20
Latin Nouv. acquis 1293, fols 59–61^{v} 2
Latin Nouv. acquis, 1293, fols 118^{r}–122^{v} . . 11
Fonds franç. 2012, (Colbert 4447), fols 49^{r}–70^{r} 9
Fonds franç, nouv. acquis, 4114, pp. 1–9. 7
Fonds franç. nouv. acquis. 4114, pp. 13–63 8
Fonds franç. 14797, pp. 157–177 25
Greek 2419, fols 279–287^{v} 25

Prag 1765 (IX.E.9), fols 58^{v}–63^{v} 25
1984 (X.H.6.), fols 24^{r-v}; 29^{v}–30^{v} 3, 30
2056 (XI.E.9), fols 135^{r}–142^{v} 29

Turin 1488 (K^{2}.IV.6) 30

Vatican Latin
1043, fols 397^{r}–402^{r} 5
4091, fols 42^{r}–47^{v} 8
4092, fols 1^{r}–8^{r} 25
4092, fol. 124^{v} 21
4425, fols 277^{v}–278^{r} 19
5377, fols 137^{r}–138^{r} 3
Barberini 273, fol. 210^{r} 20
Palat. 1144, fols 74^{r}–78^{v} 11
Palat. 1248, fols 114^{v}–123^{r} 23
Palat. 1330, fols 56^{r}–60^{v}, 73^{r}–91^{v} 25
Palat. 1330, fols 60^{v}–72^{v} 2
Palat. 1330, fols 92^{r}–101^{v} 15
Palat. 1339, fols 146^{r}–154^{v} 18
Regin. 1106, fol. 1 5

Venice, San Marco
VI.214 (XVI, 3), fols 39^{r}–52^{v} 22
VI.214 (XVI, 3), fols 180^{r}–189^{v} 2
VI.215 (XVI, 4), fols 19–26 24
fondo antico 323, fols 241^{r}–272^{v} 25
Nani Cod. volg. 27 25

Vienna 5315, fols 128–133 3
5477, fols 1^{r}–16^{v} 25
5489, fols 1^{r}–48^{v} 25
5509, fols 249^{r}–251^{v} 30

Wiblingen Benediktkloster 29

Wolfenbüttel
672, fols 37–60 5
676 (627 Helmst.), fols 1–24^{v} 7
676 (627 Helmst.), fols 25–34 25
676 (627 Helmst.), fols 91–130 7
3721, fols 221–252^{v} 25

VIII

AN ALCHEMICAL TRACT ATTRIBUTED TO ALBERTUS MAGNUS

THE listing of an alchemical treatise under the name of ALBERTUS MAGNUS, the noted thirteenth-century Dominican scholar, may well be regarded as another manifestation of that common medieval practice of issuing such writings under the names of prominent ecclesiastics in order to lend them authority and credence. Whether or not this accounts for the present ascription, it is difficult to say. For while there is no contemporary evidence for ALBERTUS MAGNUS ever having composed such works, his lively interest in scientific subjects and especially in mineralogy and even in alchemy as reflected in the third book of the *De mineralibus* might easily lend support to his authorship of some such writings.[1] Externally in the present instance the authority for the ascription is extremely doubtful, despite the fact that ALBERT's name is attached to all three known manuscripts of the work, since the earliest is from the fifteenth century, some two hundred years removed from ALBERT. None the less it is interesting to note, as will be seen in the ensuing analysis of its contents, that the present treatise bears a close relationship to several of the arguments and statements regarding the Hermetic art in the *De mineralibus*. One is therefore led to wonder whether an impostor or alchemist in preparing his tract had before him a list of ALBERT's chief arguments against alchemy which he then set out to show could be avoided by the learned operator in the art; or whether by chance we have here a copy of some of ALBERT's own jottings on the subject from alchemical texts which he used in greatly modified form in the *De mineralibus*.[2]

Unfortunately the present text offers little assistance in the way of internal evidence. Its authorities are the same as several of those named by ALBERTUS, such as CALLISTHENES, Hermes, GEBER, and AVICENNA. There is no mention of any Latin writers. The alchemical doctrines expressed are those commonly current in the thirteenth and fourteenth centuries. The most outstanding of these is the sulphur-mercury theory of the composition of metals which was popularized especially in the works ascribed to GEBER.

Aside, however, from speculation regarding its authenticity or spurious character as a work of the distinguished thirteenth-century Dominican author, the present composition has an intrinsic interest as a reflection of scientific or pseudo-scientific practice and thought manifest at least sometime before 1500. The work is singularly free from the mystical and fantastic characteristics so frequently associated with such writings especially from the fourteenth to the sixteenth century. There are none of the usual admonitions to secrecy. Instead the author, following the same lead as that of ALBERTUS in the *De mineralibus*, describes here on the authority of GEBER, the tendency to obscurity of aims and objectives on the part of operators of the art, as the mark of deceivers, and as not characteristic of the aim of true philosophy. He attributes to GEBER, whom he describes as a Spaniard (Hispanus), the statement which in the *De mineralibus*, ALBERT utters as his own, that he has examined certain alchemical books and has found them to be without distinction, and with their intention hidden under the guise of allegory.[3] The references to the influence of the heavens in the alchemical processes which appear in the *De mineralibus*[4] are not repeated here, although the work follows the current practice of using the names of the seven planets as synonyms for the metals.[5] Emphasis in the

[1] In this regard see especially, J. R. PARTINGTON, "Albertus Magnus on Alchemy," *Ambix* I (1937), 9–13; LYNN THORNDIKE, *A History of Magic and Experimental Science* (New York, 1923), II, 569–73; GEORGE SARTON, *Introduction* (II, 937, 1931); and my recent study, "Alchemical Writings Ascribed to Albertus Magnus," *Speculum* XVII (1942), 499–518.

[2] That ALBERT did rework portions of his writings from time to time has already been suggested by FRITZ PANETH, "Ueber eine alchemistische Handschrift des 14. Jht. u. ihr Verhältnis zu Albertus Magnus Buch 'De Mineralibus,'" *Archiv für die Geschichte der Naturwissenschaft und der Technik*, XII (1929), 33–45; 408–413.

[3] BM Sloane 3457, fol. 40r; ALBERTUS MAGNUS, Lib. III Mineralium, Tract. I, cap. vii; in A. BORGNET'S edition of the *Opera omnia*, V, 1890, 68. There are some changes in ALBERT'S wording, however. Thus he has *plurimos libros* for *quosdam libros*; and *verba metaphorica* in place of *verba alegorica*.

[4] *Ibid.*, III, I, ix; I, vi, *loc. cit.*, V, 71, col. 1–2; 66, col. 2.

[5] Cf. *ibid.*, III, I, vi, *loc. cit.*, V, 66, col. 2: according to ALBERT, Hermes was the one who introduced this practice. See D. W. SINGER, *Catalogue of Latin and Vernacular Alchemical Manuscripts*, 1928, I, 42 ff., no. 37.

tract is laid upon such attributes of scientific procedure as careful observation, patience, and perseverance even in the face of continued failure. There is repeated insistence upon the principle that alchemy imitates nature and hence particular stress is laid upon the necessity for observing carefully and closely natural processes and nature itself. The operator in alchemy is cautioned against becoming discouraged if his first and second or even frequent trials fail, and he does not at once see the effect for which he had hoped. He should continue to repeat the operations noting carefully the progress of the work until he sees the reason for his error. Then he may try another means.[6] Such alchemical processes are utilized and described as sublimation which is used almost synonymously with distillation, liquefaction or dissolution, congelation over warm ashes, calcination or pulverization in fire, separating and recombining of substances.

In the following brief analysis of the contents of the tract the plan and order of the author have in general been followed, that is, first, the definition of the alchemical art, its possibility, purpose, aims, methods of procedure, and accomplishment; next, the nature of substances (*corpora*) and spirits (*spiritus*) which are first defined, with the three humidities of which they are constituted; the nature of sulphur and mercury, which are said to be the principles of the generation of all metals, and the methods of their preparation; the nature of the elixir or "stone" and its preparation; the methods of preparing the substances and spirits; the common alchemical processes; the action or reaction of the elixir; and, finally, the characteristics and means of preparation of the metals useful for the art of alchemy. Throughout the description of the contents an effort has been made to present the point of view of the author of the treatise in so far as that is possible, without superimposing modern scientific concepts. Wherever possible, too, an attempt has been made, either in the text or footnotes, to indicate the parallel discussions of similar topics by ALBERTUS MAGNUS in the authentic *De mineralibus*.

The tract opens with a statement from CALLISTHENES similar to that cited by ALBERTUS in the *De mineralibus*.[7] According to CALLISTHENES, who is named as one of the founders of the art, alchemy is the science that imparts to inferior metals the nobility of the superior, by purging them of their turbid character and leading forth in them the brilliance and rarefied quality of the superior metals.

The author apparently accepts, in general, the theory which ALBERTUS attributes to the alchemists, that metals other than gold represent imperfect stages in the ascending scale toward the species gold which represents perfection. Moreover, each imperfect substance is seeking to be perfected and completed, and the perfection or completion of each imperfect metal takes place in the same way in both nature and art.[8] The aim of the alchemist is therefore to imitate nature as closely as possible.

The author accepts the possibility of the transmutation of the metals, although he indicates that it is a very difficult process and that alchemists frequently err or are anxious to deceive.[9] Every alteration or operation in alchemy, he states, involves the separation of the metals into their first principles, then their purging, and finally the recombining of the parts released and purged. In this way art achieves that which nature accomplishes by itself.[10] It is further stated that since the first principles of all metals are mercury and sulphur,[11] every alchemical operation implies either the concealing or exposing of substances and spirits in metals and their transmutation. Occult or hidden substances are made apparent through dissolution and liquefaction, those which are manifest or exposed are concealed through congelation over ashes. Complete transmutation of the natures of substances and spirits is said to be possible, however, only through that in which there is the tinting and transmuting spirit (elsewhere the elixir).[12]

Several arguments are advanced to show that mere change in color, either to white or yellow, which GEBER (and later Albertus) had stated was the aim of most alchemists, does not constitute the true and complete transmutation that art in imitation of perfect nature can achieve.[13] In this way the author of the present work would meet ALBERT's criticism of alchemical gold and its failure to stand up as does natural gold by suggesting that the former is an imperfect product. Perfect gold and silver, he contends, can be made by the learned artisan much as the physician produces health, not

[6] Sloane 3457, fol. 45r.

[7] Sloane 3457, fol. 40r; Lib. III Mineral. I, vii, BORGNET V, 68, col. 1.

[8] Sloane 3457, fol. 41v; Lib. III Mineral. I, vii, BORGNET V, 68, col. 1.

[9] Sloane 3457, fol. 44v.

[10] *Ibid.*, fol. 40r.

[11] Sloane 3457, fol. 40r. ALBERT cites for this view AVICENNA in the *Physics* and in the *Epistola ad Hasen philosophum:* Lib. III Mineral. I, iv, BORGNET V, 63, col. 1.

[12] Sloane 3457, fol. 40r–v.

[13] Sloane 3457, fol. 40v. GEBER's statement is repeated by ALBERTUS without giving any authority for it: Lib. III Mineral. I, viii, BORGNET V, 70, col. 2; see also *ibid.*, Lib. III, I, ix, BORGNET V, 71, col. 2.

through his own skill alone, but with the aid of nature, the physician, minister, and director of the art.[14] For art is the servant and handmaiden of nature. ALBERTUS MAGNUS in the *De mineralibus*, while arguing that lead which the alchemist claims he has made into gold is probably something similar to gold but not gold, also states that art alone cannot give the substantial form.[15] ALBERT too had granted, as does our author, that learned alchemists work as do learned physicians. The latter by purgative medicines purge matter which is either corrupted or easily corruptible and which impedes health, the aim of the physician. In the same way the learned alchemist works in transmuting metals, since his first act must be to purge the sulphur and mercury which are present in metals.[16] Hence our author asserts that he is a deceiver who without the necessary purging speaks of tinting alone, for he is ignorant of the art and does not recognize nor understand the true nature of spirits and substances as experience has proved.[17] The best of all alchemical operations is said to be that which proceeds from the same basis as does nature. The best operator is the one who works from the same things that nature does, that is from sulphur and mercury. These must first be well purged by decoction and immersings in very strong caustic waters and then appropriately sublimated. When the sublimated matter is mixed with the prepared metal it will tint it with a permanent tint and will introduce the brilliant and fitting form.[18]

The true course of the Hermetic art according to the present work will be determined therefore by the supervision and the skill with which the principal operations are performed. These include sublimation, dissolution, distillation, and calcination, with washings, immersings, purgings, and the above mentioned separating. Thus one substance may be deprived of or corrupted in its species and, with the aid of its component principles acting with those of another metal, another species may be introduced by the hand of the operator who is an imitator of nature. This is due to the mutual similarities and affinities in disposition toward each other which all metals have in their nature.[19] These statements may be contrasted with the cautious conclusion of ALBERTUS in the *De mineralibus* wherein he states that he does not believe that enough proof has been advanced for the acceptance of the view that the elixir is able to corrupt the species which was originally in the metal and then with the parts of the metal produce another species, just as nature is aided by the industry of the physician.[20]

In the next section of the treatise (chapt. II, in the late manuscripts) the substance or body (*corpus*) is defined as that which does not evaporate in fire, the spirit (*spiritus*) as that which flies from fire, burns and is combustible, and does not tint.[21] Every spirit and substance is said to have a triple mixed humidity, aqueous, airy or oily, and the natural basic or earthy humidity which, when joined with dryness, liquefies in fire, does not run nor burn but returns to its earlier state, when it has been congealed with dryness.[22] The alchemical art requires that some means be discovered whereby the spirit does not escape, is not consumed or burned, but instead penetrates and is mixed with all parts of the metal, so that it may tint with a permanent tincture.[23] To accomplish this the artisan endeavors to free the bodies and spirits from the first two humidities, the superfluous aqueous humidity which escapes in cremation and the superfluous airy humidity which burns and blackens and is blackened.[24] Since sulphur and mercury are the matter and the principles of the generation of all mineral bodies, it is essential that they be cleansed of the first two superfluous humidities. That which remains is the liberated earth cleansed and separated from its impedimenta. This should be conserved. The means by which sulphur and mercury are cleansed and separated from their aqueous humidity which evaporates and escapes in cremation, is sublimation (that is distillation). The airy or consumable and blackening humidity is cleansed from them by immersion in very strong caustic waters. What remains is the virtue of sulphur and mercury which is useful for the accomplishment of the work. The artisan is cautioned never to place a simple tincture in the elixir unless he is certain it has been separated from the aqueous or evaporating humidity which escapes from fire and the oily and fatty humidity which is consumable in fire. For if he does, the tincture itself will run with the aqueous humidity at the first fire or with the oily humidity will be burned and blackened. He is further warned or urged to note that there are various gradations of warmth, the extreme

[14] Sloane 3457, fol. 40v; Lib. III Mineral. I, ix, BORGNET V, 71, col. 2.

[15] Lib. III Mineral. I, viii, BORGNET V, 70, col. 2.

[16] *Ibid.*, I, ix, BORGNET V, 71, col. 1.

[17] Sloane 3457, fol. 41r. Cf. ALBERTUS, Lib. III Mineral. I, ix, BORGNET V, 71, col. 2.

[18] Sloane 3457, fol. 41r. Cf. ALBERTUS, *loc. cit.*

[19] Sloane 3457, fol. 40v–41r. Cf. ALBERTUS, *loc. cit.*

[20] Lib. III Mineral. I, vii, BORGNET V, 69, col. 1.

[21] Sloane, 3457, fol. 41r.

[22] *Ibid.*, fol. 41r–v, 41v–42r.

[23] *Ibid.*, fol. 41r.

[24] *Ibid.*, fol. 42r.

which corrupts and consumes matter, the weak which leaves matter undigested and impure, and a third kind which foments and vivifies matter and does its work smoothly and easily. The latter is the heat for the alchemists.[25] The virtues or qualities of the waters used should also be carefully noted. It is important, moreover, to note that there are two kinds of dryness, the dryness of powder, and the dryness of immersed lime.[26]

The preparation of the stone, that is the elixir, is the next subject taken up (chapt. III). Hermes in his "Secrets" is quoted for the statement that the stone rises from the earth into heaven and once again descends from heaven to the earth. For its nurse is the earth, and the wind carries it in its stomach.[27] According to our author, the stone is the combination of sulphur and mercury, which can be made naturally and artificially. It exists in potentiality, not in activity. It rises from the earth to the heavens when by assaying and sublimation it assumes the quality of fire and hence is able to resist fire and to descend once again from heaven to earth when it takes on the quality of earth by inhumation. The stone may be revived after it has been mortified by calcination and combustion, the process which had reduced it to a powder. The wind carries it in its stomach when it is placed in an alembic. Then by evaporation of its aqueous and evaporating humidity as well as of its combustible humidity it is lightened to the texture of air and is distilled finally from the mouth of the alembic as a liquid of oil and water. This fluid has in it the qualities of the primary elements and the effect of the perfected work for producing gold (ad solem) and silver (ad lunam).

All this nature likewise performs in the viscera of the earth without error because nature's work is that of the divine intelligence. Art, however, does this with great effort and much error since its action is the act of human intelligence. Nature has its own waters and vessels in the earth. Art also has its places suitable for the generation of metals as well as the ingenious aids of waters, fires, and vessels. It achieves the same as nature, therefore, because it imitates nature perfectly. Indeed, art is said to be the sole imitator of nature. Moreover, nature does not generate any metallic substance in the interior of the earth except through the natural sublimation of sulphur and quicksilver which acts in the earth as in a suffocating vase. By making the vapor go upward, then down again, it converts the whirling vapor into the sublimated thing. The artisan should conduct the work as does nature, in a vessel with waters, which have been prepared, first by decoction, then immersion, dissolution, and sublimation.[28] More detailed directions then follow for the preparation or separation and purification of sulphur and mercury. They must first be washed and then immersed in caustic waters and then decocted in them until the water runs yellow from the sulphur and clear (or white) from the quicksilver. Next these should be sublimated, then preserved, and then joined so that they tint and are tinted. The section closes with a detailed description of the process of sublimation.[29]

The preparation of the bodies and spirits is the next topic discussed [30] (chapt. IV in the late manuscripts). The defects of imperfect substances and spirits, from which they must be rid by the alchemist before they can become perfect bodies, are listed, then the means by which this is accomplished. Thus the aquosity and windiness of the spirits are carried off by sublimation; the combustible humidity by lightly assaying over a slow humid fire; the dregs removed by washings and decoctions in caustic waters; the dryness which causes brittleness is removed by waxings and immersions in oil extracted from sulphur and mercury, both of which have first been cleansed and prepared; and the compression which removes the shrill sound and adds weight is achieved by very bitter constricting waters.

Sulphur which makes a very powerful tincture for reddening and arsenic which makes a tincture for whitening are both said to be prepared more quickly from mineral substances than from more remote substances such as human blood, hair, eggs, marrow, and certain parts of animals. Various books, however, do present a multiplicity of ways and means to produce artificial sulphur and quicksilver. Many of these are said to err because they deny the principles and intentions of the alchemical art.[31]

Next come descriptions of the common processes (chapt. V) of the alchemist's art, such as liquefaction or dissolution, coagulation, congelation, and calcination to which particular attention is given. Calcination is said to take place when the substances have been reduced to very fine particles by fire and are completely soluble in liquid. Another method of

[25] Sloane 3457, fol. 42r.

[26] Sloane 3457, fol. 42v.

[27] *Ibid.*, fol. 42v; cf. ALBERTUS, Lib. III Mineral. II, 1; BORGNET V, 75, col. 1–2; D. W. SINGER, *Catalogue of Latin and Vernacular Alchemical Manuscripts*, I, 43, 49–50, 143.

[28] Sloane 3457, fol. 42v–43v.

[29] Sloane 3457, fol. 43v–44r.

[30] *Ibid.*, fol. 44r–44v.

[31] Sloane 3457, fol. 44v.

calcination is accomplished by washing the substances on thin sheets of metal smeared with common unprepared oil. Then sulphur and arsenic are sprinkled over them and they are placed in a vessel of calcination made from very fine strong clay of wisdom (lutum sapientiae).[32] The vessel should be closed on all sides and placed on a strong fire. Thin sheets of copper (venus) sprinkled with common oil may be taken and sprinkled with powdered arsenic and then placed in a vessel of calcination. The copper should then be immersed in very strong caustic waters and finally sublimated with sal ammoniac five or seven times. After it is liquefied it may be congealed over slow ashes. Thus copper (venus) will be purged and ready for silver (ad lunam) making. Likewise lead may be calcined by sprinkling sulphur over it. Finally the lead may be covered with wax and immersed in caustic waters, then sublimated with water of sal ammoniac. Next it is put under dung for liquefaction, then finally the solution is congealed over slow ashes. Thus is lead (saturnus) prepared for the red elixir. To these substances of copper and lead may be added some tincture made from surphur and mercury. Then the species will be converted into a joyous thing. The method of mixing the elixir with the prepared substances is accomplished by liquefying or dissolving them.[33]

The reason for the heaviness or weightiness of gold (sol) and lead (saturn) is said to be due to the great compression of their parts and their depth. Silver is said to be easily prepared for gold because its substance is very close to that of gold. All that is necessary is the change in weight and color.[34]

The elixir to which the following section is given over [35] (chapt. VI) is said to penetrate the prepared substances just as a medicine penetrates the veins. It enters, colors them, and is mixed entirely with them. It does not escape, nor burn, gives them weight, and makes them solid, and may be fixed in fire. The elixir, it is stated, cannot be made from sulphur alone nor from mercury alone. It is the child of the union of sulphur, the father or male principle, and mercury, the mother or female principle. Neither one, as in human procreation, can generate without the other.[36] In the preparation of the above elixir, great care must be taken lest it be too dry and therefore easily broken. The author reports that he has seen many good works which were almost completed break at the blow of a hammer because of their brittleness.[37]

The remaining portions of the tract are devoted to descriptions of the specific metals and their preparation. First sulphur (chapt. VII) which is said to contain much aqueous and evaporating humidity mixed with the dry spirit which is not well incorporated, generally flies from fire, and burns and blackens metals over which it is projected without having first been prepared. It is said to be easier to extract oil from sulphur than water from mercury, though, in general, waters are more easily extracted than oils. In oils and waters extracted from sulphur and mercury by distillation, there is said to be great efficacy. They are the ones that the wise men of the alchemist's art seek. The entrance of the tincture and its fixation is said to be aided by these waters and oils. The waters are reddish yellow, black, green, and red, according to the degree of their distillation. These waters or oils may be extracted either from sulphur or mercury or from the things used in place of sulphur and mercury. The method of preparation of these waters and oils, the author states, he will pass over since numerous books contain this information.[38]

Mercury is said to be prepared in the same way as sulphur, first by washing, then by decoction in caustic waters, and sublimation with sulphur or by sulphur, as some books state. These operations should be repeated seven times or more until the mercury is well separated from its aqueous evaporating humidity as well as from its combustible humidity, the first of which causes it to fly into the fire, while the second causes it to be burned and blackened. When it is seen not to fly nor to be burned nor blackened, it must be liquefied at once under the dung, then the solution should be mixed with the red tincture from sulphur, and finally, congealed over warm ashes. This is said to be the sublimation of the work. A second method of cleansing mercury is then set forth. Thus mercury may be taken, washed, and covered with wax, then immersed in caustic waters, or it may be covered with sheets of metal, either of white or red marchasite, and then immersed in water of sulphur which has been prepared with one part of

[32] Sloane 3457, fol. 45r–v. Cf. ALBERTUS, Lib. IV, Mineral. I, vii, BORGNET V, 93, col. 1: "tenaci luto, quod *sapientiae lutum* vocant alchimici . . . lutum autem sapientiae de quo fiunt testae, fit ex testa contrita et iterum commixta et decocta . . . Tamen alio modo in alchimicis praeparatur lutum sapientiae sed illud hic sufficiat quo aurifices utuntur."

[33] Sloane 3457, fol. 45r–v.

[34] Sloane 3457, fol. 46r. Cf. ALBERTUS, Lib. III Mineral. II, 6, BORGNET V, 82, col. 2.

[35] Sloane 3457, fol. 46r–v.

[36] *Ibid.*, fol. 46v; cf. ALBERTUS, Lib. IV Mineral. I, i, BORGNET V, 83, col. 1–2.

[37] Sloane 3457, fol. 46v.

[38] Sloane 3457, fol. 46v–47r.

both arsenic for whitening and of sulphur for reddening, and one part of vitriol with a third part of green copper. This should be distilled and the mercury extracted from it. It may then be buried and afterward congealed.[39]

Attention is called to the fact that all spirits, especially sulphur and marchasite, when raw and unprepared, blacken and burn the substances over which they are projected. When prepared, however, they whiten and redden. Care must be taken not to putrefy substances which are intended to be liquefied. The stages and numbers of the operations must be carefully observed, since these are the signs which wise and experienced men have noted for their guidance. Others, however, through their ignorance of the stages in the art, are led astray and they believe that it is the art that has deceived them.[40]

The nature of mercury is then further described. It may be produced either by nature or by art, and can never stand in conjunction with any substance unless it has been mortified and restrained. This is accomplished by the appropriate sublimation and immersion in caustic waters and through the vapor of sublimated and prepared sulphur. When mercury has been sublimated and prepared, it will at once be congealed and brought to hardness and to the metallic form. When in sublimation or in the midst of the other preparations the mercury begins to be glandulous, then it has been converted to the desired species.[41] Mercury when sublimated with sulphur and sal ammoniac will be converted into a bright red dry powder. It may then once again be burned in the fire. Then it will return to its humid and fluid texture. And that which proceeds from it into the neck of the vase which is called an aludel is converted into the likeness of a stone called alabaster. Alchemical mercury is further carefully distinguished from a medicinal mercury which is found and extracted from certain stones. This mercury is very cold and calms the nerves in paralysis but it is not useful in the alchemical process.[42]

The final section of the treatise is given over to a brief account of each of the other metals useful for the alchemical art, that is gold (fol. 49r–v), silver (fol. 49v–50r), tin (fol. 50r), and lead (fol. 50v). The descriptions parallel much that is found in the *De mineralibus* on the same topics.

The treatise whose contents have thus been briefly indicated is extant in three manuscripts; two of them in the Sloane collection at the British Museum have already been described by Mrs. DOROTHY WALEY SINGER in her *Catalogue of Latin and Vernacular Alchemical Manuscripts in Great Britain and Ireland* (Brussels, 1928, I, No. 180). One of these, Sloane 3457, fols. 40r–50v, according to the Roman numerals on the manuscript itself, which I follow (new numbering, 46r–56v), is a fifteenth-century manuscript; the other, Sloane 3120, fols. 174r–192v (new numbering pp. 1–38), dates from the seventeenth century. The third manuscript from the collection of the University of Bologna, No. 270 (457), Vol. III, pp. 77–97, is of the sixteenth century. It is identical, judging from the identity of incipits, explicits, and opening words of chapters, with the seventeenth-century Sloane manuscript.

A transcription of the text found in Sloane 3457, fols. 40r–50v, is given in the following pages. It has been made from a photostat of the manuscript. Variants in the text of Sloane 3120, fols. 174r–192v, of which a photostat has also been obtained, have been indicated in the footnotes.[43] Collations with the text of Bologna 270, pp. 77–97, have been made from my notes on the manuscript taken in the summer of 1937. Both late manuscripts are divided into chapters of which there are eight, while the fifteenth-century text has no such well-marked divisions. The two late manuscripts also omit the first chapter, as they indicate by their opening words, and they close several paragraphs before the fifteenth-century text. Each of the late texts has, however, a brief postscript enumerating the various terms for alchemical processes with their synonyms. Also throughout these late texts there are omissions of sentences, phrases, or words, which are found in the Sloane 3457 text.

The writing in Sloane 3457 is small and very difficult to decipher, and the text is much abbreviated. In most cases in the transcription the medieval

[39] *Ibid.*, fol. 47r–v.

[40] Sloane 3457, fol. 47v–48r. This is chapter VIII in the late MSS.

[41] *Ibid.*, fol. 48r–v; Lib. IV Mineral. I, ii, BORGNET V, 85, col. 2.

[42] Sloane 3457, fol. 48v–49r; Lib. IV Mineral. I, ii, BORGNET V, 85, col. 2.

[43] Photostats of the two Sloane manuscripts were obtained for me through the courtesy of the Manuscript Division of the Library of Congress, in cooperation with the Mediaeval Academy Rotograph Service. The photostats were sent by the Manuscript Division of the British Museum in the summer of 1940 at the time when the British were enduring the horrors and devastation of total air attack. Such attention to what must after all be considered a detail of minor importance in a time of grave national peril is indeed commendable. I am further indebted to the reference department of the Columbia University Library for facilitating my use of the photostats.

The photostats are now bound and housed in the Library of Congress under the heading *Modern Language Association*, Add. 42.

spelling has been retained, except in some cases of *u* and *v*, or *i* and *j*, where modern usage makes reading somewhat easier. Sentence divisions and paragraphing have also been introduced where the sense requires. In noting variations between the two Sloane texts no attempt has been made to list such minor variants as *igitur* for *ergo*, *itaque* for *igitur*, *vero* for *etiam*, and the like. Differences of word order have also not usually been indicated where these seem to be of minor significance.

Calistenus [1] unus de antiquioribus post Hermetem artis nostre inventoribus dicit quod alchimia est scientia que inferioribus metallicis corporibus inducit nobilitatem[1a] superiorum purgando turbidum et inducendo splendidum et sublime superiorum in eis. Geber Hispanus dicit Inspexi quosdam libros huius artis et inveni libros istos absque sublime et inconnixi quibusdam experientiis et celare intentionem suam per verba alegoria quod numquam fuit consuetudo philosophie vere celare secretum in quo est veritas, laus et conservatio nobilitatis artis. Itaque non deceptionis causa sit. Scias itaque quod omnis intentio et operatio est prima principia corporum separare et purgare et purgata coniungere ita ut ex eis fiat per artem quod natura facit per se ex eis.

Principia vero prima omnium metallorum corporum sunt argentum vivum et sulphur. Ideoque omnis operatio alchimie vel est occultatio vel manifestatio nostrorum corporum et spirituum et transmutatio ipsorum. Nunc ut occulta corporum manifestant aut manifesta occultant aut naturas corporum et spirituum transmutare volunt omnia capitula [fol. 40v] huius artis. Et scias quod manifestatio occultorum in corporibus et spiritibus non fit nisi per eorum solutionem. Et occultatio manifestorum non fit nisi per congelationem ipsorum super cineres ut scis. Scias tamen quod transmutatio completa in naturis corporum et spirituum non sit nisi per illud in quo est spiritus tingens et transmutans ut totum obtineat omnes partes transmutati virtute et commixtione sue substantie quod fieri non potest nisi per solutionem et liquefactionem. Quo autem modo verius et brevius illud fiat Geber declarat dicens vix unquam inveni artificem in toto corporum et spirituum substantialiter operantem sed potius citrino et albo tingentes ut in igne evangelico permaneret color ad horam et penetraret totum corpus tinctum. Sed ista non est vera et completa transmutatio quam ars perfectem imitans naturam facere potest. Sed periti artifices ita facere possunt aurum et argentum sicut medicus sanitatem. Sanitas autem quam facit est forma effectiva primo per se et artem per consequens. Nam nature ministra est et ancilla. Non ergo ars facit aurum per solam manum artificis sed natura medente ministerio et magisterio artis, processus itaque verissimus huius artis est in eo magisterio et ingenio operationum principalium que sunt quatuor: sublimatio, solutio, distillatio et calcinatio, cum lotionibus et inbibitionibus, purgationibus et separationibus premissis. Corrumpitur unum corpus [fol. 41r] a sua specie et cum iuvamento earum que in materiis sunt et que natura per manum artificis immitatur aliam speciem inducit que non erat prius in illa materia. Idcirco quod in naturis omnium metallorum cum suis dispositionibus adinvicem sunt similitudines et propinquitates et quorundam ad quedam. Optima ergo et propinquissima est operatio illorum qui operantur ex eisdem principiis mediatricis separatis et per se acceptis ex quibus operatur natura. Hec autem sunt sulphur et mercurius quibus nunc principaliter per decoctionem et bibitionem in aquis acutissimis et per sublimationem debitam quando bene purgata fuerunt prius ingrediuntur et permiscentur et tingunt fixe materias preparatas ita ut eorum virtute mox inducitur in materias forma speciosa et aptata. Qui vero absque purgatione debita precedente cum ceteris que supra diximus tincturam solam dicit deceptor est artis nostre et inscius non cognoscens corporum et spirituum naturam. Quidem experti sumus in hiis tincturis simplicibus opus quidem aliquando quinque vel sex peras [1b] purgatorias sustinuit et ultima septimam non transivit. Bonum verum opus permanet usque in finem.

Scias [2] itaque quod in arte nostra corpus vocatur omne illud quod non evaporat ab igne, spiritus vero omne illud quod evolat ab igne et adurit et aduritur et non ingreditur et non tingit. Ut inveniamus modum faciendi ut ipsum [3] non evolet et non aduratur et ingrediatur et permisceatur cum toto totum et pars cum parte et tingat ipsum tinctura fixa et permanente.[4] Ideoque de natura ipsorum dicemus omnium itaque spirituum [fol. 41v] et corporum fixe et non fixe [5] commixtio est ex subtili terreo et aereo cuius natura [6] est

[1] BM Sloane 3120, 17th cent., fol. 174r (henceforth to be designated as B) begins with the heading: Incipit tractatus Alberti qui sic incipit: Calixtenes unus philosophus, capitulum primum est hic obmissum. The whole first section is then omitted. The text begins: "Principia immediata sunt sulphur et mercurius, quoniam ipsa per decorationes et imbibitionem in acquis acutissimis, et per sublimationem debitam, quando bene purgata prius fuerint, ingrediuntur et permiscentur, et tingunt fixe materias preparatas. Ita quod eorum virtute, etc., . . ." Similarly Bologna 270 (457), III, 15th–16th cent., pp. 77–97 (henceforth designated as C), opens, Incipit tractatus Alberti qui sic incipit, Callixtenes unus philosophus cuius capitulum primum est hic obmissum. Then begins: "Principia immediata sunt sulphur et mercurius . . ." as in the B text.

[1a] Not *notabilitatem* as in D. W. SINGER, No. 180.

[1b] That is stone (Du Cange).

[2] Capitulum secundum, B, C. The wording differs in order and somewhat in context. Both texts read: "Scias igitur quod in arte nostra spiritus vocatur omne id quod evolat ab igne, et adurit et aduritur et intentio nostrae artis est scire quid et qualis res sit, hoc quod evolat et adurit et aduritur, et non ingreditur et non tingit, et inveniamus ingenium faciendi . . ."

[3] B, fol. 174v.

[4] manente, B.

[5] fixe dispositionis commixtio, B.

[6] natura est mollis et superflua, B. The rest of the sentence is omitted. The new sentence begins: Itaque humiditas . . .

in sulphure et ex subtili aqueo et aereo pinqui cuius natura est in oleo. Superflua itaque humiditas aquea est que evolat in crematione et superflua humiditas aerea est que adurit et denigrat [7] et denigratur. Et superflua [8] humiditas calcis est que obstat penetrationi et permixtioni et tincture adherenti et facit [9] stridens et frangibile. Lavando igitur et decoquendo [10] et inbibendo et cibando, sublimando et soluendo spiritus penetrat corpora mundata et colorat [11] et vivificat ea faciens quod mortuum fuerit resurgeri ad vitam mortificando illud quod male vivebat. Imperfectionis autem sulphuris et mercurii causa est quod ipsa sunt universalis materia et principia generationis omnium [12] corporum mineralium. Omne autem imperfectum contingit perfici et compleri. Perficitur autem et completur utrumque ipsorum eodem modo a [13] natura et ab arte ut prius dicetur. Quodlibet autem corpus est per se totum illud quod ipsum est quia quelibet pars auri [14] intra et extra est aurum et in ceteris. Et nota sicut quidam imperiti mentiuntur dicentes quod aurum in suo occulto est plumbum [15] et plumbum in suo occulto est aurum, sed materie eorum sunt propinquius in eis [16] adinvicem alie cum aliis sicut materia veneris [17] et ferri ad lunam et materia saturni et lune ad solem. In omni itaque spiritu et corpore secundum magis et minus est triplex humiditas inmixta scilicet aquosa que evolet [18] unctuosa adustibilis que adurit et aduritur et denigrat et denigratur. Et humiditas naturalis et radicalis [fol. 42r] que cum sicco [19] compacta liquescit in igne et non evolat nec adurit [20] sed potius ignem suo priori statu [21] in suo sicco congelata redit. Primas duas humiditates a sulphure et mercurio ars nostra querit removere et tertiam liberatam et mundatam et separatam a suis impedimentis conservare. Separa ergo a sulphure et mercurio humiditatem ipsorum aquosam per sublimationem et humiditatem [22] adustibilem et denigrantem per imbibitionem aquarum acutissimarum et cibationes et incerationes rerum quas tibi infra dicemus de sale armoniaco et tutia et marcasita et remanebit tibi virtus sulphuris et mercurii que utilis est ad finem operis tui. Et numquam curabis tincturam [23] simplicem et solam ponere in elixir nisi prius certus sis quod humiditas aquosa et evanida que ignem fugit et humiditas unctuosa et pinguis [24] aduritur et consumitur in igne et quod [25] ambe sint a spiritibus predictis separate alioquin ipsa tinctura quamvis splendida et [26] cum humiditate aquosa ad primos ignes evolat vel cum humiditate unctuosa aduritur et denigratur. Scias ergo quod triplex est calidum nostrum scilicet calidum excellens quod corrumpit et incinerat materiam et calidum deficiens quia [27] relinquit materiam indigestam et impuram. Et calidum fovens et vivificans materiam [28] quod leviter et suaviter facit opus suum et ipsum est [29] calidum ignis nostri qui est calidus et humidus. Vide ergo diligenter de igne tuo quoniam ignis [30] calidus et siccus vehementer incinerat omne opus tam nature quam artis. Item [31] inspice etiam [fol. 42v] diligenter virtutes [32] aquarum nostrarum quoniam ipse sunt aque que virtute non actu habent in se naturas et operationes [33] omnium elementorum corporum et spirituum. Natura etiam per resudationem ex venis a viis terre adducit aquas [34] salsas et aluminosas ad loca sulphuris et mercurii [35] et inbibit et exsiccat ex eis sulphur et mercurium ad opus suum. Cum vero preparabis tibi aquas ingenio et arte quibus facies opus tuum, scias etiam quod siccum nostrum est duplex. Est enim siccum [36] pulveris cuius partes per se non continuantur [37] sed permanent separate nisi quod ab eis per fortissimam combustionem eduxeris [38] illud per quod tamquam per aerem videbis. Est [39] ut siccum calcis inbibite cuius partes postquam totum solutum fuerit in igne calido ex [40] humido ad se recolliguntur et totum congelatum efficit tuum corpus.

Cum [41] ergo sulphur natura vel arte predictis [42] iuvamentis separatum et mundatum [43] fuerit mox mercurius [44] sibi adaptat substantialiter partim vaporabiliter. Ingreditur et alterat ipsum et [45] tenet eum et facit eum stare cum [46] ad similitudinem nature ingenium et artis adhibueris. Hoc autem summum ingenium [47] huius artem Hermes pater antiquissimus et optimus huius artis docet in *Secretis* suis, dicens suavitur et [48] magno ingenio, ascendit a terra in celum et iterum descendit de celo in

[7] denigrat et aduritur et denigratur, B.

[8] superfluitas calcis, B.

[9] facit corpus stridens, B.

[10] Words between here and spiritus penetrat are omitted, B.

[11] B, fol. 175r, colorabunt et vivificabunt ea, faciendo . . .

[12] omnium metallorum et corporum universalium, B.

[13] modo et a natura et ab arte, sicut praeterea dicetur, B.

[14] intus est aurum et extra et sic de aliis et non [fol. 175v] est sic sicut quidam, B.

[15] The sentence ends here in B. Then follows, Sed materie . . .

[16] propinquiores, with in eis, omitted, B.

[17] cupri, B.

[18] elevatur, B.

[19] suo sicco, B.

[20] aduritur, B.

[21] Sed post ignem sub priori, fol. 176r, B.

[22] omitted, B.

[23] fol. 176v, B.

[24] pinquis que, B.

[25] et quod, omitted, B.

[26] splendida cum est in igne aduritur et denigratur, with the intervening words omitted, B.

[27] quod, B.

[28] omitted, B.

[29] fol. 177r, B.

[30] omitted, B.

[31] omitted, B.

[32] libros, B.

[33] naturas operativas, B.

[34] aquas acetosas salsas, B.

[35] The rest of the sentence down to "ad opus suum" is omitted, B.

[36] fol. 177v, B.

[37] recontinuantur, B.

[38] eduxeris [humidum] illud, B.

[39] et etiam, B.

[40] et, B.

[41] Caput tertium, B, fol. 177v; C, p. 81.

[42] predictis rebus et, B.

[43] emundatum, B.

[44] mercurius similiter sibi adaptatur, B.

[45] fol. 178r, B.

[46] quando, B.

[47] magisterium huius artis docet in Secretis suis Hermes dicens . . . with the intervening words omitted, B.

[48] et cum magno ingenio lapis noster ascendit, B.

terram nutrix enim [49] eius est terra et portavit eum ventus in ventre suo. Lapis enim noster scilicet sulphur et mercurius [49a] naturaliter et artificialiter factus est. Lapis in potentia est non in actu et iste ascendit a terra [fol. 43r] in celum quando per assationem et sublimationem induit virtutem ignis ut possit igni resistere et iterum descendit de celo in [50] terram quando induit virtutem terre per inhumationem. Tunc enim revivificatur et refovetur quando prius in eo fuerit mortificatum per calcinationem [51] et combustionem, illam operationem que in pulverem reducit.[52] Ventus enim portavit eum [53] in ventre suo quando positus fuerit in alembicum. Tunc etiam evaporando suum humidum aquosum et evanidum et suum humidum adustibile levigatur ad virtutem aeris et distillat ultimo ab ore alembici existens simile liquori aque et olei habens in se virtutes elementorum primorum et effectum perfecti operis ad solem et ad lunam.[54] Et natura quidem operatur hec omnia similiter in visceribus terre licet multo operetur sine errore quia nature opus est intelligencie divine. Ars vero facit hoc cum multis laboribus et errore quia opus artis est intelligencie humane. Et natura quidem habet per se suas aquas et sua vasa in terra, scilicet loca apta generationi metallorum. Ars vero habet suffragia mendicata ingeniosa aquarum et ignium et vasorum. Facit tum idem quod natura quando naturam perfecte imitatur. Ars enim est sola imitatrix nature. Oportet [55] ergo te non latere quod natura non generat [56] aliquod corpus metallicum nisi in visceribus terre nisi per naturalem sublimationem sulphuris et argenti vivi in loco terre tanquam in vase prefocante et faciente vaporem [57] desursum ab [58] deorsum [fol. 43v] redire et ibi circumvolutum vaporem convertit in rem sublimatam. Scias quod [59] natura sublimat nec convertat rem ad eorum crudum sed prius per aquas acutas ex venis terre resudantes ex locis salsis et aluminosis decoctum et inbibitum. Tu ergo fac ad similitudinem nature opus tuum [60] in vase tuo cum aquis tuis, prius decoquendo et inbibendo et soluendo et protinus sublimando, et magnificabis [61] opus tuum. Probatus autem modus [62] separationis et purificationis sulphuris et mercurii est ut prius laventur et protinus inbibendo [63] aquis acutis et decoquentur postmodum in eis donec aqua citrina egrediatur de [64] sulphure et aqua clara [65] de argento vivo. Deinde sublimentur sublimata vero conservantur, tunc [66] coniungantur sic ut tingant et tingantur in hora optima.[67] Sublimationis vero modus est: [68] fac tibi vas amplum et rotundum inferius admodum inferioris partis medii [69] caldarii quod sulphur et [70] argentum vivum quodcumque illorum [71] separata prius purgata, inbibita et decocta [72] ac soluta recipiat. Deinde super illud vas aliud [73] vas admodum superioris partis medie angustum habens collum longum et strictum bene et super illius colli orificium coopertorium ex valde subtili et bene preparate luto sapientie in quo coopertulo [74] sit foramen strictum valde et parvissimum ad instar puncti unius et locum conjunctionis vasis inferioris et superioris, diligenter limes [75] et claudes luto sapientie subtili valde et tenaci et vas [76] superius sit sicut alembicus cecus carens naso quia nichil distillatur [77] ab eo. Deinde inhumabis fundum vasis [fol. 44r] inferioris in [78] cineribus super patellam et suppones ignem lentum. Et meliora sunt ad hec vasa vitrea. Et est primi vasis dispositio sicut urinalis vel medie partis inferioris inferioris [79] caldarii. Et [80] secundum vas stans super illud recipiat totum vaporem resolutum ex ipso. Vapor ergo qui recipiendus [81] est et servandus est dirigitur sursum in collum longum [82] et ibi [83] circumvolutus in se revertitur deorsum et convertitur in rem sublimatam et fixam. Sed [84] aquosus vapor et adustibilis per foramen illud [85] parvum supremum evolat. Et propter hoc diligentissime observabis ut [86] prius sis in hora sublimationis quia necessarium est valde propter diversa particula ut priusquam evolavit per illud foramen supremum vapor aquosus primo cuius vapor [87] est albus. Deinde vapor adustibilis cuius fumus erit [88] niger et [89] viridis et rubeo mixtus, statim claudas ipsum foramen ut [90] vapor naturalis et convertendus repellatur deorsum ad conversionem et perforationem. Quia in illa re conversa erit tinctura et fixio. In ceteris autem generaliter scias quod in preparationi corporum et spirituum invenies [91] artem.

[49] omitted, B.
[49a] vel naturaliter factus, vel artificialiter, B.
[50] fol. 178v, B.
[51] B, adds: "assationem. Etiam vocamus calcinationem et combustionem."
[52] deducit, B.
[53] eum, omitted, B.
[54] B, omits the following sentences down to "Oportet ergo te . . ."
[55] B, 178v, resumes.
[56] fol. 179r, B.
[57] written *vapore* in Sloane 3457, fol. 43r.
[58] ad, B.
[59] etiam quod natura non convertit nec sublimat aliquod corpus eorum, B.
[60] opus tuum, omitted, B.
[61] magnificabitur, B.
[62] fol. 179v, B.
[63] postea inbibantur, B.
[64] a, B.
[65] alba ab, B.
[66] et, B. There is a figure of a vessel in the left margin of Sloane 3457, fol. 43v.
[67] opportuna, B.
[68] est iste. Fac, B.
[69] omitted, B.
[70] vel, B.
[71] tunc volueris. Separata, B.
[72] decocta prius et, B.
[73] vas [fol. 180r] aliud habens collum et strictum bene, with the intervening words omitted, B.
[74] operculo, B.
[75] lutes, B.
[76] vas erit superius, B.
[77] distillabitur, B.
[78] inferioris super palea et suppones, B.
[79] inferioris inferioris, omitted, B.
[80] fol. 180v, B.
[81] capiendus, B.
[82] in longitudinem colli, B.
[83] omitted, B.
[84] Sed vapor et aquosus et adustibilis, B.
[85] illud evaporat. Et propter, with intervening omitted, B.
[86] et presens sis in hora sublimationis ut postquam evolaverit per illud foramen, with the intervening words omitted, B.
[87] fumus, B.
[88] est, B.
[89] cum, B.
[90] fol. 181r, B.
[91] intentio artis est aquositatem eorum evaporari, B.

Est primo evaporari et humidum assari et feculentum purgari et siccum impugnari et porosum et dispersum constringi et grossum subtiliari [92] ut penetret et penetretur et non adherens facere permisceri et adherere et permixtum totaliter ingredi et colorare et tincturam non aduri et coniuncta non separare. Hiis habitis querentes artis finem se credunt habere propositum.

[fol. 44v] Omnis itaque [93] aquositas et ventositas [93a] spirituum tolluntur per sublimationem, humiditas adustiva per levem assationem super ignem humidum et calidum et lentum, fetulenta per lotiones et decoctiones in aquis acutis. Siccum vero quod facit corporum frangibilitatem tollitur per incerationes et inbibitiones olei extracti a sulphure et mercurio mundatis et preparatis. Constrictio vero que aufert stridorem et addit pondus corporibus fit per aquas amarissimas et constrictivas quando ex eis calces incerantur et inbibuntur. Grossorum vero subtiliatio et penetrabit et penetrabitur per [94] inbibitionem aque extracte de sulphure sublimato per mixtionem vere perfectam totius cum toto et cuiuslibet partis inter se. Facit solutio cum ex spiritibus preparatis partes de singulis solueris et aquas permisceris sicut nosci. Tincturam enim in rubeum facit sulphur potissime ad hoc preparatum, in album vero arsenicum promptissime in his operationibus que fiunt ex mineralibus. In his vero que fiunt ex [95] rebus remotioribus sicut ex sanguine humano et pilis et ovis et medullis et partibus animalium quorundam. Illud quod est loco sulfuris et illud quod est loco arsenici facit ad rubeum et ad album. Operantes enim in his [96] nichil querunt nisi sulphur artificialiter extractum ab [97] illis rebus et similiter mercurium extractum. Harum ergo omnium viarum et modorum diversitas capitula et libros huius artis multiplicat et artem in errorem [98] multorum duxit [99] tum nescientes principia et intentiones ac finem artis et [100] multis modis intermediis erraverunt quod etiam multis peritis vidimus accidisse [101] [fol. 45r] propter quod experientia continua [102] specie tamen prima est utendum nec desperandum si aliquibus vicibus non statim effectum quem sperabas vidisti. Sed [103] gradus operis notandi sunt in reiterandi donec videas que causa fuerit impedimenti et erroris ut eam vitare scias et ad [104] aliam declinare. Hiis habitis breviter ad operationes communes transibimus ut generaliter ipsarum patefiat via et modus verus et artificialis.

Scias [105] ergo quod corpora et lapides generaliter non liquantur aut soluuntur sine appositione materie que humiditatem virtute [106] et effectu habeant, habeans in se quales sunt nature aquarum et salium. Non potest etiam fieri coagulatio nisi virtus siccitatis naturalis intret [107] virtutem humiditatis naturalis agens in ipsam et patiens ab ea ut siccitas humiditatem contineat ne defluat et humiditas partes sicci contineat et colligat ne in pulverem dispergantur. Adhibe ergo liquefactioni ad [108] res siccas et leviter exsiccantes virtute pocius quam actu. Liquefactio vero corporum metallicorum generaliter est ex [109] eo quia quecumque [110] frigido congelantur a frigido et humido vel a calido et humido dissoluantur ut sales et attramenta et alie vitriose [111] substantie vel vitriollum et similia. Calcinatio vera corporum ad hoc fit ut in [112] partes subtilissimas dissoluta per ignem possit [113] in fundum substantie sue recipere imbibitionem et cibationem competentem ad opus nostrum. Omnibus [114] corporibus calcinandis facilior modus [fol. 45v] est [115] corpora laminata laminis attenuatis ungantur oleo communi non preparato et sulphur et [116] arsenicum superaspergantur [117] et in vas calcinationis inmittantur. Quod quidem factum sit de subtili et forti luto sapientie et vas undique [118] claudatur et sic in ignem [119] fortem mittatur. Si ergo veneris laminas acciperis tenues [120] in oleo communi unctas [121] et desuper sparseris arsenicum pulverisatum et predicto modo in vas [122] calcinationis miseris. Accipiesque calcem istam et cum aquis acutissimis imbibes et ultimo cum sale [123] armoniaco sublimato et soluto quinque vel septem vicibus inbiberis et siccaveris et demum ad soluendum posueris sub fimo; solutum vero postmodum congelaveris [124] super cineres lentos. Erit [125] bonus optime purgatus ad lunam. Similiter plumbum calcina desuper spargendo sulphur [126] et calcem imbibitam aquis acutis. Ultimo incerabis [127] cum aqua salis armoniaci sublimati sub fimo. Pones ad soluendum et

[92] From *subtilio* (to rarefy, alchem. 1267 A.D.: *Medieval Latin Word-List*, 1934).

[93] Capitulum quartum, B, fol. 181v; C, p. 84.

[93a] unctuositas, B.

[94] penetrent et penetrentur, fol. 182r, fit per inbibitionem, B.

[95] sunt in, B.

[96] in illis nichil, B.

[97] fol. 182v, ab illis rebus. Harum itaque omnium, with the intervening omitted, B.

[98] erroribus, B.

[99] inducit, dum B.

[100] In multis viis ac modis, B.

[101] accessisse, B.

[102] continua (cum ratione tamen) primo est utendum non desperandum, si, B.

[103] secundum quem gradus operis notandi sunt ac iterum variandi donec, B.

[104] et alias declinare. The remainder of the paragraph is **omitted, B.**

[105] Capitulum quintum, B, fol. 183r; C, p. 86.

[106] humiditatem virtutem et effectum habeat in se, B.

[107] inter, B.

[108] liquefactioni res humidas et humefacientes et coagulatione leviter exsiccantes tam virtute ipsius quam actu, B.

[109] fol. 183v, B.

[110] a frigido congelantur a calido dissoluuntur et sales, with the intervening words omitted, B.

[111] aliae vitriolosae substantiae et, B.

[112] ut partes subtillissimae dissolutae, B.

[113] possint ad profundum, B.

[114] Omnibus itaque corporibus, B.

[115] ut corpora, B.

[116] vel arsenicum, B.

[117] aspergatur et sic, B.

[118] undique bene, B.

[119] fol. 184r, B.

[120] et intingas in oleo, B.

[121] omitted, B.

[122] vase mittendo calcinaveris, accipias calcem, B.

[123] cum aqua salis armoniaci sublimati quinquies vel septies. Imbibetis et dessicabitis deinde ad soluendum sub fimo ponatur. Solutum . . . , B.

[124] congeletis, B.

[125] Est, B.

[126] sulphur rubeum, B.

[127] cerabis, B.

solutum congelabis [128] super cineres lentos. Erit saturnus sic optime preparatus ad elixir rubeum.

Predictis corporibus veneris et saturni appone [129] de tinctura quam fecisti de sulphure et mercurio et videbis speciem tuam in gaudium conversam.[130] Verumtamen modus permiscendi elixir cum corporibus preparatis [131] utrum liquefícatione vel solutione fiat diligenter videbis [132] et forsan est unus modus in omnibus capitulis secundum precedentes operationes sed diversus. Causa vero malleabilitatis in corporibus artis vel nature est quando humidum eorum non evolans nec adustibile, sed naturale vehementer est suo calce imbibitum [fol. 46r] et inclusum ita [133] quod neutrum dimittit suum socium sed secum vadit quocumque uterque trahantur [134] vel dividantur. Unde [135] ergo diligenter in compositione elixiris videas [136] calcem tuam oleo sulphuris sublimati recte et sufficienter inbiberis et inceraveris ex eo ne vincat humidum super calcem aut calx ab [137] humido distilletur et dispergatur ne cohereant sibi [138] invicem partes eius. Causa vero gravitatis seu [139] ponderositatis in corporibus solis et saturni est multa constrictio partium ipsarum et [140] profundatio earum ad centrum totius. Cum ergo pondus augere volueris corporibus,[141] calcem ipsorum [142] aquis acutissimis fortissime, imbibes et incerabis ex eis que constrictive [143] sunt ut ex aquis sorbarum et prunorum et pomorum silvestrium. Sic enim calcem lune in solem tingendum preparabis quia materia eorum sunt valde propinque et non oportet mutari nisi pondus et colorem mundificatione lune et calcis eius debito modo precedente.

Compositionis [144] conditiones elixiris quas ars nostra in ipso querit [145] sunt nunc ut ipsum scilicet penetret et ingrediatur corpora preparata [146] sicut medicina venas et ut coloret ea et permisceatur totaliter cum ipsis et non evolet nec aduret [147] et consolidationem faciat et pondus et fixum sit in igne. Ideoque scias [148] quod humidum unctuosum naturale [149] purum et subtile, quod [150] non relinquit suam calcem in igne quod [151] extrahitur a [152] sulphure et arsenico ut sicut venenum ignorantie et media [153] veritatis non constituet cum per [154] se illud quod intendit in finem nisi cum corporis [fol. 46v] preparati materia miscueris sicut medicina non facit sanitatem nisi corpori conveniens [155] et commixta. Ideoque et medicina per se preparata et corpore similiter [155a] indigebis. Et scias quod ex solo sulphure vel eius quod est loco sulphuris [156] vel ex solo argento vivo vel eius quod est loco ipsius numquam potest fieri elixir sed ex natura sulphuris agente in mercurio et ingrediente in ipsum substantialiter et vaporabiliter sicut videbis in modis [157] sublimationum mercurii vel cum sulphure vel sine sulphure. Et in modis [158] cibationum mercurii [cum] sulphure vel [159] marcasita vel limaturis [160] metallorum. Sulphur enim pater est et mercurius mater metallorum. Pater enim non potest generare sine matre in quam agat ut mittat [161] virtutem seminis formantis materiam generationis que est in femina. Sulphur ergo vel quod loco eius est immitte; [162] mercurium vel suo simili. Si vis generationem perficere [163] qui aliter operabitur errabit. In compositione ergo [164] elixiris caveas [165] ut non facias multam appositionem alborum vel [166] citrinorum corporum siccantium virtute sua [167] sed bene inbibitorum et inpregnatorum aquis et rebus subtiliatis quales supradiximus nam prevalebit siccitas in eis et erunt frangibilia et non [168] ductibilia propter quod ego vidi multa bona opera et pene [169] completa ad ictum mallei [170] scindi vel frangi [171] propter angustiam siccitatis eorum absque humiditate pingui et [172] naturali etc.

Hiis [173] prehibitis ad intelligendum intentionem et [174] finem artis nostre [175] de natura spirituum et corporum. Et primo de principalibus spiritibus scilicet sulphure et mercurio qui ad usum nostri operis sunt perstringamus. [fol. 47r] Scias itaque quod licet in sulphure sit humiditas [176] aquosa et evanida mixta cum multo spiritu sicco sed non bene incorporata propter quod fugat [177] ignem valde cum [178] humiditas sua unctuosa adustibilis et adustiva multo maior est propter quod valde adurit [179] et denigrat corpora quando non prepa-

[128] fol. 184v, B.
[129] apponitur, B.
[130] esse versam, B.
[131] preparatis ut ex eo tingantur ut liquefactione vel solutione, B.
[132] Non enim forsan, B.
[133] fol. 185r, B.
[134] trahatur, with the next two words omitted, B.
[135] vide, B.
[136] ut, B.
[137] omitted, and B continues, humido destituatur[sic] et . . . .
[138] erga, B.
[139] et, B.
[140] in profundo ipsorum in centro totius, B.
[141] In the margin is written, *nota.*
[142] eorum, B.
[143] fol. 185v, B.
[144] Caput sextum, B, fol. 185v; C, p. 89.
[145] quaerit et intendit sunt istae, B.
[146] perfecta, B.
[147] aduratur, B.
[148] fol. 186r, B.
[149] naturaliter, B.
[150] omitted, B.
[151] eo quod, B.
[152] de, B.
[153] materia, B.
[154] tibi, B.
[155] adveniens, B.
[155a] simpliciter, B.
[156] eius nunquam potest fieri elixir, with the intervening words omitted, B.
[157] in modo subli[fol. 186v]mationis, B.
[158] modo cibationis, B.
[159] In the margin is written, *Nota bene*, and two lines below, *Nota hic.*
[160] limatura, B.
[161] et immittat, B.
[162] immittes mercurio, B.
[163] perficere materie qui autem aliter, B.
[164] cuiuscumque, B.
[165] caveas tibi ne facias, B.
[166] et, B.
[167] fol. 187r, B.
[168] non bene, B.
[169] bene, B.
[170] written malei, in Sloane 3457.
[171] vel frangi, omitted, B.
[172] omitted, B.
[173] Caput septimum. Hiis praehibitis est intelligendum, B, fol. 187r; C, p. 91.
[174] et vim et finem, B.
[175] omitted, B.
[176] fol. 187v, B.
[177] fugit, B.
[178] tamen, B.
[179] aduritur preparata, B.

ratum [180] super ipsa proicitur et cito calcinatur cum ipso.[181] Unde est etiam quod facilius extrahis oleum de sulphure [182] quam aquam de mercurio, vero facilius extrahis aquam quam oleum quia plus habet de humiditate aquosa quam unctuosa. In ipsis vero oleis et aquis extractis per distillationem a sulphure et mercurio est magna virtus operis nostri quoniam ipsa sunt illa [183] que querunt sapientes artis [184] nostre et adiuvetur per ea ingressio et tinctura et fixio. Sed modos preparationis eorum [185] multi libri habunt unde non oportet hic dicere de eis.[186] Ipse enim sunt aque [187] flave, nigre, virides et rubee que secundum gradum distillationis sue sive de sulphure et mercurio sive de rebus receptis loco sulphuris et mercurii extrahantur.[188] Et scias quod sive per modum aquarum sive per modum sicce substantie in spiritibus predicti [189] operis oportet super sulphur mercurium commisci substantia vel virtute vel utroque modo. Sulphur enim in compositione elixiris habet se ad mercurium sicut sperma viri ad semen mulieris. Est enim calidum et siccum et [190] formator et figurator mercurii ad generationem communis filii ipsorum. Et sicut diximus de sulphure [191] prius, ita oportet etiam mercurium rectificare primo lavando et coquendo [192] in aquis acutis quas nosti. Postea [193] sublimando et cum sulphure vel a sulphure sicut alii libri dicunt et operationes ad sublimiores [194] gradus super reiterare vel septem vicibus vel pluribus donec a sua humiditate [fol. 47v] aquosa et evanida et ab humiditate adustiva optime separetur quare prima facit ipsum in igne fugere, secunda facit ipsum aduri et denigrari. Et cum ipsum videris nec effugere nec aduri nec denigrari, tunc festina ad solutionem eius sub fimo sicut scis et tinctura rubea ex sulphure tingens ipsum solutum [195] in aquis sub fimo permisceris ambas aquas et congelabis super cineres lentos et hec est sublimitas operis huius. Alium quoque modum [196] vidimus nos quia mercurius lotus et inbibitus et inceratus aquis acutis vel limaturis [197] metallorum, vel marcasita alba vel rubea, cum aqua sulphuris inbibitur sic [198] fit quia recipitur una pars arsenici ad album vel ad rubeum sulphuris et [199] pars vitriolli cum tertia parte viride eris et ponitur ad distillandum et ex ea inbibitur mercurius et conburitur et postmodum congelabitur [200] sicut scis.

Communiter [201] autem de omnibus spiritibus [202] et precipue de sulphure et arsenico teneas quod ipsi crudi et indigesti [203] et non preparati denigrant et adurant corpora supra que preiciuntur; preparati vero albificant et rubificant. Calces [204] vero et atramenta et tartarum dealbant. Borax vero et alumina et olea inpinguant. Aque vero ingrediuntur et penetrant et permisceri faciunt et inducunt et profundant tincturam. Cum autem indigebis hiis effectibus cogita de rebus et non oblivisceris earum operationes quoniam [205] omnium istarum rerum sunt in duobus gradibus aut cum permutant aut corrumpunt. Permutant ergo quamdiu [206] saluata humiditate et siccitate naturali et substantiali illarum [fol. 48r] rerum in quas agunt. Unde [207] calcinatio non corrumpit sed permutat tantum. Si enim corrumperet [208] numquam corpora calcinata et aquis inbibita calce [209] et demum soluta sub fimo et iterum congelata super ignem redirent [210] ad speciem corporis metallici. Igitur in calcinatione saluata est humiditas naturalis que beneficio imbibitionis [211] iterum resuscitatur. Corrumpit autem quando separavit humiditatem naturalem a suo sicco quod in eius [212] gremio latitabat quod fit duobus modis scilicet per combustionem que incinerat metalla et per putrefactionem que extrahit eorum humiditatem et convertit in superficie ad florem quem vocamus communiter eruginem quod enim est putredo in corporibus mollibus. Hec est rubigo vel erugo in metallis.[213] Unde quando res adurentes ut sulphur et sales, proiiciuntur super corpora statim erumpit flos eorum [214] scilicet rubigo vel erugo. Hoc autem [215] totum diximus hic.

Ideo ut non lateat vos error qui accidit multis operantibus quoniam credentes [216] se soluisse, putrefecerunt res solutas non observantes [217] gradus et numeros [218] operationum qui signis cum a [219] sapientibus et expertis sunt notati et cum ignorantia graduum sunt decepti credunt

[180] non bene, B. [181] cum eo, B. [182] a sulphure, B.
[183] ista, B. [185] huius, B.
[184] fol. 188r, B. [186] ipsis, B.
[187] sunt foetulentae et nigrae, viridae, rubeae et albae secundum gradus, B.
[188] omitted, B.
[189] in praedictis spiritibus operetur opus semper sulfuris et mercurii oportet commisceri substantialiter vel virtute, B.
[190] written calidus et siccus, Sloane 3457; fol. 188v, B.
[192] decoquendo eum, B. [191] fulgure, B.
[193] Postmodum sublimationes et cum sulphure vel sine sulphure sicut, B.
[194] et operationes subtiliores et gradus super ipsum reiterare oportet septem vicibus aut pluries, B.
[195] fol. 189r, solutum, soluatur etiam in aqua sub fimo, B.
[196] modum sublimum, B.
[197] limatura, B.
[198] quae sic fit. Recipe unam partem, B.
[199] ad rubeum quintum partem sulfuris et 7 partes vitrioli cum tertia parte viridi, B.
[200] congelatur, B.
[201] Capitulum octavum, B, fol. 189v; C, p. 93.
[202] omitted, B.
[203] id est, B.
[204] Omitted down to Borax vero, B.
[205] autem, B.
[206] fol. 190r, quamdiu operantur salvata sua humiditate, B.
[207] unde phisica calcinatio, B.
[208] comburerentur, B.
[209] et calx demum, B.
[210] rediret, B.
[211] imbibitionis aquarum et solutionis iterum resuscitatur corrumpunt, B.
[212] quae in, B, fol. 190v.
[213] metallis duris, B.
[214] ipsorum, B.
[215] dicimus ideo hic et non lateat vos, B.
[216] quando credentes se calcinavisse combusserunt corpora in cinere et credentes se [fol. 191r] soluisse putrefecerunt, B.
[217] observando gradus, B.
[218] modos operationis, B.
[219] signis suis raro a, B.

quod ars decepit ipsos.[220] In hoc libro antequam de reliquis artis nostre rebus necessariis aliqua dicamus, de natura mercurii quedam utilia preponemus. Scias ergo quod mercurius sive in terra per opus nature sive extra per opus artis nunquam veniet neque stabit in coniunctione cum aliquo corpore nisi mortificatus et retentus. Mortificatur autem et retinetur [fol. 48v] per sublimationem debitam et per imbibitiones aquarum acutarum et cibationes limaturarum sibi pertinentium et per vaporem sulphuris sublimati et preparati precipue congelatur et perducitur ad duritatem et ad formam metallicam. Sublimior vero eius cibatio est marcasita alba ad album et rubea ad rubeum. Et scias quod hoc probatum est. In sublimatione vero ipsius tantus sis et expertus quoniam vidi quod quando sublimatur[221] in vase vitreaco cum longo collo ad hoc preparato super manet ad ipsum quotienscumque sublimatur et non plus siccatur nec induratur nisi habeat respiraculum sursum per quod humiditas sua evanida et aquosa undet. Cum autem in sublimatione vel inter alias preparationes suas incipit fieri glandulosus tunc scias quod convertitur ad speciem quam intendis et secundum hoc observabis ipsum et procedes igitur in opere tuo secundum viam rectam. Ipse quoque mercurius inter operationes et preparationes suas in singulis gradibus suis habet multa speciala utilitates ad varias et ad diversas. Nam cum sulphure et sale armoniaco[222] sublimato mixtus convertitur in pulverem rubeum siccum et splendidum et iterum combustus in igne, redit ad substantiam suam humidam et fluentem. Et illud quod prefocatur de ipso in collo vasis quod vocatur aludel convertitur in similitudinem lapidis qui vocatur alabastrum qui dum sursum ponitur in ignem et assatur redit in argentum vivum. Et expertus sum quod quotienscumque[223] mercurius sublimatur per se solum nunquam residebit de pulvere in fundo vasis sed redit ad speciem priorem et nullus defectus invenitur in ponderi quia sua humiditas viscosa ita retinet suam calcem secum quod non vaporat in sublimatione. Fert ipsum totum secum [fol. 49r] ad collum aludel et ibi prefocatus spiritus eius revertitur in eadem specie totali ad fundum vasis. Et scias quod non omne argentum vivum est utile, non induratum nec variatum in pondere vel colore. Et scias quod non omne argentum vivum est utile ad opus nostrum. Est[224] enim quoddam argentum vivum quod invenitur et extrahitur de lapidibus quibusdam in terra. Et hoc est frigidissimum et resoluit nervos in paralisi et illud non est utile ad opus nostrum. Et est signum cogitationis eius quia est nigrius et humidius argentum vivum quam et ceteris.

Diximus in precedentibus de intentione et via et fine et possibilitate artis nostre et de sulfure et mercurio et de modis communibus et specialibus preparationibus ipsorum quia ipsa sunt principia omnium corporum tingendorum. Nunc de natura singulorum corporum arti nostre utilia breviter comprehendamus. Aurum enim primum propter nobilitatem gradum tenet inter omnia corpora quia ipsum est temperatissimum propter maximam depurationem sulphuris et mercurii que eveniunt in compositione ipsius et habet multum de substantia mercurii et parum de virtute eius et multum de virtute sulphuris et parum de substantia eius propter quod ratione mercurius est ponderosum et ratione virtutis sulphuree multe est rubeum propter fortissimam comparationem sui sulphuris et mercurii in sua calce non est ita humidum in tactu et unctuosum sicut cetera corpora. Ideo non facit limaturas nigras vel limaturas quando protrahitur super purgamentum sicut faciunt cetera corpora. Sed si admiscetur ei argentum vel aliud metallum tunc facit limaturas nigras quia unctuositas corporis sibi admixti tendit ad superficiem [fol. 49v] et facit ipsum albescere et humescere. Et quia partes multum profundantur ad centrum ideo est ponderosum magis quam propter vivi argenti sicut plumbum vero ponderosum est magis propter suum argentum vivum quoniam propter consoliditationem partium, est enim plumbum magis ceteris corporibus ponderosum propter consolidationem partium sibi debiliter adherentium et ideo minus inter omnia corpora sonororum. Aurum vero propter fortem et tenacem coherentiam partium suarum inter omnia acutioris soni est. Aurum vero non aduritur ab igne sibi proportionato. Vehementissimus enim ignis consumit omnia sub globo lune posita. Non aduritur etiam ab hiis rebus que cetera corpora adurunt sicut a sulphure et arsenico. Cementum

[220] eos. The rest is omitted down to "Nota quod . . ." B.

[221] Cf. ALBERTUS MAGNUS, Lib. IV Mineral. Tract. I, ii, BORGNET V, 85, col. 1.

[222] Cf. ALBERTUS, Lib. IV Mineral. I, ii, BORGNET V, 85, col. 2.

[223] *Ibid.*, *loc. cit.*, V, 85, col. 2.

[224] Texts B and C resume: Nota quod mercurius est duplex, quidam mercurius invenitur et extrahitur de lapidibus quibusdam in terra et ille est frigidissimus et est de genere ventorum, et resoluit nervos in paralisim. Ille non est utilis ad opus nostrum. Et est signum cognitionis eius, quia ipse nigrior est et humidior mercurio vivo communi. Finis. In both B and C there then follows a postscript on alchemical processes and their synonyms:

B, fol. 191v: Calcinatio, mortificatio, interfectio, putrefactio, separatio, vivificatio, distillatio, destitutio, unum sunt. Unde versus: Calcino, sublimo, tero, solvo, coagulo, fixo. Sic intelligendum est secundum maiorem artem universalem sublimatio, fixio et constrictio, unum sunt. Intelligitur unaquaeque dictio sub uno nomine cum suis sequentibus scilicet secundum sensum particularem. Intelligitur calcinatio quatuor modis: uno modo per ignem, sicut plumbum quod convertitur in cinerem. 2° modo sicut cuprum quod convertitur per arsenicum in pulverem [fol. 192r] per ignem. Tertio modo in cellario, vel in loco humido per sales. Quarto modo per aquas corrosivas.

Solutio, distillatio, assatio, sublimatio, fixio, quantum ad particularia unaquaeque est per se, sed ad universalem etc. Sciendum est quod calcinatio dicitur, quando durum in cinerem convertitur. Solutio dicitur quando durum in aquam convertitur. Coagulatio quando aqua convertitur in cinerem vel in lapidem. Sublimatio est quando de fundo ascendit ad superiora. Fixatio, est quando fumando non recedit [fol. 192v] ab igne, quoniam illud permanens erit, ut argentum liquescens sine fumo. Distillatio est quando distillatur sicut aqua rosacea. Imbibitio, inceratio, impastatio, est quando aliquid liquidum funditur super siccum. Finit alchimia Alberti Magni.

aut pingeret solem ut ipsum artifices ad extremum splendorem et ruborem per lateres et salem quando conburitur cum illorum compositione.

Argentum vero habet de substantia sulfuris multum et de virtute eius parum, de substantia mercurii parum et de virtute multum, ideo est album quia color sequitur multitudinem virtutis, virtus vero in vapore locata est. Materia eius vicinior est materie auri quam aliqua materia metallica. Ideo facilius in aurum quam alium corpus mutatur. Non enim indiget alio labore nisi ad transmutandum colorem et adendum pondus. Litargirus [225] etiam argenti pre omnibus rebus valet ad tincturam albam quia materia eius valde propinquioram dispositionem habet ad argentum. Quando autem est fetulentum tunc decoque cum sale de tartaro et albescit valde. Hermes [226] antiquissimus pater [fol. 50r] alkymie dicit quod si lamine argenti liniantur cum sale armoniaco et aceto forti et suspendantur super alembicum quod est genus vasis transeuntur in colorem lazurii. Et tunc si calcinentur ille lamine cum sulphure et rorabuntur super illam calcem de aceto et zerus quod est herba que vocatur ypericon fermentabitur totum simul et complebitur lazurium optimum quod erit rarioris pretii quam argentum de quo est extractum.

Stannum vero male commixtum est ex primis suis componentibus scilicet sulphure et mercurio quia humidum suum naturale est paucum et non bene ligatum cum suo sicco quod est multum. Propter quod etiam frangibilius est omnibus corporibus et facit frangibilia omnia corpora quibus miscetur. Habet autem humidum aquosum et humidum unctuosum adustivum valde et multum propter quod in tactu humescit. Non est autem sonorum per se quia non habet partes bene consolidatas et non admiscetur vapore in campanis nisi propter hoc quod temperet acuitatem sonoritatis cupri ut sit sonus eius gravior. Cito enim putrescit quia non est bene mixtum ex suis componentibus. Quanto autem plus liquescit in igne tanto efficitur frangibilius. Quia secundum Avicennam ipsum est balbutientis [227] commixtionis que in omnibus partibus mixti non equaliter fit sed alia pars est plus mixta alia vero minus. Sicut homo dicitur balbutientis lingue que verba quedam in omnibus litteris et syllabis perfecte attingit et quedam imperfecte fit autem minus se ipso in qualibet combustione quia suum humidum naturale [fol. 50v] quod liquescit in igne consumitur defacili propter hoc quod non bene mixtum est suo sicco et de facili in igne dimittit ipsum.

In compositione vero plumbi [228] modicum intrat sulphur secundum substantiam et virtutem, ideoque frigidissimum et ponderosum est valde. Avicenna dicit de ipso quod si ex plumbo factus obulus latitudinis duorum digitorum circa renes ponatur et levius camphora purgatur extinguit totam libidinem. Sed si in hiis infrigidaverit renes particulosum eris quia convertit hominem in maniam vel epilensium. Secundum Hermetem vero tinctura ad solem optima fit ex saturno quoniam fortissime comburitur cum thutia rubea ita quod totum humidum suum aquosum evolat et humidum suum unctuosum fuerit compositum. Hec [229] est finis magni Alberti.

[225] i.e. lithargyrus. Cf. ALBERTUS, Lib. IV Mineral. I, v, BORGNET V, 89, col. 2.

[226] The same passage is quoted by ALBERTUS MAGNUS in Lib. III Mineral. II, iii, BORGNET V, 78, col. 2. The herb is there given as *Zeruph*, and is merely referred to as a certain herb (herba quedam, fermentabitur simul et complebitur azurium). According to the above text, however, it is also called *ypericon*, which is probably the same as *hypericon*, noted by PLINY (*Hist. Nat.*, Bk. 26, chap. 53–54).

[227] Cf. ALBERTUS, Lib. III Mineral. II, 1, BORGNET V, 76, col. 1; Lib. IV, I, 4, BORGNET V, 87, col. 2.

[228] Cf. ALBERTUS, Lib. IV Mineral. I, iii, BORGNET V, 86, col. 1–2.

[229] Not *et* as in D. W. SINGER, No. 180.

IX

FURTHER MANUSCRIPTS CONTAINING ALCHEMICAL TRACTS ATTRIBUTED TO ALBERTUS MAGNUS

SINCE the publication in 1942 of my preliminary survey of the alchemical writings ascribed to Albertus Magnus,[1] several more manuscripts containing such treatises or excerpts of them have come to my attention. These manuscripts are of interest not only because they give additional evidence of the currency of such works but also because the texts in two of them appear to have been written in the late thirteenth or early fourteenth century, that is, shortly after the death of Albertus Magnus. Both of these early manuscripts are miscellanies. That at the Vatican library, Palatine 978,[2] comprises, in addition to the *De alchimia* or *Semita recta*, so consistently attributed to Albertus,[3] several other tracts that are both non-alchemical and alchemical in content.[4] Among the former are an incomplete text of Albert's *Liber mineralium*,[5] and Chalcidius' preface, here anonymous, to his translation of and commentary on the *Timaeus*[6] while the latter group includes an alchemical tract attributed to Rasis and Avicenna,[7] the *Summa* of Avicenna or the *Epistola ad Hasem*,[8] the work usually attributed to

[1] SPECULUM, XVII (1942), 499–518. See above VII.

[2] This manuscript was inadvertantly omitted from my earlier article, although it had been examined and noted by Professor Thorndike in his "Alchemical Writings in Vatican Palatine and Certain Other Continental Latin Manuscripts," SPECULUM, XI (1936), 373–374. The volume was also recalled to my attention by the late Monsignor Pelzer in 1951 at the Vatican Library. The codex, of vellum and paper, is written in several different hands. In the vellum portion, in which the *Semita recta* appears at fols. 33r–46v, with additions to 52v, there are decorated initials. The first 25 fols. are in a hand which appears earlier than that which follows. But both are unusually clear, probably Italian hands. Fols. 53 on are on paper in a fifteenth-century hand. On one of the flyleaves at the beginning is the statement that "the volume was bought by Thomas Ray(mond?), prior to the Augustinians from a bookseller (*bibliofilo*) of 'Annipolitanorum' in the year 1516."

[3] SPECULUM, XVII, 511–515. See also the recent English translation, under the title, *Libellus de alchimia*, by Sister Virginia Heines, S.C.N. (University of California Press: Berkeley, 1958). Above VII 511-515.

[4] These have already been indicated by Professor Thorndike, SPECULUM, XI, 373.

[5] The work here opens in Tract. II, cap. 13, "Orites habet tres species quarum una niger et rotunda . . . ," which coincides with the text printed in Borgnet, *Opera omnia*, V, 42, col. 2.

[6] Fols. 59r–62v, in a fourteenth-century hand, (incipit), "Socrates in suis exhortationibus virtutem laudens . . . Primas partes Tymei Platonis aggressus non solum transtuli sed etiam partis eiusdem commentarium feci . . ."; and closing (fol. 62v) ". . . omnium que pervenient videt et ex hiis que accidunt que sit facta. Explicit liber Deo gratias." The work has been edited several times. See especially B. W. Switalski, "Des Chalcidius Kommentar zu Plato's Timaeus. Eine historisch-kritische Untersuchung," *Beiträge zur Gesch. d. Philosophie des Mittelalters*, Bd. III, Heft 6 (1902), 1 ff.

[7] Fols. 25v-32v, "Incipit Rasis qui etiam Avicenna dicitur. De quo facerit Albertus mentionem in Alchimia sua. Cum Rasis multiloquium . . .." For other examples of this work see Thorndike and Kibre, *A Catalogue of Incipits of Mediaeval Scientific Writings in Latin* (Mediaeval Academy of America, 1937), col. 155. (This work will henceforth be referred to as TK). In addition, see J. Corbett, *Catalogue des manuscrits alchimiques Latins* (Brussels, Union Académique Internationale, 1939 [I] and 1951 [II]), I, 188; and the catalogue of alchemical books in the Palermo MS. 46–72 (cf. SPECULUM, XVII, 504, n. 2).

[8] Fols. 52v–58v, following the *Semita recta*. For other examples of the Epistola, (incipit) "Tractata sunt inter me et Hasim . . .," see TK, 724; and under "Pertracta sunt . . ." TK, 484; also Corbett, I, 51, 183; the Palermo MS. 46–14; and Bologna University MS. 139 (105), fourteenth-century, fols. 313–338.

Morienus Romanus and Khalid Rex,[9] the *Rosarius* of Arnald of Villanova,[10] and several other treatises of like nature.[11]

In the Vatican manuscript the *Semita recta* or *De alkimia* is clearly attributed to Albertus, "Dominus Albertus Magnus super alkimiam." It has the characteristic incipit, "Omnis sapientia a domino deo est et cum illo . . . , " and is in content similar but not identical with the text printed by Borgnet (*Opera omnia*, XXXVII, 545). For example, the manuscript reading "Cum igitur multas regiones . . . " appears in Borgnet as "Cum in regiones et plurimas. . . . " Also on folio 34r of the manuscript, there is a list of the various alchemical signs utilized in the text that does not appear in Borgnet. However, the desinet, at folio 41v, "vel tertia examinatione simul et tinctura separatim sunt,"[12] coincides roughly with the close of the text, exclusive of the additions, in Borgnet (XXXVII, 372).

The second early manuscript, dating probably from the close of the thirteenth century, was called to my attention by Mr T. C. Skeat, deputy keeper of the manuscripts at the British Museum. In this codex, Additional 41486, folios 7 to 8, there is a selection that Mr Skeat identified as two chapters, here anonymous, from the *De alchimia*. The excerpt is entitled "Regula theoricae" and begins "Nota quod quidam philosophus dicit quod metalla differunt sola accidentali forma et non substantiali forma. Spoliatio in metallis accidentium . . . , " and closes "Non credo quod metalla possint transubstantiari nisi reducantur in primam materiam (naturam) id est in talem calcem et tunc possible est hoc concedo." It coincides roughly with another fragment without titles or ascription in a Vatican manuscript: Palatine 1339, folio 15, that was also collated by Mr Skeat. However, as he points out, the selections in these two manuscripts differ considerably from the comparable sections in Borgnet (*Opera omnia*, XXXVII, paragraphs 2–3).[13]

[9] Fol. 58r–v, opening here without the pious beginning found in D. W. Singer, *Catalogue of Latin and Vernacular Alchemical Manuscripts in Great Britain and Ireland*, 3 vols. (Brussels, 1928–31), I, No. 66. (This reference will henceforth be referred to as DWS). The opening words in the present MS. are "Moriene querere libet primum quare. . . ." The tract closes incomplete at fol. 58v. For this and other examples, see TK, 414; Corbett, I, 32, 94, 165; Bologna University MS. 168(180), fifteenth-century, fols. 61r-69r; and DWS, I, No. 66(iv).

[10] Fols. 66r–76v, here entitled "Liber abbreviatus comprobatus verissimus thesaurus thesaurorum Rosarius. Dividitur quelibet pulvericum. . . ." For references other than those cited at TK, 386; and TK, 373, under "Iste nameque liber . . .," see Corbett, I, 155; and II, 37; also DWS, I, No. 233. The MSS are very numerous.

[11] At fol. 63r, "In nomine domini Amen. Ad huius artis notitiam integre perveniendum . . ."; at fol. 63v," Incipit nobilium et variorum nimie et eximie laudis doctrina. Dicit enim Hermes de philosophorum floribus . . . ." (For similar examples of this latter work see below note 35; also DWS, I, No. 13 (TK, 290); No. 18 (TK, 465); and Nos. 20 and 23). Separate recipes appear to continue to fol. 65v.

[12] The text continues here with additions to fol. 46v, comprising sections entitled (fol. 43v) "De calcinatione corporum"; "De reductione calcis"; (fol. 44r) "De sublimatione spirituum"; (fol. 45r) "Preparatio salis communis"; (fol. 45v) "De solutionibus spirituum"; (fol. 46r) "De calcinatione corporum"; with the "Finis operis," at fol. 46v. Then follow recipes for goldmaking, for distilling, for congelation, with illustrations of an alembic at fol. 52r, and so on.

[13] See below, note 19, for a somewhat similar excerpt in Cambrai 919 (818). For the "Practica alkimiae" attributed to Albertus Magnus in Vatican Palatine manuscript 1339, see SPECULUM, XVII (1942), 509, item 18. See above VII 509.

British Museum MS. Additional 41486 also contains at folio 1, an alchemical tract, the opening words of which, "In nomine domini dei omnipotentis incipiam scribere auctoritates et operationes meliores et leviores magnorum virorum philosophorum quamplurimorum probatas et veras de scientia alchimiae . . . , " resemble the prologue found in some of the other manuscript texts of the *Semita recta* or *De alchimia.*[14] A further selection from this manuscript at folio 196v, entitled "Modus solutionis et congelationis," and beginning "Caretur corpus . . . , " coincides with the text printed by Borgnet (*Opera omnia*, XXXVII, 561–562), as an addition to paragraph 36 of the *De alchimia.*

Further manuscripts that contain among other tracts, texts of the *De Alchimia*, or *Semita recta*, date from the fourteenth to the sixteenth century. At the Vatican, MS. Palatine 1335,[15] has a copy of this work without the heading but with the usual incipit, and with an explicit similar to that found in some other manuscripts,[16] but varying from the Borgnet text. Accompanying the *Semita recta* in this manuscript is a copy of the so-called Aristotelian letter to Alexander, which is alchemical in content and which is elsewhere attributed to Albertus;[17] as well as a number of other alchemical tracts that have already been noted by Professor Lynn Thorndike.[18] Furthermore, a manuscript at Cambrai, 919(818), of the fifteenth century, has at folios 127v–142v what appear to be excerpts "extracta de libro qui Semita vocatur recta."[19] And there are several codices in the Magliabechian collection in the Biblioteca Nazionale at Florence that contain the *Semita recta.* Some of these last named manuscripts were briefly noted earlier,[20] but they had not yet been examined. Hence they may be included here in their numerical order. Thus Cl.XV.2(II.IV.230), at folio 42r(old 75), under a variant title, has an Italian translation of the *Semita recta:* "Liber status Alberti ordinis predicatorum. Incipit qui vocatur semita iustico. Omne sapientia da dio e cum quello . . . "; CL.XVI.15, of the fourteenth to fifteenth century, at folios 1r to 13r, has the Latin text, with the usual heading;[21] CL.XVI.24, at

[14] Cf. DWS, I, No. 178; and SPECULUM, XVII (1942), 514. See above VII 514.

[15] This fifteenth-century MS. was also earlier noted by Professor Thorndike in his "Alchemical Writings in Vatican Palatine Manuscripts," SPECULUM, XI (1936), 375, item 9. In the summer of 1957, while at the Vatican Library, I took the opportunity to look at the manuscript again.

[16] The text closes, "Et hec est elixir quod transformat omnia metalla in solem et lunam in una hora. Explicit Semita recta magistri Alberti ordinis predicatorum. Sit laus deo." For other examples with similar explicits, see SPECULUM XVII (1942), 512–513, citing Bologna University MS. 139 (105); and Florence, Riccardian 921 (L. III. XIV). The same explicit is found in Vienna 5477, and in Lucca, Bibl. Pubblica 1430, for which see below. See above VII 512-513.

[17] Fol. 119v, "Aristoteles ad Alexandrum scripsit sic. Recipe lapidem animalem vegetabilem et mineralem. . . ." It is ascribed to Albertus in Florence, Riccardian MS. 940 (L.I.XV), of the fifteenth-century, at fols. 105 to 112v, "Albertus ad Alexandrum" (incipit) "Iuvit te divina potentie . . .;" and is also similar to the letter in Montpellier, Bibl. de la Faculté de Médecine 490, fifteenth-century, fols. 68v–69v (Corbett, II, 117–118).

[18] SPECULUM, XI (1936), 375.

[19] Corbett, II, 39. The selection begins "De differentia metallorum dicit. Albertus de ordine predicatorum in libro qui per eum intitulatur de Semita alkymie. Sic metalla different inter se accidentali forma."

[20] SPECULUM, XVII (1942), 512–513. See above VII 512-513,

[21] "Incipit alchimia fratris Alberti de ordine predicatorum. Omnis disciplina a domino deo est . . ./. . . ad cuius opus preparatum venit perfectum et fixum."

folios 1r–23r, has the text without a title, but with the well known opening words and a slightly variant explicit;[22] CL.XVI.37, of the fourteenth century, has the text at folios 28r to 37v, with the customary titulus and incipit, but a divergent ending;[23] CL.XVI.110, a dated manuscript of the year 1533, has the text at folios 37v to 44v, with a slightly erroneous title, "Incipit Practica mineralium Alberti Magni Episcopi de Saxonia," the usual incipit, but a variant explicit, "Finit liber Semita recta Alberti Magni de Saxonia. Nota in totum verum hec in totum album vel falsum vel malum. Finis. Finitus die tertius Febr. M.D. XXXIII."[24]

Also at Florence are still other manuscript texts of the *Semita recta.* At the Biblioteca Nazionale, Palatine MS. 955, of the sixteenth century, has another Italian version, described as "Comincia Semita recta della archimia d'Alberto Magno. Ogni sapientia da dio. . . . "[25] And at the Riccardian Library, MS. 119 (L.III.XIII), of the fifteenth century, has a copy with the customary titulus and incipit;[26] while MS. 1164(L.III.XXXII), of the same collection has a variant incipit.[27]

Moreover, outside Florence, additional examples or excerpts of the *Semita recta* have turned up at such widely separated depositaries as Lehigh University (Bethlehem, Pennsylvania), and the Yale Medical Library (New Haven, Connecticut), in the United States; as well as in the European libraries of Lucca, Milan, Montpellier, Munich, and Padua. Among the foregoing, the manuscript text at Lehigh University, MS. 57, and the selection from the *Semita recta* contained in the Fritz Paneth manuscript now housed at the Yale Medical Library (Historical Section) have already been described: Lehigh University MS. 57 by Dr W. J. Wilson;[28] and the Yale MS by Fritz Paneth, the former owner of the

[22] "Omnis sapientia a domino deo est . . ./. . . Explicit practica Alberti Magni permanens."

[23] "Magister Albertus. Semita recta. "(Incipit) "Omnis scientia a domino deo est . . ." (Explicit) ". . . fiat de sicca in sole inter duos pannos et reserva ad usum tuum. Explicit."

[24] Another tract in this same collection: CL.XVI.75, fols. 42r–43v, described as "Hec sunt secreta secretorum magistri Magni Alberti episcopi Ratisponensis que tractant de invisibilitate," and opening "Modus sive forma qualiter hoc opus est . . ." is not alchemical. It belongs rather to the several "Experimenta" that follow in the manuscript.

[25] Fols. 51v–65r. The MS includes other alchemical tracts among them (fol. 65r) the *Lumen luminum;* (fol. 70v) a recipe "a fare lapis philosophorum"; and "Galen[sic], De perfectione magisterii," etc.

[26] Fols. 127v–134v, "Liber qui dicitur Semita recta metallica philosophie editus a fratre Alberto ordinis predicatorum feliciter." This MS was noted earlier (SPECULUM, XVII, 513) but it had not yet been examined. See above VII 513.

[27] Fols. 81r–103r, "Incipit liber Fratris Alberti Allemania de Colonia de ordine predicatorum super alchimia. Prohemium. In nomine dei patris omnipotentis. Incipiamus scribere secreta secretorum multis incognita vera et completa . . ." Chapter II begins "Cum igitur ego Albertus Theutonicus de ordine predicatorum delexerim scientiam. . . ." The work ends unfinished at fol. 103r. For a somewhat similar text see the references in note 14 above.

Although G. Lami's catalogue of Riccardian manuscripts lists another codex, L.III.XIIIbis (Lami, p. 122), "Liber Alberti Magni qui dicitur Semita recta," this is no longer found in the collection. From the title, however, it would appear to be the same as the preceding item, that is 119(L.III.XIII).

[28] The MS was copied at Naples by Arnaldus de Lishout de Bruxella, between about 1472 and 1490. "Incipit liber quem composuit Albertus Magnus et vocatur Semita recta in alkimia. Omnis sapientia a Domino Deo est. . . ." See W. J. Wilson, "An Alchemical MS by Arnaldus de Bruxella," *Osiris,* II

codex.[29] On the other hand, there are several hitherto unnoted texts among the manuscripts in the European collections. Of these the Lucca, Biblioteca Pubblica MS. 1430(L.142.rubro 82),[30] which I have examined in microfilm has a slightly variant titulus, "Incipit opus Alberti ordinis predicatorum super artem veram," but is identifiable by the usual incipit. And it conforms in general with the text in Borgnet, although there are some variations in arrangement and wording. Moreover, at the close, there are in the MS two additional sections, "De tribus lapidibus principalibus" and "De scorpione," which are not in the Borgnet text, but which are referred to in the Palermo inventory of the fourteenth century.[31]

Similarly not earlier noted, is the copy of the *Semita recta* in a manuscript at Milan in the Trivulziana collection. The nineteenth-century cataloguer of these manuscripts, which were formerly in the Trivulziana Palace, but which are now housed in the Castello Sforza, described the codex containing the *Semita recta* merely as "Tractatus de alchimia" (N. 245), with no further indication of the contents.[32] In this manuscript which has since been renumbered (E. 27), the text appears without the titulus but with the usual incipit, after some random

---

(Bruges, 1936), 221; also "Catalogue of Latin and Vernacular Alchemical Manuscripts in the United States and Canada," *Osiris*, VI (Bruges, 1939), 475–476.

[29] The work is at fols. 769–772, in a fourteenth-century hand, "De metallis et alchimia queritur utrum verum est quod dicunt quidem Aristotelem dixisse cum secundum rei veritatem. . . ." See Fritz Paneth, "Ueber die Schrift Alberts des Grossen, De Alchimia," *Archiv für Gesch. der Math. d. Naturwiss. und d. Technik*, XII (1930), 408–413; XII (1929), 1–13, and 33–45. I had an opportunity to examine the manuscript at the Yale University Medical Library, Historical Section, while engaged in examining manuscripts and incunabula for the revision of *A Catalogue of Incipits*, under a grant from the American Philosophical Society.

[30] The leaves are unnumbered. This MS, too, was called to my attention by Professor Thorndike. It is in several hands. The section in which the *Semita recta* occurs appears to be of the late fifteenth or early sixteenth century.

[31] Palermo 4 Qq. A. 10, fourteenth century, items 35–36. Cf. SPECULUM, XVII (1942), 513–514. The work closes ". . . a hoc est elysir quod transmutat omnia metalla in hora una in aurum et argentum. Amen deo gratias." Cf. SPECULUM, XVII, 512, for the similar explicit in Paris, Bibl. nationale 7162; and SPECULUM, XVII, 513, for that of Florence, Riccard. 921. See also note 16 above. Following the *Semita recta* in the Lucca manuscript are recipes for "De coagulatione in candela quae ardet in aqua," for "Separatio elementorum in herba celidoniae," and for an "Elixir vitae." Next, there is a tract headed "Incipit liber qui dicitur lumen luminum," the opening words of which, "Notandum quod septem sunt metalla sicut et septem sunt planetae . . .," do not, however, coincide with the *Lumen luminum* frequently ascribed to Rasis (cf. TK, 133, 160, 619). They appear rather to be similar to those of the treatise usually ascribed to Hermes, under the title "Secreta" or "De salibus et corporibus." Cf. TK, 513, and the "Incipiunt secreta magistri Jacobi secundum Hermetem philosophum inventorem metallorum secundum transformationem naturam," (incipit) "Primo dicendum est quod septem sunt planete . . ."; also TK, 519, to which may be added Florence, Riccardian 921 (L.III.16), fols. 113r-115v; Palermo 46–16; Lucca 1939, fol. 78; Vatican Palatine 1339, fols. 72r–74v, both fourteenth century; and a fifteenth-century manuscript at the Armed Forces Medical Library in Cleveland, fols. 31r–34r. In addition, the tract may be similar to the "Inventor transformationis . . ." of TK, 366; and possibly also to the "Septem sunt planete septem metalla . . ." of TK, 663. See above VII. The last part of the codex is in Italian and in a hand much later than the preceding portion.

[32] Giulio Porro, *Catalogo dei codici manoscritti della Trivulziana* (Turin, 1884), p. 443, "cod. membr. in 4° de sec. XV." This catalogue was kindly loaned to me by Professor Thorndike.

notes at the beginning of the volume.[33] It is then followed by a number of other alchemical tracts,[34] and at folio 91v, by a "Libellus alkymie extractus de semita recta. Primo dicam de dispositionibus nominum sive specierum ipsarum. Secundo de rebus pertinentibus ad opus. . . . "[35]

Of the other manuscripts, that at Montpellier, MS. 493 of the Bibliothèque de la Faculté de Médecine, has an incomplete copy of the *Semita recta*.[36] Preceding the text in this manuscript, there is a rubric, at folio 23r, that reads: "Semita recta hoc opus intitulatus secundum Albertum." However, the usual prologue incipit is missing and the work begins with "Nunc ergo qualiter ad tanti laboris opus accedere debeatis . . . " (the first chapter of the Borgnet edition). Toward the close of the work the Montpellier text diverges somewhat from that in Borgnet, although it resembles the text in the Lucca manuscript noted above.[37] On the other hand the text contained in a manuscript at the Bayerische Staatsbibliothek at Munich, CLM 27105, lacks the customary titulus but is identifiable by the usual incipit.[38]

Also at Padua, in the University library, there is a hitherto unnoted text of the *Semita recta* in Italian translation. In this manuscript, 1369,[39] the work opens "Incomincia il libro de alkimia del Reverendo padre Maestro Alberto nel qualli

[33] The work closes, at fol. 25r, ". . . habebis effectum. Illud quem nos perducat. Qui est benedictus in secula seculorum. Amen. Explicit semita recta alkimie Alberti."

[34] At fols. 25r–34r is an hitherto unnoted tract, "Incipit tractatus alkimie extractus de omnibus libris bonis repertis et expertis per me dominum Malcum de Artisiodoro. In primis ad lunam faciendam. Recipe somarie partem unam. . . ." It closes, at fol. 34r, ". . . Et nota quod idem facit de calce lune et iovis et aliorum corporum et cetera."

Next, at fol. 34r, is the work entitled "Incipit liber qui nominatur benedictum lilium," which opens "Gloriosus deus . . ." and is similar to the text at TK, 279, opening "Gloriosus dictus. . . ." See also DWS, I, no. 350. Following the explicit of the "Blessed lily," at fol. 37r, "Explicit benedictum lilium inter spinas," there is a "De balneis," beginning "[B]alneum Marie sic fit. Recipe ollam quasi plenam . . ." and closing, at fol. 37v, "sicut sol pondere et colore." Other examples of this work are noted in TK, 77. Next, at fol. 37v, is an "Elixir solis verum. Hermes ad solem verissimum experimentum," beginning "Fabro quodam erario in terra Maurorum. . . ." The close appears to merge with a number of selections on "Aquae," which continue to fol. 91v. For other texts of the "Fabro quodam . . ." see TK, 259, and DWS, III, 1162, to which may be added Corbett, I, 81, 105; also B. M. Add. MS. 41486, fols. 14v–15; and Bologna University 474(830), fifteen century, fols. 63v–64r.

[35] It is not entirely clear where the work ends. At fol. 103r, after the words, ". . . et sic lapis in vesica hominis potest molificari," there follow "Hec sunt nomina philosophorum in magistriis suis et in suis rebus occultis," to fol. 104r. Next, at fol. 104v, another, "De diversis oleis . . . ," opening "Accipe unum talentum olei olive . . . "; and at fol. 106v, "Incipit liber secretus de floribus philosophorum. Hermes dicit in primis corpus solutum in aquam . . . ," which appears to coincide with the tract noted above in note 11. Other brief tracts or excerpts and recipes follow to fol. 108r.

[36] Fifteenth century, fols. 23r–38r. The explicit reads: "et hec est verum elixir quod transmutat omnia metalla. Amen. Explicit." Corbett, II, 120–121.

[37] See note 31 above.

[38] The MS is fifteenth century, and the tract is at fols. 48r–58r, "Circa principium alchimiae de nobilissima scientia alchimiae. Omnis scientia a deo est. . . ."

[39] The codex is of paper and the leaves are unnumbered. The hand is an unusually clear one. I examined this manuscript in 1951 while abroad on a fellowship from the John Simon Guggenheim Memorial Foundation for my study on "Scholarly Privileges in the Middle Ages."

si tracta de belissimi secrete sperimentali per el detto Reverendo padre con multa diligentia. Proemio. Ogni disciplina viene da Dio nostro signore. . . . " It closes " . . . apri il pignato et sciogli la pezza pian, pianno, che troverar la calcina dentro gía fatta, et bella à maraviglia."[40]

Additional texts[41] of the other alchemical works attributed to Albertus Magnus may similarly be noted at this time. At Padua, also in the University library, MS.1380, of the fifteenth century, at pages 243 to 278, has the *De alchimia* (not the *Semita recta*), earlier edited from other manuscripts.[42] The work is here entitled "Magni Alberti illustri philosophi alchimiae artis liber," and is identifiable by the usual incipit, "Calistenus unus de antiquioribus post Hermetem. . . . " At the close the text varies slightly from the examples earlier noted, and reads: "humidum aquosum evolet, et humidum suum unctuosum fuerit consumptum. Explicit liber Alberti Magni in arte alchimiae." Then follows in the same manuscript the text of the *Alkimia minor*, similarly edited earlier from other manuscripts.[43] In the version before us, the treatise is entitled "Practica Fratris Alberti de necessariis scientiae huius," but again is recognizable by the incipit "Dilectissimo in Christo Patri — Ex cunctis nostrae scientiae libris et philosophorum secretorum abditis. . . . " It appears, too, to follow the usual text of the work, but here has a variant ending at page 301: " . . . videbis ea in corporibus humanis et metallorum substantia mirabilia apparere. Explicit. Finis practicae."[44]

[40] After several blank leaves in the manuscript there begins an Italian translation of Nicholas di Conti: "Incomincia il libro del'archimia de magistro Nicolò di Conti della Marca Trivisana. Una cossa é in medicina de tutte le cosse, la rosera. . . ." It closes ". . . pexi de venere equesto fa in tre fusione e sera bene purgada senza alguna rotura over frazione." This tract does not appear to have any similarity to the alchemical texts attributed to Nicolaus de Comitibus in Lynn Thorndike, *History of Magic and Experimental Science* (1934), III, Chapter X.

[41] Note might also be taken here of a selection from the *Semita recta* indicated by Dr Dorothea Waley Singer in Edinburgh University MS. 131 (old numbering D 6 V 17), of the fifteenth century, fols. 112 to 115. The tract is here anonymous, and after the heading, "Notabilia pulchra circa artem," opens with the "Alkimia est ars ab alchimo inventa . . ." of Chapter II in the text printed by Borgnet.

[42] See SPECULUM, XVII (1942), 504, item 1; edited *Isis*, XXXV (1944), 303–316. See above VII 504.

[43] SPECULUM, XVII (1942), 504, item 2; edited *Isis*, XXXII (1949), 267–300. See above VII 504.

[44] For other tracts entitled *Practica*, which do not, however, coincide with the above, see SPECULUM, XVII (1942), 509, items 18–19; and SPECULUM, XI (1936), 377.

The *Practica* is followed in the Padua manuscript, at pp. 309–333, after two blank leaves, in a hand different and probably later than the preceding, by the "Liber lucis Fratris Johannis de Rupecissa ordinis minorum," opening "Consideravi tribulationes philosophorum. . . ." (For other texts of this work see TK, 117). Next, at pp. 331–336, "Sequuntur excerpta ex libro de quinta essentia. Modus extrahendi quintam essentiam . . . gloriosus Deus et sublimis ita ordinavit. . . ." (For further examples of this work on the fifth essence, see TK, 155, 215, 329; and L. Thorndike, *History of Magic and Experimental Science*, III, appendices 22–23).

The remainder of the manuscript is in Italian in what appears to be a sixteenth-century hand. After two blank pages (337–339), there follows, at p. 340, an Italian text of Antonius del Abbatia, on the Fifth essence: "Questa e opera et dottrina del Reverendo Sacerdoto Messer Patre Antonio dall'Abbatia, qual tratta di far la quinta essentia. In prima piglia del meglior vino negro di portrai . . . ," closing, at p. 358, ". . . Laudemo Dio sempre." (For Antonius de Abbatia, see L. Thorndike, *op. cit.*, IV, 333, 356). Then, after another blank page (359), there is an alchemical tract in Italian attributed to Giovanni Pico della Mirandola. "Del Signor Ioan. Pico della Mirandola. La theorica. Al nome sia

Several examples of "Aquae," in addition to those indicated earlier,[45] that were sometimes attributed to Albertus Magnus, have further been noted. Among these, two versions may be distinguished. The first, "Liber duodecim aquarum," (incipit), "Libelli huius series. Prima aqua ovorum vitelli equaliter . . . , " does not, in the following instances, bear Albert's name: Florence, Riccardian 940(L.I.XV), folios 1r–2v; Cambridge University Library 1388(Ff.VI.50), folios 144–145r; and Vienna 5489, folios 57r–58r, all of the fifteenth century.[46] The second version, however, which, with some variations, had previously been noted in two manuscripts: Vienna 5315, and Vatican 5377,[47] is also clearly attached to Albertus in a Vatican manuscript, 4847, of the fifteenth century. The work begins, at folio 256r, "Incipiunt experimenta aquae vitae. Inter caetera domini Alberti Magni experimenta haec aqua describitur ab ipso ut a summis quondam philosophis virtuosa approbata . . . haec descripta aqua sit descripta ab Aristotele et ab aliis summis philsophis et probata. De aqua composita calida in finibus. Aqua composita quem ad frigidas et ad calidas passiones. . . . "[48]

Among the remaining treatises associated with Albertus Magnus, there is a further copy of the *Compositum de compositis*,[49] in Cambrai 918, dated in the year 1426. From the incipit, "Talentum mihi . . . , " and explicit of this text, it appears to be similar to that in Vatican MS.4091.[50] There is a reference too, to the latter work in a Montpellier manuscript, 493, in a collection of notes and short extracts, "Item pondera ad album sunt haec secundum Albertum libro de compositis."[51]

Moreover, a further alchemical tract or excerpt bearing Albert's name is found in a fifteenth century manuscript in the Riccardian collection at Florence, MS.940(L.I.XV). The work begins at folio 73v, "Ad opus nostrum debet esse mineralis et antequam malgameter debet purgare et extingui. . . . " Albert's name appears toward the end of the work (fol. 83r), " . . . in sulphure et sic fit ut dicitur est. Metra Alberti Magni." Next, follows, "Arsenicum fore dicit. . . . "[52]

To the foregoing may also be added a few clarifications based on further studies of items noted or omitted in 1942. The "Dona Alberti Receptae Alchemicae

---

del'omnipotente Dio, Padre, Figlio. . . . " Then, at p. 366, is "La praticha. Hora veniamo alla praticha . . . "; which in turn is followed, at p. 392, by an alchemy attributed to Marsilio Ficino, also in Italian and in a hand difficult to decipher: "Di Marsilio Ficino. Sopra la parola che dice. . . . " It closes at p. 400. For other alchemical tracts attributed to Ficino, see TK, index. An alphabetical index of the contents of the manuscript is found at p. 403.

[45] SPECULUM, XVII (1942), 504–505, item 3. See above VII 504-505.

[46] See the reference in the preceding note; also TK, 385; and TK, 478.

[47] SPECULUM, XVII, 505; also TK, 361. See above VII 505.

[48] This manuscript was called to my attention by the late Monsignor Pelzer in the summer of 1957, while I was at the Vatican examining mediaeval scientific manuscript texts for the revision of *A Catalogue of Incipits of Mediaeval Scientific Writings in Latin*, under a grant from the American Philosophical Society.

[49] SPECULUM, XVII, 506–507, item 8. See above VII 506-507.

[50] *Corbett*, II, 32; and SPECULUM, XVII, 506, for the explicit in Vatican 4091. See above VII 506.

[51] Corbett, II, 123.

[52] I have not yet been able to identify this work.

etc." in Digby 71, at folios 56–60, of the Bodleian Library at Oxford, proved on examination to belong to a collection of excerpts, of which those belonging to Albertus are not alchemical but pertain rather to the *De mirabilibus mundi*.[53]

The "Notabilia alchymica ex Alberti Magni, Avicennae, Democriti aliorumque operibus," earlier listed among the unidentified items,[54] in Vienna MS. 5509, continues: "Albertus Magnus. Sciendum est quod vitriolum in se habet sulphur album inadjustibile et ar. vi. . . . " and is a kind of miscellany.

There is also another selection from Albertus among other alchemical tracts in a Munich University manuscript, Folio 673, of the fifteenth century.[55] The selection begins at folio 81r, "Nota supra punctum Alberti quod acetum debet septies distillari . . . , " and closes at folio 82r, "et corpus metallicum auge in medicina."[56]

The translation of the "Propositiones" in Chantilly 419(919), is in Italian: "O qui cosa pura. . . . "[57]

The "Regimen operis," in the Riccardian Library, MS. 119(L.III.XIII), of the fifteenth century, at folios 177r–180v, opens "Nota quod est lapis humidus. . . . "[58]

The "Trifolium novellum," in Lyons, Bibliothèque de la Ville 317(253), of the year 1556, begins (fol.3) "Subsequenti libri effectus XII continet singularissima documenta de trifolio novello. Primum est quomodo fit elexir magnum. . . . "[59]

It is very probable that further search will augment the number of alchemical manuscripts containing tracts of this nature attributed to Albertus.[60] For the present, the several additional manuscripts here presented will serve as further testimony for the renown which the noted Dominican savant, Albertus Magnus, enjoyed from the close of the thirteenth to that of the fifteenth century, as an adept in the alchemical art.[61]

HUNTER COLLEGE

[53] For the *De mirabilibus mundi*, see Thorndike, *History of Magic and Experimental Science*, II, Chapter lxiii.

[54] SPECULUM, XVII, 517. See above VII 517.

[55] Among the other works in this MS is the "Liber perfecti magisterii Aristotelis (fol. 4r, incipit) "Cum ergo studium solenti indagine. . . . " For this work, also attributed to Rasis, cf. TK, 160, "Cum studii solertis. . . . "

[56] The selection from Albertus is followed by the "Opus Gilberti Cardinalis," (incipit) "Recipe aluminis plume vitrioli salis petre. . . . " Cf. TK, 613; and DWS, item 159, for this work.

[57] Corbett, II, 62.

[58] Cf. SPECULUM, XVII, 511, item 22. See above VII 511.

[59] Corbett, II, 69, correcting SPECULUM, XVII, 516, item 26. See above VII 516.

[60] Thus for example, an "Albertus Magnus, Alchimia," is noted among the manuscripts of the Zentralbibliothek at Zurich, although I have not yet had an opportunity to examine the manuscript. See "Katalogisierung der Mittelalterlichen medizinischen und alchimistichen Handschriften der Zentralbibliothek Zurich," in *Gesnerus: Vierteljahrsschrift herausgegeben von der Schweizerischen Gesellschaft für Geschichte der Medizin und der Naturwissenschaften*, Jahrgang 2, Heft 3 (1945).

[61] In a manuscript at Paris, Bibl. nat. 15173, of the thirteenth to fifteenth century, the "Tabula de Alberto Magno posita in choro Fratrum Predicatorum Parisius," at fols. 84r–86v, lists the "Librum de scientia alchimiae," among his works. The explicit of Raymond Gaufridi, "Verbum abbreviatum," in the Riccardian MS 847 (L.II.XIII), fol. 34r (old. 57r), attests the fact that "Rogerius⟨Bacconis

APPENDIX

The manuscripts noted in the foregoing account are:

Bethlehem, Pennsylvania, Lehigh University 57.
Bologna University 139(105), 168(180), 474(830).
Cambrai 918; 919(818).
Cambridge University Library 1388(Ff.VI. 50).
Chantilly 419(919).
Cleveland, Armed Forces Medical Library.
Edinburgh University 131.
Florence, Biblioteca Nazionale, Magliabechian CL.XV.2, CL.XVI.15, CL.XVI. 24, CL.XVI.37, CL.XVI.75, CL.XVI. 110; Palatine 955.
Florence, Riccardian 119(L.III.XIII), 847 (L.II.XIII), 921(L.III.XVI), 940(L.I. XV), 1164(L.III.XXXII).
Fritz Paneth, see New Haven.
London, British Museum, Additional 41486, Stowe 1070.
Lucca, Biblioteca Pubblica 1430, 1939.
Lyons, Bibliothèque de la Ville 317(253).
Milan, Castello Sforza (Trivulziana N.245) E.27.
Montpellier, Bibliothèque de la Faculté de Médecine, 490, 493.
Munich, Bayerische Staatsbibliothek, CLM 27105; University Library, Folio 673.
New Haven, Connecticut, Yale University Medical Library, Codex Fritz Paneth.
Oxford, Bodleian, Digby 71.
Padua University Library 1369, 1380.
Palermo 4 Qq.A.10, item 35–36; 46-14, 46-16, 46-72.
Paris, Bibliothèque Nationale 7162, 15173.
Vatican, 4091, 4847, 5377;
Vatican Palatine 978, 1335, 1339.
Vienna Nationalbibliothek 5315, 5477, 5489, 5509.
Yale University Medical Library, see New Haven.
Zurich, Zentralbibliothek.

---

anglicus)fuit discipulus fratris Alberti ordinis predicatorum." Also in the "Secret of Secrets of Philosophers' Art," Albertus is cited by Hugh of England in a list of alchemical authors among whom are Hermes, Plato, Morienus, Geber, Aristotle, Vergil, Avicenna, Alphidius, Pope Innocent, Friar Robert Lombard, Friar Bacon, Arnold of Villanova (of the New Town), William Frances, Ptolemy, and others. See DWS, I, item 21, from British Museum MS. Stowe 1070, fifteenth century, fols. 32–37.

X

TWO ALCHEMICAL MISCELLANIES: VATICAN LATIN MSS. 4091, 4092

Two manuscripts of primarily alchemical tracts at the Vatican Library are of interest chiefly because their miscellaneous contents provide examples of several well known works along with a number of alchemical recipes. The two manuscripts: Vatican Latin 4091 and 4092[1], so far as can be ascertained, bear no certain relationship to each other, aside from the fact of their consecutive shelf marks. The first of them, Vatican 4091, of both paper and parchment, in varying hands of the 14th to 15th centuries, consists of one hundred and twenty-seven folios[2]. It opens with an acephalous tract, designated in the margin as "Liber qui dicitur textus". This is further identifiable by the incipit, "Studio namque florenti phisico quandam philosophie partem secretam videlicet scientiam famosam inclitam gloriosam in sapientibus occultam . . .", as a tract elsewhere anonymous[3], but attributed in the variant

[1] Both MSS. were examined at the Biblioteca Apostolica Vaticana, in July of 1937. They were again checked in 1951, and have since been verified by microfilms of the two MSS.

[2] The fols. are numbered I-III + 127, with numeration in the lower corner. At the close are two blank flyleaves. Fols. 101–126 are on parchment of the 14th century; the remainder are on paper of the late 14th or beginning 15th century. Fols. 1–100, 220 × 280 mm., is written in long lines in a semicursive hand. The ink is yellowed and the MS. is without ornamentation. The hand changes at fol. 54. Fols. 101–126, 185 × 28 mm., are in a 16th-century hand except for fols. 113, 122v., and 123v., which are part of a more recent restauration. The first initial (fol. 101) is in black ink with ornaments. There are numerous glosses except at fols. 54–98. The binding is in parchment without ornaments. I am indebted for assistance in the above description to Mlle Marthe DuLong.

[3] A gloss beginning in the top margin and running along the right and lower margins reads: "Et scias quod glosator huius libri . . .".

For a description of the nature and contents of the work as well as other examples, see Lynn Thorndike, *History of Magic and Experimental Science* (New York, 1934), henceforth cited as Thorndike, III, 182, and Appendix 12, pp. 688–691, for headings of the tract in Paris, Bibl. Nat. 7149. Further MSS. may be noted in the work of Lynn Thorndike and Pearl Kibre, *A Catalogue of Incipits of Mediaeval Scientific Writings in Latin* (Mediaeval Academy of America, Cambridge, Mass., 1937), henceforth to be indicated as TK, under

(continued on page 176)

printed version to a Magister Valentinus[4]. As in other examples of this tract which have already been noted elsewhere, the text following the prologue begins, "Cum enim uniuscuiusque rei principium . . ."[5]. It is here further followed by a list of seventy-eight rubrics of the tract[6].

The text of the above work in this manuscript is obviously a variant. It does not coincide with any other copies already noted of the work[7]. But they too differ from each other. A more careful comparison with the available manuscript copies of the work would appear to be essential before the order of the sections is determined. Until that is done, however, it may be of interest to note other characteristics of the text in this manuscript. Part one of the first book here closes with the pious ending ". . . et quod de ea in suis libriš occultaverit et sermonibus philosophi nichil enim prodest occultatio philosophorum: in sermonibus ubi doctrina Sancti Spiritus operatur. Sit igitur nomen domini nostri Ihesu (*sic*) Christi benedictum et gloriose Virginis matris eius in eternum et ultra per infinita secula seculorum. Amen". This ending elsewhere, with some slight verbal differences, appears as the close of the treatise[8]. In this manuscript three blank folios intervene before the text resumes with the heading, "Liber primus, pars secunda de lapide minerali", with the opening words, "Quatuor autem species sunt neque plus neque minus que ad huiusmodi elixir conveniunt componendum . . ."[9]. The work closes apparently incomplete, ". . . sed non oportet quod illa vasa, in quibus fixantur, habeant colla longa, sicut vasa in quibus mercurius fixatur. Et sic finit opus Ieber

[4] Lazarus Zetzner, *Theatrum chemicum* (Strasbourg, 1651–1661, 6 vols.), IV (1659), 941–954.

[5] Vatican 4091, fol. 1v.; and see TK 136, and the other references noted above in note 3.

[6] Vatican 4091, fols. 3r.–4v. Following the close of the list of rubrics, the work continues. "Ait enim Archelaus in fine . . ."

[7] See the references in note 3 above.

[8] That is the close of part one, Vatican 4091, fol. 13r, is similar although not identical with the explicit of the entire work in Corbett I, 67, 198; and II, 44; also Zetzner IV, 954.

[9] Fols. 13v.–16v. are blank. The text resumes at fol. 17r. A similar incipit "Quatuor autem sunt spiritus et non plures . . ." for a "Textus alchimie abbreviatus", is indicated as in Montpellier 479, 16th century, fols. 84v.–89v., by Corbett II, 104; and in Zetzner IV (1659), 912–934, with a different explicit, but entitled, "Practice vera alkimiae per magistrum Ortholanum", and dated 1386.

quod multi experti probaverunt, nec potuerunt illud fine debito terminare. Amen"[10].

The second treatise in the manuscript entitled "Tractatus domini fratris Alberti Episcopi Ratisponensis ordinis predicatorum", is also identifiable by its incipit "Talentum mihi traditum negotiationis domini non abscondam ne maledictionem consequar . . ." as the "Compositio de compositiis", which is found in numerous examples and is usually attributed to Albertus Magnus[11].

Following the explicit of the preceding tract is a series of alchemical verses, designated as "Centum versus", but actually comprising one hundred and twelve of them, of which the first three lines and the explicit read as follows:

Fili doctrinam sanam tibi porrigo binam
Summum thesaurum tene mente dum foris aurum
Sic amplexare tibi ne dominetur avare
. . . ./. . .
Ars complementum sub versibus hiis, cape centum, Explicit capitulum. Deo gratias. Amen[12].

Among the remaining tracts in the manuscript, as already noted by Dr. A. G. Little, there are transcribed in a hand later than that of the other works, several tracts under the name of Roger Bacon. They comprise the "De arte experimentali. Idem de potestate artis et naturae. Idem de retardanda senectute. Idem de magnete"[13]. The second of these tracts is the only one

[10] Vatican 4091, fol. 42r. The work is obviously incomplete. A note in a hand slightly later than the preceding adds that the text continues at fol. 17, but this no longer appears to apply.

[11] Vatican 4091, fols. 43r.–48v. For other notices and MSS. of this work of which I am preparing an edition, see my article "Alchemical writings ascribed to Albertus Magnus", *Speculum* XVII (1942), 506–507; and "Further Manuscripts containing alchemical tracts attributed to Albertus Magnus", *loc. cit.*, XXXIV (1959), 245. See also Corbett I, 56, where the work is erroneously confused with the *Semita recta*; also Corbett II, 32, 123. The work was printed in a somewhat variant version in Zetzner IV (1659), 825–841.

[12] Vatican 4091, fols. 48v.–49r. For other examples of these verses see TK 265; also Bologna Univ. 270 (457), X, 3, pp. 1 ff.; Florence, Laurenziana Ashburnham 1451 (1374), fols. 58v.–61r.; Munich, Stadtbibl. CLM 276, 14th century, f. 92. There are some verbal differences between the text in the Vatican MS. and that noted by DWS no. 824.

[13] Vatican 4091, fols. 50–52 are blank. At fol. 53r., in a hand of the 16th century the above titles are indicated. Below the titles is the statement: "excripsit ex opere pergameno" and below the title: "Liber rarus".

For the "De arte experimentali", fols. 54r.–67v., ⟨inc.⟩ "Positis radicibus sapientie . . ." see TK 495; A. G. Little (ed.), *Roger Bacon Commemoration*

of alchemical content. It has been summarily noted by Dr. Little[14]. But, since he gives few details for this variant version, a more detailed description may not be amiss. After the above title, the work opens, "Vestre petitioni respondeo in primis quod hec scientia currit(?) modo speculative fit(?) experimentalis revolvendo omnis sensus et modos librorum magicorum et fraudes eorum . . .". It thus differs after the first three words from other examples, although in general the context appears the same. The explicit: "contra febres et passiones animis (*sic*) et cordis vilior quocumque hec tibi rescribit habebit clavem qui aperit et nemo claudit et cum clauserit nemo aperiet etc." also differs verbally from that found elsewhere but the context is similarly the same[15].

On the last of the folios containing the works of Roger Bacon, there is a list of the titles and some incipits of the separate books of the "Liber Septuaginta[16]" attributed to Geber, and here following in the manuscript, although without any author's name attached. The first book opens: ⟨rubric⟩ "Incipit liber Divinitatis qui est unus de septuaginta, ⟨incipit⟩ Laudes sint Deo habenti gratiam et bonitatem et pietatem et misericordiam, qui donavit nobis rem quam

[14] See in preceding note.

[15] For other examples of the work, see TK 771; also Cambridge Univ. 1255 (Ff.IV.12), a. 1528, fols. 257v.–275v. Although the text printed in Zetzner V (1660), 844–861, "Epistola Fratris R. Baconis, De secretis operibus artis et naturae et de nullitate magicae", varies considerably from that in the MS., the explicit is practically the same. See also Little, *loc. cit.*, pp. 395–396.

[16] Vatican 4091, fols. 99r.–101r. On fol. 99v. there is a fragment of a letter sent to a "Reverendissimo in Christo patri et domino meo singularissimo domino P divina Dei providentia sancte romane ecclesie tituli sancti Marchi presbytero cardinali". Only the last line of the letter remains: "scriptum Ruthene non manu propria XXI die mensis Novembris". The blank sections of the fols. contain the list of books of the *Septuaginta*.

---

13 *continued*

Essays (Oxford, 1914), 384–385; and the *Opus maius*, pars VI, *Opera hactenus inedita Rogeri Baconi*, 1928, IX, xvi.

The "De potestate artis et nature eiusdem", ⟨inc.⟩ "Vestre petitioni respondeo . . .", Vatican 4091, fols. 67v.–76r., was noted by Little, *op. cit.* (1914), pp. 395–396; and *Opera hactenus inedita*, 1928, IX, xvi.

For the *De retardanda senectute*, ⟨inc.⟩ "[H]omines (for Domine?) mundi qui ex nobili bona stirpe . . .", Vatican 4091, fols. 76r.–93r., col. 1, see TK 218; Little, *op. cit.* (1914), 399–400; and *Opera hactenus inedita*, (1928) IX, xvi, the short version of the "Epistola". Chap. I here opens "Mundo senescente . . .".

The De magnete, ⟨inc.⟩ "Amicorum intime quandam magnetis lapidis . . .", Vatican 4091, fols. 93v.–98r., is Pierre de Maricourt, De magnete. See TK 39; *Opera hactenus inedita* (1928), IX, xvi.

non meruimus apud eum et tribueret nobis . . ."[17]. After a section which was restored at the close of the 14th or the beginning of the 15th century, and on which were recopied some sections that were lacking[18], the work closes abruptly in the "Liber fiducie"[19], ⟨incipit⟩ "Iam preterierunt libri apud nos ad appropinquandum tempus preparationis lapidis maioris . . ./. . . ⟨explicit⟩ distilletur cum oleo propter fortitudinem ignis evagentem (*sic*) ei et eorum convenientia".

Also interpolated in the above folios ⟨at folio 124⟩, there is a recipe in thirty-eight lines entitled "Liber rebis", and opening: "Recipe rebis qui nascitur in duobus montibus . . . et aqua predicta rectificat omnes lapides id est plumbum iovem et lunam"[20].

The second manuscript: Vatican 4092, is largely of paper, with the exception of two folios at the beginning which are in parchment. It belongs to the late 14th or early 15th century and is numbered, after folios 3 to 27, in Roman numerals contemporary with the manuscript[21]. The folios 3 to 26 contain a table of the contents ⟨from folio VIII of the early numeration, to folio CCL⟩. The end of the table is lacking. However, included in the table is a list of all

[17] Vatican 4091, vols. 101r., col. 1–126r., col. 2. The work here is on parchment in a hand, possibly English, of the first part of the 15th century. For Geber, *Liber Septuaginta,* translated by Gerard of Cremona, see the edition by Berthelot from Paris, Bibl. Nat. 7156, in *Archéol. et hist. des sciences* (1906), 310–363; also J. Ruska, *Lippmann Festschrift* (1927), pp. 39–47. See also DWS nos. 74–102; TK 383; Corbett I, 73, 98; and British Museum Add. 41486, fols. 21–26.

[18] Vatican 4091, fols. 120–126 were restored probably at the beginning of the 15th century, with pieces of parchment, on which were recopied the parts that were missing. The text continues from 123v. to 125r.

[19] For the "Liber fiducie qui est 9 (14, or 29) de 70", see DWS I, nos. 80, 91; TK 308.

[20] No other examples of this recipe have so far appeared.

[21] It is numbered fols. I-II, 3–27, then I-CCLXXXXIII; 215 × 295 mm. Fols. 3–282v. are all in the same hand (probably North Italian), in two columns. Fols. CCLXXXXIIII to CCLXXXXII are in another hand in two columns. The gatherings are of 24 fols.; the first are marked by a letter in the lower margin of the first page toward the right (A to F). There is no indication of provenance. The binding is in calf. On the back are the arms of Pius IX and of Cardinal Lambruschini.

The preliminary material at fols. I-II, in parchment of the 14th century, comprises a legal formulary. There is reference to property at Mutina or Modena and there are a number of Italian proper names. At the upper margin of the first of the leaves (in a 15th-century hand) is written "Magister Iohannes Andreas de pi . . . gnariis de Pad. emi hunc librum a domino Pol. pro d. ribus presente magistro Francesco de Pensauro 1444".

the recipes with reference to the folios, but not always in the order in which they now appear in the manuscript.

Following after the table of contents the codex comprises several well-known works: the *Semita recta*, or *De alchimia*, attributed to Albertus Magnus, with the usual incipit: "Omnis sapientia a Domino Deo est et cum ipso fuit semper et est ante aevum . . ." but differing in the explicit from other examples: ". . . et cum labor in damno. Iam satis dictum est de preceptis. Serva et custodi"[22]. Next in the manuscript is an alchemical tract attributed to Roger Bacon and elsewhere identified as the "Breve breviarum". It is here entitled, "Liber fratris Rogerii Baconi de naturis metallorum et transformatione ipsorum", and opens as do other examples, but has a variant explicit: "Ars alchimia duo principaliter considerat, videlicet corpora metallorum infirma . . ./. . . ⟨explicit⟩ et mutationis optinet principatum quare de ipso principaliter est agendum etc."[23].

Next there is an extract from a commentary on Book IV of the Meteorology by Albertus Magnus[24]: "Tractatus Alberti Magni ad literam in libro Metaurorum quarto et capitulo eiusdem octavo. ⟨Incipit⟩ Non enim negavimus hoc quot (*sic*) dicunt alkamici (*sic*) scilicet quot de omni re trahatur oleum vitrum (*sic*) . . ./. . . ⟨explicit⟩ quiescere erit incineratum, et eius cinis erit albus et similis calci".

The above extract is followed in turn by the "Liber perfecti magisterii et primo racio huius artis; audi et intellige et sis sollicitus"[25]. This work which is elsewhere variously attributed to Aristotle, Geber, Rasis, and even Albertus Magnus[26], is here suggested as by "Arnoldus" in a hand later than the rest of

[22] Fols. I.ra.-VIIIr.a. The title is in the margin in a humanist hand. For other copies of the work, of which I am preparing an edition, *Speculum* XVII (1942), 511–515; and *Ibid.*, XXXIV (1959), 238–244; also Zetzner II (1659), 423–458, may be consulted.

[23] Fols. VIIIr.a.-XVIIr.b. For other MSS. which appear to vary especially in the explicit, see TK 60; Little (1914), 396–397; DWS no. 191, v; also Corbett I, 184. See also TK 62, under "Ars principaliter duo . . .".

[24] Fols. XVIIr.b.-XVIIIIr.a.; *Opera omnia* (ed. Borgnet, Paris, 1830), IV, 738–761, col. 2, Lib. IV, tract. II, cap. 8–761, col. 2, in cap. X.

[25] Fols. XVIIIIr.a.-LXXXr.b.

On fol. LXVIIIv.b, there is a recipe: "Sublimatio arsenici citrini secundum fratrem Thomam de Aquino".

[26] TK 160, under the incipit "Cum studii solertis indagine . . ."; Corbett I, 28–30, 97, 109; II, 100; DWS 114; Thorndike III, 651; also Geneva 82, 16th century, fols. 134r.–144v.; and anon. Florence, Bibl. naz. Pal. 981, 15th century, fols. 21r.–36r.; Munich Stadtbibl. CLM 405, fols. 67v.–73r.; and Vatican Pal. 1328, fols. 35r.–39r., with incipit "Quoniam studii solertiis . . .".

the text. The incipit "Cum solerti indagine universarum rerum artificia filosofia comperierit sedulitate, tamen, karissime fili . . ." is similar, although not identical with other examples, but the explicit "et incorporentur quot sit unum. Finit hic etc. etc.(?)". varies considerably[27].

Less well known than the above is the next tract on alchemical processes: "Incipit doctrina magistri Leonardi de reductionibus corporum calcinatis(*sic*)[28]. ⟨Incipit⟩ Cum enim calcem ☉ ⟨solis⟩ vel ☽ ⟨lune⟩ que remanet . . ." Part II then follows: "Incipit secunda pars que tractat de incineratione spirituum corporum et salium. ⟨Incipit⟩ Ex salibus est inscidar sublimatus . . ."

The succeeding folios in the manuscript are made up of a series of recipes which are of interest because of the names of individuals associated with them. The first of these recipes may be a selection from some longer work since it opens: "In nomine Dei comnipotentis eterni amen. Nota bene. Hoc est capitulum cuiusdam maximi secreti in scientia nostra alkimie ad veram et probatam congelationem mercurii quam attulit ultra mare frater Nicolaus de ordine Hospitaliorum Sancti Iohannis . . ."[29]. Then follow: "Congelatio . . . per me Iohannem"[30]; "Fixio mercurii secundum dominum Gasparum . . ."[31]; "Torquena(?) perfecta probata per magistrum Rugerium de Brandellis ad album"[32]; Albatio Odowardi[33]; a recipe "secundum dominum Antonium de Anccona"[34]; Dulcuratio ☉ ☽ ⟨solis lune⟩ secundum magistrum Abraham Ermenum"[35]; "Receptum probatum per egregium dominum Gasparrum doctor(*sic*) iuris Parisiensis"[36]; Opus magni(*sic*) domini Johannis Gnamundi"[37]; "Opus regis ungarie"[38]; "Capitulum Raymundi fratris Guanfredi minister(*sic*) generalis ordinis minorum ad ☉ ⟨solem⟩ et ad ☽ ⟨lunam⟩"[39]; "Dealbatio

[27] See the above references especially DWS 114; and Corbett I, 28–30.

[28] Vatican 4091, fols. LXXXr.b-LXXXIIIIr.a. No other examples of this work have so far been located.

[29] Fols. LXXXXIVv.b–LXXXXVr.a.

[30] Fol. CVIIIIv.a.

[31] Fol. CVIIIIv.b.

[32] Fol. CXXr.b.

[33] Fol. CXXVIIIr.b.

[34] Fol. CXXXIIIv.a.

[35] Fol. CXXXIIIIv.a.

[36] Fol. CXLIIIv.a.

[37] Fol. CXLVIv.b.

[38] Fol. CXLVIIIr.b.

[39] Fol. CXLVIIIIr.b.

quam habuit verus a familia regis Anglie"[40]; "Albatio domini Jacobi de Palermo"[41]; "Alia secundum fratrem Johannem de Mantoa ordine(*sic*) minorum"[42].

Next there follow two more longer treatises. The first is a work of Friar Helias, "Incipit liber fratris Helie intitulatus Vade mecum"[43], with opening words similar to those found elsewhere: "Cum infrascriptis aquis distillationibus . . ." but with a somewhat different explicit, ". . . quorum effectu si non ignoras satis nosti". The second is an *Alkimia* elsewhere attributed to Pseudo Aristotle, but here anonymous: "Incipit liber pietatis notabilia etc. ⟨incipit⟩ Audi aure cordis que dico et in corde tuo quasi in libro scribe . . ./ . . . ⟨explicit⟩ semper ylarus (*sic*) iuvenemque reddit ei faciem et benedictus sit Deus vivus verus qui dedit sapientiam sapientibus"[44].

Several more recipes follow[45]. They are ascribed as before to various individuals: "secundum magistrum Odowardum cementum"[46]; "secundum magistrum Odowardum tinctura super ☉ ⟨solem⟩ et pondus"[47]; "super ☉ ⟨solem⟩ probatum et verum secundum Aristotilem"[48]. "Augumentatio ☉ ⟨solis⟩ probatum per fratrem Iohannem Teutonicum"[49]; "capitulum faciens rubeum et ponderosum secundum Rogerium filosofum"[50]; "ad ☉ ⟨solem⟩ secundum magistrum Iohannem de Monte Nigro[51]"; "pulcrum negocium verum probatum per quendam nobilem de Francia[52]". "Recepte quas habui ab egregio domino G. de Insule Paridis"[53]; "receptum domini G. de insule Paridis"[54]; "Experimentum

[40] Fol. CLIIIv.a. It appears again at fol. CLVIIv.a.

[41] Fol. CLXVIIIv.a.

[42] Fol. CLXXXIIr.b.

[43] Fols. CLXXXIIIv.a.–CLXXXXIr.a. It is not clear whether the series of recipes that follow the incipit are actually part of the work of Helias or not. On Helias, see Thorndike, III, 347; DWS I, no. 172; III, no. 1131; and TK 133, under "Cum de infrascriptis . . .".

[44] Fols. CLXXXXIr.a.–CLXXXXVIIr.a. See further TK 71; also anon. in DWS no. 675; and in Cambridge Univ. 1255 (Ff.IV.12), a. 1528, fols. 38r.–43r.

[45] Fol. CLXXXXVII.

[46] Fol. CCXXIXv.a.

[47] *Idem.*

[48] Fol. CCXXXr.a.

[49] Fol. CCXXXIVv.b.

[50] Fol. CCXXXVIIr.a.

[51] Fol. CCXLIIIIv.a.

[52] Fol. CCXLVIv.b.

[53] Fol. CCXLVIIIIr.b.

[54] Fol. CCLIr.a.

domini Marchionis de Tolusio verum super ☉ ⟨solem⟩"[55]; "Opus magistri Rudicum(?) filosofi moderni"[56],; "Opus magnum domini Johannis diastiri[57] de Anglia"; "Opus magnum regis Friderici siculani"[58]; "aliud domini abbatis"[59]; "Crocis ☽ ⟨lune⟩ verum et probatum per dominum Gasparum de Padoa"[60]. The collection closes with a recipe for "sal armoniacum"[61].

Still another series of recipes of which some are in Italian, follow in the manuscript. The first is alchemical[62]; the second is a formula or conjuration to apprehend a thief[63]; and a third in Italian is probably medical[64].

The foregoing recipes are succeeded by other tracts: a "Synonima alkimie ⟨incipit⟩ Aer ventus, aqua liquor, adeps est illud . . ./. . . ⟨explicit⟩ Zoar id est Saturnus. Zohra id est venus"[65]; a table of signs of Albumasar for the zodiac; and for the planets, together with the corresponding metals, and the signs used for these and other metals[66].

At the close of the manuscript there is still another recipe, in a cursive hand, "Experimentum ad fixandam lunam quod ego probavi in Castello . . ."[67].

It may thus be concluded that the tracts contained in the two manuscripts described above are for the most part well known alchemical works whose alleged authors belong largely to the preceding centuries. These are, for example, for Latin authors, the *Compostio des compostiis*, and the *Semita recta*, attributed to Albertus Magnus; two alchemical tractates of Roger Bacon; the *Vade mecum*, ascribed to Friar Helias; and the incomplete text of the work best known by its incipit, "Studio namque florenti . . .". In addition there is included a tract on alchemical processes by an otherwise unknown Leonardus.

[55] Fol. CCLVv.a.

[56] Fol. CCLVIIIv.a.

[57] Fol. CCLVIIIIv.a.

[58] Fol. CCLXIIr.a.

[59] Fol. CCLXIIv.b.

[60] Fol. CCLXVIv.a.

[61] Fol. CCLXXXIIv.a.

[62] Fol. CCLXXXIIv., of the end of the 14th century, or beginning 15th century.

[63] Fol. CCLXXXIIIr.-v.

[64] Fol. CCLXXXIIIv. There is a proper name that is not entirely legible: "Maestro Berto Geno. in Zenee(?)".

[65] Fols. CCLXXXIIIIr.a.–CCLXXXXIv.a.

[66] Fol. CCLXXXXIIr.a. Fol. CCLXXXXIIv. is blank.

[67] Fol. CCLXXXXIIIr.

Especially, too, in the second manuscript, there are a large number of alchemical recipes with proper names, for the most part, of European persons. Of non-Latin authors, presumably, are the several books of the *Septuaginta*, usually attributed to Geber; the here anonymous *De perfectu magisterii*, also elsewhere attributed to Geber, Rasis, or to Pseudo Aristotle, and another alchemical tract, here anonymous, although elsewhere attributed also to Pseudo Aristotle. The two manuscripts are therefore good examples of alchemical miscellanies, made up of works current in the 14th to the early 16th centuries, and collected apparently by some enterprising alchemist for his own information and use.

List of Incipits included in the Two MSS.: Vatican 4091 and 4092

(numbering references are to notes covering the incipits)

Aer ventus aqua liquor . . . n. 65
Amicorum intime quandam . . . n. 13
Ars alchimia duo principaliter . . . n. 23
Audi aure cordis qui dico . . . n. 44
Cum enim calcem solis . . . n. 28
Cum enim uniuscuiusque rei . . . n. 5
Cum infrascriptis aquis . . . n. 43
Cum solerti indagine . . . n. 26–27
Domine mundi qui ex nobili . . . n. 13
Fili doctrinam sanam tibi . . . n. 12
Homines (for Domine?) mundi . . . n. 13
Iam preterierunt libri . . . n. 19
In nomine dei omnipotentis . . . n. 29
Laudes sint deo habenti . . . n. 17
Mundo senescente . . . . . n. 13
Non enim negavimus hoc quod . . . n. 24–25
Omnis sapientia a domino . . . n. 22
Positis radicibus . . . n. 13
Quatuor autem species . . . n. 9
Recipe rebis qui nascitur . . . n. 20
Reverendissimo in Christo . . . n. 16
Studio namque florenti . . . n. 3
Talentum mihi traditum . . . n. 11
Vestre petitioni . . . n. 13,15

(continued from 167)
the text incipit, 136, and for the prologue, 703. See further TK 246, 343 (Thorndike, IV, 335); 720; Dorothea Waley Singer, *Catalogue of Latin and Vernacular Alchemical Manuscripts in Great Britain and Ireland* (Brussels 1928-31, 3 vols.), henceforth to be cited as DWS, I, no. 339; James Corbett, *Catalogue des manuscrits alchimiques Latins*, I (Brussels, 1939), *Manuscrits des bibliothèques publiques de Paris*; II (Brussels, 1951), *Manuscrits des bibliothèques publiques des départements français*: these volumes henceforth to be cited as Corbett, I, 66, 125, 197; also *Ibid*., I, 193, for a compendium of the work; and *Ibid*., II, 43. There is also what appears to be a commentary on the work by Johannes Mohen in Cambridge Univ. 1256 (Ff. IV. 13), a. 1528-29, fols. 105v.-165v. It there has a prol. "Studio namque florenti phisico. Investigavi radices principii ...". The text that follows opens: "Presens tractatus in theoricam et practicam dividitur ...".

XI

A FOURTEENTH CENTURY SCHOLASTIC MISCELLANY

Of likely interest to editors of Thomist opuscula and other investigators of medieval scholastic philosophy is a collection of short tracts and extracts by Thomas Aquinas, Albertus Magnus, Robert Kilwardby, Avicenna and Ps. Aristotle contained in a fourteenth century manuscript at the New York Academy of Medicine. The contents of the manuscript were noted in the recent *Census of Mediaeval and Renaissance Manuscripts in the United States and Canada,*[1] but the brevity of the description makes it impossible to adequately determine the nature of the treatises included. The *Census* further failed to take note of some of the shorter tracts or extracts. The Aquinas compositions included are the *De ente et essentia,* the metaphysical tract on "Being and Essence," which has recently been edited as well as translated into English; [2] and the *De eternitate mundi,* which in this recension has a different ending from that of the version in Aquinas' collected *Opera.*[3] A second tract on the eternity of the world, a prominent subject of discussion in the Paris studium in the thirteenth century, is also found in the codex without author or heading.[4] Although a note in the lower margin of the folio on which this selection begins states that it is from the second part of a work of Albertus Magnus, presumably the second part of the *Summa theologiae,* where the subject of eternity and the eternity of the world is discussed, the extract differs from the text printed in Borgnet's edition of Albert's collected works.

In addition to the foregoing, two other authentic philosophical works of Aquinas are found in the manuscript, namely that on the "Unity of the Intellect against the Averroists"; [5] and the tract "On the Motion of the Heart." [6] In general these texts agree with those of the printed editions. Two further tracts assigned in the codex to Thomas Aquinas, the *De sensu communi,*[7] and *De potentiis animae interioribus,*[8]

---

[1] Compiled by Seymour de Ricci with the assistance of Dr. W. J. Wilson, New York, 1937, II, 1312, no. 6.

[2] Item 1 below.

[3] Item 2 below.

[4] Item 4 below. The work was omitted from the *Census* description.

[5] Item 11 below. Also omitted from the *Census* description.

[6] Item 12 below.

[7] Item 6 below. Also omitted from the *Census* description.

[8] Item 7 below. Cf. Fr. Pelster, "Neue philosophische Schriften Alberts des Grossen," *Philosophisches Jahrbuch,* XXXVI, 1923, 161 *et seq.* This

are also found in other manuscripts under the authorship of Albertus Magnus. In context, moreover, they resemble closely the discussion of these subjects in the second part of the *Summa de creaturis* attributed to Albertus Magnus and printed with the collected works in the Borgnet edition. There are discussed the common sense and the five inner senses, imagination, fantasy, judgment, memory, and reminiscence. The subjects of these two tracts are also treated in brief in the second book of the *Compendium theologicae veritatis.* Extracted from the *Summa theologiae* of Albertus Magnus is another selection which appears in the manuscript without author or title.[9] Concerned primarily with the processes of digestion and nutrition the work begins with the statement from the authors of natural science regarding these topics. Its main purport is, however, theological in nature since it is introduced as one of the supporting arguments in the thesis, "the verity of human nature which is descended from Adam." [10] The stomach, liver, heart, and other organs, especially the cerebrum are said to participate in the process of digestion.

The manuscript also includes what appears to be an abbreviated version of the tract on the origin and classification of sciences, *De ortu scientiarum*,[11] attributed to the English Dominican, Robert Kilwardby, who in 1272 was named to the archbishopric of Canterbury. The text here included varies considerably from others described in recent accounts of the work. There is in this manuscript no differentiation into chapters of which the usual number is given as sixty-three. No one of the manuscript texts has as yet been published in its entirety. In the field of science there is further the *De congelatione*, relating to mineralogy which is usually assigned to Avicenna, although it here appears anonymously without heading or rubric.[12] Probably on this account it was overlooked by the compilers of the *Census*. The text agrees generally with that published by E. J. Holmyard and D. C. Mandeville. In this

---

work is to be distinguished from the other treatise, *De Potentiis animae*, and which begins, "Sicut dicit Damascenus impossibile est . . ." which also appears under Albert's name. Cf. D. O. Lottin, "L'authenticité du de Potentiis animae d'Albert le Grand," *Revue néo-scolastique de Philosophie*, 1930, XXXII, 321-338.

[9] Item 8 below. Not indicated in the *Census*.

[10] See the passage from the Borgnet text noted below with the item.

[11] Item 5 below.

[12] Item 3 below. Not indicated in the *Census*.

manuscript the tract is followed by a list of the seven metals and the four minerals or spirits, mercury, sulphur, arsenic, and sal ammoniac.

The remaining tracts in the manuscript are all on the subject of moral ethics. Included is a "Flower of Ethics" (Flos ethicorum), or *De laudabilibus bonis,*[13] in which are noted the laudable virtues prudence, courage, temperance, gentleness, continence, justice, liberality, and magnanimity, with their opposites or vices, imprudence, cowardice, covetousness, intemperance, incontinence, injustice, and greediness. This work which Albertus Magnus cites as by Aristotle in the second part of the *Summa theologiae,*[14] is a medieval Latin translation of the short tractate, *De virtutibus et vitiis,* which frequently appears with the ethical writings of Aristotle, although it is believed to be spurious and of a period later than Aristotle.[15] The translation of the *De virtutibus* here included is probably that of Robert Grosseteste since it appears elsewhere with a collection of Grosseteste's translations of the Aristotelian Ethical writings together with the translation of the work that follows.[16]

---

[13] Item 9 below.

[14] *Summa theologiae,* II, tract XVI, Quest. 103: "Aliquando dividitur secundum subjecta et sicut dicit Aristoteles in libro *de laudabilibus bonis,* anima triplicis partis assumpta est a Platone, scilicet rationalis, irascibilis et concupiscibilis. Et sic rationalis virtutis est prudentia, ut dicit. Irascibilis est mansuetudo et fortitudo. Concupiscibilis vero temperantia et continentia. Totius autem animae justitia, liberalitas, et magnanimitas . . ." and again, "Illa qua est in libro *de laudabilibus bonis,* datur penes subjectum quod est potentia animae, quam perficit virtus ad actum. Et ideo prudentia est in rationali cum omnibus sibi adjunctis virtutibus . . . ," Borgnet XXXIII, 263, 264. Cf. notes on the text below. The work is also listed in the 1410-1412 catalogue of the Amplonian collection at Erfurt: ". . . librum de bonis laudabilibus Aristotilis . . . ," Paul Lehmann, *Mittelalterliche Bibliothekskataloge Deutschlands und der Schweiz,* München, 1928, II, 19.

[15] See *Virtues and Vices* (De virtutibus et vitiis). The Works of Aristotle, translated [from the Greek] into English under the editorship of W. D. Ross, Oxford, pp. 1249-1251; also Aristotle, *The Athenian Constitution, The Eudemian Ethics; On Virtues and Vices* (Greek text) with an English translation by H. Rackham, Cambridge, Mass., 1935, pp. 484-503 (Loeb Classical Library).

[16] See F. M. Powicke, "Robert Grosseteste and the Nicomachean Ethics," *Proceedings of the British Academy,* 1930, XVI, 92-93; and S. H. Thomson, "The 'Notule' of Grosseteste on the Nicomachean Ethics," *Proceedings of the British Academy,* XIX, 1933, 199, note 1. Both cite the earlier work of Pelzer, reporting on the Milan, Ambrosiana MS. E. 71 sup., in *Revue néo-scolastique de philosophie,* Louvain, 1921, XXIII, 336-38, note.

The brief selection on the passions of the soul which here appears without author or title is probably also a Latin translation by Robert Grosseteste of the *De passionibus animae,* attributed, incorrectly it is believed to Andronichus of Rhodes, the Peripatetic philosopher of the first century before Christ.[17] In this brief composition are listed and defined the four irrational passions, sadness, fear, voluptuousness, and covetousness, as well as the four cardinal virtues, temperance, justice, fortitude, and prudence. The last selection in the manuscript opens without heading or author with a quotation from Seneca's *De beneficiis beneficium.*[18] It relates chiefly to the moral effects of giving and receiving. A short paragraph on what must be considered in choosing a friend, and some jotted notes in a hand later than the rest of the manuscript close the codex.

As described in the *Census* the manuscript, a small octavo (17 x 13 cm.), is on vellum with modern vellum binding. It is part of the E. C. Streeter collection purchased by the Academy of Medicine. Of its earlier provenance nothing is known. Quite probably it was originally part of a larger volume since its present 71 folios show an earlier foliation numbering from 80 to 150 with a preliminary leaf added. The writing, apparently of Italian origin, is abbreviated and somewhat difficult to decipher due to the wrinkled character of some parts of the vellum. On the verso of the first leaf is an astrological diagram with the signs of the zodiac, also the degrees, ca[lidus], sic[cus], fri[gidus], etc. On the upper margin is written: "Nota quod luna qualibet die movit per 13 gradus. . . ." The contents of the manuscript are as follows:

[1] fols. 2r(old numbering 80)-15r, col. 1, Liber de essentia et esse . . . fratris Thome de Aquino. Quia parvus error in principio magnus est in fine . . . / . . . diffinitio propter suam simplicitatem in quo sit finis et consummatio huius sermonis. Amen.[19]

---

[17] See the notes accompanying item 10 below and also the references in the note above.

[18] Item 13 below.

[19] For other manuscripts of the *De ente et essentia* see Lynn Thorndike and Pearl Kibre, *Catalogue of Incipits of Mediaeval Scientific Writings in Latin,* Cambridge, Mass., 1937, col. 570; M. Grabmann, "Die echten Opuscula," *Beiträge zur Geschichte der Philosophie des Mittelalters,* XXII, 2nd edition, 1931, 302-303; and P. Glorieux, *Répertoire des Maitres en Théologie de Paris au XIII siècle,* Paris, 1933, I, 87. Recent editions of the *De ente et essentia* include the *Opera omnia,* Paris, 1875, XXVII, 468-479; M. D.

[2] fols. 15r(old number 94)-21r, De eternitate mundi D. Thomas. Supposito secundum fidem catholicam mundum ab eterno non fuisse . . . / . . . per fidem perfectum per deffectum alterius perfectionis qui superaddi debent imperfectum dictum et sic patet ad obiecta.[20]

[3] fols. 21r(old 100)-24v, [Avicenna, *De congelatione*]. *The text begins without heading or rubric*: Terra pura lapis non fit quia contumacionem non facit . . . / . . . erat permutetur. Hec autem per liquefactionem non fit sed accidunt ei ex hec res quedam extranee.[21]

After a short space there follows a list of metals and minerals. Septem sunt metalla: aurum, argentum, ferre, ferrum, cuprum, stannum, et plumbum. Quatuor spiritus: argentum vivum, sulphur, auripigmentum quod est idem quod arsenicum, et [sal?] ammoniacus.

[4] fols. 24v(old 103)-26r, [Albertus Magnus?]. *In the lower margin is written*: Istud est de secunda parte Alberti ubi multa loquitur de eternitate in principio libri. *The work begins without heading or rubric*: Quia ergo de eternis et eternitate mundi aliqua mota et prescripta sunt secundum philosophos modernos. Voluimus hic submittere paucula. De quiditate ipsi eternitatis secundum sui substantiam et esse. Et primo queritur quid sit eternitas de

---

Roland-Gosselin, "Le 'De Ente et Essentia' de S. Thomas d'Aquin. Texte établi d'après les manuscrits Parisiens," *Revue de sciences philosophiques et théologiques*, 1926, VIII, and an edition by Carolus Boyer, Rome, 1933. An English translation is that of George Leckie, *Thomas Aquinas, Concerning Being and Essence*, New York [c. 1937]. See also John Goheen, *The Problem of Matter and Form in the 'De ente et essentia' of Thomas Aquinas*, Harvard University Press, 1940; and the review of the last named by Frances E. McMahon in *The New Scholasticism*, 1940, XIV, 414-416.

[20] M. Grabmann, *loc. cit.*, p. 301, indicates a different ending for the close of the tract. It is printed in the *Opera omnia*, Paris, 1875, XXVII, 450-53. Other manuscripts and editions are listed by P. Glorieux, *op. cit.*, I, 96. See also *Controversia de Aeternitate Mundi, Textus antiquorum et scholasticorum*, collegit M. Gierens, Rome, 1933.

[21] Not noted in the *Census*. For other manuscripts see Thorndike and Kibre, *op. cit.*, cols. 718-19; and James Corbett, *Catalogue des manuscrits alchimiques latins*, Brussels: [Union Académique Internationale], 1939, pp. 175-176. The above text agrees with that published by E. J. Holmyard and D. C. Mandeville, *Avicennae de congelatione et conglutinatione lapidum, being sections of the Kitâb al-Shifâ*, the Latin and Arabic texts edited with an English translation of the latter with critical notes, Paris, 1927.

qua sic loquuntur maximi philosophi. Postea de fine eviterno. Tertio de tempore. Queretur ergo primo quid sit eternitas secundum substantiam . . . / . . . esse evum vel eviternitatem unde medium est inter utrumque et convenit cum utroque. Explicit.[22]

[5] fols. 26r(old 105)-27v, Robert [Kilwardby], De ortu scientiarum. Scientiarum quedam divina est scilicet que deo auctore tradita est quedam humana scilicet que humanis rationibus est inventa. Prima est theologia. Secunda duplex est quia quedam licita est et dicitur philosophia scilicet que divino lumine intervis illustrante . . . quedam illicita et dicitur magica scilicet que ex humana perversa voluntate et malignorum spirituum instinctu duxit originem . . . (fol. 27r, col. 1-2, cites Hugo de St. Victor) Hec Hugo de magicis docet et sunt in XI artes scilicet nigromancia, geomantia, ydromancia, aerimancia, piromancia, aruspicium, augurium vel auspicium, horoscopia, sortilegium, maleficium, prestigium. Ex omnibus igitur philosophie dictis manifestatum est quod semper quelibet pars est utile ad omnes alias et quod principaliter sermocinales ordinantur ad reales et ille ulterius ad ethicam et ethice partes ad moralem ethicam ordinantur et ita omnes ad virtutem et per virtutem ad beatitudinem.[23]

[6] fols. 28r(old 107)-31r, Thomas de sensu communi.[24] Queritur de sensu communi et primo queritur que sit necessitas ponendi sensum communem (Borgnet XXXV, 306) . . . (fol. 28v; Borgnet

[22] The last word is marked through with red and beside it is written: "Epilogus libri de ortu scientiarum a Roberto A(?)," which relates to the next tract. The subject of the eternity of the world is treated of in Albert's *Summa theologiae*, II, 1; Borgnet XXXII, 91 *et seq.* The account differs, however, from that given above.

[23] For other manuscripts and secondary accounts of the *De ortu scientiarum* of Robert Kilwardby, see D. E. Sharp, in *The New Scholasticism*, 1934, VIII, 1-30; L. Thorndike, *History of Magic and Experimental Science*, 1932, II, 81-82; and E. Sommer-von Seckendorff, "Robert Kilwardby und seine philosophische Einleitung: 'De ortu scientiarum,'" *Historisches Jahrbuch*, 1935, LV, 312-324. No one of the manuscript texts has as yet been published in its entirety.

[24] Both this and the following tractate frequently appear in the manuscripts under the name of both Thomas Aquinas and Albertus Magnus. Both selections appear, however, to be derived from Albertus Magnus' *Summa de creaturis*, Part II, Questio xxxv, De sensu communi, Questio xxxvii, De potentia imaginativa: Borgnet, *Opera omnia*, XXXV, 306 *et seq.*

XXXV, 310) Secundo queritur quid sit sensus communis? Dicit enim Avicenna. Sensus communis . . . (fol. 29v, col. 2; Borgnet XXXV, 314) Tertio queritur de organo sensus communis . . . (fol. 30r, col. 1; Borgnet XXXV, 315) Quarto queritur de objecto sensus communis Ad quod sciendum est quod sensibile distinguitur ab Aristotele tripliciter. Quorum quidam dicimus duo . . . fol. 30v, col. 2) Patet ergo quid sit sensibile proprium et erigantur ad hoc quod aliquid sit sensibile proprium. Nomina autem sensibilia que ad presens inquirimus quorum hec objecta 5 sunt sensus communis scilicet motus, status, figura, magnitudo, numerus et unumquodque tantum ad numera reducitur et si aliqua alia . . . / . . . (fol. 31r, col. 2; selection ends) Et notandum quod sensus communis proprius est. Est sui sensibile quod est suum sensibile per se sed communis dicitur quia per posterius sentit omnia sensata propria.[25]

[7] fols. 31v(old 110)-39v, Tractatus Sancti Thome de quinque potentiis anime interioribus.[26] Sunt autem secundum quosdam philosophos

---

P. Glorieux listed the works among the doubtful treatises under Albert's name: *Répertoire des Maitres en Théologie de Paris au XIII siècle*, Paris, 1933, I, 72. M. Grabmann, "Die echten Opuscula," *Beiträge zur Geschichte der Philosophie des Mittelalters*, XXII, 2nd edition, 1931, 350-51, while reporting on several thirteenth century manuscripts which contained the two works under Thomas Aquinas' name, came to the conclusion that the second especially belonged more likely to Albertus. The subject of the two tracts is also treated in brief in the second book of the *Compendium theologicae veritatis* ascribed to Albertus Magnus: Borgnet, *Opera omnia*, XXXIV, 64-67; Cap. 36, De sensu communi, to Cap. 40, De memoria, where is considered the difference between memory and reminiscence. Cf. Fr. Pelster, "Zur Forschung nach den echten Schriften des hl. Thomas von Aquin," *Philosophisches Jahrbuch*, 1923, XXXVI, 35-49; and the same author's "Neue philosophische Schriften Alberts des Grossen," *loc. cit.*, pp. 150-168.

[25] The Borgnet text ends differently (XXXV, 318): ". . . accipit enim omne id quod accipit sensus proprius et per posterius, et praeterea suum sensatum per se et illa objectio quae facta est in contrarium, non tenet nisi de sensu proprio." Then follows, Questio XXXVI, De actu sensus communis, which is not included in the above selection. There are also some verbal differences; thus for the 4th article, Borgnet XXXV, 315, has: "Quarto, quaeritur de objecto sensus communis. Enumerantur enim a Philosopho in II *de anima* quinque sensibilia communia, scilicet motus, quies, figura, numerus, et magnitudo. . . ."

[26] The heading is written in the lower margin. See the preceding note. This tract appears to agree in general, except for some verbal differences,

partes anime sensibilis que sunt quinque scilicet ymaginatio, phantasia, estimativa, memoria, et reminiscentia. Et primo de ymaginatione dicenda sunt 4 scilicet quid sit et quid sit objectum eius et quid sit organum et quis actus eius . . . (fol. 32v, col. 1; Borgnet XXXV, 326) Secundo videndum est quid sit objectum eius . . . (fol. 32v, col. 2; Borgnet XXXV, 327) Tertio videndum est de organo ymaginationis . . . (fol. 33r, col. 1, Borgnet XXXV, 328) Quarto videndum est de actu ymaginationis. Et sciendum quod ymaginationis sicut sentire est actus sensus et intelligere intellectus. Et hec quod accipit ex verbo Aristotelis in principio 3. de anima [27] . . . (fol. 33v; Borgnet XXXV, 329) Deinde dicendum est de fantasia et queruntur quinque. Quid sit et quid obiectum eius et quid organum eius et quis actus eius et quis modus corruptionis ipsius . . . (fol. 33v; Borgnet XXXV, 330) Quid sit Phantasia . . . (fol. 34r; Borgnet XXXV, 332) Tertio queritur de organo fantasie ad quod notandum est [28] quod tres sunt cellule capitis scilicet anterior, posterior, et media . . . (fol. 35r) De diffinitione Avicenne extracte secundum opinionem Algazeli [29] . . . (fol. 37r; Borgnet XXXV, 347) De objecto memorie. Secundo queritur quid sit objectum memorie . . . (fol. 37r, col. 2; Borgnet XXXV, 349) De organo memorie. Tertio queritur de organo memorie. Et dicitur communiter ab omnibus philosophis quod eius organum . . . (fol. 38r; Borgnet XXXV, 350)

---

with the text printed in the *Opera omnia*, ed. Borgnet, XXXV, 323-356: *Summa de creaturis*, Pt. II, Questio 37, De potentia imaginativa, to Questio XLI, De reminiscentia. Questio XXXVII, "De potentia imaginativa. Deinde transeundum est ad partes animae sensibilis quae sunt apprehensivae deintus, quae secundum Philosophos sunt imaginatio, phantasia, aestimatio, memoria, et reminiscentia, de quibus primo agendum est sigillatim, et postea in communi. Primo ergo quaerendum est de imaginatione. Et quaeruntur quatuor, scilicet quid sit? Et secundo, quid sit eius objectum? Et tertio, quid organum. Et quarto, quis actus? . . ."

[27] The text in Borgnet XXXV, 328 reads: Art. IV. "Quis sit actus imaginationis? Quarto et ultimo, quaeritur de actu imaginationis. Et videtur quod imaginari sit proprius actus imaginationis, a simili in aliis potentiis: quia sentire est actus sensus, et intelligere actus intellectus. Hoc etiam accipitur ex verbo Aristotelis in principio tertii de Anima. . . ."

[28] Borgnet XXXV, 332-33 includes arguments pro and con which are omitted in the MS. On p. 333 is the "Solutio. Dicendum quod tres sunt cellulae capitis, scilicet anterior, posterior, et media. . . ."

[29] Borgnet XXXV, 339: "Et videtur secundum Avicennam et Algazelem. . . ."

De actu memorie. Actus memorie est . .. (fol. 38r, col. 2) Capitulum de diffinitione reminiscentie.[30] Diffinitio reminiscentie. Primo ab Aristotele sic. Reminiscentia . . . (fol. 38v, col. 1) Differentia memorie et reminiscentie in tribus consistit. Unum est . . . (fol. 39r, col. 2) De impedimentis eius est dicere quod fit aut ex parte reminiscentie aut ex parte organi. Ex parte reminiscentie primo dupliciter . . . / . . . ex signis et nocibus sunt et hec melius et frequencius. De causa autem reminiscendi bene vel male patet sufficienter per ea que dicta sunt de complexione organi memorie, est enim in subiecto eodem vel eadem cum memoria.[31]

[8] fols. 39v(old 118)-41r, *without heading or author.* Auctores scientie naturalis [32] dicunt quod chymus qui primam digestionem accipit a stomacho non trahitur nisi per aliquid epatis ad ipsum epar. Humor enim qui est in epate et virtutem epatis habet . . . (fol. 40v, col. 2) Est ergo 4 digestio stomachi, epatis, cordis, et omnium membrorum et maxime cerebri a quo fit decisio seminis principaliter [33] . . . / . . . sicut omni prudenti experto patet per omnia tractatus sequens applicetur.

[9] fols. 41r(old 120)-44v, Flos ethicorum.[34] (*In the lower margin is*

[30] Borgnet XXXV, 351-54 is much fuller than the text in the MS.

[31] Borgnet XXXV, 356 ends differently: Art. IV. " qui sunt bene reminiscibiles, et qui mala? " . . . " et similiter caliditas et frigus facit: Calidum enim fortiter facit spiritus discurrere et fluere formas; frigidum autem fortiter tenet impressas."

[32] This tract or excerpt is not indicated in the *Census.* Most of it may be found to be similar to a passage in Albertus Magnus, *Summa theologiae,* II, tract XVII: Borgnet XXXIII, 311-319. Questio CX, De veritate humanae naturae quae propagata est ab Adam. (pp. 311-12) " Ad solutionem autem objectorum oportet praenotare, qualiter nutrimentum fiat et semen generationis in homine. Dicimus igitur secundum auctores scientiae naturalis quod chymus qui primam digestionem accipit in stomacho, non trahitur ad hepar nisi per aliquid hepatis. Humor enim qui est in epate. . . ."

[33] Borgnet XXXIII, 318: " Solutio. Dicendum, quod propter istas rationes quidam dixerunt quod in veritate ex superfluo nutrimenti quod convertitur in veram naturam hominis secundum omnia similia, ex quorum nutrimento et augmento nutriuntur et augentur membra dissimilia, ut dicunt physici, fit generatio. Et illi tenent viam superius positam, quod scilicet nutrimentum primo accipit virtutem hepatis, secundo cordis, tertio virtutes omnium membrorum, et maxime cerebri, a quo fit decisio seminis principaliter. . . ." The Borgnet text then diverges entirely from the manuscript.

[34] This is a medieval Latin translation, probably by Robert Grosseteste of

the alternative title: Tractatus qui dicitur flos ethicorum dicitur etiam sive intytulatur de laudabilibus bonis eo quod sic incipit.) Laudabilia sunt bona quidem (fol. 41r, col. 2) vituperabilia autem turpia. Et bonorum quidem estimativa virtutes. Turpium autem malicie. Quare laudabiles quidem virtutes laudabiles . . . Triplicis autem partis anima assumpta est secundum Platonem. Rationalis quidem virtus est prudencia. Irascibilis autem est mansuetudo et fortitudo. Concupiscibilis vero temperacia et continentia. Tocius autem anime justicia liberalitas et magnanimitas[35] . . . (fol. 43r, col. 2) Consequitur autem magnanimitati simplicitas et virilitas et viriditas. Hic est finita pars huius tractatus prima et incipit secunda sic inprudentia est malicia. In ibi agit de viciis oppositis virtutibus iam dictis. Inprudentia est malicia irrationalis . . . / . . . que omnia videlicet laudabilium sunt. Malicie autem sunt contrarie huic. Omnia autem que malicie et consequencia ipsi vituperabilia sunt.

[10] fols. 44v(old 123v)-45r, *without title or heading*.[36] Quid est passio. Passio est irrationalis anime motio et preter naturam homini appropinquans. Generales omnes autem passiones sunt quatuor tristicia, timor delectatio, concupiscentia. Et tristicia quidem est anime (fol. 45r) irrationalis constrictio vel opinio presens mali presencie . . . Species autem virtutis quatuor. Temperancia,

---

De virtutibus et vitiis ascribed to Pseudo-Aristotle. See notes 14-16 above. Cf. Cambridge, Peterhouse MS 116, 13th century, fols. 241-242, Aristotiles de Virtute. Laudabilia quidem sunt bona vituperabilia autem turpia . . . / . . . omnia autem que malitie et consequencia ipsi vituperabilia sunt." M. R. James, *A Descriptive Catalogue of the Manuscripts in the Library of Peterhouse*, Cambridge, 1899, pp. 134-135. Also cited by the references given above in note 16.

[35] See note 14 above for the exact quotation from this section of the tract by Albertus Magnus.

[36] Not indicated in the *Census*. This tract corresponds to the *De passionibus anime* ascribed to Pseudo-Andronichus in the Latin translation apparently by Robert Grosseteste (d. 1253). Cf. Cambridge, Peterhouse MS 116, 13th century, fols. 241-242, Andronici peripatetici de passionibus. Quid est passio. Passio est irrationalis . . . / . . . fortitudo autem scientia durorum et non durorum et neutrorum: M. R. James, *op. cit.*, pp. 134-135. The work was also edited from the Milan MS by Bruno Roesener, *Bemerkungen über die dem Andronikos von Rhodos mit unrecht zugewiesenen Schriften*, IV Teil, Schweidnitz, 1893, pp. 13-16. See also the references cited above in note 16.

justicia, fortitudo, prudencia. Prudencia est scientia bonorum vel malorum vel neutrorum . . . / . . . Temperantia est scientia virtutum et non virtutum et neutrorum. Fortitudo est scientia durorum et non durorum et neutrorum.

[11] fols. 45r(old 124r)-67v, [Thomas Aquinas, De unitate intellectus contra Averroistas]. *The work begins without title or heading.*[37] Sicut omnes naturaliter scire desiderant veritatem ita naturale desiderium inest omnibus fugiendi errores . . . / . . . per quos eius errori resistetur vel ignorantie consuletur.[38]

[12] fols. 67v(old 144)-70v, Sanctas Thomas de Aquino de motu cordis. Quoniam omne quod movetur necesse est habere motorem. Dubitabile videtur quid moveat cor et quare motus eius sit. Non enim videtur eius motus esse ab anima . . . / . . . et huiusmodi ex quibus cor calescit et infrigidatur. Explicit de motu cordis.

[13] fol. 71r(old 150), *in a different hand from the rest of the manuscript, without heading.*[39] Sicut vult Seneca quarto de beneficiis beneficium dare et invicem gratiam referre . . . / . . . vis reddere beneficium benigne accipe . . . quo benefactori recompensata fuerit optima.

Then follows a short paragraph on the choice of a friend: In amico eligendo considerandum est quod sit discretius alioquin nec consulere nec reprehendere . . .

A few manuscript notes at the lower margin close the codex.

---

[37] Also omitted in the description in the *Census*, this work is classed among Thomas Aquinas' authentic writings. See Grabmann, "Die echten Opuscula," *Beiträge zur Geschichte der Philosophie des Mittelalters*, XXII, 2nd edition, 1931, 292-293. It is printed in the *Opera omnia*, Paris, 1875, XXVII, 311-335, and was recently published in a critical edition by Leo W. Keeler, Rome, 1936. For other editions and manuscripts see Glorieux, *Répertoire des Maitres en Théologie de Paris au XIII siècle*, Paris, 1933, I, 95. See also F. Picavet, "L'Averroisme et les Averroistes du xiii s. d'après le *De unit. Intell.*," *Revue de l'hist. des religions*, 1902, XLV, 56-69.

[38] Printed in the *Opera omnia*, Paris, 1875, XXVII, 507-511. For other editions and manuscripts see Thorndike and Kibre, *Catalogue of Incipits*, 1937, col. 569, under "Quia . . ." and Grabmann, "Die echten Opuscula," *Beiträge z. Geschichte d. Philos. des Mittelalters*, XXII, 2nd edition, 1931, 306. See also Glorieux, *Répertoire* . . . , 1933, I, 96.

[39] This selection on moral ethics, I have been unable to identify further.

XII

ARTS AND MEDICINE IN THE UNIVERSITIES IN THE LATER MIDDLE AGES

The association of arts and medicine in the middle ages revealed in the terms 'university of Arts and Medicine' at Bologna, and Padua, or in the hierarchy of the Faculties of Arts and of Medicine at Oxford, Paris, and the universities established on the Parisian model such as Cologne and Louvain, and in the frequently encountered titles, 'Doctor of Arts and Medicine', or 'Master of Arts and Doctor of Medicine', is rooted in the distant past. Indeed the linking of arts and medicine coincides with the tradition, that goes back to classical Greek antiquity, of medicine itself as an art [1], distinguished by its intellective qualities as well as by those of a more practical nature, and the belief that the exponent of this art, the physician, must of necessity be a person of scholarly status, characterized by rationalism [2], breadth of knowledge and skill in practice. Such or similar views were already expressed by Plato in his *Dialogues*, particularly in the *Gorgias* and the *Phaedrus*. In the former, he distinguished medicine or *physica* as an art, from an empirical knack like cookery which he characterized as irrational because the one exercising it lacks a concern for the reasons for the pleasure he evokes and is guided only by experience and routine. On the other hand, in the practice of medicine, the physician with a due regard for cause and effect, proceeds rationally, following a prescribed course of action in accordance with fixed rules and principles related in general to the human body and

[1] For a recent summary discussion and bibliography on the comprehensive term arts, see Henri I. Marrou, 'Les arts libéraux dans l'antiquité classique', *Actes du quatrième congrès international de philosophie médiévale* (Montréal-Paris, 1969) (henceforth cited as *Actes*), pp. 5-27, and especially pp. 6-8. The term liberal arts appears not to have been utilized before the Roman adaptation of Greek learning. I presently have underway a study of 'Arts and Medicine in the Middle Ages'.

[2] The term rationalism here is intended to convey the idea of the reliance 'upon accurate observation and accumulated experience' and the conclusion 'that disease and health depended on the environment and on the supposed constituents of the human frame'. See *Hippocrates with an English Translation* by W. H. S. Jones, Loeb Classical Library (Cambridge, Mass., 1962), general introduction, p. xiv.

the particular nature and constitution of the patient[3]. Plato had, moreover, in the *Phaedrus* attributed to Hippocrates of the line of Aesculapius, the assertion that the study of medicine as an art is dependent upon the study of the nature of the human body which in turn cannot be comprehended without an investigation of the nature of the universe[4].

The precepts of medicine as an art and of the necessity for the physician to be versed in a broad spectrum of subjects before coming to the study of medicine were transmitted to the Latin west and were made more explicit through the translation into Latin of the works of Hippocrates of Cos, the greatest of the representatives of classical Greek medicine, and of his later disciple, Galen, together with their commentaries and other accompanying introductory matter compiled by representatives of the Alexandrian school of medicine. Thus the famous Hippocratic *Aphorisms*, the most widely circulated of the Hippocratic writings, which was translated from Greek into Latin probably at the close of the fifth or the beginning of the sixth century, contained in the often quoted opening phrases: '*Vita brevis, ars vero prolixa(or, longa)*...' the contrast between the brevity of human life and the longevity of the medical art[5]. And in the preface to the accompanying commentary, frequently attributed to Oribasius, the fourth century physician to Emperor Julian the Apostate[6], the specific arts that should be studied before coming to medicine, were named. They comprised grammar, rhetoric, dialectic, arithmetic, geometry, music, and with occasional exceptions, astronomy or astrology, or philosophy. For good measure too, according to some recensions, there were added as subjects for preliminary studies, herbs, minerals, medicines, and the four elements[7].

[3] *Gorgias: Plato with an English Translation* by W.R.M. Lamb, Loeb Classical Library (Cambridge, Mass., 1967), (463-465, 501) pp. 313-321, 447.

[4] *Plato's Phaedrus*, translated by H.N. Fowler, Loeb Classical Library (Cambridge, Mass., 1971), (270) pp. 547-551.

[5] For the *Aphorisms*, see Lynn Thorndike and Pearl Kibre, *A Catalogue of incipits of Mediaeval Scientific Writings in Latin*, revised and augmented edition (Cambridge, Mass., 1963), (henceforth cited as TK, with column number), 1704; and my 'Hyppocrates Latinus', *Traditio*, 32 (1976) 257-292.

[6] For Oribasius (A.D. 325-400), see *Oribasius latinus*, edited by Henning Mosland (Oslo, 1940).

[7] See for example, manuscripts Bern, Stadt und Hochschule, Cod. 232, tenth century, fol. 4v; Paris, Bibliothèque Nationale, 7029, twelfth century, fol. 32r; and other manuscripts described in 'Hippocrates Latinus', *Traditio*, 32 (1976), 263-267.

Also in the widely known so-called *Epistle* of Hippocrates to King Maecenus, already current in Latin manuscripts of the ninth century[8], reference was made to the need for those studying the art of medicine to consider the nature of the human body. Following these specific prerequisites to the study of medicine as an intellective art, there were outlined in the so-called Oribasian commentary to the *Aphorisms* the tracts making up the program of medical studies, beginning with the ethical and moral precepts of the famous *Oath* or *Sacramentum*, and following with the *Aphorisms*, Galen's *Ars medica* or *Tegni*, and so on[9].

Galen himself had aided in the perpetuation of the concept of medicine as an art and the need for the physician to be both a philosopher and a technician[10]. His *Ars medica* (*Tegni*, or *Ars parva*), which provided a general outline of medicine, and together with the *Introduction* or *Isagoge* by Johannitius, that is Hunain ibn Ishaq, the late ninth century Bagdad translator from the Syriac and Arabic[11], formed part of the anthology or collection of medical tracts, known as the *Ars medicinae* or *Articella*[12] which later became the basis of the university medical curricula. In the opening words of the *Isagoge*, '*Medicina dividitur in duas partes id est theoricam et practicam...*' Hunain drew attention to the twofold aspect shared by medicine as an art with other arts. The precept '*Omnis ars duplex est...*' was expanded and interpreted for medicine in the twelfth century at Chartres and by the Victorines at Paris, as theory and practice. That is theory corresponding to the speculative side of medicine, which was intended to impart knowledge of the subject but not how to practice it, and practice (*practica*), related to the practical, was intended to show the reasons

[8] TK 817.

[9] For Oribasius, see the reference in note 6 above; also for the Oribasius or Pseudo-Oribasius' Commentary, see TK 113; and manuscript London, British Museum, 12E. XX, twelfth century, fol. 116v, and in *Traditio*, 32 (1976), 266-268.

[10] See Owsei Temkin, *Galenism: Rise and Decline of a Medical Philosophy* (Ithaca, 1973), 38, 69 ff., 100-101; and Richard Walzer, 'New light on Galen's moral philosophy (from a newly discovered Arabic source)', *The Classical Quarterly*, 43 (1949), p. 82; also Lynn Thorndike, *A History of Magic and Experimental Science* (New York, 1964), I, 123-124.

[11] TK 856; Temkin, *Galenism*, pp. 105ff.

[12] Temkin, *Galenism*, p. 100ff.; Arnold C. Klebs, *Incunabula scientifica et medica: Short Title List* (Bruges, 1938), p. 62; and see Alexandre Birkenmaijer, 'Le rôle joué par les médecins', *Studia Copernicana*, I (Warszawa, 1970), pp. 73-101 (especially 77ff.), for Maurus of Salerno's commentary on the *Ars medicinae* in the twelfth century.

for which the knowledge acquired was being put into practice. But it did not describe the actual practice itself[13]. Such manual activity or practice had, however, been earlier described in a commentary on the early text of the *Aphorisms*, where *practica* was specifically defined as that which the physician performs manually[14]. Moreover, actual practice or experience, under a trained physician was part of the statutory requirements for the license in the medical faculty in the fourteenth century at Paris and elsewhere[15]. And a fifteenth century commentator on the *Aphorisms*, Matheolus of Perugia at Padua, especially emphasized the importance and necessity for such practical experience[16].

From the foregoing brief sketch, intended primarily to make clear the hoary antiquity of the association of the liberal arts with the art of medicine, and of the concept of the physician as both scholar and technician, which continued to be manifest throughout the middle ages[17], we may turn to our present theme, the nature of the association of arts and medicine in the later middle ages and the measures taken particularly in the University of Paris and the universities established on the parisian model, such as Cologne and Louvain, to ensure the continued adherence to the concept of the physician as scholar and technician.

At Paris scholarly activities had continued through the later fourteenth and fifteenth centuries in the face of greater than usual calamities. That is despite the deliterious and cumulative effects of the devastation caused by the Hundred Years War between the French and the English, the recurrent Black Death, the Schism, and the attendant social, political and economic ills[18], the Arts Faculty, with only

[13] Richard W. Hunt, 'The Introduction to the "Artes"', *Studia mediaevalia in honorem admodum Reverendi Patris Josephi Martini* (R.J. Martin, O.P.) (Brugis Flandrorum [1943]), pp. 85-98.

[14] See the commentary on the *Aphorisms* in MS Glasgow, Univ., Hunt. 96, ninth century, fol. 98^{v}: 'Medicina partitur secundum minorem partionem in partes duas id est theurica (*sic*) et practica. Theurica est quod intellectum medico subcumbit. Practica enim quod operantur manibus a medico sit...': *Traditio*, 32 (1976), 262; Luke Demaitre, 'Theory and Practice in Medical Education at the University of Montpellier in the Thirteenth and Fourteenth Centuries', *Journal of the History of Medicine and allied Sciences*, 30 (1975), 105.

[15] See below.

[16] See Pearl Kibre and Nancy Siraisi, 'Matheolus of Perugia's Commentary on the Preface to the *Aphorisms* of Hippocrates', *Bulletin of the History of Medicine*, 49 (1975), especially pp. 414-417 et passim.

[17] I presently have underway a study of 'Arts and Medicine in the Middle Ages'.

[18] Pearl Kibre, *Scholarly Privileges in the Middle Ages* (Cambridge, Mass., 1962), pp. 151 ff.; 179 ff.

occasional interruptions, had continued to function and to provide the basis and foundation for not only medical studies but also for the other two higher faculties of law and theology[19]. According to the statutes reiterated in the second half of the fourteenth century and again in the fifteenth century, all members of the Faculty of Medicine were required to have first qualified in arts. And this dictum was apparently followed at both Cologne and Louvain[20]. Indeed, as the records show, masters or licentiates in medicine at Paris were, with few or no exceptions already masters or licentiates in arts[21]. And at Louvain, one of the first scholars summoned to teach medicine, was Johannes Van Eel or de Neele de Breda, master of arts and doctor of medicine from Paris, and the first candidate promoted to the doctorate in medicine at Louvain in 1433, Johannes Stockelpot, was already a master and professor of arts[22].

Hence, mindful not only of the statutory requirements for a prior training in arts, but also of the apparent compliance with them by those who became members of the medical faculty, we may with probable profit examine briefly the nature and content of the requisite program in arts, in order to determine the extent to which it contributed to the ideal of the physician as scholar and technician. Although the documentary provisions on the content of the arts curriculum are meagre, their outlines have become clearer as a result of the earlier studies of such scholars as Louis John Paetow, Mgr. Martin Grabmann, F. Van Steenberghen, Mgr. Palémon Glorieux, M.-D. Chenu, O.P.,

[19] See James A. Weisheipl, O.P., 'The Place of the Liberal Arts in the University Curriculum during the XIVth and XVth Centuries', *Actes* (1969), pp. 209 ff.

[20] *Chartularium universitatis Parisiensis*, edited by H. Denifle and E. Chatelain, 4 volumes (Parisiis, 1891-1899, reprinted Paris, 1964) (henceforth cited as *Chart.*), II, no. 1185, p. 678, where the specific subjects are named. These are designated as 'scientiae inferiores, sc. grammatica, logica, physica, etc.' and they are characterized as the 'via et fundamentum ascendendi ad superiores...', *Chart.*, II, no. 1037, p. 501; no. 1187, p. 688; and see Mgr. de Ram, 'Anciens statuts de la faculté de médecine de Louvain', *Académie royale de Belgique*, *Commission royale d'histoire*, *Bulletin*, third series, 5 (Bruxelles, 1863), 391-418 (especially p. 391). The statutes of the medical faculty at Louvain were largely based on the statutes drawn up in 1393 by the faculty of medicine in Cologne (F.J. Bianco, *Die alte Universität Köln und die spätern Gelehrten-Schulen dieser Stadt*, I (Köln, 1855), p. 24 of the Appendix).

[21] See for example the 'Rotulus doctorum in medicina universitatis Paris.', *Chart.*, II, no. 1164, pp. 629-630.

[22] For Johannes de Neele de Breda, and Johannes Stockelpot, see Mgr. de Ram, 'Anciens statuts', p. 392; also E. Reusens, *Documents relatifs à l'histoire de l'université de Louvain (1425-1797)* (Louvain, 1893-1902), tome I, 'L'université en général', pp. 72-78; for Johannes de Neele, and for Johannes Stockelpot of Louvain, pp. 79 ff., p. 131.

Astrik L. Gabriel, James A. Weisheipl, O.P., J. Paquet, R. Josef Martin, O.P., and a host of others[23]. In general the arts program at Paris and at the other continental universities following the example of Paris, comprised a fairly broad spectrum of subjects under the three philosophies, rational, natural, and moral, introduced at Paris probably in the second half of the thirteenth century with the incorporation of the entire Aristotelian Corpus of writings[24]. In the first or rational philosophy, there were included in theory at least, the disciplines of the old trivium, that is grammar, rhetoric, and logic or dialectics. In grammar until the year 1366, when reform statutes were adopted at Paris, those seeking the license in arts were expected to demonstrate their competence in the subjects covered by the late classical grammarians Donatus and Priscian who had provided guidance in Latin grammar and usage in schools from the sixth century in western Europe[25]. Both authors had used examples drawn from classical writers to illustrate grammatical usage and had indeed helped to preserve knowledge of those authors, although there was no provision in the statutes for the reading of such works themselves. Nevertheless, it would appear that the candidate for the license who had had to master the contents of Donatus and Priscian could have had a good command of the Latin language, at least on its grammatical side. However, in the fourteenth century at Paris, there was a tendency, whether from the calamitous situation of the city or not, is not clear, to waive or modify the requirements relating to Donatus and Priscian, with an apparent decline in grammatical competence[26].

[23] For a general survey of the Faculty of Arts at Paris, with previous bibliography on the subject, see the introduction of Mgr. Palémon Glorieux, *La faculté des arts et ses maîtres au XIIIe siècle* (Paris, 1971); and the various essays on the subject in the *Actes du quatrième congrès international de philosophie médiévale* (Montréal and Paris, 1969); also R.M. Martin, O.P., 'Travaux récents relatifs à la faculté des arts aux XIIIe et XIVe siècles', *Revue d'histoire ecclésiastique*, 31 (1935), 359-368; and Jacques Paquet, 'Statuts de la faculté des arts de Louvain (1567-1568?)', *Bulletin de la Commission royale d'histoire*, 136 (1970-1971), pp. 179-271, with helpful references and bibliography for the fifteenth century.

[24] *Chart.*, I, no. 246, p. 677, March 19, 1255.

[25] *Chart.*, II, no. 1185, p. 673; no. 1165, pp. 632-648; no. 1184, pp. 661-671; notes 24a, 33, and 1156, pp. 621-622, note 10. For the texts see the references in the following note, also Wayland Johnson Chase, *The Ars minor of Donatus*, English translation with introduction, University of Wisconsin Studies in the Social Sciences and History, 11 (Madison, 1926).

[26] *Chart.*, II, no. 1185, p. 678, especially items (14), and 4; also III, Introduction, xi-xiii. For the texts of the grammarians, see Henricus Keil, *Grammatici Latini* (Leipzig, 1864), volume IV.

Hence under the reform statutes of 1366, at Paris, for reasons that are not entirely clear, that is possibly because of antipathy toward the pagan content of the time honored grammarians or perhaps for the more likely reason that members of the faculty wished to utilize more up-to-date texts, Donatus and Priscian were replaced by the more recent grammarians Alexander of Villadieu and Eberhard of Bethune. The former, a Franciscan friar, had earlier been a student at Paris and had composed his grammar or *Doctrinale* in about 1199, while the latter had written his *Graecismus* in about 1202. Both so-called new grammars were composed in metrical form in hexameters, and unlike the works of Donatus and Priscian, their authors used as illustrative examples, passages from earlier medieval Christian authors. However, both authors based their grammatical structure on the earlier works of Donatus and Priscian. They thus presupposed a grounding in the works of those authors, that is preliminary grammatical training which was presumably to have been acquired by students either before coming to Paris, or in the special preparatory grammar schools maintained and supervised by the Faculty of Arts[27]. Under the new reform statutes of 1366, the grammar requirement encompassing the *Doctrinale* and the *Graecismus* could not be waived. Similar requirements were also incorporated into the statutes of the newly founded universities of Cologne and Louvain. At Oxford, however, Donatus and Priscian continued to be included under the statutory requirements[28].

As for the second component of the trivium, rhetoric, there is no mention in the Paris statutes. However, this lacuna does not mean, that at Paris there was no teaching of rhetoric, a subject which Peter of Abano in the early fourteenth century, on the authority of Galen and Alpha-

[27] L.J. Paetow, *The Arts Course at Medieval Universities with Special Reference to Grammar and Rhetoric*, The University Studies, 3, no. 7 (Urbana-Champaign, Ill., 1910), chapters 1 and 2; also A.L. Gabriel, 'Preparatory Teaching in the Parisian Colleges during the Fourteenth Century', *Garlandia: Studies in the History of the Mediaeval University* (Frankfurt am Main, 1969), chapter 4. See also H. Roos, 'Le *trivium* à l'université au XIIIe siècle', *Actes* (1969), 193-196.

[28] *Chart.*, III, Introduction xi-xiii; also no. 1319, January 5, 1366; on Louvain, see Henry De Vocht, *History of the Foundation and the Rise of the 'Collegium Trilingue Lovaniense', 1517-1550*, tome I, *The Foundation*, Recueil de travaux d'Histoire et de Philologie — Publicaties op het gebied der Geschiedenis en der Philologie, series 3, no. 42 (Louvain, 1951), pp. 80-82; E. Reusens, 'Statuts primitifs de la Faculté des Arts de Louvain', *Académie royale de Belgique, Commission royale d'histoire, Bulletin*, third series, 9 (Bruxelles, 1867), 152, 156, 175-176, 178; and for Oxford, *Statuta antiqua universitatis Oxoniensis*, edited by Strickland Gibson (Oxford, 1931), XCII, 32, 33-34, a. 1340, and a. 1409, and thereafter, pp. 200-201.

rabi, had deemed essential for the physician. Peter of Abano had gone on to explain that the physician needed to know rhetoric so that he might persuade his patients to follow the course of treatment prescribed, and also, following Galen's lead, so that he might understand medical metaphors such as the brain rules the body, as the king has the highest place in a city, and the heart is the seat of bravery or fear, hence a coward is said to lack heart[29]. Rhetoric indeed was being offered in the later fourteenth century according to contemporary reports. For example, Nicholas of Clemanges, rector of the University of Paris in 1393, rose to the defense of Paris against Petrarch's assertion that rhetoric and the poets were taught to a far greater extent in Italy than elsewhere. Nicholas replied that he had seen and heard lectures being given in the Paris studium on the *Rhetoric* of both Aristotle and Cicero, and that the best of the poets, Virgil, Horace, Terence, Ovid, and so on, were indeed being taught and read[30]. And Pierre d'Ailly, chancellor in 1389, and later Cardinal in 1411, corroborated this. He described the program encompassing those authors who were being lectured on in the last decade of the fourteenth century at Paris. He reported that in the first school of philosophy (that is under rational philosophy), he found the doctors according to their Faculty, offering the rudiments of grammar in Priscian; the logicalia of Aristotle; the rhetorical blandishments of Tullius Cicero and others, the poets and prose writers, Virgil, Ovid, Fulgentius, Horace, Orosius, Juvenal's *Satires*, Seneca's *Tragedies*, Terence's *Comedies*, Sallust, Sidonius's *Epistolae*, Cassiodorus's *Formulae*, Martial's *Epigrams*, Titus Livy's *Decades*, Valerius Maximus, and others[31]. Moreover, the humanist tastes of Jean Gerson, chancellor in 1395, as revealed in his sermons, and demonstrated by the recent researches of Gilbert Ouy[32], and the manifest interest in rhetoric of Guillaume Fichet, at Paris in 1449, and rector of the university in the year 1467, portrayed by Jacques Monfrin[33], were, in all likelihood, reflected in the teaching

[29] Cf. H. Roos, 'Le *trivium*', *Actes* (1969), p. 197; and see Peter of Abano, *Conciliator differentiarum philosophorum et praecipue medicorum* (Venetiis, 1496), Diff. 1, fol. 5a; also Diff. 135; 66.

[30] Nicholas of Clemanges (1365-1437), *Chart.*, III, no. 1650, pp. 589-590.

[31] Pierre d'Ailly (c. 1350-1420), *Chart.*, III, xi.

[32] For Jean Gerson (1363-1429), see J.L. Connolly, *John Gerson, Reformer and Mystic* (Louvain, 1928), especially pp. 141-143, and the forthcoming account by Gilbert Ouy.

[33] On Guillaume Fichet (1433- c. 1480), see the forthcoming account by Jacques Monfrin.

in the Faculty of Arts. A similar conclusion may in all probability be drawn for Cologne and Louvain. At Louvain, for example, Antonius Haneron, the forerunner of Carolus Viruli and the humanists of the age of Erasmus, was active as a professor of the Latin language between 1430 and 1438. His handbook based on the work of Alexander of Villedieu and classical sources was utilized until the close of the fifteenth century[34]. However, unlike the absence of provisions in the statutes for teaching rhetoric at Paris, Cologne, and Louvain, there was statutory provision for rhetoric in the curriculum of the fourteenth and fifteenth century at Oxford[35].

On the other hand in regard to logic, the third subject of the traditional trivium, there is no doubt whatever that it was both taught and required in the arts curriculum, and that it continued, as earlier, to be considered of utmost importance to the physician. The afore mentioned Peter of Abano at the beginning of the fourteenth century, following the earlier tradition, had asserted that it is impossible to understand the art of medicine without the art of dialectics[36]. And the university statutes demonstrated the continued agreement with this view. Candidates for the license in arts were required to have studied the logical works of Aristotle comprised under the 'Old Logic', that is the works introduced and known before about 1128, and the works of the 'New Logic', those introduced after 1128, especially the *Prior and Posterior Analytics*, which were deemed of particular importance from the standpoint of methodology[37].

Under the second division of the curriculum of the Faculty of Arts, or natural philosophy, *mathematica* included the old quadrivial subjects of arithmetic, in all likelihood, covering as was true earlier, both the theory of numbers, embodied in the Boethian or Nicomachean arithmetic, as well as more elementary and practical numeration, and

[34] On Antonius Haneron, and other aspects of humanism in Louvain, see Jozef IJsewijn, 'The Coming of Humanism to the Low Countries', in *Itinerarium Italicum, presented to P.O. Kristeller*, edited by H.A. Oberman and Th. Brody, Studies in Medieval and Reformation Thought, 14 (Leiden, 1975), pp. 193-301.

[35] See the references in note 28 above.

[36] Peter of Abano, *Conciliator*, Diff. 1, fol. 2^r^; also Diff. 135. For an example of the importance attached earlier to the relation of logic to medicine see especially E.F. Hartung, 'Medical Regulations of Frederick Second of Hohenstaufen', *Medical Life*, 41 (1934), 587-601; also F.R. Packard, *History of the School of Salernum*, printed with *The School of Salernum*, the English version by Sir John Harrington (New York, 1920), pp. 34-36.

[37] *Chart.*, III, no. 1319, pp. 143-148, January 5, 1366.

calculation in the algorisms and treatises transcribed from the Arabic; also geometry based on Euclid; music largely from Boethius's *De musica*, and astronomy or astrology[38]. Of these astronomy was held to be particularly important to the physician, as Peter of Abano and others made clear. Peter of Abano had himself translated the Pseudo-Hippocratic tract on astrological medicine from which he drew the statement that 'he is not a true physician who does not know the stars and their relation to disease and health'[39]. However, although the statutes of the Faculty of Arts at Paris, included the requirement of one hundred lectures in mathematics, this was liberalized and was considered to have been met by the study of one complete work such as the thirteenth century *Sphere* of John Sacrobosco, and one other work not specifically named[40]. Furthermore the candidate for the license in arts was to have attended lectures on the Aristotelian treatises in natural philosophy, such as the *Physica*, the *De generatione et corruptione*, *De anima*, *De caelo et mundo*, the *Meteorologia* and the tracts on animals, their locomotion, parts, and generation, as well as the tracts of the *Parva naturalia*, the *De sensu et sensato*, *De sompno et vigilia*, *De memoria et reminiscentia*, *De longitudine et brevitate vite*; and also on *the Metaphysica*, since metaphysics was considered the third division of natural philosophy[41].

Finally candidates for the *magisterium* in arts were also required to have attended lectures on the '*libri morales*' that is especially the *Ethica* and on at least the first three books of the *Liber Meterorum*. All dispensations from the above provisions were forbidden[42].

Although there was at Paris, and in the other universities organized on the Parisian model, an effort to maintain the institutional separation of the faculties of arts and medicine, there nevertheless continued

[38] *Ibidem*, also Pearl Kibre, 'The Quadrivium in the Thirteenth Century Universities', *Actes* (1969), 176 ff.; and for Oxford, James A. Weisheipl, O.P., 'Curriculum of the Faculty of Arts at Oxford in the Early Fourteenth Century', *Mediaeval Studies*, 26 (1964), 168 ff. Peter of Abano's explanation of the relation of the quadrivial arts to medicine is contained in *Conciliator* (Venetiis, 1496), Diff. 66 and 93.

[39] *Ibidem*, Diff. 7; and see also Lynn Thorndike, 'The Three Latin Translations of the Pseudo-Hippocratic Tract on Astrological Medicine', *Janus*, 49 (1960), 116; and my 'Hippocrates Latinus', *Traditio*, 33 (1977), 283 ff.

[40] *Chart.*, II, no. 1185, p. 678 : Item quod audivistis centum lectiones de mathematica ad minus. (Istud per facultatem sic est interpretatum quod sufficit audivisse unum librum totalem mathematice, sicut tractatum de sphaera (Sacrobosco) et alium librum actu...).

[41] *Chart.*, III, no. 1319, pp. 143-148, January 5, 1366.

[42] *Ibidem*.

to be a close relationship between the members of the two faculties. For, although students, who had attained the licentiate in arts before matriculation in medicine, would have completed their work in the foregoing subjects of the arts curriculum, and would be expected henceforth to devote their attention exclusively to the subjects of the medical curriculum, there were others who had attained the baccalaureate but not the licentiate in arts before their matriculation in medicine. These students were permitted therefore to continue their arts training along with their medical studies. Also since many members of the medical faculty, in the fourteenth and fifteenth century, as earlier, had taught in the Faculty of Arts before going on to the Faculty of Medicine, they continued to have an interest in the former faculty. At Paris, however, once they were members of the medical faculty, they were forbidden to lecture on subjects in arts with the exception of the Aristotelian *De animalibus* and the *Meteorologia*, both of which were considered of singular importance to the physician[43].

Turning now to the medical program, the length of time to be spent on it, the subject matter and chief authorities studied, we may draw attention first to the fact that there appears to have been little change in the curriculum since the later thirteenth century, except regarding the length of time required. Also before noting the details, we should emphasize that here as in the case of the earlier provisions regarding the arts curriculum, the statutory requirements undoubtedly referred to minimum coverage. In any event in the first half of the fourteenth century, the stipulations of the statutes of 1270-1274[44], requiring candidates for the examination in medicine, who were already licensed in arts, to have attended lectures in medicine for five and a half years, or for six years, if they were not so licensed, were modified and the length of time was slightly increased. That is the five and a half years were changed to fifty-six months, which not counting vacations, would roughly equal six years, and the six years for those who were not licensed in arts was changed to sixty months[45], the equivalent

[43] Ernest Wickersheimer, *Commentaires de la faculté de médecine de l'université de Paris (1395-1516)* (Paris, 1915), Introduction, pp. xix ff. See also Vern L. Bullough, 'The Medieval Medical University at Paris', *Bulletin of History of Medicine*, 31 (1957), 197-211 (especially pp. 201-203).

[44] *Chart.*, I, no. 453, p. 517 : statuts de la faculté de médecine, 1270-1274.

[45] *Chart.*, II, no. 933, pp. 379-381, for June 22, 1331.

roughly of six and a half years.[46] However, as suggested earlier, members of the faculty of medicine were, with almost no exception, also masters or licentiates in arts.

The course of medical instruction as seen in the prescribed texts was based largely upon Greek medical theory, both in the Latinized versions of Greek physicians and in Arabized form through the works of Muslim authors who were for the most part indebted to Greek medicine. Among the Latinized Greek authors and texts were the Hippocratic *Aphorisms*, the tracts *On Acute Diseases*, and the *Prognostics*; also Galen's *Ars Parva*, or *Liber Tegni*, with the *Introduction* or *Isagoge*, by Johannitius or Hunain ibn Ishāq. The preceding texts, together with the work of the sixth century Byzantine authors, Philaretus, *On pulse*, and of Theophilus, *On Urines*, were all usually comprised in the anthology or collection of medical treatises known as the *Ars medicinae* or *Articella*[47]. Furthermore, besides the works of Greek or Byzantine origin, the candidates were to have studied and lectured on Avicenna's *Canon*[48], which covered the entire field of medicine and was largely based on Galen. Some notion of the nature of the content may be gleaned from the topics covered. That is there were treated the general fundamentals with which the physician must be acquainted, namely the physiological constituents of the body that are essential for the maintenance of health; those things that are involved in the curing of disease, the signs and symptoms of diseases, listed in descending order from head to toe; also the methods of care, diet, and regulation of the air. In addition to Avicenna, there was prescribed the medical treatise of Averroes, entitled *Colliget* or *Correctorium*[49] and the ninth book of the *Almansor* by Rasis, the tenth century physician of Haron al-Raschid[50]. This work too contained a listing with their cures of diseases arranged from head to toe.

[46] The vacations were of about 11 weeks, that is the time between June 29, feast of St. Peter, and September 14, feast of the Elevation of the Holy Cross. See *Chart.*, II, no. 923, pp. 356-360, August 1331.

[47] See the references in note 11 above. To the collection of works brought together in the twelfth century were added others from time to time, such as the Sixth Book of the Epidemics by Hippocrates, also the tract on Acute diseases of Hippocrates with Galen's commentary. See further the program for Paris in Wickersheimer, *Commentaires*, p. xxiv.

[48] TK index for MSS and editions of Avicenna's *Canon*.

[49] TK index for MSS and editions of Averroes' *Colliget*.

[50] TK index for MSS and editions as well as commentaries for Rasis, *Nonus Almansoris*, that is the ninth book of the *Liber Almansoris*, in ten books (TK 272).

At Paris, too, there were assigned several other works. Among them the treatise entitled *Viaticum*[51], translated from the Arabic into Latin by Constantinus Africanus, dealt with a great variety of subjects, including states of mind as well as physical ills. Other texts were on more specific topics, such as the long work on *Diets* by Isaac[52], or Ibn al Daschazzar, and the *Antidotarium* of Nicholas of Salerno[53]. The latter contained a listing of medicines with the various uses to which they could be put. It was often accompanied by the *Quid pro quo*, that is the list of acceptable substitutes[54]. In addition there was prescribed at Paris, the tract on urines in verse by Aegidius of Corbeil, physician to King Philip Augustus of France at the close of the twelfth century[55]. In general it might be said that as in the arts curriculum the texts stipulated in the statutes in all probability represented only a modicum of those actually utilized or read. However, they did represent the basic authorities.

Although the advent of the fifteenth century saw few changes in either the arts or the medical curriculum at Paris, the conditions in the city itself had grown steadily worse. The Faculty of Medicine had had to defer lectures and disputations because of the misery resulting from the wars, the lack of food, and the raging pestilence. Because of the multitude of the sick the regent (teaching) masters were so occupied with medical practice they could not perform their teaching duties[56]. Hence largely as a result of the difficulties of subsistence in the city of Paris and of travel in and to the French kingdom, many students from outside the kingdom withdrew from or failed to enter the studium at Paris. This was one of the bases for the establishment of the University of Louvain by former members of the University of Paris[57]. The University of Cologne (Köln) had earlier been established (that is in 1388) by scholars migrating from Paris[58]. In both Cologne

[51] TK 187, for MSS and editions.

[52] TK index under Isaac for MSS and editions.

[53] TK index for *Antidotarium Nicolai*, for MSS and editions.

[54] TK index under *Quid pro quo*, for editions and MSS.

[55] TK index for MSS and editions of the text and commentaries.

[56] *Chart.*, IV, no. 2115, pp. 351-352, for the year 1418. For earlier reports of similar conditions, see *Chart.*, III, no. 1284, p. 107, for the year 1363, for the studium in general.

[57] In this regard see especially E. Reusens, *Documents relatifs à l'université de Louvain (1425-1797)* (Louvain, 1893-1902), I, p. 2ff.; and especially p. 2, n. 1: 'Anno 1422 Karolo sexto defuncto succedit Karolus septimus in Francie regno omnium malorum et calamitatum tempestatibus repleto; nulli tutum iter erat ex Brabantie duci, subjectis, qui studii causa Parisii universitatem adire non metueret...'.

[58] For Cologne (Köln), founded in 1388, see F.J. Bianco, *Die alte Universität Köln*

and Louvain, the curriculum followed that of Paris for the most part. As far as provisions regarding the content of the medical curriculum for both universities are concerned the statutes are extremely brief. At Cologne, however, one may gather from the extant inventory of the collection of books deeded to the university by Bernard de Loen, a professor of medicine in the first half of the fifteenth century, and the fact that Amplonius Ratinck (Ratinger), whose famous collection of manuscripts is still extant in Erfurt, was professor of medicine at Cologne in 1399 to 1435, that there was no dearth of texts[59]. Among the works included, for example in the collection of Bernard de Loen, those of Hippocrates and Galen, for the Greeks, and of Avicenna, Isaac Judaeus, Rasis, for Arabic medicine, were prominent both in the texts and as subjects of commentaries. Included also were the works of more recent Latin authors such as Arnald of Villanova (d. 1309), Gentile da Foligno (d. 1348), Marsilius of Santa Sofia (d. 1405), member of the famous Santa Sofia family at Padua, Petrus de Tossignano or Tussignano, professor of arts and medicine at Bologna toward the end of the fourteenth century, Thomas del Garbo, son of the equally well known Dino del Garbo, and William of Varignana, a member of another prominent medical family of Bologna[60]. In general there appears to have been a fair distribution between ancient and more recent or contemporary authors. At Louvain, however, although there may well have been a similar distribution among the authorities, there appears to have been a greater emphasis at least in the statutes upon the more ancient. Thus in the medical College statutes and in those of the medical faculty, the general requirement was that the candidates for the license in medicine have a thorough grounding in the principles and precepts of Hippocrates and Galen[61]. Also in the ceremony for licensing the candidates were to recite the Hippocratic *Oath*, in an abbreviated fashion, however[62].

und die spätern Gelehrten-Schulen dieser Stadt, I (Köln, 1855); also Friedrich Moritz, 'Aus der medizinischen Fakultät der alten Universität Köln', *Festschrift zur Erinnerung an die Gründung der alten Universität Köln im Jahre 1388* (Köln, 1938), pp. 237-288.

[59] Moritz, p. 247 ff.

[60] Moritz, p. 239 ff. For MSS and editions, where available, of the authors named see TK index.

[61] A. Van Hove, 'Statuts inédits du collège de la faculté de médecine de l'université de Louvain (1607)', *Académie royale de Belgique, Commission royale d'histoire, Bulletin*, 84 (1920), p. 95. These refer back to those issued earlier and published by de Ram, 'Anciens statuts', p. 395.

[62] de Ram, 'Anciens statuts', p. 409, note; Van Hove, p. 102. The *Oath* that was to be taken by licentiates but not for the doctorate, included the following: '...numquam revelabit, neque umquam dabit toxicum vel abortivum, et in morbis periculosis et acutis, procurabit egrotantibus confessionem, quantum in eo erit'.

Furthermore in addition to their study of the medical authorities, candidates for degrees or for the license to teach, which in most cases permitted them to practice as well as to teach medicine, had to comply with the requirement of competence in supervised practical experience. For the license in medicine, each candidate was to have practiced medicine for two summers outside of Paris, or continuously for two years in Paris under the direction of his master, a practicing physician[63]. On the subject of practice one might add, in order to counter the too frequently repeated criticism that the medieval physician emphasized his scholastic skills rather than engaged in actual practice, that such criticism has no validity, as far as the fourteenth and fifteenth centuries are concerned. Not only, for example, did the physicians respond, on the occasion of the outbreak of the Black Death in October 1348, to King Philip VI's request that they prepare a brief compendium showing the causes, both universal and remote, particular and immediate, together with the possible remedies for the Epidemic, but also they went directly to the aid of those stricken with the dread disease. They did so in 1348[64], as well as in the recurrent outbreaks of the plague through the remaining fourteenth and into the next century. This was done, one may add regretfully, perhaps, at the expense of their lectures, which in many instances had to be suspended temporarily while they treated the sick and the dying[65]. In addition professors of medicine very often served as physicians to princely personages[66].

Although the renown of the physicians at Cologne and at Louvain does not become apparent until after the close of the fifteenth century, we may nevertheless conclude that these two universities together with their alma mater, Paris, did much to ensure the continuance of the time honored linking of arts and medicine. And through this association, by statute and precept, they furthered the tradition of the physician as a literate, rational person, distinguished by his breadth of knowledge as well as skill in practice.

[63] *Chart.*, II, for the year 1335.

[64] *Chart.*, II, no. 1159, p. 623; also Anna M. Campbell, *The Black Death and Men of Learning* (New York, 1931), p. 14ff.

[65] For medical practice during later outbreaks of the plague, see the references in note 56 above.

[66] For example, Jean l'Aventage at the time of the death of John, Duke of Burgundy was physician to Duke Philip of Burgundy: *Chart.*, IV, no. 2105, p. 344; and Pierre Bechebien, member of the Faculty of Medicine in 1420, was physician to the Count of Virtus: *Chart.*, IV, no. 2126, p. 361.

XIII

THE FACULTY OF MEDICINE AT PARIS, CHARLATANISM AND UNLICENSED MEDICAL PRACTICES IN THE LATER MIDDLE AGES

The rôle of the medical faculty of the university of Paris [1] in matters affecting the health of residents of the city of Paris was an active and important one. Not only did the faculty respond to the requests for aid in the periodic outbreaks of pestilence and plague from 1348 onward,[2]

[1] Material for the present article, read in part before the New York Society for Medical History, and constituting part of a larger study now in progress on "The Rights, Privileges, and Immunities of Mediaeval Universities and University Scholars," was gathered during a year abroad under a Fellowship Grant from the John Simon Guggenheim Memorial Foundation for 1950-1951.

A list of the extended titles for those works frequently cited in abbreviated form in the notes will be found at the close of the article.

[2] In 1348 King Philip IV asked for aid from the university faculty of medicine: *Chart. univ. Paris.*, II, no. 1159, p. 623; A. M. Campbell, *The Black Death and Men of Learning*, New York, 1931, pp. 14-17; and cf. *ibid.*, p. 97. In the fifteenth century so many masters, because of the great multitude of the sick, were occupied with practice that they were unable to carry on their teaching: *Chart. univ. Paris.*, IV, pp. 351-352. See also *ibid.*, III, p. 107, no. 1284. In the year 1500 when the provost of the city of Paris asked the faculty's aid in combating the plague, the faculty requested in return the provost's assistance in combating illegal medical practice by charlatans and empirics: Wickersheimer, *Commentaires*, Paris, 1915, introduction, particularly, pp. lxxxviii-xci; also pp. 425 (1499-1500), and 448 (1500-1501).

but on its own initiative it undertook the less spectacular task of attempting to stamp out charlatanism and medical practice by empirics. It also endeavored, " in the public interest," to establish an effective surveillance over apothecaries, herbalists, and surgeons. To realize these aims, the faculty relied not only on the issuance of regulations and statutes but even more particularly upon the active prosecution, with the aid of the bishop's court, of those who engaged in illicit practices. The regulations and the records of the court proceedings in specific instances, in the fourteenth and fifteenth centuries, which have been utilized in the present study, reveal the steps taken to punish charlatans and empirics and the difficulties of enforcing the university regulations.[3]

The university's right to prosecute unlicensed persons who were practicing medicine was based, it asserted, upon a regulation issued at some earlier date by the bishop's court at Paris. The intent of this regulation which, in 1311 and 1322, was said to have been made some two hundred years before, was to prohibit from engaging in medical practice in Paris anyone who had not been examined and approved by the faculty. Both the authenticity and dating of such a statute appear doubtful since so far no text of such a pronouncement seems to have been found. There is also no apparent evidence that an organized faculty of medicine was functioning in Paris before 1200.[4] It is of course possible that the term " two hundred years " was a mere figure of speech to establish the hoary antiquity of the faculty's jurisdiction.

There were some precedents outside of Paris for the principles of examination and licensing of practicing physicians but no records of such regulations appear to be extant before the first quarter of the twelfth century. Such regulations would appear therefore to be a distinctly medieval phenomenon. No legal restrictions on practicing physicians prevailed in antiquity, despite the emphasis of the Hippocratic school of physicians upon adherence to a strict code of professional ethics. And although this code of ethics, preserved in the Hippocratic Oath, persisted into the middle

[3] The most interesting collection of materials for this purpose is that contained in the seventeenth century manuscript in the Paris Archives nationales: MM 226: " Extrait sommaire des divers procès de contestatione de la faculté de medecine depuis contra divers particulaires exercant illicitime la medicine. Pour l'utilité publique et d'histoire . . . ab anno 1311 ad annum 1395." Most of the materials in this collection have already been published in the *Chart. univ. Paris.*, which at II, xxi, reports on it.

[4] Medicine along with Civil Law was being taught at Paris between 1175 and 1190 and very probably earlier, but it is doubtful that the medical faculty was organized at that early period: *Chart. univ. Paris.*, I, pp. 55-56, no. 54.

ages,[5] there were no laws against medical practice by ignorant and untrained persons who might never have heard of the Hippocratic oath. Thus Pliny the Elder caustically remarked that there " is no law which punishes ignorance, no example of redress for this capital crime, that they (the physicians) learn by endangering our lives and carry on experiments by causing deaths, to such an extent that the greatest impunity is given to a physician for having killed a man." [6] Only in the fourth century of the Roman Empire do we encounter any legislation in this regard. But the laws made under Valentinian I and Valens providing for the examination of those preparing to practice medicine pertained only to the chief physicians, the *archiatri* or the physicians associated with the royal or imperial person. The Theodosian Code further added that after the prospective *archiatri* had submitted to an examination by a college or royal council of the chief physicians, they must have the emperor's consent before they could practice in the palace.[7] It was apparently to this royal council of chief physicians that Cassiodorus addressed his *Formula comitis archiatrorum,* in the early sixth century.[8]

But even such scanty legislation became a dead letter with the breakdown of Roman imperial authority in western Europe. From the sixth century onward, medical learning and skill, transmitted from antiquity together with the code of medical ethics embodied in the Hippocratic oath, were obliged with other classical learning to take refuge in monastic centers. There under ecclesiastical supervision medical study and practice were at first encouraged and cultivated probably for purely practical reasons and in accordance with the clear admonitions of the " Book of Ecclesiasticus " [9] that the physician and medicine are to be honored because they are created by God. Cassiodorus in his monastic retreat at Vivarium urged the monks to become acquainted with the medical works that he had collected for their use; [10] and Rabanus Maurus two centuries later, in both

[5] In this regard see especially L. C. MacKinney, " Medical Ethics and Etiquette in the Early Middle Ages: the persistence of Hippocratic Ideals," *Bulletin of the History of Medicine*, 1952, vol. 26, 1 *et seq*., and the references there cited.

[6] Pliny, Nat. Hist., lib. XXIX, cap. 8 (*Bibl. classica latina,* 1829, vol. 79: viii, p. 198).

[7] See H. Conring, *De antiquit*., pp. 57-59, 259-261, citing " Const. Valentiniani et Valentis "; and *The Theodosian Code and Novels and the Sirmondian Constitutions, a translation with Commentary, Glossary, and Bibliography*, by C. Pharr, Princeton University Press, 1952, p. 388.

[8] Variarum, liber VI, paragraph xix (Migne, vol. 69, cols. 700-701).

[9] Liber Ecclesiasticus, 38, 1-11 (*Biblia Sacra Vulgatae Editionis Sixti V Pont. Max*., 1922, p. 655) : " Honora medicum propter necessitatem: etenim illum creavit Altissimus . . . Altissimus creavit de terra medicamenta. et vir prudens non abhorrebit illa."

[10] De inst. divin. lett., cap. 31 (Migne, vol. 70, cols. 1146-47).

his encyclopedic "De universo" and in his "Commentary on the Book of Ecclesiasticus," urged that out of necessity medicine should be cultivated and honored rather than spurned.[11]

By the twelfth century, however, the increasing tendency of members of monastic orders to engage in medical practice to the neglect of their religious duties was cause for alarm and regulation by the ecclesiastical authorities. Prohibitions of such practice, at first directed only to monks who practiced medicine for gain, were later extended to any or all medical practice or study outside the monasteries by members of the orders.[12] In the thirteenth century Pope Honorius III renewed the prohibitions and extended them to all clerics regular or secular.[13] But by the middle of the fourteenth century such restrictions were being set aside by papal dispensations, and clerics, regular or secular, were given permission to study, to lecture, and to practice medicine at Paris or elsewhere in accordance with the university regulations.[14]

Direct regulation of those who wished to teach medicine and to practice among the populace first appeared in southern Italy where the school of Salerno was already a flourishing medical school in the eleventh century. Legislation relating to the examining and licensing of prospective physicians is extant, however, only from the twelfth century.[15] On the other

[11] De universo, liber XVIII, cap. 5 (Migne, vol. 111, col. 501): "Medicinae curatio spernanda non est quia et sanctos viros ea uti legimus . . . Eccl. Honora medicina propter necessitatem." Comm. in Ecclesiasticum, liber VIII, cap. 13, De medico honorando (Migne, vol. 109, col. 1030).

[12] This was done at the councils of Reims in 1131 and at the Lateran council in 1139: E. Lesne, *Histoire*, pp. 679, 688. For the prohibitions of 1163 and 1179 (1180), see *Chart. univ. Paris.*, I, pp. 3 (no. 1); 78, note.

[13] For the prohibitions of Pope Honorius III in 1213 and 1219, see *Chart. univ. Paris.*, I, pp. 77-78; 90-93; and for those of 1227-1268, see *ibid.*, I, pp. 478-479.

[14] On January 9, 1364, clerics were permitted to enter the faculty of medicine and to be given a license; and on November 1, 1380, pope Clement VII granted to Guibertus de Celceto, a canon of the church of S. Germain and master of medicine, the right to lecture on and to practice medicine at Paris. A similar dispensation was given to Guibertus de "Saliceto," physician of Charles V, on September 25, 1377, by Gregory XI: *Chart. univ. Paris.*, III, pp. 109-110; 292, no. 1452; 331, 339, no. 1501; Arch. Nat. MM 266, p. 166. See also *Chart. univ. Paris.*, IV, pp. 55, 138, 197, 209, 578, 604, for such dispensations in the fifteenth century; Wickersheimer, *Commentaires*, introduction, pp. xlv-xlvii.

[15] For Salerno and Naples, see H. Conring, *De antiquit.*, pp. 60-61, 104, 106-107; H. Rashdall, *The Universities of Europe in the Middle Ages* (new ed. by F. M. Powicke and A. B. Emden, 3 vols.), Oxford, 1936, I, 76 *et seq.*; 83-85; also F. R. Packard, *History of the School of Salernum*, New York, 1920, pp. 34-36. The English translation of the ordinances was published by E. F. Hartung, "Medical Regulations of Frederick the Second of Hohenstaufen," in *Medical Life*, 1934, vol. 41, pp. 587-601.

hand ecclesiastical supervision of those who wished to teach medicine in the university is revealed at Montpellier in 1220, when Cardinal Conrad, the papal legate, made a ruling in this regard. He stated that although the science of medicine had flourished for a long time at Montpellier, henceforth no one ought to be free to teach medicine publicly there unless he received the license to teach (licentia docendi) from the bishop of Maguelone after he had been examined and recognized as qualified.[16] Earlier, in January, 1181, Guilhem VII, lord of Montpellier, had declared that the teaching of medicine in the schools of Montpellier should be free from outside interference.[17]

Although many of the provisions enacted by the medical faculty at Paris, for the examination and licensing of prospective physicians, resembled the imperial legislation at Salerno and Naples, the action of the faculty of the northern university provides a distinct contrast to the other centers. For unlike either Salerno or Montpellier, the initiative for the active prosecution of those practicing without a license came not from the imperial, ecclesiastical, or royal authorities but from the university medical faculty itself. In 1271 and 1272, the faculty at Paris took occasion to define more clearly the requirements for obtaining the license which was conferred by the chancellor of the Cathedral of Notre Dame.[18] At the same time the faculty proceeded to legislate against persons who were practicing illegally without a license and without the approval of the faculty, or more explicitly against those who "by shameful and brazen usurpation," assumed the office of medical practitioner at Paris. The members of the faculty denounced those empirics, who, without the approval and counsel of the more learned members of the profession, were administering to all comers medicines which they had concocted out of their own heads. They were declared by their treatment of the sick, based only on the whims of chance and fortune, to be guilty of criminally handing over many to suffering and even to death. The faculty pointed out that by practicing without authorization such persons were imperilling the safety of their own souls and were daily incurring the penalty of the ban of excommunication which would be launched by the official of the bishop of

[16] *Cartulaire de l'université de Montpellier* (2 vols.), *Montpellier*, 1890, I, pp. 180-183.

[17] *Ibid.*, pp. 179-180. See also E. Nicaise, introduction to his edition of *La Grande Chirurgie de Guy de Chauliac*, Paris, 1890, pp. li *et seq.*

[18] *Chart. univ. Paris.*, I, p. 517, no. 453; English translation by L. Thorndike, *University Records*, pp. 81-82. For other documents on license requirements, see *Chart. univ. Paris.*, I, nos. 444, 451-456; II, nos. 921, 996; IV, no. 2659. See also Wickersheimer, *Commentaires*, introduction, pp. xi-xvii, xviii *et seq.*

Paris against them. By their practices these empirics were said to constitute a distinct threat to the welfare of the residents of Paris as well as a serious discredit to the good name and repute of the more learned members of the medical profession. The faculty went on further to assert that it had been urged to take action to correct the existing critical situation by clergy and laymen alike. To prevent the continuation or perpetuation of such errors, perils, and resulting scandals, the faculty drew up, therefore, the regulations which were, it insisted, in confirmation of a statute made long ago, a statute which was said to be supported by letters of the official of the bishop of Paris, by royal authority, and the oaths taken by the individual members of the faculty of medicine.[19]

The regulations of 1271 were directed particularly against "certain manual operators," who made or possessed various medicaments which they administered without knowing the relation which these medicines had to diseases. Under every penalty allowed by civil and canon law for noncompliance with the law it was provided that no surgeon, male or female, no apothecary nor herbalist, was to exceed or overstep the limits or bounds of his craft, either secretly or publicly. The surgeon was to engage only in manual practice, the apothecary and herbalist were only to mix drugs which were to be administered exclusively by masters in medicine or under their express license. No one of the aforementioned was to visit any sick person nor "to administer to him any alterative medicine or laxative or anything else" that pertained to a physician, nor was he to advise that it be administered except by a master in medicine. Surgeons, apothecaries, and herbalists, were to be bound by oath to obey these provisions. Furthermore, bachelors in medicine,[20] that is those who had been permitted to lecture but were not yet licensed as masters in the medical faculty, under penalty of having their promotions withheld, were strictly forbidden to visit patients or to administer to them any drugs unless they were accompanied by or were in the presence of a master of the medical faculty. Information regarding anyone acting contrary to this statute was to be revealed secretly and under oath to the dean or to some teaching master in the medical faculty. The one to whom such information was given was to be obliged to shield the informer.[21]

[19] *Chart. univ. Paris.*, I, p. 488-490, no. 434. The document is translated into English by L. Thorndike, *University Records*, pp. 83-85.

[20] For the use of the term "baccalarius," or "bachelarius," in medicine, see Wickersheimer, *Commentaires*, introduction, p. xviii and note.

[21] *Chart. univ. Paris.*, I, pp. 489-490; Thorndike, *op. cit.*, pp. 84-85; Wickersheimer, *op. cit.*, introduction, pp. lxxii *et seq.*

Thus armed with laws of its own making, the faculty through its dean undertook the more difficult task of securing their enforcement. In 1311, a charlatan or empiric against whom the dean of the faculty brought charges of illegal practice demanded to know by what right the faculty dared to trouble him in his medical practice. To this demand the faculty made the reply noted above that their authority dated back to a statute of the official of the bishop of Paris made two hundred years earlier. By this statute, it was asserted, the right to practice medicine in Paris was denied to anyone who was not a master or who had not been licensed in the faculty of medicine.[22] The case, in 1312, of Clarice de Rothomago, wife of a certain Peter Faverel, revealed the steps taken against unlicensed persons. In this case, which ran from January 17 to June 15, 1312, Clarice was accused of practicing medicine illegally in Paris and was arrested at the instance of the dean of the faculty of medicine. She was then put under ban of excommunication by the official of the bishop's court at Paris. From this penalty she appealed to the official of the bishop of Senlis, the so-called conservator of the apostolic privileges of the university.[23] Her appeal was, however, of no avail since the dean of the medical faculty was able to obtain from the bishop of Senlis a reaffirmation of the sentence of excommunication against Clarice and against her husband as well. They were both to be denounced in all the churches and anyone who associated with them was to be subject to the same penalty.[24]

The effectiveness of this ban of excommunication and oral denunciation, applied against Clarice and her husband, as a means of frightening off other unlicensed persons from medical practice, appears to have been slight. Numerous cases of illegal practice continued to come to the

[22] Pajon de Moncets, *De l'origine des appariteurs des universités et de leurs masses*, Paris, 1782, pp. 122-123. Wickersheimer, *op. cit.*, pp. lxxii-lxxiii, indicates that it was probably toward 1220 that the faculty of medicine obtained from the diocesan official a sentence reserving the right to practice medicine at Paris and in the faubourgs to those who had obtained the master's degree in medicine with the approval of the chancellor of the university.

[23] The conservator of apostolic privileges of the university had the general power of protecting the university in its enjoyment of the privileges granted to it, and to secure respect for these privileges by punishing those who infringed upon them by ecclesiastical censure: Rashdall, *The Universities of Europe in the Middle Ages*, 1936, I, 342-343; 417-419.

[24] Paris, Arch. Nat. MM 266, pp. 3-13; *Chart. univ. Paris.*, II, pp. 149-153, nos. 693, 693a-c. The husband of Clarice, Petrus Faverel, was excommunicated as "empeiricus" on June 13; *ibid.*, pp. 150-151. He had sent no witnesses and had failed to appear himself after the appeal. He was therefore judged contumacious and the costs of the case were adjudged against him. The sentence against Clarice was issued on June 14, 1312; *ibid.*, pp. 151-152.

attention of the faculty. One of the most interesting of these was the case of Jacqueline Félicie de Almania. Her involvement began with her citation on August 11, 1322, for illegal practice, before the official of the bishop of Paris by the proctor of the dean of the medical faculty. She was duly excommunicated and, like Clarice, appealed against this sentence.[25] In the course of her trial, the proceedings of which continued for several months, a great many witnesses were called to testify on each side. Among the witnesses for the prosecution, on the side of the faculty, was the military knight and surgeon, John of Padua, who had been, as early as 1301, surgeon to the king of France, Philip IV.[26] John asserted that the penalities of prohibition and excommunication had been in operation for more than sixty years against ignorant and illicit empirics practicing in Paris and its environs. These penalties had been applied with the full approval of the venerable official of the bishop's court at Paris as well as with that of the illustrious kings of France. Yet contrary to these well known facts the defendant in question had persisted in acting as a physician although she was totally ignorant of the art of medicine. She was not lettered, nor had she been approved as competent in those things which she presumed to treat.

Furthermore, John pointed out, as it was forbidden by law that a woman practice law or be a witness in a criminal case,[27] so it was of far greater moment that she be likewise barred from the practice of medicine. Such practice required her to prescribe for patients foods and drinks for internal consumption and to apply clysters when in truth she knew neither the causes of the diseases from which they were suffering nor understood the letter or art of medicine. How much more serious therefore, John argued, was the danger that she might thus kill a man by these potions and clysters than that she might lose a civil suit through ignorance of the law. For through lack of knowledge in the former she might commit murder, and such a death would be a mortal sin over which the church would have jurisdiction. Hence in John of Padua's opinion the admonition

[25] *Chart. univ. Paris.*, II, pp. 255-256, no. 811; Arch. Nat., MM 266, pp. 13, 22, 23. Of this case Wickersheimer, *Commentaires,* introduction, p. lxxv, states: "C'est dans les pièces du procès intenté en 1322 à Jacqueline Félicie que nous trouvons les détails les plus intéressants pour l'histoire du charlatanisme à Paris au moyen âge."

[26] For John of Padua, see *Chart. univ. Paris.*, II, p. 256, note 1; also *ibid.*, II, no. 812, note; and Wickersheimer, *Dictionnaire,* II, 459.

[27] For the prohibition against the admission of women to the corporation of barristers or lawyers, see Paul Fournier, *Les Officialités, au moyen âge. Etude sur l'organisation, la compétence et la procédure des tribunaux ecclésiastiques ordinaires en France, de 1180 à 1328,* Paris, 1880, pp. 32-33; and for the prohibition against their appearing in civil courts as accusers, *ibid.*, p. 238.

and decree of excommunication launched by the official of the episcopal court at Paris should be binding.[28]

Equally emphatic were the arguments put forth by the defending counsel. He pointed out that Jacqueline Félicie had treated and cured many sick persons; that she had brought them comfort when other physicians had failed to do so; and that she had visited and cared for her patients assiduously until they were cured. This was corroborated by several witnesses who were brought to give testimony in Jacqueline's behalf. To each of these witnesses in turn the court put the questions of how they had learned about Jacqueline; whether she had acted as if she were a qualified physician; whether she had attempted to extort money from them; and finally, whether they knew that she had not been approved in any *studium generale*,[29] at Paris or elsewhere, or if they had seen her at Montpellier. In each instance the replies were similar. They had learned of her through a friend; she had proceeded as did most physicians in examining a patient; she had consistently refused to take any money until the patient had been cured; and they had not inquired into the matter of her qualifications. Among the witnesses for the defense was John of St. Omer. He testified that he had been cured of an illness by Jacqueline who had visited him several times and had done more for him than had any of the other physicians who were called in during his illness. She had given him a drink of some kind of clear liquid, which she or some one else had first sampled. Matilda, the wife of John of St. Omer, also attested the cure and added further that Jacqueline had applied poultices to John's chest.[30] Another witness, John Faber, asserted that Jacqueline had cured him by administering certain potions, one of them green in color, the other clear and colorless, but of what they were made, he did not know.[31]

An even more telling witness was a woman named Yvo Tueleu, a servant at the bishop's court in Paris. She related that she had been ill of a fever for which she had been visited by several physicians, none of whom had been able to cure her. Then at her request Jacqueline had come to her bedside, had given her a glass of the very clear liquid which had acted as a purge, and had successfully cured her of the fever.[32] Various other

[28] *Chart. univ. Paris.*, II, p. 256, no. 812; Arch. Nat. MM 266, p. 14.

[29] The usual term for the place in which the university associations were established; for its use see especially, Rashdall, *The Medieval Universities*, 1936, I, pp. 6-8.

[30] *Chart. univ. Paris.*, II, pp. 257-262; 261-262; Arch. Nat. MM 266, pp. 17-21.

[31] *Chart. univ. Paris.*, II, p. 259.

[32] *Ibid.*, II, p. 262.

persons who had been treated by the defendant testified to her ability and skill. One of them, Dominus Odo de Cornessiaco, a friar of the Hotel Dieu at Paris, stated that he too in his illness had been visited by several prominent physicians including John de Turre,[33] and the physicians Martin, Herman, and others. But none of them had been able to cure him. Then Jacqueline had come and had brought him back to health. Her course of treatments had included steam baths, massages with oil, and applications of herbs including leaves of camomile, melilot, and others. He stated that she had worked incessantly until he was entirely cured. Another former and grateful patient, Johanna, the wife of a certain Dionysius, stated that she too had been ill of a fever for which she had been visited by several physicians, including a certain Friar de Cordelis, the masters Herman, Manfred, and several others. All of them had given her up for certain death. Then Jacqueline had come and saved her. And still a further former patient, Johanna de Monciaco, a storekeeper or haberdasher, testified that she had been ill of an affliction of the kidneys, and that she had been for eleven days at St. Sulpice where she too was visited by the physicians, Guilbert, Herman, Manfred, and Thomas, none of whom had been able to help her. Then Jacqueline had succeeded in doing so by administering a glass of the clear liquid mentioned earlier.[34]

Also pointed out, in Jacqueline's defense, was the fact that there were many persons, practicing daily in Paris, who had not been approved in any university either at Paris or elsewhere and these persons similarly were without licenses either from the chancellor, the bishop of Paris, or from the said dean and masters of the medical faculty.[35] The defense then went on to attack the legality of the university statute.[36] This law, it was claimed, which had been invoked by the medical faculty had no legal validity, since it had never been approved by those whom it affected.

[33] *Ibid.*, II, pp. 259-260. Jean de Turre is probably to be identified with the son of the physician of Montpellier, Jourdain de Turre, who is noted by Wickersheimer as dedicating two of his works to his son in 1318: Wickersheimer, *Dictionnaire*, II, 497, 513-514.

[34] *Chart. univ. Paris.*, II, pp. 260-262; Arch. Nat. MM 266, pp. 18-19. Of the physicians named, Martin, Herman (Lombardus), Manfred, and Thomas (of Saint Georges), were all masters in the faculty of medicine, between 1310 and 1332: *Chart. univ. Paris.*, II, pp. 141, 350; 262, note 15; p. 394, note; Wickersheimer, *Dictionnaire*, II, 535, 766.

The various uses of the herbs camomile, or "camomilla" and melilot or "mellilotum" are noted in *The Herbal of Rufinus*, edited by L. Thorndike, Chicago University Press, 1945, pp. 71-72, 185-186.

[35] *Chart. univ. Paris.*, II, pp. 257-262, no. 813; Arch. Nat. MM 266, pp. 17-21. For the list of several other empirics condemned along with Jacqueline, see below.

[36] *Chart. univ. Paris.*, II, pp. 263-265, no. 814; Arch. Nat. MM 266, pp. 23-26, November 2, 1322.

It was merely an admonition by mandate of the venerable official of the bishop of Paris, an admonition, however, which was directed against ignorant, foolish, and unskilled persons merely simulating the medical art, yet totally ignorant of its precepts. Surely, it was argued, Jacqueline, an expert in the art of medicine and one who was well instructed in the precepts of medicine, could not be said to belong to this group. Moreover, if the university claimed that it was acting according to the law made some two hundred years earlier, the defense would direct attention to an even earlier law that states, " what touches all ought to be aproved by all." [37] Yet in this statute by which the faculty claimed to be proceeding, it does not appear that there was a summons of the masters, doctors, bachelors, and scholars of each faculty of the university then living at Paris, nor was there a summons of the bishop, archdeacon, dukes, barons, citizens, and burghers of Paris, whom such a decree also concerns and interests. Certainly none of these are named in the statute. In sum therefore, the defense argued, since those for whom the statute presumably was made had not been called, it was not valid, in their absence, and consequently it could not be binding on Jacqueline or on any other person.[38]

As a final argument, the defense counsel declared, it was better and more fitting that a wise and sagacious woman, experienced in the art of medicine should visit another woman, to examine her and to inquire into the hidden secrets of her being, than that a man should do this. For a man is not permitted to do these things, that is to inquire into her innermost secrets and to touch the various parts of her body. Indeed a man ought ever to avoid and shun the secrets of women and fly from their intimate association as much as he can. Besides, the defense counsel continued, it was often true that a woman would rather die than reveal the secrets of her infirmity to a man out of a sense of modesty and even of shame. For this reason many women have died in their illnesses since they were unwilling to have a physician who might learn their innermost secrets. In the case of Jacqueline, the court was reminded, members of both sexes had confided in her and she had been able to cure those whom other doctors could not. In conclusion the defense counsel asserted, the decree or statute invoked by the faculty of medicine could not be binding since it had been shown to be contrary to the public good.[39]

[37] For the use of this famous maxim, from the Roman Civil Code of Justinian, in the thirteenth and fourteenth centuries, see P. Kibre, *The Nations in the Mediaeval Universities* (The Mediaeval Academy of America), Cambridge, 1948, p. 39, note 64.

[38] *Chart. univ. Paris.*, II, pp. 263-265, no. 814; Arch. Nat. MM 266, p. 24.

[39] *Chart. univ. Paris.*, II, pp. 263-265, no. 814; Arch. Nat. MM 266, pp. 24-26.

Most of the above arguments the university members characterized as trifling. They answered the objection to the statute on the basis of its conflict with the earlier law, that what touches all ought to be approved by all, with the assertion that the statute in question was not made by the cathedral chapter of Paris, that it was not such a statute as would require that the persons named by the defense be called. The present dictum, the university insisted, provided a sufficient basis for the official of the bishop of Paris, the minister and executor of the law, to act upon. He could discern by this statute that such a person as the defendant was not qualified to practice the medical art. The final verdict against Jacqueline Félicie, issued on November 2, 1322, found her and several others named at the same time, guilty of willful disobedience. She and the others were prohibited by a solemn reiteration of the original sentence of excommunication from practicing medicine or from exercising the functions of a physician under the further penalty of a fine of sixty Parisian pounds.[40]

Despite the specific character of this condemnation, it is quite apparent that illegal practice by charlatans and empirics continued. In the search for a remedy the medical faculty turned to the pope for aid and humbly beseeched him to take some action. On June 21, 1325, Pope John XXII wrote to Stephen, bishop of Paris, to urge his cooperation in preventing those ignorant of the art of medicine from practicing in Paris or its suburbs. The pope stated that he had been informed in a petition drawn up by the masters and scholars of the university that persons ignorant of the medical art, old women particularly, and even more to be detested, soothsayers, as well as others, were presuming to practice medicine in the city and environs of Paris, and that these charlatans were causing many deaths. In complying with the university's petition, the pope further asked the bishop of Paris to make careful inquiries into the reports, and, if necessary, to endeavor to find out the truth by calling a council of men learned in medicine whose advice he should then follow.[44]

Whether from inaction of the bishop of Paris or because the bishop's efforts had no greater success in securing an elimination of illegal practice

[40] *Chart. univ. Paris.*, II, p. 267, no. 816; Arch. Nat. MM 266, p. 23. The list of other persons condemned at the same time as Jacqueline for practicing illegal medicine included several women: Domina Jacoba, Johanna Conversa, wife of John Liblous who was also condemned for illegal practice of medicine (cf. Wickersheimer, *Dictionnaire*, II, 505; *Chart. univ. Paris.*, II, pp. 256, 267); also Margarita de Ypra, surgeon, and Belota Judea. Others included were Stephanus Burgundus or Etienne Burgondus, empiric, and Master Jacob Lépelé.

[41] *Chart. univ. Paris.*, II, pp. 285-286, no. 844.

than the earlier efforts of the university itself, Pope John XXII again found it necessary, some five years later, on January 1, 1330, to address the new bishop of Paris, Hugh, on the subject of those illegally practicing medicine in the city and suburbs. His information regarding the presence of several such persons in the city had once again come from the university. He urged the bishop to make every effort to see that henceforth no one was permitted to practice medicine in the city or suburbs of Paris unless he was a master or was licensed in the art, or was otherwise known to be qualified by having been approved by a council consisting of the dean of the medical faculty and two of the masters then lecturing on medicine in the university. Those who should disobey this dictum must, he said, be subjected to ecclesiastical censure.[42]

Between 1330 and 1332 the medical faculty was involved in a dispute with the chancellor over the granting of licenses. In the course of the quarrel the faculty sought for and obtained the support of the pope, of the king, and also of the provost of Paris. The final settlement reaffirmed the faculty's right to determine the qualifications necessary for the licensing of candidates for medical teaching and practice. The chancellor would henceforth be obliged to confer the license on anyone whom the faculty declared worthy and qualified.[43]

Throughout the fourteenth century papal support for the faculty's supervision of medical practice continued. Clement VI, in 1340, threatened with excommunication not only those who should attempt to practice in Paris without the approval of the medical faculty but also those who should utilize the services of such physicians. Nevertheless illegal practice continued.[44] In 1347 (January 27), the dean and the faculty of medicine were obliged to petition the pope further for aid against those who were practicing illegally. Their petition again reported that there were at Paris men and women audaciously usurping the office of physician and engaging in the practice of medicine about which they knew little or nothing. To remedy this situation it was urged that the pope ask the bishop of Senlis, the conservator of the university's apostolic privileges, to use his authority to forbid anyone to practice medicine unless he was a master of the art or science of medicine or had at least been licensed in

[42] *Ibid.*, II, pp. 336-337, no. 900; and cf. no. 844 for a similar letter. In Arch. Nat. MM 266, p. 160, 'ad an. c. 1331,' are noted several illicit practitioners at Paris (*Chart. univ. Paris.*, II, p. 337, note).

[43] *Ibid.*, II, nos. 918-943, for the entire conflict. For the instrument of composition of the difficulties, see *ibid.*, II, pp. 397-399, no. 943.

[44] BN fonds franç. 22110, fol. 387r.

another university. He was also to announce to all transgressors that they would be punished by ecclesiastical censure.[45] Three years later, on April 2, 1350 (1351), the faculty was still trying through one of its representatives, Adam of Francovilla, at the papal court to obtain articles with the pope's signature against illegal practice.[46] Restrictions on student doctors were also tightened on February 3, 1375, by the measure requiring all bachelors in medicine or those not yet licensed to take an oath that they would not practice medicine nor visit the sick, unless they were accompanied by one of the masters in the faculty.[47]

The university made further efforts too to subject the apothecaries to specific regulation. In addition to the provisions relating to the dispensing of medicines contained in the statutes of 1271, the medical faculty had, on February 28, 1322, drawn up new articles, " in the public interest," which required that all apothecaries and dealers in drugs appear each year before the assembled faculty to take the oath that they were doing everything in their power to carry on effectively their work as apothecaries and herbalists. They must also swear that they were keeping on hand for easy reference a corrected copy of the *Antidotarium* of Nicholas of Salerno; [48] that they were using true and accurate weights tested according to those used at the fairs; that they would not use for filling prescriptions any medicines that had been corrupted; and that if they could not obtain the simples called for in their recipes they would use no other substitutes than those provided for in the *Quid pro quo*.[49]

The ordinances provided also that the dean of the medical faculty and one apothecary chosen by the faculty would make periodic visits to the apothecary shops to look over the stocks of medicines. The apothecaries were prohibited from dispensing any medicinal laxatives or opiates which

[45] *Chart. univ. Paris.*, II, pp. 602-603, no. 1138.

[46] To defray the expenses incurred by Adam of Francovilla, the faculty was obliged to levy a tax on all its members: *Chart. univ. Paris.*, III, pp. 7-8, no. 1197; Arch. Nat. MM 266, p. 161.

[47] *Chart. univ. Paris.*, III, pp. 217-218, no. 1396.

[48] *Ibid.*, II, pp. 268-269, no. 817, and note. For Nicholas' Antidotarium, see also *ibid.*, I, p. 517, note 4. Nicholas probably flourished at Salerno in the twelfth century and is unknown except as author of the Antidotarium. See further for the work G. Sarton, *Introduction to the History of Science* (3 vols., Baltimore, 1927-48), II, 239-240.

[49] The Quid pro Quo (*Chart. univ. Paris.*, II, p. 569, note 6), which frequently appears with the Antidotarium of Nicholas, is probably by him. It gives an alphabetical list of medicinal simples or drugs with their substitutes. In the oath taken in 1422 by the apothecaries, they had to swear that they would not substitute one drug for another in the prescriptions except by the permission of the master who had given the original prescription; see below, note 51.

they had not first shown to the dean and the aforementioned apothecary, and had indicated the use to which they were to be put. They were further prohibited from selling or dispensing any laxative medicines, aborticides, poisons, or any other dangerous drugs, to any person without the advice of a physician who had been officially approved in the university of Paris, or in some other recognized university. Anyone who wished to become an apothecary must first read and swear to obey these regulations.[50]

The faculty ordinances relating to dispensers of drugs were later strengthened by royal mandate. On May 22, 1336, King Philip VI of France addressed the provost of Paris and his lieutenant to the effect that they must enforce the law requiring apothecaries to take the oath to obey the ordinances of the medical faculty. The apothecaries were also to be required to swear that they would take care to see that their subordinates and the herbalists took the same oath to uphold and observe the ordinances. The provost was asked to make certain that the regulation requiring the showing of the medicinal laxatives and opiates to the masters of the faculty of medicine were enforced, and that care was taken to ensure that the medicines were fresh and good and that they had not been permitted to become spoiled or soiled.[51]

Despite the foregoing measures, King John of France, in December of 1352, asserted that according to information received from the dean and masters of the faculty of medicine there were many unauthorized persons of both sexes dispensing drugs and medicines freely in Paris. Included in their number were old women, monks, rustics, apothecaries, and numerous herbalists, also students of the medical faculty not yet licensed,

[50] *Chart. univ. Paris.*, II, pp. 268-269, no. 817. For statutes of the corporation of herbalists (épiciers) at Paris, see *Les métiers et corporations de Paris*, ed. by Lespinasse, Paris, 1886, pp. 500, 503; *Chart. univ. Paris.*, II, 269, note 2.

[51] *Ibid.*, II, 269, note 2; p. 462, no. 1001; *Ordonn. des Rois*, II, p. 116. The mandate of Philip VI referred directly to the university statute of Febr. 1322; similarly King John's ordinance regarding the apothecaries in 1353, also agrees in large part with the faculty provisions of 1322: *Ordonn. des Rois*, II, 532. The earlier ordinances were also confirmed by Charles VI in 1390 (Aug. 3); and by Charles VII, on November 30, 1437: *Chart. univ. Paris.*, III, p. 534, no. 1586; IV, 601-602, no. 2515. See also the "Oaths required of Apothecaries at Paris," October 2, 1422, by the faculty of medicine: *Chart. univ. Paris.*, IV, pp. 406-407, no. 2196; translated by L. Thorndike, *University Records*, pp. 298-299. At this time (1422) the apothecaries were required to swear that they had on hand a corrected copy of the Synonyms (of Simon a Cordo of Genoa, physician to Pope Nicholas IV (d. 1292), and chaplain to Pope Boniface VIII (d. 1303): G. Sarton, *Introd.*, II, p. 1085), and of the Circa instans of Platearius, a pharmaceutical work, probably of the late twelfth century. See further Wickersheimer, *Commentaires*. Introduction.

The oldest statute regarding apothecaries at Montpellier, appears to date from the year 1340: *Cartulaire de l'université de Montpellier*, I, p. 344, no. 12.

or coming from other localities to practice in Paris. Such persons, although they were ignorant of the science of medicine, were unacquainted with the complexions and constitutions of men, and lacked knowledge of the virtues of medicines as well as of the time and method for administering them, were nevertheless administering them freely. The king found this a highly offensive proceeding, as well as a very dangerous one. For, his report continued, in such medicines, particularly laxatives, if administered unduly, lurks peril of death. Furthermore according to the reports, not only were these charlatans dispensing drugs about which they knew nothing, they were also applying clysters, and practicing phlebotomy, without calling in the aid of a qualified physician. Such shameful practices were resulting in "clandestine homicides and abortions on every hand and sometimes publicly." Accordingly, the king in his desire to provide for the welfare of his subjects, forbade anyone of either sex or of any condition whatsoever, "to administer any medicine, alterative, laxative, sirup, electuary, laxative pills, or clysters of any sort," for symptoms that he did not understand. No one was to administer opiates or offer medical advice or otherwise exercise the office of a physician in any way unless he was master or a licentiate in the science of medicine at the university of Paris, or in another university, unless he was acting under the advice and direction of a master of the university, or had been otherwise approved by the faculty of medicine as qualified to practice. The provost of the city of Paris was to have the power to enforce this edict by imposing pecuniary and other civil penalties upon those who should disobey it.[52]

In addition to the foregoing provisions, the king further decreed, in August 1353, that the pharmaceutical establishments of the city of Paris and of its environs must be visited twice each year, namely about Easter and at the feast of All Saints (November 1), by a commission made up of representatives of masters of the apothecary art together with two masters of medicine. Apothecaries were also prohibited from delivering any medicinal remedies without an express commission from a physician. Any apothecaries or pharmacists who violated the royal ordinances were to be punished severely.[53]

[52] *Chart. univ. Paris.*, III, pp. 16-17, no. 1211. The document is translated into English by L. Thorndike, *University Records*, pp. 235-236. See also *Chart. univ. Paris.*, II, p. 462, no. 1001; and *Les métiers et corporations*, ed. by Lespinasse, Paris, 1886, p. 504. For near deaths caused by illegal practitioners, see also *Chart. univ. Paris.*, II, p. 337, note.

[53] *Ibid.*, III, p. 20, no. 1215. The king was said to have confirmed certain ancient ordinances of the university (*Ordonn. des rois*, II, 532; and cf. *Chart, univ. Paris.*, II, p. 268).

It does not appear that the royal edicts were any more efficacious in stamping out charlatanism than were those of the university. On August 3, 1390, another royal ordinance indicated the continued persistence of illegal practice. Charles VI on that date reported to the provost of the city of Paris and to his other justices that the king's attention had been called to the fact that in Paris persons without approval or license were engaging in medical practice as well as in surgery. Such persons were said to be visiting patients and to be promising to effect cures which they were unable to accomplish. The king therefore demanded that the provost and other justices investigate these charges and take appropriate action against those who were found to be unqualified and who were practicing without the approval of the medical faculty.[54]

There was also at Paris, as in Naples and Salerno, an attempt made to regulate the practice of surgery, although this was at first primarily a municipal concern rather than that of the university.[55] The separation of manual surgeons from the medical faculty was rigorously maintained through the fourteenth and early fifteenth centuries.[56] The masters in medicine were, however, on occasion called in for consultation at the trials of unauthorized persons operating as surgeons. This is illustrated in the case of Perretta Petonne who, at the instance of the masters of the surgeons, was arrested in 1411 for operating as a surgeon although she had not been approved by either the physicians or surgeons. Her case was already before the Parlement in 1410. She had first been interrogated, on June 9 of that year, by masters in medicine who had tried to find out if she could read. Their conclusion was that she did not know an "*a* from a fagot," and furthermore that she did not know what were the

[54] *Ibid.*, III, pp. 534-535, no. 1586; *Ordonn. des rois*, VII, 353.

[55] As early as 1307 a municipal statute provided that barbers who practiced surgery were forbidden to do so unless they had been examined by six masters of surgery who had been named by the provost of Paris and who had been sworn in and made responsible for the loyalty and qualifications of the surgeons (BN fonds fr. 11709, fols. 14r, 13v; 86r-v). The ordinance was renewed in 1311 by Philip IV who put master Jean Pitard, his surgeon, in charge of the examining masters of surgery (*Chart. univ. Paris.*, II, p. 149, no. 692, and note) and by succeeding monarchs (*Chart. univ. Paris.*, III, p. 14, no. 1205; also *ibid.*, III, pp. 42, 70-71, 113; IV, pp. 423, 618). See also Wickersheimer, *Commentaires*, introduction pp. lxxvi *et seq.*

[56] Thus on June 9, 1408, the faculty of medicine in its congregation considered the case of Johannes de Pisis, a surgeon, who before his acceptance into the faculty had manually operated. This master was summoned before the faculty and was required to promise under oath that he would no longer operate manually in public surgery at Paris: *Chart. univ. Paris.*, IV, p. 156, no. 1853. Cf. E. Wickersheimer, *Commentaires*, pp. lxxvi, 5, 47.

properties of herbs in prohibited remedies, such as " ache " and " ysope." At a second interrogation, on June 16, when the sick persons treated by Perretta were summoned to testify, Perretta declared that she was working " for God." She asserted that it was unjust that she should be molested when several other women were engaged in the practice of surgery at Paris, yet they were not being interrogated. The chief objection to Perretta, as the learned editors of the *Chartularium* noted, was not her sex, but the fact that she was practicing without the approval of the commission of municipal surgeons.[57]

In 1436 the surgeons were admitted as actual scholars in the faculty of medicine. They were allowed to attend lectures but could not proceed to the degree. However, they were as scholars to enjoy all " the privileges, franchises, liberties, and immunities conceded to the university." The reasons set forth by the university for the admission of the surgeons to the faculty of medicine, were that " in recent times," against the good of the public, many unapproved, false, or fictitious surgeons, who were corrupting and destroying the venerable science of surgery were making of it a public horror and scandal to the detriment of the people. The reference was to the struggle that was being carried on between the surgeons and the inferior class of barbers. The latter were claiming that they could operate surgically in certain cases although they had not been approved by the commission of municipal surgeons.[58]

Some seven years later, in 1443, the surgeons and the medical faculty also united to make common cause against a group of illicit medical practitioners called " cabusatores et cabusatrices." But not long thereafter, in 1446, a conflict broke out between the surgeons and the medical faculty when the surgeons did not respond to the call to a faculty convocation. The faculty had demanded that the surgeons take an oath in the presence of the faculty that they would refrain from going outside their proper

[57] *Ibid.*, p. 60; *Chart. univ. Paris.*, IV, pp. 198-199, note 1, no. 1912. It would appear that medical and surgical studies were not considered unsuitable for women. This is illustrated by the plan of education outlined, in 1309, by Pierre Dubois. In his treatise " On the Recovery of the Holy Land," Pierre Dubois stated that " to educate the girls in medicine and surgery, it will be advisable that two girls more highly trained than the others in medicine and surgery and their experiences remain to teach the others both theory and practice ": selection translated by L. Thorndike, *University Records*, pp. 148-149. See further on women physicians in the middle ages, E. Nicaise, introduction to his edition of *Guy de Chauliac*, pp. lxiii *et seq.*, p. 16.

[58] *Chart. univ. Paris.*, IV, pp. 594-595, no. 2496; Wickersheimer, *Commentaires*, p. 162. For the litigation between the surgeons and barbers, see *Chart. univ. Paris.*, IV, pp. 442-443, no. 2253; also *ibid.*, IV, pp. 675-676, no. 2621.

field of activity and that they would not prescribe digestive and laxative medicines or sedatives. This the surgeons refused to do.[59]

On January 11, 1494, the medical faculty opened its lectures to the corporation of the barbers. Up to that time the barbers had apparently taught each other. At one time a student in the medical faculty had acted as their teacher, but he had been obliged by the faculty to discontinue.[60] The surgeons requested that the faculty once again close its doors to the inferior barbers, and finally, in 1495-1496, reached an accord with the faculty. Not long afterward, however, in 1498, the medical faculty again complained that the surgeons were prescribing alterative and laxative medicines. It was not until 1506 that amicable relations were finally restored between the surgeons and the medical faculty.[61]

That the combined efforts of the medical faculty, the popes, the kings of France, as well as of the municipal magistrates, were unable to succeed in stamping out illegal practices in medicine, surgery, or in the sale and preparation of medicaments and drugs,[62] is amply illustrated by the continued reiteration of measures against these practices. In the first quarter of the fifteenth century, Henry V of England, as one of the first of his acts as regent of France, reaffirmed the statutes of the French monarchs against such evils. He threatened with imprisonment anyone found to be practicing without authorization or a license from the medical faculty of the university.[63] Nevertheless the university was obliged, from the year 1423 on, for some ten years, to carry on a long and wordy suit in the Parlement of Paris against a certain Jean de Domremi who designated himself physician, surgeon, and visitor of the surgeons of the kingdom, although apparently he had no official authorization whatever.[64]

Numerous other instances could be cited for the continuation of unauthorized and unlicensed medical practice both before and after 1500

[59] Wickersheimer, *Commentaires*, pp. 171, 179, 210.

[60] *Ibid.*, pp. 331-332; 353.

[61] *Ibid.*, pp. 365, 368, 390, 397, 403, 404, 474-478, 483.

[62] On December 7, 1437-1438 the medical faculty assembled to hear the response of the herbalists on the question of whether they would take the required oaths or not. The herbalists did not bother to appear and were declared, after they failed to heed a second summons, contumacious and hence subject to excommunication: Wickersheimer, *Commentaires*, p. 163.

[63] *Chart. univ. Paris.*, IV, p. 423, no. 2227; E. Nicaise, introduction to his edition of *Guy de Chauliac*, p. lxiii, cites a manuscript for the ordinance of Henry V in 1420.

[64] *Chart. univ. Paris.*, IV, pp. 424-428, nos. 2228-2231; *Journal de Clement de Fouquebergue, Greffier du Parlement de Paris, 1417-1435*, ed. by A. Tuetey (Société de l'histoire de France, 3 vols., Paris, 1903-1905), II, 168, 223, note 1, 224; *Wickersheimer, Commentaires*, pp. 129-149.

and even into our own time. The medical faculty of the university of Paris had thus been unsuccessful in its contest against such practice, and the university records of the fourteenth and fifteenth centuries reveal the obstacles encountered in the attempts to enforce the approved license requirements and to prosecute those who practiced without them. On occasion our sympathy may go out to such an empiric or natural healer as Jacqueline Félicie appears to have been. But there seems little doubt that the enforcement, by licensing, of specific requirements and qualifications was, then as now, in accord with the public interest. The continued instances of charlatanism, quackery, and illegal practice even into our own day illustrate the inherent difficulties of the problem. The efforts, therefore, of the medical faculty of the university of Paris in initiating in Paris the contest against these practices and in enlisting against them successively the aid of ecclesiastical, municipal, and royal authorities would appear worthy of our interest and earnest consideration.

LIST OF FREQUENTLY CITED WORKS

Chartularium universitatis Parisiensis, edited by H. Denifle and E. Chatelain, 4 vols., Paris, 1889-1897.

Conring[ius], H., *De antiquitatibus academicis dissertationes septem,* Gottingae, 1739.

Lesne, E., *Histoire de la propriété ecclésiastique en France*: Fasc. 50, Tome V, 1940: " Les écoles de la fin du VIIIe siècle à la fin du XIIe."

Migne, J. P. (editor), *Patrologiae cursus completus,* Series latina, 221 vols., Paris, 1844-1864.

Ordonnances des roys de France de la troisième race jusqu'en 1514, recueillies par ordre chronologique, 22 vols., Paris, 1723-1849.

Thorndike, L. (editor and translator), *University Records and Life in the Middle Ages* (Records of Civilization, Columbia University Press), New York, 1944.

Wickersheimer, E. (editor), *Commentaires de la faculté de médecine de l'université de Paris (1395-1516),* Paris, 1915.

Wickersheimer, E., *Dictionnaire biographique des médecins en France au moyen âge,* 2 vols., Paris, 1936.

MANUSCRIPTS

Paris: Archives Nationales:

M 70, no. 11 bis, Histoire de la faculté de Médecine, 1395-1434; no. 12, Chirurgiens, fols. 1r-3r, copied in the 17th century.

MM 226, 17th cent.

Bibliothèque Nationale:

fonds français 11709, 14th-15th centuries.

fonds français 22110, Actes concernant le pouvoir et la direction de l'université de Paris, fols. 3 et seq.

XIV

"ASTRONOMIA" OR "ASTROLOGIA" YPOCRATIS

Variously entitled in manuscripts as "Astronomia", "Astrologia Ypocratis", "De Iudiciis infirmitatum secundum dispositionem lune ad planetas", and so on, this tract on astrological medicine circulated in Latin form under the name of the famous physician, Hippocrates of Cos, in the high Middle Ages and early modern era[1]. It appears to have commanded considerable attention in the fifteenth and sixteenth centuries in the very era in which Copernicus made his remarkable astronomical discoveries. The latter as has frequently been shown, appear to have had little effect in discouraging continued adherence to the precepts of astrology among learned as well as unlearned segments of the population. Astrology was especially honored in the Italian universities where there were separate chairs in the subject[2]. Professors, of whom Giovanni Garzoni (1419—1505) of Bologna is an example, not only in Bologna, but also in Padua, and Florence, delivered orations and pronouncements extolling the study and efficacy of a knowledge of astrology[3]. And those who predicted the future on the basis of their increasingly elaborate and detailed knowledge of the positions, orbits, and motions of the heavenly bodies, won plaudits and renown not only from their academic peers but also from the chief potentates of Europe[4].

---

[1] For earlier discussions of this work see especially L. Thorndike, *A History of Magic and Experimental Science*, New York, 1923—1958, repr. 1966, Vol. I, pp. 178—179 (hereafter cited as Thorndike); also his "The Three Latin Translations of the Pseudo-Hippocratic Tract on Astrological Medicine", *Janus*, XLIX (1960), pp. 104—129; and P. Kibre, "Hippocratic Writings in the Middle Ages", *Bulletin of the History of Medicine*, XVIII (1945), pp. 399—400. The present essay is related to her more extensive study: *Hippocrates Latinus: Repertorium of Hippocratic Writings in the Latin Middle Ages, Traditio*, 1975.

[2] See for example C. Malagola, *Statuti delle Università dei Collegi dello Studio Bolognese*, Bologna, 1888, pp. 453—454, who cites examples in 1387 and 1389; and for earlier examples, M. Sarti et M. Fattorini, *De Claris Archygymnasii Bononiensis Professoribus*, Bologna, 1888—1896, Vol. I, pp. 523—584.

[3] P. Kibre, "Giovanni Garzoni of Bologna (1419—1505), Professor of Medicine and Defender of Astrology", *Isis*, LVIII (1967), pp. 504—514. See below XIX.

[4] In this regard see Thorndike, IV—VIII, indices et *passim*.

This adherence to astrology or to the belief in the rule of the stars, that is the supposed influence of the heavenly bodies on human affairs, and especially upon the states of health and disease of the human body, was not, however, a novel phenomenon of the later Middle Ages and early modern era. It was rather part and parcel of earlier medieval thought, as well as, very probably, of antiquity. As one distinguished medievalist has remarked, the rule of the stars in the Middle Ages was thought of as a universal law of nature[5] and astrologers based their confidence in divination of the future on the acceptance of this law. They thus defended astrology, which they believed to accord with well defined and seemingly predictable results, on the premise that knowledge of the operation of that law would lead men to avoid the specific pitfalls that had been predicted or forecast, just as one who listens to a weather forecast is prepared for changes in the weather. Hence the study of natural astrology, which involved the pursuit of knowledge of the shapes, sizes and motions of the heavenly bodies, which in turn led to the more accurate charting of the stars, to weather predictions, and to other developments involving navigation and so on, went hand in hand with the study of the stars in relation to human affairs and human health and disease, and to the forecasting of these effects or to judicial astrology.

It was in this milieu and particularly in accord with the belief in the influence of the stars on health and disease, that Hippocrates' name carrying with it the authority and prestige of the famed physician of Cos, was presumably invoked as the supposed author of a treatise on the prognostications of the course of health and disease according to the positions of the moon in each of the twelve houses or signs of the zodiac. It is highly improbable that this work bearing the name of Hippocrates, emanated either from the master himself or from any of his immediate disciples. Indeed, there is no indication that such a work was ever ascribed in antiquity to Hippocrates, although attention might be drawn to the fact that this improbability does not follow from evidence of Hippocrates' stated aversion to a belief in astral influence. On the contrary, in the work on *Airs, Waters, and Places,* which is generally accepted as authentic, Hippocrates gave expression to his belief in the effects on disease and health, not only of meteorological changes but also of the position of the stars. "For knowing the changes of the seasons, and the risings and settings of the stars, with the circumstances of each of these phenomena, he will know beforehand the nature of the year that is coming... If it be thought that all this belongs to meteorology, he will find out, on second thoughts, that the contribution of astronomy to medicine is not a very small one but a very great one indeed"[6]. The work on *Airs, Waters, and Places,* it might also be recalled, was among the earliest of the Hippocratic writings to be translated into Latin, that is probably in the sixth century[7].

---

[5] *Ibid.*, II, 973, et *passim.*

[6] Kibre, "Hippocratic writings", p. 400, n. 183, where is cited *Hippocrates* with an English translation by W.H.S. Jones (Loeb Classical Library, 1923, 4 vols.), I, 73.

[7] *Op. cit.*, p. 393, notes 187–188.

Although the work on astrological medicine, which circulated under the name of Hippocrates, is not found in its complete form in extant Latin manuscripts before the thirteenth century, it is highly probable that the text was derived from an earlier Greek or Byzantine source. Recent research indeed appears to have located this source in the work of a Byzantine scholar, Imbrasius of Ephesus, of the sixth century of our era. Dr. Richard Durling has reported on the finding of such a text under Imbrasius' name in the Bodleian Library at Oxford[8]. This text coincides with the *Prognostication of Disease by Astrology*, that is, on lunar prognostications in medicine, attributed to Galen, a tract printed with his collected works. The Galenic text is very similar although not identical with that appearing under Hippocrates' name[9]. Possibly also derived from the earlier Byzantine or Greek text are several fragments or abbreviated versions relating to lunar and other prognostications in medicine, which are extant in manuscripts of the ninth century onward[10].

However, the aim of this study is not to deal with questions of authorship nor to consider further the antecedents of the text current under Hippocrates' name. Rather the intention here is to focus on the work itself as it appeared to and was accepted by medieval and early modern European scholars; furthermore to take note of the availability or currency of the work primarily in Latin but also in vernacular renditions, and the views stated regarding the work by some representative scholars of the thirteenth to the sixteenth centuries. In so doing, the aim is to throw further light on the continued interest in astrological medicine and the name of Hippocrates.

The manuscript texts containing the tract on astrological medicine under Hippocrates' name are numerous as the listing of those so far noted in the Appendix to this article demonstrates. They also present considerable verbal differences. These have already been shown by Lynn Thorndike to fall into three major groupings. Two of these are assigned to the well known translators from the Greek, who were authors in their own right, namely William of Moerbeke, archbishop of Corinth in 1277, and Peter of Abano professor and physician in Paris and Padua, who is reputed also to have spent some time in Constantinople (d.c. 1316)[11]. The trans-

---

[8] Durling notes under items 2027 and 2527 of *A Catalogue of Sixteenth Century Printed Books in the National Library of Medicine*, compiled by R. J. Durling (Bethesda, Md. Washington, Superintendent of Documents, 1967), regarding the "De diebus decretoriis [Quem Petro Aponensi attribuunt] per Lucam Gauricum castigatus", that "The latter treatise appears to be a version of the *Prognostica de decubitu,* translated by Peter of Abano and attributed in a Bodleian manuscript to Imbrasius of Ephesus". The work is said, on the other hand, to have been compiled in Egypt probably during the Ptolemaic period. See further S. Weinstock, "The Author of Ps. Galen's *Prognostica de decubitu*", *Classical Quarterly*, XL (1948), pp. 41–43, where further bibliography is provided on the subject.

[9] Thorndike, I, 178–179, citing the edition by C. G. Kühn, *Claudii Galeni opera omnia*, Leipzig, 1821–1833, Vol. XIX, pp. 529–530.

[10] See Appendix below, under IV.

[11] Thorndike, "The Three Latin Translations"; and for Peter of Abano, Thorndike, II, 893–894.

lator of the third group is anonymous. It is possible that, upon a more detailed comparison of the texts, this group might fall into more than one division, since the individual items are more numerous and verbally more heterogeneous than the preceding two. Also whereas the first two appear to have been translated from the Greek, the third group of texts may have been translated from the Arabic, since they frequently appear with Arabic authors, such as Haly, who is named as the author of the prologue of the tract in at least one manuscript[12].

The individual groups are distinguishable from each other by the incipit of the prologue which was probably written by a presumed commentator or translator of the work. The first group of texts in the translation by William of Moerbeke, which comprises some thirty-five manuscripts of the thirteenth through the sixteenth century, has the distinctive incipit: "Sapientissimus [Ypocras] et omnium medicorum peritissimus ait..." whereas those in the translation by Peter of Abano, contained in only twelve manuscripts of the late fifteenth through the seventeenth century, have the incipit: "Cum legerem libros Ypocratis [compositos] medicorum optimi inveni hunc parvum sed magne utilitatis librum..." On the other hand, texts of the third group by an anonymous translator, are much more numerous, comprising some sixty manuscript copies of the thirteenth through the sixteenth century. This version, as indicated earlier, is closely related to the translation by William of Moerbeke, from which it is, however, differentiated by the opening words of the prologue. However, the incipits in this group vary among themselves. The most frequently encountered are: "Dixit [Dicit] Hypocras..."; "Dixit Hippocras medicorum optimus. Cuiusmodi medicus est...;" "Dixit [Dicit] Ypocras qui [cum] fuit medicus et magister optimus..."; "Sicut dicit Ypocras qui fuit medicus et magister optimus..." and so on.

Furthemore, in addition to the above three groupings, there are others, as noted below in the Appendix. These comprise Commentaries, Epitomes, and fragments, dating from the ninth to the sixteenth century, as well as translations into the three vernaculars, English, French, and Spanish. In practically all of these Hippocrates is named as author, thus justifying our continued association of his name with this tract, despite its spurious character.

In general, despite their verbal variance and differences in arrangement, the content of the work is similar in all the versions. That is, following the introductory passage of more or less extended length, there is the comparison of the physician who lacks a knowledge of astronomy or astrology to a blind man. This section is abbreviated in some texts and made more descriptive in others. For example, in some texts such a physician is likened to a man deprived of his sight, the noblest sense given to man, tapping his way hither and yon with his cane on which he must depend, not daring to move forward or to venture into new lanes. No one, the author

---

[12] That is in Munich CLM 182, 15c, ff. 331*ra*–333*ra*, "Astron. Ypocratis. Haly in librum Ypocratis, De esse egrorum. Dixit Ypocras..." This is Haly Abbas or Ali ibn 'Abbas (10th century).

continues, would put himself into the hands of such a physician. Recognizing therefore the necessity for the physician to learn astronomy, the author asserts that while reading the works of Hippocrates, the wisest and best of physicians, he found this small but very useful book, essential for the physician. For if he knows the content of this book he will be able to pronounce judgement on the health, life, and death of his patient. The author then directs the physician to observe the moon when the patient has taken to his bed; and he provides the physician with a brief account of the nature of each of the zodiacal signs in the presence of the moon[13]. He next urges the physician particularly to observe the moon when it is full, because at such time the blood and marrow in men and beasts rise in accord with the rising of the sea and all earthly things. The author further requests that the physician observe and ascertain whether the moon is going out of conjunction, for then the infirmity of his patient increases until the moon is in opposition[14]. And when it is in opposition, he should ascertain whether it was with an evil planet or in an evil place and if it was facing the lord of the house of death or not and if the illness will be of long or short duration[15].

A further selection chosen from the texts will suffice to illustrate the tenor of the tract. Following the earlier instructions, the physician is next told that

> when illness betakes anyone and the moon is in Aries with Mars and the Sun, the patient will suffer from a malady of the head because of the lack of heat... yet he will have hot fevers which will not subside. He will also suffer anxiety and will scarcely be able to speak. He will have pains in the chest and lungs and will have a rapid pulse[16].

The treatment for this affliction then follows. The patient should be bled and should use cold applications and should take cold food, and drink to minimize the heat. This illness, the author continues, may develop into frenzy. And if Saturn and Mars should be with the moon in Aries, the patient will die from the malady

---

[13] See for example Paris BN 7432, 15c, f. 264*r*, cited in the Appendix I, under the translations by William of Moerbeke.

[14] *Ibid.*; also Vatican 4085, 14c, f. 135r (William of Moerbeke translation): "Quando igitur infirmus decumbit in letto est necessarie videre si luna exeat a combustione [elsewhere coniunctione] quia tunc crescit infirmitas quosque veniat ad compositionis gradum. Et quando fuerit in oppositione vide si fuerit in planeta malo aut in malo loco aut si aspexerit dominum domus mortis. Et in hoc poteris scire si infirmus debet mori vel non vel si habebit longam infirmitatem vel curtam i.e. si longi temporis vel brevis patietur".

[15] W. Hartner, *Oriens-Occidens*, Hildesheim, 1968, pp. 447—460, provides a useful description of astrological terms.

[16] Vatican 4085, f. 135 r: "Luna cum fuerit in signo arietis cum marte aut cum sole erit infirmitas in capite propter nimiam caliditatem solis et dolebit pulsus capitis infirmi. Habebit quoque febren calidam et non recedit ab eo caliditas solis et dolebunt. Patitur quoque anxietate et vix loquitur. In pectore quoque nimium calorem et dolorem patitur in pulmone et habet vehementissimum pulsum. Scias tamquam necesse est eum minuere de vena cordis et uti rebus frigidis et cibo et potu minuentibus calorem. Et enim scias quod hec passio deveniet in frenesim quando cum luna fuerit mars aut saturnus et morietur ex hac infirmitate infra 15 dies s. ea die qua fuerit luna cum sole per quartum aspectum vel plus hoc erit si luna addat suo lumini".

within 15 days from the day in which the moon was with the sun through the fourth aspect. From Aries, the author proceeds to Taurus and so on through the twelve signs of the zodiac[17].

We may now turn from the tract itself to some views regarding it expressed by physicians and other scholars of the thirteenth century and thereafter. In the university milieu, attention has already been drawn to Peter of Abano who appears as a translator of the work and who was himself convinced that the science of astronomy or astrology was both useful and essential to the physician or medical practitioner. By knowledge of this subject, he asserted in his *Conciliator*, changes in the weather could be foretold and treatment of an individual case regulated accordingly. Like the pseudo-Hippocrates, whom he accepted as the ancient master, and cited along with Haly, he held that the physician should keep his eyes especially upon the moon[18].

Another articulate thirteenth century spokesman on the subject of the importance of astrology or astronomy for the physician was Roger Bacon, a member of the Franciscan Order and student and master of arts in both the Universities of Oxford and Paris. While Bacon does not quote directly from the so-called Hippocratic *Astrologia* he does name both Hippocrates and Haly in relation to this recommendation regarding the need for the physician to study astronomy, or astrology. He thus asserted that infirmities, health and the like, as well as the times the diseases occur and also how they may be cured should be understood through astrology, that is, by an astrological consideration of the hours of conception and nativity of individuals, the domination of the celestial forces might be known for those hours. He then went on to lament the fact that

> few physicians of this time know astronomy, and therefore many of them neither understand their own authors nor can they understand them and for this reason they neglect the better part of medicine[19].

Moreover, the ill-fated Cecco d'Ascoli (d. 1327), in his *Commentary on the Sphere of John of Sacrobosco*, quoted from the pseudo-Hippocratic tract in the opening sentences of the Prohemium to the commentary. He repeated the admonition from the Hippocratic work that the physician must of necessity know and consider the nature of the stars and their conjunctions.

> The physician cannot perform his duties well without a knowledge of the stars. He is like a blind man who must be led yet very often loses his way, without such knowledge. Thus spoke Hippocrates the best of physicians in the book of the aspects of the stars toward the moon: the physician that is not perspicacious in the science of the stars, will discover that no one will entrust himself to him, because as a blind man, he is unable to serve his patients with skill[20].

---

[17] See the last part of the passage quoted in the previous note.

[18] Thorndike, II, 893–894, citing Peter of Abano's *Conciliator*, Diff. 10, 104, 105, and 113.

[19] The *Opus Maius* of Roger Bacon, trans. by R. B. Burke, New York, 1962, Vol I, pp. 273–274.

[20] L. Thorndike, *The Sphere of Sacrobosco and Its Commentators*, Chicago, 1949, p. 344

A further example of the continued reliance on the work of pseudo-Hippocrates in the fourteenth century comes from the work of Augustine of Trent, an Augustinian friar. Between 1336 and 1347, he addressed a treatise to the Bishop of Trent, Nicholas Abrein, who was bishop during those years, in which he drew attention to the work of Hippocrates on the influence of the moon in the twelve signs of the zodiac as a source of information for particular diseases. Augustine referred also to Hippocrates as a great astrologer in that tract: "Fuit Ypocras magnus astrologus in illo libello". Augustine described Hippocrates' method of observing the moon in the signs of the zodiac as one procedure for the prediction of the outcome of disease in an individual[21].

In the following century too, there is evidence for the continued regard for the Hippocratic *Astronomia* or *Astrologia.* Thus Franciscus Florentinus or Paduanus, both a Minorite and an inquisitor, based a work that he wrote on the pestilence in 1456 upon numerous authorities in astrology, among whom he included Hippocrates and Galen. Although Franciscus acknowledged the fact that professors of astrology sometimes made mistakes, he attributed this to improper training. He granted that it is useful to know the hour of death in advance in order to prepare for it and he went on to cite "Hippocrates the primate of physicians", to the effect that one should not entrust himself to a doctor who is unskilled in astrology[22].

Furthermore, an outspoken exponent of astrological medicine in the fifteenth century, Conrad Heingarter of Zurich, was connected with the court of John II, duke of Bourbon, and with Louis XI of France. In his work prepared for the duke of Bourbon he quoted from among his many authorities in favor of astrology "Hippocrates in his *Prognostics* and his book on the judgements of the stars, that is on the influence of the moon in the zodiacal signs". Conrad also held that "medicine cannot be separated from natural philosophy or from astronomy"[23].

Toward the close of the fifteenth century, a copy of the *Astrologia Ypocratis* was given to Charles VIII by his physician, Jean Michel, on 17 July 1498, even though a few years before the work had been among the books belonging to Simon de Phares that were sent to the Parlement of Paris for examination by the faculty of theology and was condemned. However, this condemnation has been interpreted as a result of the continued quarrel between the university faculty and the king in the late fifteenth century[24].

There were continued exponents of astrological medicine and supporters of the Hippocratic tract on the subject in the sixteenth century as Lynn Thorndik- has ably illustrated. And it was not until the third quarter of the seventeenth century that the astrological medical tract was rejected finally as spurious. François

---

[21] Thorndike, III, 227–228.
[22] *Ibid.*, IV, 313 et seq., 319.
[23] *Ibid.*, IV, 367–368.
[24] *Ibid.*, III, 277, and IV, 549–550.

Bayle succeeded in doing this in 1677[25]. However, an earlier French classical scholar, Claude Saumaise or Salmasius, 1648, had held that "the tract on astrological medicine according to the position of the moon in the [zodiacal] signs should not be assigned to Hippocrates"[26].

In summation one must still ponder the question whether the long adherence to and continued support of the tradition of Hippocrates as author of a tract on medical astrology was merely the expression of a deep-felt veneration for the doctrine of the rule of the stars and hence a manifestation of the desire to unite this precept with the most venerated of the physicians of antiquity, or was the result of a conscious effort on the part of the proponents of medical astrology to lend respectability and plausibility to their belief by using the name of Hippocrates. Although there is no resolution of this question in the foregoing account, the brief review of instances of the use to which the work on medical astrology was put and the listing of the many manuscripts containing the work in the various recensions will serve perhaps to illuminate an aspect of the role that both Hippocrates and the stars played in late medieval medical thought.

APPENDIX
The "Astronomia" or "Astrologia Ypocratis" Manuscripts

The following manuscripts containing the above work are arranged roughly by centuries under each of the major versions of the tract. That is first, under the two well known translators, William of Moerbeke and Peter of Abano, respectively; next under the anonymous translator or translators. Following these are the various abbreviated and fragmented Latin versions and those in the vernacular tongues. In each instance the manuscripts not previously noted are indicated by an asterisk(*). Those earlier noted by Lynn Thorndike, either in his "Manuscripts of the Writings of Peter of Abano", *Bulletin of the History of Medicine*, XV (1944), p. 218; or his "The Three Latin Translations of the Pseudo-Hippocratic Tract on Astrological Medicine", *Janus*, XLIX (1960), pp. 104–129, or both. These have been included to provide a more complete overview of the currency of the tract than might otherwise be the case.

The abbreviations utilized are, with some obvious exceptions, those adopted by Lynn Thorndike and Pearl Kibre for *A Catalogue of Incipits of Mediaeval Scientific Writings in Latin*, revised and augmented edition (Cambridge, Mass.: The Mediaeval Academy of America, 1963), which is hereafter referred to as TK with column number.

---

[25] *Ibid.*, VIII, 293.
[26] *Ibid.*, VII, 103–104.

I

William of Moerbeke's translation from the Greek, distinguished by the *incipit*: "Sapientissimus Ypocras [et] omnium medicorum peritissimus ait: Cuiusmodi medicus est qui astronomiam ignorat. Nemo quidem in manus illius se committere debet quia imperfectus est et cecus et ideo non merito talis medicus reputatur..." The *desinit* varies insofar as some texts close without the section on fixed stars: "De stellis fixis". In such instances, the closing words are: "...et si fortuna aspexerit eam [eum] evadit [vivat], et sin [si non] morietur". With the added section, it closes: "...dabunt cum labore et difficultate".

XIV Cent.

Cambridge: *CU 1705 (Ii. I. 13), 14c, ff. 126r—132, fragments, of which f. 129*r—v*, contain the "Astronomia Ypocratis. Sapientissimus Ypo. et omnium..."

*Cuc 424, 14c, ff. 7r—9v. "Sapientissimus Ypocras et medicorum optimus ait: Cuiusmodi medicus.../...cum labore et difficultate. Explicit pronosticatio Ypocratis infirmitatum".

Cues: Hospital zu Cues 208, 14c, ff. 32*r*—33*v* (T).

Hospital zu Cues 307, 14c, ff. 167r—168v. "Hippocratis Astrologia. Sapientissimus Ypocras et omnium medicorum peritissimus ait: Cuiusmodi medicus [est] qui astronomiam ignorat. Nemo quidam manibus eius committere se debet, quia imperfectus est et quia cecus..."(T).

Erfurt: *Ea Q. 386, c. 1359, ff. 52v—53v (Col. R 72. 9). "Sapientissimus Ypocras et omnium medicorum peritissimus.../...cum labore et difficultate. Expl. astro. Y".

Leipzig: *Univ. 1143 (1499), before 1400, ff. 186v—189r, printed by Sudhoff, without identification, *Archiv f. Gesch. d. Medizin*, XVI (1925), pp. 95—102. "Sapientissimus Ypocras et omnium medicorum peritissimus ait: Cuiusmodi medicus est, qui astronomiam ignorat.../...et quicquid dant, dant cum labore et difficultate. Explicit liber de pestilencie" (*sic*).

Milan: Ambros. M. 28 sup. 14c, ff. 75r—78v (T).

Munich: *CLM 267, 2°, 14c, f. 80ra, beginning missing; des. "...si fortuna eam aspexerit vivet si non morietur".

Oxford: BLas 345, late 14c, ff. 31v—37v. "Ut ait Galienus [Gulielmus?] sapientissimus Ypocras omnium medicorum..." The third or anon. translation is at ff. 6—12*v*, in the same manuscript. See below (T).

Paris: BNna 625, 14c, ff. 89va—93rb. "Incipit tractatus Ypocratis de iudiciis infirmitatum ad dispositionem lune ad planetas. Sapientissimus Ypocratis omnium medicorum et peritissimus ait: Inscius medicus est qui astronomiam ignorat. Nemo quidem se committere.../...et si fortuna aspexerit eum evadet et si non morietur. Explicit tractatus Ypocratis de iudiciis infirmitatum secundum dispositionem lune ad planetas".

Vatican: VA 4085, 14c, ff. 135r—139r. "Liber Hippocratis de pronosticationibus egritudinum secundum motum lune tractatus a Domine fratre Guglielmo de

Morbeccha archiepiscopo corintio ordinis predicatorum. Sapientissimus et omnium medicorum peritissimus Ypocras ait: Cuiusdam medicus est qui astrologiam ignorat nec quisquis in manus eius committere se debet... Legens ergo in libris Ypocratis medicorum optimi inveni hunc librum parvum sed maxime admodum utilitatis quia valde necesse est... Luna cum fuerit in signo Arietis cum Marte..." Proceeds through the twelve signs, ending with "Luna in piscibus... Luna in stellis fixis... Scias quod per eum non perficiunt, dabunt cum labore et difficultate. Finis".

XV Cent.

Florence: FL Bisc. 13, c. 1400, ff. 60r—71v (T).

*FL Plut. 29 cod. XIII, 15c, ff. 170—173 (Bandini II, 33). "De signis infirmitatum. Sapientissimus Hippocras et omnium medicorum peritissimus ait.../...dabit cum labore et difficultate". In a collection of astrological texts of Arabic authors.

*FL Ashb. 1448, 15c, ff. 130—135v. "Liber excellentissimus pronosticorum secundum viam astronomie Ypocratis". Followed at ff. 136*v*—137, by a "Tractatus de natura et ordine XII signorum. Aries est primum signum et est igneus masculinus diurnus..." (TK 131).

*Gerona BC 75, ff. 113v—116. "Sapientissimus Ypocras..." (G. Beaujouan, "Manuscrits médicaux du Moyen Age conservés en Espagne", [in:] *Mélanges de la Casa de Velasquez, publié avec le concours du C.N.R.S.*, T. VIII, Paris, 1972, p. 187).

*Glasgow: Hunt. 461. 2., 15c. "De virtute lunae. Sapientissimus Ypocras et omnium mediocrum peritissimus...

*Kraków: Jagiel. 601, 15c, ff. 72r—74r. "Predicere egritudinem urina non visa. Sapientissimus omniumque medicorum peritissimus Hypocras ait: Cuiusmodi est medicus qui astronomiam ignorat.../...cum labore et difficultate nimia. Finitur deo gratias". F. S. Benjamin, Jr. and G. J. Toomer, *Campanus of Novara and Medieval Planetary Theory*, Madison, 1971, p. 101.

London: *BMsl 434, 15c, ff. 96*v*—101. "Tract. de sign. zodiaci nat. Sapientissimus Ypocras omnium medicorum peritissimus..." BMsl 636, 15c, ff. 98(96)v—102v. Without heading. "Sapientissimus Ypocras omnium medicorum peritissimus ait: Inscius medicus est qui astronomiam ignorat... Cum luna est in Ariete cum Marte.../..." Ends incomplete in the sign Aquarius (T).

Munich: *CLM 31, 15c, ff. 199vb—202va. "Sapientissimus Ypocras et omnium medicorum peritissimus ait: Cuiusmodi medicus est.../...cum labore et difficultate. Explicit est libellus Ypocratis de virtute lune... Deo gratias. Laus deo". This tract is said to have been written or transcribed by "dominus doctor Johannes Lochner" in the fifteenth century. However, the rest of the manuscript is dated in the fourteenth century: "scriptus fuit iste liber sub anno domini MCCCXX".

Oxford: BLd 29, 15c, ff. 167r—172v. "De observandis signis planetarum in morborum curatione. Dixit sapientissimus Ypocras omnium medicorum peritissimus..." (T).

Paris: *BN 7292, 15c, ff. 287va–289ra. "Sapientissimus Ypocras omnium medicorum perfectissimus ait: Quis medicus est qui astronomiam ignorat. Nemo in manibus illius se committere debet.../...et quicquid dederunt dabunt cum labore et difficultate. Explicit astrologia Ypocratis".

BN 7337, 15c, pp. 78a–84b, in a fine humanist hand. "Liber de pronosticationibus egritudinum secundum motum lune traductus a domino fratre Guglielmo de Morbecha archiepiscopo Corinthio ordinis predicatorum. Sapientissimus et omnium medicorum peritissimus Ypocras ait: Cuiusmodi medicus est qui astrologiam ignorat nec quisque in manus eius committere se debet quia imperfectus est cecus talis medicus.../...dabunt cum labore et difficultate. Finis". There then follows "Notabilia medicandi. Notandum quod cum ceperimus curare egrotantis oportet quod luna sit in aspectum bonorum et cave ne sit in oppositione..." which apparently continues to p. 87*r* (T).

*BN 7432, 15c, ff. 264r–266r, 266r–268. "Incipit liber Ypocratis viri peritissimi de illo celesti de quo in pronosticis sermonem facit dicens: Est quoddam celeste quod oportet ipsum medicum considerare cuius si tanta est prudentia mirabilis est minimum que stupenda. Cap. primum de eo quo intendit et est prologus. Sapientissimus Ypocras et omnium medicorum peritissimus ait: Cuiusmodi medicus est qui astronomiam ignorat. Nemo quidem in manus illius se committere debet quia imperfectus est et ideo cecus non inmerito talis medicus reputatur. Est quidem huiusmodi medicus ut homo sensu sui nobiliori scilicet visu viduatus qui non ire cognoscit herens baculo stat et non prius se movere audet ea parte qua vult ire donec cum baculo huc et dextrorsum atque sinistrorsum munitum solliciteque viam pretendere attemptet et tamen post baculi examinationem insecutus timidisque passibus vix ire audet semperque timet ne alium maximeque se ledat. Porro sic medicus ignorans astronomiam se per omnia habet. Propter quod quia ad perfectionem cognitionis morborum et curationis eorundem scientia astronomorum est necessaria. Ideo hanc habere sollicitus fui. Legens igitur in libris Ypocratis medicorum principis inveni hunc librum parvum sed magne utilitatis qui valde est necessarius omnibus medicis quem qui bene vocaverit sanitatem vitam mortemque infirmitatis prenuntiare poterit. Iubet itaque Ypocras omnis medicus aspiciat lunam quia cum plenam est lumine tunc crescit sanguis in homine et in omnibus in terra et in mari degentibus et in cunctis mundanis rebus suum crescit complementum. Cum igitur infirmus succumbit in lecto opus est videre si luna exeat a combustione quia tunc crescit infirmitas quousque veniat ad oppositionis gradum". In the succeeding chapters, consideration is given to the moon in each of the twelve signs of the zodiac beginning with "in Ariete" and ending with "in Piscibus", and with the selection on fixed stars, des. "...et quicquid dederint dabunt cum labore et difficultate. Finit".

Then follows (ff. 266r–268r) "Incipit tractatus de pronosticis et componendis atque mensurandis medicinis. Magna utilitas atque laus medico in veris pronosticis consistit..."

Vatican: *VA 2487, 15c, ff. 225ra–226va. A commentary by "Marsilius de

Sancta Sophia, Super Ypo. Liber de infirmitatibus que eveniunt luna existente in quolibet XII signorum coeli. Sapientissimus Ypocras et omnium medicorum peritissimus ait: Cuiusmodi est astronomia necessaria.../...luna fuerit in vergine et...dabunt cum labore et difficultate. Deo gratias. Explicit liber parvus magne utilitatis...repertus est in libris Ypocratis excellentissimi physicorum et astrologorum". VA Barb. 328, 15c, ff. 2r—(7r), although it contains the statement in the title that it was translated by "Frater Guglielmus de Morletta [Morbeka] ordinis fratrum predicatorum archiepiscopus de Corinto", is the text of the third translation. See below. VAp 1229, 15c, ff. 377r—382v. "Sapientissimus et omnium medicorum peritissimus Ypocras ait: Non medicus est qui astronomiam ignorat nec quidam in manibus illius qui committere se debet.../...[the last sign Pisces is here followed by the 28 mansions of the moon, des.] si non morietur. Quemadmodum diximus in precedentibus" (T). VA Urb. 1398, 15c, ff. 11v—17v. "Incipit astrologia Ypocratis. Sapientissimus Ypocras omnium medicorum peritissimus ait: Cuiusmodi medicus qui astronomiam ignorat nemo quidem in manus illius committere debet quia imperfectus est.../...dabunt cum labore et difficultate. Finis. Explicit astrologia Ypocratis" (T).

The above text is followed by another "Incipit Astronomia Ypocratis. Coniunctio est aspectus perfecte amicicie manifeste. Sextilis occulte amicicie.../...tempus in quo luna fit uncta planetis malis vel saltim a bonis separata. Explicit Astronomia Ypocratis". Two further selections on astrological medicine without any author's name follow to f. 20*r*.

Venice S. Marco VII. 28, 15c, ff. 3r—7v. "Sapientissimus Ypocras omnium medicorum peritissimus ait quod..." (T).

Vienna 5216, 15c, ff. 47v—50v, anon. "Non est medicus qui astronomiam ignoret..." This text is followed at ff. 51r—53r by "De predicandis aegritudinibus ex urinis. Dixit Hermes non est medicus sapiens in pronosticis signis.../...crisum et malum sexta die revelabit". (TK 919; F. J. Carmody, *Arabic Astronomical and Astrological Sciences in Latin Translation. A Critical Bibliography*, Berkeley and Los Angeles, 1956, p. 81—5, indicates MSS Vienna 5307, 15c, f. 150r—v, fragments; and Wolfenbüttel 2841, 15c, ff. 380v—382.

Vienna 5239, 15c, ff. 1r*—3r*. "Sapientissimus Ypocras omnium medicorum.../...dabunt cum labore et difficultate. Explicit astrologia Ypocratis". The third translation occurs in this same MS at ff. 32*r*—35*r* (T) *5503, a. 1506, ff. 188r—194r. "Versio libelli de infirmitatibus secundum locum lune. Traductio Guilhelmi de Moerbecha archiepiscopi Corinthi ordinis predicatorum. Sapientissimus et omnium medicorum peritissimus aut Ypocras [ait]: Qui medicus et astronomiam nescit nemo quidem se in manus illius committere debet quia non medicus diceret medicus sed metodicus quia imperitus est et cecus... (paragraph 2) Legimus (Legens ergo in libris: VA 4085) igitur libros Ypocratis medicorum optimi inveni hunc librum parvum sed magne (maxime admodum: VA 4085) utilitatis... infirmus decubuerit in lecto opus est videre si luna exeat combustionem... Nunc videamus naturas omnium signorum iuxta presentiam lune in eius. Aries..." followed by the remaining signs (des. f. 194) "...de natura complexionis nati aut sub eo nati tamen omnia cum labore et difficultate fit".

Vienna: *5511, 15c, ff. 12r—17v. "Sapientissimus Ypocras et omnium medicorum peritissimus ait: Cuiusmodi medicus est qui ignorat astronomiam. Quasi cecus... Nunc videamus... Cuicumque infirmitas accidit cum luna fuerit in Ariete... [and the last] Cum luna fuerit in Pisces addens suo lumine... malorum morietur". Then follow versus: "Jupiter atque Venus boni sunt a capute draconis... Mercurius cum luna sunt mediocres... Explicit tractatus astronomie Ypocratis de casibus medicinalibus".

Wiesbaden: *63, 15c, ff. 114v—117. "Sapientissimus Ypocras et omnium medicorum peritissimus.../...dabunt cum labore et difficultate".

Wolfenbüttel *2841, 15c, f. 380vb. Carmody, 1956, 81—5.

II

Peter of Abano's translation from the Greek. For this briefer version, see the earlier cited notices of L. Thorndike, "Manuscripts of the Writings of Peter of Abano" and "The Three Latin Translations of the Pseudo-Hippocratic Tract on Astrological Medicine". Incipit "Cum legerem libros Ypocratis medicorum optimi..." Cap. 1. "Nunc videamus naturam omnium signorum..."

XV Cent.

London: *BMadd 34603, included in an astrological manual compiled by Marcus Schnagel of Cracow, c. 1500, ff. 80—85*v*. "Libellus de medicorum astrologia", and again at ff. 305*v*—306*r*, incomplete. "Cum legerem libros Hippocratis medicorum optimi inveni hunc parvum sed magne utilitatis librum...Iubat ergo Hippocras ut medicus aspiciat lunam...Signum Arietis.../...et per nocumentum malorum morietur. Hipp. libellus de medicorum astrologia fuit a Petro de Abbano in latinum traductus". At ff. 305*v*—306*r* (old numbering 314 in upper margin), without heading. Incipit as above; incomplete at the close, "...et sedeat plane ubique et sic velit et da ei aquam bibere frigidam..."

This text agrees with that of the edition printed as an appendix to [Firmin de Bellavali] *Opusculum repertorii pronosticon in mutationes aeris*, Venice, 1485, ff. 46—49r (Klebs 406.1). BMsl 780, 15c, ff. 55v—58v, without heading. "Cum legerem libros Ypocratis compositos medicorum optimi inveni hunc parvum sed magne utilitatis librum.../... [ends incomplete in the sign Pisces] dolebunt si membra cum luna fuerit..."

At f. 166v of this manuscript there is an English translation of the Peter of Abano text.

Milan: *Ambros. Y 131 sup. misc., 15—16c, ff. 107—110v. "Hypocratis libellus de medicorum astrologia incipit a Petro de Abbano in latinum traductus. Cum legerem libros Hyppocratis... (cap. 1) Nunc videamus naturam omnium signorum..." (A. L. Gabriel, *Catalogue of Microfilms of One Thousand Manuscripts in the Ambrosiana*, Notre Dame. Indiana. 1968, no. 951).

Munich: CLM 2841, 15—16c, ff. 58r—65v. Hippocrates", De infirmitatibus ex aspectibus planetarum versus lunam provenientibus". Without introductory matter. Inc. cap. 1. "Nunc videamus naturam omnium signorum et primo de Ariete. Cum cuiquam infirmitas occidat.../...malorum morietur. Hippocratis libellum de medicorum astrologia finit a Petro de Abbano in Latinum traductus" (T).

Oxford: BLcm 46, 15c, ff. 140r—144r. "Cum legerem libros Hippocratis medicorum optimi..." (Thorndike, 1960, 116).

Vatican: 6280, 15—16c, ff. 174r—175v. "Hippocrates. De medicorum astrologia. Traductus Petro de Albano. Cum legerem libros Ypocratis medici optimi... Cum incidit infirmitas... ending with Cum luna fuerit in piscibus.../...per nocumentum malorum morietur. Hippocratis libellus finitus. Laus deo opt. max." (T).

6971, 16c. Ital. tr. by Pietro d'Oliva di Ventimiglia (Kristeller, *Iter* II).

Vienna 5498, 15c, ff. 53r—59v. "Cum legerem libros Ypocratis medicorum optimi inveni hunc parvum sed magne utilitatis librum..." (T).

XV—XVI cent.

Genova: Bibl. Civica Beria 1.2.37, cart. misc. 16—17c, ff. 1—23v (numbering irregular). "Hyppocratis libellus de medicorum astrologia a Petro de Abbano in latinum traductus. Cum legerem libros Hyppocratis..."

Astronomia or Astrologia Hippocratis
Peter of Abano's translation: Printed editions

Appendix to [Firmin de Bellavale] Opusculum repertorii pronosticon in mutatione aeris. Venice, Ratdolt, 1485, ff. 46r-49 r (Klebs 406.1; NYAM 96, Streeter Collection). "Cum legerem libros Hypocratis medicorum optimi ..."

With Jo. Ganivet, *Amico medicorum*, Lugd. 1550; Francof. 1614, ff. 80—85v. "Cum legerem libros Hippocratis medicorum optimi inveni hunc parvum.../...et per nocumentum malorum morietur. Hypocratis libellus de medicorum astrologia fuit a Petro de Albanno [sic] in Latinum traductus" (NYAM).

With Tomaso Sefirielle Bovio, *Melampio ouero confusione de medici safisti*, Verona appresso Girolamo Discipoli, et fratelli, 1585. "Hippocrates, Libellus de medicorum astrologia. A Petro de Abbano in Latinum traductus. Cum legerem libros Hyppocratis medicorum optimi inveni hunc parvum sed magne utilitatis librum et valde necesse est omnibus medicis. Qui hunc bene scierit santiatem, mortem, vel vitam infirmitatis poterit pronunciare. Iubet ergo Hyppocras ut medicus aspiciat lunam..."

III

Third translation possibly from the Arabic, for which see Thorndike (1960), 111—116; Kibre (1949), 399; Thorndike II, 924—925; TK 453—454; Diels (1906), 50.

This version is differentiated from that of William of Moerbeke, and of Peter of Abano, chiefly by the incipit. There is, however, a close relationship with that of William of Moerbeke. The incipits of this version also differ from each other. The three types encountered most frequently are: 1) "Dixit Hippocras medicorum optimus. Cuiusmodi medicus est..."; 2) "Dixit [Dicit] Ypocras qui [cum] fuit medicus et magister optimus. [Ille] Cuiusmodi medicus non est qui astronomiam ignorat [quod] nullus homo debet se committere in manus illius qui non est medicus perfectus..." 3) "Dixit [Dictus] Ypocras non est medicus qui astronomiam ignorat nec aliquis mittat se in manus illius quia non est medicus perfectus... Nunc [autem] videamus..." The usual *desinit* is: "...et si fortuna eam aspexerit vivet, si non [autem] morietur. Explicit tractatus Hippocratis de egritudinibus cognoscendis per astronomiam".

XIII–XIV cent.

Brussels: 4863 (4862–69), 13–14c, ff. 42r–46r (Silvestre; Calcoen, p. 95; TK 1246). "De iudiciis infirmorum. Quidam sapientissimus philosophus ait: Quis medicus est qui astronomiam nesciat..."

Cambridge: CUc 37, early 14 cent., ff. 61r–65r. "Tractatus Ypocratis pro infirmitatibus per astronomiam cognoscendis. Dicit Ypocras qui fuit medicus et magister optimus... [through the twelve signs, ending in Pisces] /...et si fortuna eam aspexerit vivet si non morietur".

Erfurt: Ea Q. 215, 14c, ff. 85v–88v (T).

Ea F. 267, late 14c, ff. 189r–190v (T).

Florence: *FLa 139(208–140), pp. 197a–221a. "Dixit [Dicit] Ypocras qui [cum] fuit medicus et magister optimus.../...si non [autem] morietur".

London: BM Cotton Appendix VI, c. 1300, ff. 5ra–8rb. "Incipit Ypocras de astronomia. Dixit Ypocras qui fuit medicus et magister optimus. Cuiusmodi medicus est qui astronomiam ignorat. Nullus homo debet committere se in manus illius quia non est medicus perfectus. Cognovi quod opus erat sciendi astronomiam. Aspexi libros Ypocratis et inveni librum hunc parvum sed optimum. Dicit Ypocras quod medicus primo aspiciet lunam quando est plenam luminis... Quando infirmus cadit in leto opus est ei videre si luna exeat.../...cum luna fuerit in piscibus et mars cum ea erit infirmitas ex calore opus est ei ut minuat et si fortuna eam aspexerit vivet si non morietur" (T).

BMr 12.C. XVIII, 14c, ff. 33vb–35va. "Dixit Ypocras qui fuit medicus et magister optimus. Et medicus non est qui astronomiam ignorat.../...et opus est ei ut minuat sanguinem et si fortuna aspexerit eam vivet si non morietur. Explicit de Ypocrate". In the lower margin of the MS is the statement: "Explicit tractatus Ypocratis de egritudinibus cognoscendis per astronomiam" (T).

BMsl 3281, 14c, ff. 62ra–64ra, as above.

3282, 13–14c, ff. 89v–90r, as above; des.: "non autem morietur. Explicit".

3284, 14c, ff. 81v–85v, as above.

Madrid: 10063, 13–14c, ff. 23va–24va. "Liber iudiciorum Ypocratis gloriosi qui dicitur liber lune". "Dixit Ypocras cuiusmodi medicus est qui astronomiam ignorat.../...sin autem morietur. Explicit gloriosus liber lune" (J. M. M. Vallicrosa, *Las Traducciones orientales en los manuscritos de la Biblioteca Catedral de Toledo*, Madrid, 1942, p. 160).

Milan: Ambros. A. 183, inf., 14c, ff. 71rb–73vb, as in CUc 37 above.

Munich: *CLM 267, 2°, 14c, ff. 82v–90ra, Diels, 1905, 130. Beginning missing, but identifiable by the following: "...erit infirmitas qui exiens a balneo... et opus est ei medicina pectoris... Si vero non fuerit cum luna vel non aspexerit aliqua fortuna... Si autem luna sit in cancro et aspexerit.../...Quando luna fuerit in piscibus addens sue lumine et gradibus... et si fortuna eam aspexerit vivet si non morietur. [in the margin] Explicit liber de iudiciis egrit. secundum lunam".

CLM 28229, 14c, ff. 84v–88ra, as above (T).

Oxford: BLas 345, late 14c, ff. 6r–12v, as above (T).

BLd 28, early 14c, ff. 81v–85v, as above (T).

Paris: BN 6891, 14c, ff. 90ra–91va. "Sicut dicit Ypocras qui fuit medicus et magister optimus..." (T).

BN 7348, 14c, ff. 5rb–12r. "Dicit Ypocras quod medicus primo aspiciat lunam quando est plenam..." (T).

BN 7413, II, 13–14c, ff. 24ra–28rb (T).

BNna 693, 13–14c, ff. 107vb–109va. "Dixit Ypocras qui fuit medicus et optimus magister perfectus medicus non est qui astronomiam ignorat. Nullus debet committere se in manus illius.../...cum luna in Piscibus cum marte cum ea... infirmitas est ex calore. Opus est ei ut minuat et si fortuna eam aspexerit vivet si non morietur". Although this is designated as 13c, on the cover: "Tractatus varii astrologici Lat. 693. Codex membranaceus sec. XIII", it is more likely of the 14c, since the astronomical tables included are all of the 14c; and at the end some fragments contain the dates 1322 and 1323. The codex is further indicated as from the Library of the Earl of Ashburnham, Appendix no. CXX. May 1897 (T).

Seville: *Colombino 5-5-14, 14c, ff. 48ra–50vb. Without heading ."Sicut dicit Ypocras medicorum optimus cuiusmodi medicus est qui astronomiam ignorat. Nullus homo debet committere in manus illius quia non est medicus perfectus et quasi cecus. Cognovi ergo quia opus erit sciendi astronomiam et aspexi in libris Ypocratis et inveni librum parvum et optimum quemque bene sciverit magnus efficietur et est valde necessarius omnibus medicis. Dixit Ypo. quod primo debet aspicere lunam quando est plena luminis quia tunc crescit sanguis et medulla in omni homine et bestiis omnibus secundum augmentum in mari et in cunctis rebus mundanis.../...Cum luna est in piscibus et mars cum ea erit infirmitas ex minimo calore et opus est ei ut minuat sanguinem et si fortuna aspexerit eam vivet si non morietur. Explicit libellus Ypocratis".

Vatican: *VAp 1094, 13–14c, ff. 407ra–409ra. "Dicit Ypocras qui fuit medicus et magister optimus cuiusmodi medicus est qui astronomiam ignorat. Nullus [homo] debet committere se in manus illius qui non est medicus perfectus... Aspexi libros Ypocratis et inveni librum hunc parvum sed optimum. Dicit Ypocras quod medicus primo aspiciat lunam quando est plenam luminis quia tunc crescit sanguinis et medulla omnium hominum et medulla in omnibus bestiis fit augmentum in mari... /...Cum luna fuerit in piscibus et marte cum ea est infirmus ex calore opus est ei ut minuat et si fortuna eam aspexerit vivet si non morietur".

XV cent.

Basel: Univ. Library F. II. 10, 15c, ff. 169v—172vb. "Sicut dicit Ypocras. Qualis medicus est ille qui astronomiam nescit..." (TK 1484).

Bethesda: *National Medical Library ff. 271v—277r. "Dicit Ypocras.../...si fortuna aspexerit eam vivet, si autem non morietur. Explicit opusculum Ipocratis nobilissimi viri d.g.a."

Cambridge: *CUt O.II.40, 15c, ff. 122r—126r. "Sicut Hippocras medicorum optimus cuiusmodi medicus ait qui astronomiam ignorat nullus homo debet.../... si fortuna aspexerit eam vivet si non morietur. Explicit expositio signorum".

Catina: 85, 15c, ff. 258v—261v. Cap. 1. "Cum infirmitas cuiusquam accidit..." (TK 309).

Cues: Hospital zu Cues 212, a. 1419, ff. 235v—237v (T).

Dijon: 449, 15c, ff. 53—54v (T).

1045, 15c, ff. 180v—186v (181—187). "Pronostica secreta. Dixit Ypocras qui fuit sumus medicus..." (T).

Florence: FL Ashb. 206, 15c, ff. 64va—67va. "Incipit liber Ypocratis de pronosticatione mortis et vite secundum motum lune in signis et aspectu planetarum quem transtullit frater Gullielmus de Morbecha ordinis fratrum predicatorum. Dixit Ypocras medicorum optimus cuiusmodi medicus est qui astronomiam ignorat, nullus homo debet se committere in manus illius..." Although this text is said to have been translated by William of Moerbeke, it belongs to the texts of the third translation. Thorndike (1944), 219.

Gdańsk: *Polish Academy of Sciences 2315, a.1467, ff. 146v—154b. "Sequitur Astronomia Ypocratis. Dixit Ypocras medicorum optimus nullus homo in manus illius medici.../...a cibo et potu" (G. Günther, *Katalog der Handschriften der Danziger Stadtbibliothek*, Vol. III, pp. 250—253).

*Ghent: 5(416), 15c, ff. 154v—(157v).

Klagenfurt: Bischöfl. Bibl. XXX d. 25, 15c, ff. 11v—14v. Lacks introductory matter (Thorndike, 1960, p. 112)

London: BMadd 15107, 15c, ff. 58r—60r. "Incipit astronomia medicine Ypocratis. Dicit Ypocras qui fuit medicus et magister optimus: medicus qui astronomiam ignorat nullus homo debet se committere in manus illius quia non est medicus perfectus. Cognovi quia opus erat sciendi astronomiam. Aspexi libros Ypocratis et inveni librum hunc parvum sed optimus.../...si aspexerit fortunam vivet si non morietur. Explicit medicina astronomica Ypocratis" (T).

BMh 2375, 15c, ff. 89–93v. "Qui fuit medicus et optimus magister..." Incomplete text, ends with Aquarius (T).

BMsl 3171, 15c, ff. 104v–116r. "Dixit Ypocras medicorum optimus cuiusmodi medicus est qui astronomiam ignorat. Est enim tanquam cecus sine baculo... Inspexi libros Ypocratis... necesse omnibus medicis. Dixit Ypocras quod primo aspice lunam... Cum infirmitas cuique acciderit cum luna fuerit in ariete.../...cum luna fuerit in piscibus... cum vero luna fuerit in piscibus addens [repetition sic]... Et si fortuna aspexerit eum vivet. Si non autem morietur. Explicit". Except for the opening words, this text closely resembles that of the translation by William of Moerbeke, and includes the comparison to a blind man (T).

Madrid: *BN 3370, ff. 194–197v. "Astrologia medica. Dixit Ypocratis... (Beaujouan, 1972, p. 187).

*BN 17961, ff. 19–28v, as in the preceding item (Beaujouan, 1972, p. 187).

Milan: Ambros. N 190 sup., 15–16c, ff. 1r–12r. "Aliter dixit Ypocras non est medicus qui astronomiam ignorat.../...et si fortuna aspexerit eum vivet si autem non morietur" (T).

Munich: CLM 182, 15c, ff. 331ra–333ra. "Astron. Ypocratis". Prol. "Haly in librum Ypocratis, De esse egrorum. Dixit Ypocras medicorum optimus..." Continues as in BMsl 3171, above. This text coincides with that printed at Padua, 1483 (Klebs 518.1; CPHL, f. 2r) (T).

*CLM 8950, 15c, ff. 172v–176r. "Dixit Ypocras medicorum optimus: cuiusmodi medicus est qui astronomiam ignorat.../...si autem non morietur".

*CLM 11067, a. 1446, ff. 69vb–72rb. "Incipit Ypocratis de aegritudinibus. Dixit Ypocras medicorum optimus: Cuiusmodi medicus hic est qui astrologiam ignorat. Nullus homo debet se mittere in manus illius quia non est medicus perfectus.../...si non autem morietur. Explicit tractatus de cognitione egritudinum Ypocratis anno domini MCCCCXLVI nona die mensi Septembris". The manuscript includes other tracts on astrological medicine as well as on weather prediction.

Oxford: BLas 393, 15c, ff. 58r–59v. "Astronomia Ypocratis in acutis. Dixit Ypocras medicorum optimus quidam de medicis qui astronomiam ignorat est eum tamquam cecus.../...fortuna aspectet eam vivet si non autem morietur. Explicit astronomia Ypocratis in acutis".

Paris: *Bibl. Reg. 6944, a. 1402, item 8. "Astron. Hippocratis. Sicut dicit Hippocras qui fuit medicus et magister optimus..." This item is cited by Renzi, V, 1859, 117. However, it has so far not been located.

BN 7443, 15c, ff. 133r–137r. Without heading. "Dixit Ypocras medicorum optimus cuiusmodi medicus est qui astronomiam ignorat. Nullus homo deberet se mittere in manus illius quia non est medicus perfectus. Cognovi ergo quia opus erat sciendi astronomiam et aspexi in libris Ypocratis et inveni librum parvum sed optimum quem qui bene scierit magnus efficienter et est valde necessarius omnibus medicis.../...Dixit Ypocras quod primum aspice lunam quando est plenam.../.. Cum luna est in piscibus et mars cum ea erit infirmitas ex minimo calore interiori.

et opus est ei ut minuat sanguinem et si fortuna aspexerit eam vivet si non autem morietur. Explicit" (T).

Several other tracts on astrological medicine follow in the manuscript.

Prag Univ: *280, 15c, ff. 211–217.

*I.F.II, 15c, ff. 188a–192b. "Hippocratis Tractatus de egritudinibus cognoscendis per astronomiam. Dixit Ypocras.../...si autem non, morietur" (J. Truhlar, *Catalogus codicum*, Vol. I, pp. 96–97).

*1610 (VIII. G. 28), 15c, ff. 183v–186r. "Tractatus de iudiciis lunae secundum Hippocratem. Dixit Ypocras non est medicus.../...si non autem morietur" (Truhlar, 1, 597–598).

Vatican: *VAbarb 328, 15c, ff. 2ra–7r. "Incipit liber Ypocratis pronosticationis vite et mortis secundum motum lune per 12 signa et aspectum planetarum quem transtulit Frater Guiglelmus de Morietta [sic] ordinis predicatorum archiepiscopus Corinto. Dixit Ypocras qui fuit medicus et magister optimus: Cuiusmodi medicus est qui astronomiam ignorat. Nullus homo debet se commitere in manibus illius qui non est medicus perfectus...Cum infirmus cuique acciderit quando fuerit luna in ariete.../...Opus est si ut minuat et si fortuna eam aspexerit vivet, si non morietur. Explicit liber Ypocratis de prognosticis deo gratias". Despite the attribution of this translation to William of Moerbeke, the incipit is that of the third translation. However, except for the opening phrase and other minor variations such as "nullus homo" for "nemo quidem" and the omission of the remainder of the phrase or paragraph following "debet se committere in manibus illius qui non est medicus perfectus", contained in the texts noted by Thorndike, 1960, p. 106, lines 1–3, the work agrees with the translation of William of Moerbeke.

*VA Chigi M. VII. 146, 15c, (a. 1447) ff. 34ra–36vb. "Dixit Ypocras cuiusmodi medicus est qui astrologiam ignorat. Nullus [homo] debet se mittere in manus illius. Aspexi libros Ypocratis et inveni hunc librum parvum sed optimum.../...si fortuna eam aspexerit vivet si non morietur. Explicit".

*VAp 1116, 15c, f. 24r. "Dixit Ypocras medicorum optimus cuiusmodi medicus qui astronomiam ignorat. Nullus homo debet se mittere in manus illius quia noscet ipsum esse medicum imperfectum ut id ita statur in prologo pronosticorum. Est enim quoddam... in quo oportet nostrum medicum pervidere". The remainder of the folio is blank. It is preceded at ff. Ira *et seq.*, by Avicenna's *Canon.*

*VAp 1340, 15c, ff. 88ra–90vb. "Dixit Ypocras medicorum optimus cuiusmodi medicus.../...si non autem morietur. Explicit tractatus Ypocratis de egritudinibus cognoscendis".

VAp 1354, 15c, ff. 238va–241rb, as above (T).

VAp 1367, 14c, ff. 159va–160ra. "Incipit tractatus medicinalis astronomie. Dixit Ypocras: Cuiusmodi fuit medicus optimus et magister et qui astronomiam ignorat nullus homo debet se committere in manibus eius quia non est perfectus medicus. Cognovi quia opus erat sciendi astronomiam et aspexi libris Ypocratis adinveni hunc parvum librum sed optimum. Dixit Ypo. quod medicus primo aspiciat lunam quando est plenam luminis...in loco solis evadet infirmus sed habebit prius magnum periculum est..." [The text is incomplete].

At ff. 176va—179ra, in this same manuscript, there is another example of the above work: "Tractatus medicinalis propter transitum lune. Dixit Ypocras qui fuit medicus expertus et magister quod qui astronomiam ignorat nullus homo debet se committere in manibus eius quia non est perfectus medicus. Cognovi quia opus erat sciendi astronomiam et aspexi libros Ypocratis adinveni hunc parvum librum sed optimum. Dixit Ypocras quod medicus primo aspiciat lunam quando est plenam.../...opus est ei ut minuat sanguinem et si fortuna eam aspexerit vivet si non autem morietur". Works of Arabic authors and the heading: "Opinio experte Zaelis et aliorum tractatus Haly" follow.

VAp 1401, 14—15c, ff. 95r—(98). "Dixit Hypocras..." as above.

VAp 1416, 15c, ff. 223r—227r. Anon. "Iudicium de infirmo quam infirmitatem patitur... Item cum quis infirmatur et luna exeat de combustione tunc crescit infirmitas quousque venerit ad oppositionis gradum et quando erit in coniunctione vide si fuerit causa mala... Cum infirmitas accidat luna in ariete... Si fortuna aspexerit eam vivet si non morietur" (Campanus, 1971, p. 79).

Venice: Museo Civico Correr., Cicogna 2721 (3747), Paper fol. 15c, ff. 37ra—39rb. "Dixit Ypo. qui fuit medicus et magister optimus. Cuiusmodi medicus est qui astronomiam ignorat. Nullus homo debet se intromittere in manus eius qui non est medicus perfectus.../...et si fortuna eam aspexerit vivet, si non autem morietur. Explicit" (Campanus, 1971, p. 95). *San Marco CL VIII. cod. 74 (3577), 15c, ff. 117r—121v. "Dixit Ypocras qui fuit medicus optimus et sublimus.../...si non morietur. Explicit tractatus de cognitione infirmitates ex presentia lune in signis duodecim secundum Ypocratem".

Vienna: *VI 4295, 15c, ff. 137v—139v. "Ps. Hipp. Excerpte e libro de medicorum astrologia". "Dictus Ypocras: non est medicus qui astronomiam ignorat nec aliquis mittat se in manus illius quia non est medicus perfectus... Nunc [autem] videamus.../...si fortuna eam aspexerit vivet, si non morietur. Explicit tractatus Ypocratis de egritudinibus cognoscendis per astronomiam".

VI 5239, 15c, ff. 32*r*—35*r* (TK 309, Cap. 1: "Cum infirmitas cuiusquam accidit...").

VI 5275, 16c, f. 195*ra—b*, fragments, incomplete, ending with "Gemini".

What appear further to be commentaries on the so-called *Astrologia* or *Astronomia Ypocratis* are found in the following manuscripts.

Padua: *Univ. Libr. 1795, 15c, ff. unnumbered. "Consilium Ypocratis et iudicium super infirmos cum infirmitatibus et medicamentis ac notitia mali. Ipocras medicus integerrimus et magister perfectissimus consulendo declarat in hunc modum de medico ignorante astronomiam. Nullus hominus intromittat se in manibus medici astronomiam ignorantis quia non est medicus perfectus nec voce medica meretur decorari. Nam est tanquam cecus viam baculo cespitano deambulans et viam examinans huc et illuc miserabiliter... Cognovi ergo medico necessariam esse ut astronomiam sciret et adisceret. Unde hoc est opusculum composui necessarium medicis valde. Nam primo opus est medicus aspiciat lunam... et ad hoc ut possit denotari tale secretum dicam de naturis omnium signorum luna existente in eis. Primo cum infirmitas cuipiam acciderit quando luna fuerit in Ariete cum Marte.../...et opus est ei ut sanguinem minuat et si fortuna eam aspexeat vivet si non autem morietur. Finis".

Then follow further astrological medical selections. "Si queratur phisicus ire ad infirmum et inerit luna seperando se a coniunctione solis.../...aut infortuna quia secundum illud ut predictum est iudicandum erit. Finis". "Si aliquis inceperit egrotare luna existente in sagittario et seperando se a saturno.../...ausus nisi medicamina levia et restaurativa propinare. Quia aliter infamiam et dedecus consequeris. Tabula de egris computa quod sunt dies... Deo gratias".

Vienna 2467, 15c, f. 97r—v (TK 1011). "De eventibus infirmitatum propter motum lunae. Ut ait Ypocras in pronosticis. Oportet medicum diem principii non ignorare. Etiam ibidem est quoddam celeste sidus quod medicum non ignorare in quo invenitur res miranda necnon et nimino stupenda... Et sublunari motu sub quo moventur omnia inferiora. (f. 97*v*) Idcirco in medicina summa est utilitas scire in quo signo est luna. De bono accubitu sive malo vel communi ut patet in hac regula. Luna prima tota die bona accubitus bonus... De communibus vero actu et eventu... in iudicibus omnibus. Sciendum est quod quatuor sunt virtutes que sive vigilantibus sive dormientibus nobis semper vigilant..." At f. 98r, there is the continuation of a tract, "De elementis".

IV

In addition to the above, a number of epitomes or fragments relating to astrological medicine under the name of Hippocrates are found in the following manuscripts of the eleventh through the sixteenth centuries. The following are arranged by centuries.

*Copenhagen Kgl. S. 1653, 11c, f. 183. "Epitomium or Epitomia de infirmis. Saturnus dies que in lector [sic] acciditur.../...xxi dies convalescit" (TK 1381; Beccaria 8. 17).

*Munich: CLM 615, 13c, ff. 49*vb*—50*vb*. "Incipit epytomia [empyromium]. Saturnus est dominum planetarum ideo ab ipso est potius incipiendum.../...hic erit vicesimo primo die convalescat".

*Douai: 715, 14c, ff. 4v—8v. "Epizonium Ypocratis de infirmis..."

*Avignon: 1022 (Anc. fonds 341), 15c, f. 12. "Tract. astrol. secundum Galenum et Hippocratem. Et quoniam principalis intentio.../...si non, morietur".

*London: BMe 2433, 15c, f. 47. "Complexiones hominis astronomiae et philosophiae secundum Galenum".

*BMsl 2030, f. 132r—135v. "Epistola Ypocratis. Excerpta quedam. Mirabilis contra infirmitates. Quatuor sunt humani corporis partes et.../... (ff. 134r—135v) mensibus quare superius. Luna prima tota die bona est. Luna secunda..." etc. This resembles the tract ascribed to Galen in a ninth century manuscript:

*Berlin: Preussische Staatsbibl. Cod. Phillip 1790, 1st half 9th century, ff. 40v–41v. "Incipit lunaris liber 1. Luna I qui decubuerit si tertia die se adlevaverit.../...et contrariis rebus a medicis factus curatus evadit. Explicit dicta Galieni de lunae diebus pro infirmis" (Beccaria); also: Madrid BN 19, f. 87. "Expositio Galieni pro infirmis. Luna prima si decubuerit..." (Beaujouan, 1972, p. 184); and:

Florence: Riccard. 728 (VIII. 3), 16c, f. 155. "Math. Curtius, Lectiones super G. et Astronomia Hippocratis" (Kristeller, *Iter* I, 179).

A further tract on astrological medicine is indicated by the explicit of the following:

*Stift Heiligenkreux (*Xenia Bernardina* I, 194), ff. 115–120. "Liber Hippocratis scoratus.../...explicit, in quo docetur, quae infirmitates sunt curabiles et quae non ex motuum stellarum scientia".

Possibly related to the above are the following:

Cambridge: CUpem 204, 15c, ff. 68v–69. "Pronosticon Ypocratis qui dies mortis vel salutis ostendit. Saturni die qui in lectum ceciderit..." (TK 1381).

Paris: BN 7443, 15c, ff. 137r–138v, without indication of Hippocrates' name but following the usual astrological medicine attributed to him. "Saturni die qui in lectum ceciderit..."

Vienna: 5512, a. 1436, f. 163r–v. As in CUpem 204, above.

Possible variants of the preceding are:

Florence: Riccard. 905, ff. 38v–39r. "Solis die in lecto qui cecederit..." (TK 1517).

Vatican: Regin. (VAr) 1324, 16c, f. 66r. Pronostica Galieni or Epitomia Ypocratis. "Solis die in lecto qui cecederit si die V. Si vero die leviorem noctem habuerit xiiii die levabit". Only 12 lines.

The following texts, either by Haly or Alkindi, to whom they are ascribed in other manuscripts, are ascribed to Hippocrates in the following manuscripts:

Munich: CLM 288, 14c, ff. 163vb–164rb. "Tractatus Ypocratis de iudiciis astrorum. Saturnus in ariete sub radiis fuerit [facit] pluvias et radios siccitates.../...et bonam complexionem [conditionem] ostendit etc. Explicit tractatus Ypocratis de iudiciis astrorum" (TK 138). CLM 588, 14c, f. 113v. A text similar to the preceding with variants as noted in the brackets.

Oxford: BLcm 517, 15c, ff. 20rb–21va. "Incipit libellus de impressionibus Ypocratis feliciter. Saturnus sub radiis in ariete facit pluvias. In omnibus autem facit infirmitates ex reumatissime.../...et bonam complexionem ostendit. Finis libelli Ypocratis de impressionibus". For an analysis of the above manuscript see L. Thorndike, "Notes on Some Less Familiar British Astronomical and Astrological manuscripts", *Journal of the Warburg and Courtauld Institutes*, XXII, nos. 1–2 (1959), p. 167 *et seq.*; and for other similar texts, Carmody (1956), pp. 81–82 (TK 1383).

Further Latin manuscripts containing the *Astronomia* or *Astrologia Ypocratis* that have so far come to my attention but for which I have not yet received microfilms are:

Kraków: Jagiellonian 793, a. 1459, ff. 212—228. "Tractatus astronomie Ipocratis". W. Wisłocki, *Katalog rękopisów B. J.* (*Catalogus codicum manuscriptorum Bibliothecae Universitatis Jagiellonicae Cracoviensis*), Cracow, 1877—81, Vol. I, p. 236.

Naples: Biblioteca nazionale fonds principale VIII. C. 45, 15c, item 22, f. 80. "Hypocras de iudiciis astronomie". (I am indebted to Dr. Ronald Doviak for this item.)

Wrocław: Ossolineum 815, 15c, ff. 56-60. "Astronomia Hippocratis". W. Kętrzyński, *Katalog rękopisów Biblioteki Zakładu Narodowego im. Ossolińskich* (*Catalogus manuscriptorum Bibliothecae Ossoliniana Leopoliensis*), Lwów, 1881—1898, Vol. III, pp. 267—268. (I am indebted to. Jadwiga Kozicka, for this and the Kraków references.)

Vernacular versions
XV—XVII cent.

Cambridge: CUt R. XIV. 52, 15c, ff. 143r—145r. "This is the book of Ypocras. In this book he techith to know the planets sikenes lyfe and deth and the tymes therof. First saith Ypocras that a lithe... When the mone is in the signe of Taurus that signe is..." (and so on through the 12 signs of the zodiac, ending: "...Here endith the Book of Ypocras of lif and deth translated of astronomers the best upon Avicen".

London: BMadd 12, 195, 15c, "The boke of Ypocras for to knowe be the planetes of seknes, both of lyf and deyth, and the tymes".

BMsl 73, 15c, ff. 132v—136v, English translation probably of the Peter of Abano version.

Oxford: BLas 210, 15c, ff. 36v—42r. Astrological medicine. English and Latin. "As sayeth Ypocras best of phisicos who knows no astronomie yt no man should himself into his handys... In this sayde booke sayeth Ypocras loke when the moon hath ful his light".

"Nunc videamus naturas omnium signorum.../...vivet si non, morietur. Et sufficit de iudiciis secundum motum lune in 12 signis. Explicit. Explicit liber Ypocratis de naturis signorum iuxta presentia lune et aspectus aliorum planetarum ad ipsam in signis variis existentium".

BLas 393, 15c, ff. 32r—33r. "This is the boke of Ypocras. In his boke he tellyth how for to know by the planets lif or dethe and the tymes thereof. First he sayeth that a lethe shall take hede of the moon when he is at the full..." The tract then goes on to Aries and the other signs. It is not clear where it ends since the tract becomes interwoven with several *experimenta* or prescriptions at f. 33r.

BL Bodl. 621 (2155), late 16c, ff. 213—(239). Hippocrates, "De la significacion de la muerte et de la vida segun el movimento de la luna...el interprete Gulideolo medico" (16c), with tables and admonitions.

Paris: St. Geneviève 3151 (V. F. in 8vo. 9), 17c, in a collection of tracts on *Astronomy* and *Astrology* copied or composed by Claude Lenfant, f. 14. "S'ensuyt l'astronomye de maistre Hypocras. Maistre Hypocras et Galyen disent que c'est ung povre maistre qui sciat point d'astronomye". The tract is apparently incomplete.

There are doubtless many other examples of this tract to be found if one combs the various manuscript collections carefully, but the foregoing may perhaps give some indication of the extent to which the work was current in manuscript form.

XV

LEWIS OF CAERLEON, DOCTOR OF MEDICINE, ASTRONOMER AND MATHEMATICIAN († 1494?)

BY his astronomical tables drawn up on 16 March 1485, in the tower of London, where he had been placed at the command of king Richard III, Lewis of Caerleon called attention not only to his own plight but also to his abiding interest in astronomical phenomena.[1] Yet he has failed to receive more than passing notice from recent writers,[2] despite the several manuscripts containing the works of leading astronomers and mathematicians of both Oxford and Cambridge to which Lewis' name and notes are attached, as well as his alleged participation in the stirring events that preceded the accession of Henry VII (Tudor) to the throne of England. These considerations would appear to warrant the present effort to rescue Lewis of Caerleon from obscurity and to call attention to his extant manuscript notes on astronomy and mathematics.

According to the brief account in the *Dictionary of National Biography* (X, 128), Lewis of Caerleon, "an obscure fifteenth-century scholar," was often confused with the more distinguished and better known fourteenth-century theologian, Lewis Charlton or Cherleton (d. 1369), bishop of Hereford. The confusion is said to have arisen because of similarity of name and pursuits, and the fact of both coming from the Welsh border.[3] The account then indicates that according to Bale (p. 475), Lewis of Caerleon, "a distinguished mathematician, theologian, medical writer, and teacher at Oxford (d. 1369)," composed a number of works, the titles of which are indicated.[4] Of these works, however, it is said, "nothing else seems to be known."[5] It is interesting therefore to note that the *Catalogue of Royal Manuscripts* (II, 68), calls attention to manuscripts in the British Museum which contain works by Lewis of Caerleon similar to those noted by Bale.[6] One of these, Royal MS 12.G.1, had already been noted by

---

[1] See below, item 14, note.

[2] Cf. R.W.T. Gunther, *Early Science in Cambridge* (Oxford, 1937), p. 141; F. M. Powicke, *The Medieval Books of Merton College* (Oxford, 1931), pp. 36, 218, and *addenda*; and R. W. Hunt, "Medieval Inventories of Clare College Library," *Transactions of the Cambridge Bibliographical Society*, 1950, *2*: 123.

[3] The account in the *Dictionary of National Biography* is given under Charlton or Cherleton, Lewis. Caerleon (also written Kaerlyon, Carlion, Karlyon), is in Monmouthshire. See David Williams, *History of Monmouthshire* (London, 1796), p. 43 ff.

[4] John Bale (1495–1563), bishop of Ossory, *Scriptorum illustrium . . . Catalogus* (Basle, 1557, 1559, 2 pts, fol.), p. 475. The account given by Bale is repeated in large part by John Pits or Pitseus (1560–1616), *Relationum historicarum de rebus Anglicis* (edited by W. Bishop, Paris, 1619, 4to), 1,503. Pits also confuses the two men, putting everything under Ludovico de Caerleon, 1369. He adds, however, that the *Tabulae eclipsium Richardi Wallingfordi* are in a MS in "bibl. baronis Lumleiani." It is worthy of notice that the present Royal MS 12G.1, is a Lumley MS and in all likelihood identical with the MS noted by Pits.

The titles of the works listed are: "Super magistrum Sententiarum (lectures on theology)"; "De eclipsi solis et lunae"; "Tabulae Eclipsium Richardi Wallingfordi"; "Canones Eclipsium"; "Tabulae Umbrarum"; and "Fragmenta astronomica."

[5] *Dictionary of National Biography*, *10*, 128. This work will henceforth be cited as *DNB*.

[6] Royal 12G.1, henceforth to be cited as BMr 12G.1; Harley 7055, fol. 232; and Sloane 1697, henceforth to be cited as BMsl 1697

Tanner in his account of "Ludovicus Kaerlion," whom he carefully distinguished from the fourteenth-century theologian. Tanner, however, continued to list under the fifteenth-century "Ludovicus Kaerlion," the theological tracts belonging in all likelihood to Lewis Charlton, bishop of Hereford.[7] Still another manuscript containing tracts and notes by Lewis of Caerleon, listed by Tanner as "Norwic. Moore 820," is extant in Cambridge at the University library.[8] Others are in St Johns College library, and in Oxford in the Bodleian and Corpus Christi libraries.[9]

The confusion regarding Lewis of Caerleon had in no way been mitigated by the fact that the antiquarian John Leland (d. 1552), referred to a "Johannes Cairleon" whose *Tabulae de Rebus astronomicis*, produced at London, 1482, were extant in Clare College, Cambridge, in Leland's time. No trace of them is there today, however.[10] On the other hand, in his notes compiled from direct observation of the contents of various libraries, Bale had distinguished clearly between the works of the fourteenth-century theologian,[11] and those of Lewis of Caerleon, the fifteenth-century physician, mathematician and astronomer. The works of the latter he described as in Clare College, Cambridge, and in the Museum of Robert Recorde.[12]

Additional informative details regarding Lewis of Caerleon were provided by Anthony Wood and his editor, John Gutch, who affirmed that the Lewis of Caerleon who flourished in 1482 was a different person from Lewis Charlton of the fourteenth century with whom he is sometimes confused. The first named, Lewis of Caerleon, who was despoiled and imprisoned by Richard III for his aid to the Lancastrian cause, was said to have been the most famous mathematician of his time. He was incarcerated by Richard III because of his affection for Henry (Tudor), Earl of Richmond and the standard bearer for the Lancastrian claims.[13] Similarly, Stow in his *Annales of England* referred to a certain Welshman called Lewes [of Caerleon], "learned in physicke," and in the service of Elizabeth of York, widow of Edward IV. This Dr

Lewis of Caerleon's name is erroneously associated with the *Experimentarius* in BMr 12E.IV. It is possible that his name does appear on the flyleaf of the MS where the almost illegible name "Laur. Kear" (?) may refer to Laurentius Kearlion.

[7] Thomas Tanner, *Bibliotheca Britannico-Hibernica* (London, 1748), pp. 449–450; and see note 11 below.

[8] Cambridge University Library 1017 (Ee. 3.61), 15th cent., henceforth to be cited as CUL 1017 (Ee.3.61). Mr H. V. Pink of the Cambridge University Library very kindly verified this fact for me. He points out that "The Norwich Moore MSS. . . formed part of the library of John Moore, successively Bishop of Norwich and Ely which was presented [to the Cambridge University Library] by King George I in 1715."

[9] St Johns College Library 41(B.19), 15th cent., henceforth to be cited as CUsj 41(B.19); Oxford, Bodleian, Digby 178, no. 7, 15th cent., with marginal notes by Lewis of Caerleon at fols. 15–46, henceforth to be cited as BLd 178; also at the Bodleian, Savile 38, 15th cent., henceforth to be cited as BL Savile 38; and Corpus Christi College 234, 15th cent.

[10] John Leland, *Commentarii de scriptoribus Britannicis* (ed. A. Hall, Oxford, 1709, 2 tom.), p. 471. For a John Charleton c. 1486–1493, see note 25 below. See also R. W. Hunt, "Medieval Inventories of Clare College Library," *loc. cit.*, pp. 105–125.

[11] *Index Britanniae quos ex variis bibliothecis non parvo labore collegit Ioannes Baleus, cum aliis* (edited by R. L. Poole, with the help of Mary Bateson, Oxford, 1902), p. 284; and see R. W. Hunt, *loc. cit.*, pp. 122, 123. Bale stated that "Ludovicus Sharleton, Episcopus Herefordensis scripsit 'Lecturam Sententiarum,' li. iiii; 'Lecturam Theologiae,' li. i; atque alia nonnulla; claruit a.d. 1369: ex Collegio Regine, Oxon."

[12] Thus Bale further stated that "Ludovicus Caerlion, astronomus peritus, scripsit, 'De eclipsi solari ac lunari, li. i, Modus operandi, pro eclipsi lune;' 'Tabulas eclipsium, li. i, Altitudo lune in arcu, longitudo;' 'Canones eclipsium, li. i, Eclipsium solis, quantitatem et dur.;' 'De tabulis umbrarum, li. i, Circa compositionem tabularum umbrarum;' atque alia plura composuit, Ludovicus Caerlion, Britannus, doctor in medicinis et astronomus, Londoni claruit, 1482: Ex Aula Clarensi Cantabrigie." Bale then added as if he were a different person: "Ludovicus Kaerlion, doctor in medicinis, reliquit quedam fragmenta astronomica; et 'De eclipsium calculatione, li. i;' claruit a.d. 1480: Ex Museo magistri Roberti Recorde."

Robert Recorde (1510?–1558), described as a famous mathematician, was fellow of All Souls College, Oxford, in 1531. He also taught medicine and mathematics at Cambridge; and then returned to Oxford. See *DNB* and Gunther, *Early Science in Oxford*, vol. I, pt. ii, pp. 13–22. Gunther indicated that Recorde taught astrology and included a list of his works bearing on the early history of Oxford science.

[13] Anthony Wood, *Fasti Oxoniensis, Appendix to the History and Antiquities of the Colleges and Halls in the University of Oxford* (edited by John Gutch, Oxford, 1790), p. 26.

Lewes, or Lewis as he is elsewhere referred to, was said also to have been physician to Lady Margaret, Countess of Richmond, as well as friend and physician to her son, Henry (Tudor), Earl of Richmond. He was believed to have supported Henry when the latter sponsored or joined in the conspiracy and uprising against Richard III headed by the duke of Buckingham.[14] As related by Polydore Vergil, this "Ludovicus of Wales," because he was a man of discretion and the confidant of Lady Margaret, acted as go-between for the delivery of secret messages from the Countess of Richmond to the closely guarded Queen Elizabeth whom he also served in the capacity of physician. It was largely because he was a physician, and under no suspicion whatever, according to Polydore Vergil, that Lewis was able to carry on the negotiations between the two women.[15] Lewis of Caerleon was further credited with having done much to forward the project for the marriage of Henry (Tudor), to Elizabeth, eldest daughter of Queen Elizabeth of York.[16]

Following the capture and summary execution of the duke of Buckingham, a number of the persons alleged to have been involved in the uprising, together with Lady Margaret, Countess of Richmond, and shortly afterward Queen Elizabeth of York, were brought to London.[17] It is very probable that it was on this occasion that Dr Lewis, physician to both Queen Elizabeth and Lady Margaret and an avowed friend of Henry (Tudor), Earl of Richmond, was put under arrest in the tower of London. Although his name does not appear in the lists of those singled out for punishment by Richard III,[18] the fact of Lewis' despoilment and imprisonment in the tower of London is substantiated by the note accompanying the astronomical tables for 1482 and 1483 which Lewis revised in 1485 while in the tower. In this note he stated that "after the composition of these tables, which I had lost through the plundering of king Richard, I, being imprisoned in the tower of London, composed other tables of eclipses, which deviated from those by a few seconds, for the reason that this is in a different latitude and hence the observations differ." [19] The date of the composition of the revised tables is clearly indicated by the example of the eclipse with his observation of it made by Lewis in the tower, "in the present year 1485, post meridian, on the sixteenth day of March." [20]

The reputed friendly and professional association of the physician Lewis of Caerleon, with Henry Tudor, which probably was the chief reason for Lewis' imprisonment in the tower of London by Richard III, was amply attested by the royal favors extended to Lewis of Caerleon by Henry immediately following his accession to the throne. Thus on 24 February 1486, in the first year of his reign, Henry VII provided "a grant for life to Lewis Caerlion, doctor in medicine, of 40 marks a year out of the issues of the county of Wilts." [21] Again, on 27 November 1486, another grant for life was made "to the king's servant, Lewis Caerlion, doctor in medicine, of an annuity of 20 marks at the receipt of the Exchequer from Michaelmas, I Henry VII," [22] and, further, on 3 August 1488, there was a "Grant for life to Lewis Caerlyon to be one of the knights of the king's alms in the free chapel or church of the college of St Mary the Virgin, SS George the Martyr and Edward the Confessor in Wyndesore castle." [23]

[14] Th.Stow[e], *Annales of England* (continued to the year 1614 by Ed. Howes, London, 1615), pp. 464–465; also Sir James H. Ramsay, *Lancaster and York* (1892), vol. II, p. 505; Polydore Vergil, *Historiae Angliae libri 26* (Duaei, 1603, 8 vo., 2 tom.), vol. II, pp. 1395–1396; *Rotuli Parliamentorum, ut et Petitiones et Placita in Parliamento*, vol. VI, 250–251, a.d. 1483, I Rich. III.

[15] *Hist. Angliae*, vol. II, p. 1395.

[16] Stow[e], *op. cit.*, p. 465.

[17] *Rotuli Parliamentorum*, vol. VI, pp. 244–249.

[18] *Idem.*

[19] See note to item 14 below.

[20] BMr 12G.I, fol. 6v, "Istam est solis anno Christi in presento 1485 post meridiem 16 diei Marcii, contingentem ego observam in turre Londoni."

[21] *Calendar of Patent Rolls*, Henry VII (London, 1914), vol. I, p. 75, I Henry VII.

[22] *Ibid.*, vol. I, p. 145, 2 Henry VII.

[23] *Ibid.*, vol. I, p. 219, 3 Henry VII. This fact is also noted by Tanner *op. cit.*, p. 449, from MS Norwic. Moore 507. Mr Pink (see note 8 above) informs me that this MS is also now in the Cambridge University library (Ii.5.31). It "is made up of extracts from the Patent and Escheat

This appointment was reaffirmed on 14 September 1491, "in place of William Stocton, deceased."[24] Lewis of Caerleon apparently lived on until 1493–1494, since his name continued to appear in the treasurer's rolls through the years 1493–1494.[25]

Information regarding the academic career of Lewis of Caerleon is wanting since his name does not appear in the extant matriculation rolls of either Oxford or Cambridge. However, there appears to be ample evidence that he was associated with, or at least interested in, the work of leading astronomers and mathematicians of both universities, with a particular predilection for those of Merton College, Oxford.[26] Thus he annotated and made use of the works of the earlier Merton College astronomers Richard of Wallingford (d. 1336), abbot of St Albans;[27] and Simon Bredon (d. 1372).[28] He also transcribed and corrected the astronomical tables of John Killingworth (d. 1445) of Merton College;[29] and made use of the calendar with astronomical tables of the Oxford Minorite, John Somer (fl. 1383).[30] He discounted as untrue the alleged authorship of the table of the diversity of the ascension of signs for the whole habitable earth which had been ascribed to John Walter (or Fitzwalter, d. 1412?), fellow of Worcester College, Oxford.[31] He also gave considerable attention to the work of one of the leading Cambridge astronomers, John Holbrooke (d. 1437), master of Peterhouse, Cambridge. He noted that John Holbrooke, whose works he transcribed, was chaplain to Henry V, by whom he was held in high esteem. Lewis stated that he considered Holbrook excellent in speculative astronomy, without equal among all those astronomers that England has produced, and of ever increasing fame.[32]

Lewis further referred to the work of Roger and Thomas Suthwell. The last named, Thomas Suthwell, was the author of a scheme of nativity of Henry VI whom he served as court astrologer.[33] It is probably to this horoscope that Lewis of Caerleon referred

---

Rolls; the reference quoted by Tanner occurs on folio 67." See E. H. Fellowes, *The Military Knights of Windsor* (*1352–1944*) (Windsor, 1944: Hist. Monographs relating to St George's Chapel, Windsor Castle), p. 12. Edward III by letters patent, dated 6 August 1348, had laid the foundations for his "College within the Chapell," which was to be dedicated thenceforth "to the honour of God, the Blessed Virgin Mary, St George the Martyr, and St Edward, the Confessor" (*Ibid.*, pp. vii *et seq.*). The original primary purpose of the foundation was to provide for distinguished soldiers in their old age and poverty, and secondarily to establish a brotherhood of laymen who would meet daily in St George's Chapel to pray for the souls of the king and his successors on the throne (*Ibid.*, p. xv). Ashmole indicated, however, that some "attained admittance, probably out of devotion rather than poverty, as Lodowick Carly, the King's physician, . . . temp. Henr. VII," Elias Ashmole, *The History of the Most Noble Order of the Garter* (London, 1715), p. 98. A poor knight was "a bedesman, a pensioner or almsman, charged with the duty of praying for the souls of his benefactors," Fellowes, *op. cit.*, pp. xv–xvi.

24 *Calendar of Patent Rolls*, vol. I, p. 365, 7 Henry VII.

25 Fellowes, *op. cit.*, p. 12. For a John Charleton (c. 1486–1493), who was one of the Knights of prayers in the Collegiate church of St Mary and St George in the castle of Windsor, see *Calendar of Patent Rolls*, vol. I, p. 420, 8 Henry VII; Fellowes, *op. cit.*, p. 12.

26 See Gunther, *Early Science in Oxford* (1920), vol. I, pt. ii, pp. 10–12; (1923), vol. II, pp. 31 ff.; 43 ff.; (1937), vol. XI, pp. 41–44; and Lynn Thorndike, *History of Magic and Experimental Science* (New York, 1934), vol. III, pp. 15, 122 ff.

27 *Ibid.*, vol. III, pp. 119 ff.; Gunther, *Oxford Colleges and their Men of Science* (Oxford, 1937), p. 41; also his *Early Science in Oxford*, vol. II, pp. 32–34, 50, 337–48; and his *Early Science in Cambridge*, pp. 130–137. See also item 34 below.

28 On Simon Bredon, see Thorndike, *op. cit.*, vol. III, p. 521; Gunther, *Early Science in Oxford*, vol. I, pt. ii, p. 10; vol. II, pp. 52–55; also F. M. Powicke, *The Medieval Books of Merton College* (1931), p. 138, and item 35 below.

29 See item 30 below.

30 See items 21, and 32, below. See also *DNB*; and Gunther, *Early Science in Oxford*, vol. II, pp. 60–62.

31 See item 33 below; also *DNB*; and Gunther, *op. cit.*, vol. II, p. 66.

32 See item 29 below; also CUL 1017(Ee. 3.61), 15th cent., fols. 161v–162r. See *DNB* and Gunther, *op. cit.*, vol. II, pp. 65–67; also Thorndike, *op. cit.*, vol. IV, p. 98. A volume of John Holbrooke's astronomical tables which he presented to Peterhouse is now Peterhouse MS 267; another volume of his astronomical tables also originally presented to Peterhouse in 1426, is today at the British Museum, Egerton 889.

33 CUL 1017(Ee. 3.61), fol. 160v, "et talis est figura Rogeri et magistri Thome Suthwell," and again on fol. 162r; BM Egerton 889, 15th cent., fol. 5r: "Nativitas H. 6^{ti} secundum Suthwelles astronomum. Nativitas H. 6^{ti} anno Christi inperfecto 1421 4^{a} die decembris. . . ." See Gunther, *Early Science in Oxford*, vol. II, p. 65, "Suchwelles. Scheme of Nativity of Henry VI (astrologer royal)." He is probably the master Thomas Sothewell, clerk, in the king's service,

as being transcribed and sent on 18 July 1441 to his special masters in the king's household at Sheen, John Somerset and John Langton, both of whom had been educated at Oxford but went later to Cambridge.[34] In 1441, John Somerset, fellow of Pembroke College, Cambridge, physician to Henry VI and chancellor of the Exchequer, and John Langton, master of Pembroke and chancellor of the university of Cambridge, were both named in a patent for the foundation by Henry VI of a college in Cambridge [King's College], the members of which, headed by a rector, "were to study and pray for the good estate of the king."[35] Lewis also transcribed the work of Humphrey, duke of Gloucester, concerning whose estate John Somerset had acted as one of the executors and had negotiated for gifts of his books to Oxford University.[36]

Further evidence for Lewis' interest in the work of both Oxford and Cambridge is provided by his gifts to both universities of copies of his tables of eclipses.[37] In addition he gave as a gift, on 26 October 1490, to Merton College, Oxford, astronomical tables for the use and profit of the students there.[38] His expressed hope, that they would be of use, appears to have been realized since on 25 October 1497, "power was given to master Joh. Davys of using at the time the book of tables of master Ludowici, which said master Lewis gave to the College." It is interesting to note that as bond for the tables, master John Davis put up "a certain book of letters of Seneca."[39]

Although Lewis of Caerleon refers to himself as Doctor of Medicine, he appears to have left no writings on medical subjects. His own extant compositions relate chiefly to astronomy and mathematics. They include various redactions of astronomical tables, as well as tracts on the art of composing tables with canons for their use, and calculations of eclipses of sun and moon. In addition to his notes and corrections accompanying the works of leading Oxford and Cambridge astronomers and mathematicians, there are extant annotations and transcriptions by Lewis of Caerleon for the astronomical tables of the Picard John de Lineriis, with the canons of his disciple John of Saxony; and also of Lewis' notes on the *Geometry* of Euclid. For convenience in reference, a list of Lewis of Caerleon's compositions, arranged as far as possible alphabetically by the first important word in the title, is here included, together with the opening words of the text and the manuscripts in which they are found. This list is followed by a further listing of the authors and works found in the manuscripts which Lewis transcribed or annotated.

Lewis of Caerleon's compositions:

1. De arte componendi tabulas eclipsium

[inc.] "Si volueris componere tabulas eclipsium pro . . ."

CUL 1017(Ee.3.61), 15th cent., fols. 142r–146r.

See also "Ad opus eclipsium . . ."

2. De arte compositionis tabularum astronomie

[inc.] "Circa compositionem tabularum elevationum signorum . . . / . . . signorum prescriptorum prout volueris. Explicit."

CUL 1017(Ee.3.61), fols. 3r–7v.

3. Calculationes eclipsium solis, a.d. 1481, per diversas vias

i. Calculatio eclipsis solis contingentis anno domini 1481, 28 Maii post meridiem, secundum

---

and on the patronage rolls of the king, who appears to have died shortly before 28 Oct. 1441. See *Calendar of Patent Rolls*, p. 7, 20 Henry VI.

[34] CUL 1017 (Ee. 3.61), fol. 175v, "Completum est hoc opusculum anno domini MCCCCXLI, xviii die mensis Julii magistris meis specialibus magistro Johanne Somerset et magistro Johanni Langton in vigilia assumptionis beate Marie eodem anno mense Augusti in familia regis apud Shene per manus meas liberatum."

For John Somerset and John Langton, see *DNB* and *Calendar of Patent Rolls*, p. 296, 17 Henry VI; and pp. 521–523, 19 Henry VI.

[35] *Calendar of Patent Rolls*, pp. 521–523, 19 Henry VI.

[36] *DNB*.

[37] CUL 1017 (Ee. 3.61), fol. 147v, "sicut tabulas eclipsium quas dedi universitatibus Canteburgensis et Oxonie," and again at fol. 151v. See Gunther, *Early Science at Oxford* (1923), vol. II, pp. 44 ff.

[38] H. E. Salter, *Registrum annalium collegii Mertonensis 1483–1521* (Oxford Historical Society, 1923, no. 76), pp. 139, 215; F. M. Powicke, *The Medieval Books of Merton College* (1931), pp. 36, 218.

[39] Salter, *op. cit.*, p. 251.

tabulas Arzachelis. [inc] "Tempus vere . . ." (fol. 12v).[40]

ii. Calculatio eiusdem per tabulas novas expansas (fol. 14r).

iii. Calculatio eiusdem eclipsis per extractione radicis semidyametrorum solis et lune . . . secundum doctrinam canonis Gerardi Cremonensis super tabulum Arzachelis (fol. 14v).

CUL 1017(Ee.3.61), fols. 12v–14v, with the Canons of Johannes de Lineriis, and notes by Lewis of Caerleon to fol. 15v.

4. Canones eclipsium lune et solis

[inc.] "Postquam novas tabulas eclipsium composuerim cum singulis tabulis ad easdem pertinentibus. Convenit ut modus operandi per easdem plane declarare. Pro eclipse vero lune. Intra tabulam eclipsis lune cum argumento latitudinis lune . . . . / . . . et sic finitur calculatio eclipsis lunaris."

BMr 12G.1, fols. 5v–6v. At fol. 5v: "Circa calculationes eclipsis solis ista sunt primitus requirenda . . . / . . . (fol. 6r) et si idem tempus casus duplicaveris provenit duracio eclipsis solis et sic finitur," is followed by a note: "Require alios canones in fine proximi quaterni quas primo composui priusquam fueram incarceratus per Regem Ricardum . . . (fol. 6v) Istam est solis anno Christi in presento 1485 post meridiem 16 diei Marcii contingentem ego observam in turre Londoni et inveni principium. Hoc totum secundum dyametros Wallynfordi abbatis et geometri eximi."

BMsl 1697, fols. 31r–32r, "per me Ludovicum Caerleon alios canones conversim priusquam fueram incarceratus per Regem Ricardum tertium."

CUsj 41(B.19), fols. 5v–8v, "Explicit opus m. Lodowyci Caerlion in eclipsibus lune et solis . . ."

5. Compositione (De) tabularum diversitatis aspectus sine astrolabio

[inc.] "Invenias primo gradum ascentem et altitudinem lune . . . Lewys."

CUL 1017(Ee.3.61), fol. 143v.

6. "Demonstratio geometrice eclipsis solis apparentis anno domini in presento 1481 post meridiem 28 die mensis maii, hora ut subscribitur ex calculo et diligenti examinatione Lodowici Caerlyon in medicinis doctoris et examinatur tam arsmetrice quam geometrice secundum regulas et auctoritates Albategni, Gebri, et commentatoris super Almagestum et Arzachelis et Richardi de Sancto Albano . . ."

CUL 1017(Ee.3.61), fol. 15r–v.

7. Modo (De) calculandi eclipsium geometrice sine tabulis

[inc.] "Quicumque voluerit quantitatem et durationem eclipsis lunaris . . . / . . . Explicit opus M. Lodowyci Caerlyon in eclipsibus lune et solis."

BMr 12G.1, fols. 7v–8v; 9–15.

8. Modo (De) calculandi eclipsis solis secundum canones Arzachelis anno Christi 1339.

CUL 1017(Ee.3.61), fol. 146v.

9. "Nove radices per me Lodovicum calculate."

Oxford BL Savile 38, fol. 6r–v.

10. "Ad Opus eclipsium requiritur notitia . . ." and "De arte componendi tabulas eclipsium," citing Richard [Wallingford] of St Albans, Albategni, Geber, Arzachel, and Alfraganus,

[inc.] "Si volueris componere tabulas eclipsium . . ."

CUL 1017(Ee.3.61), fols. 142r–143v.

11. [Regula] Pro diversitate aspectus lune in longitudine et latitudine calculanda

[inc.] "Paucas premittam suppositiones. Prima est hec . . ."

BMr 12G.1, fols. 9r–10v; with tables at fol. 11r–v;

CUsj 41(B.19), 15th cent., fol. 9r–10v; with tables at fol.10v.[41]

12. Tabula angulorum et diversitatis aspectus ad eclipses per calculationem Ludowyci Caerlyon in medicinis doctoris . . . secundum doctrinam Albategni et Richardum de Sancto Albano.

Canones [inc.] "Nota quot requiruntur hic ad habendum archum primum . . ."

Exemplum componendi tabulas [inc.] "Altitudo capitis arietis in predicta . . ."

CUL 1017(Ee.3.61), fol.106r–v; 107r–v.

13. "Tabula cordanum medietatum M. Symonis Bredonis, expansa ad singulas medietates per me Lodowycum, et est preciosior quam Tabula Albategni quia calculatur pro singulis 15 minutis, usque ad 8. Sed hic non posui nisi 4 verificata pro singulis 15 minutis i.e. Opus Lodowyci Caerlyon in Eclipsibus Lune et Solis etc. sc. ct.H.6."

BM Harley 7055, fol.232, "Catalogue of the manuscripts of the library of Sir Henry Spelman," sold by auction by John Harding who bought them 20, 21, 22 December 1709 (fol.3). For the "MS olim penes Henr. Spelman," see Tanner, *op. cit.*, p. 449.

14. "Tabula eclipsis lunaris secundum dyametros Ricardi Abbatis de S. Albano, libro suo primo de compositione Albionis questione 18, 19, et 21, Ad sciendum longiorem cum . . . / . . . noviter facta et expansa ad singularem argumentum latitudinis lune . . . per me Lodowycum [facta] anno Christi 1482 cui finaliter adheret."

BMr 12G.1, fol.1–2v;

BMsl 1697, fol.25r–26v;

CUsj 41(B.19), fol.1r–2v.

A note at the bottom of the first page of the table reads: "Nota quod post compositionem istarum tabularum quas amiseram per exspoliationem regis Ricardi, ego existens incarceratus

---

[40] On the use of the tables of Arzachel, see Thorndike, *History of Magic and Experimental Science*, vol. III, pp. 122 ff.; 197 ff.; 284; and Gunther, *Early Science in Oxford* (1923), vol. II, pp. 44, 384.

[41] See Gunther, *Early Science at Oxford* (1923), vol. II, pp. 52–55.

in turre Londoniarum composui alias tabulas eclipsium que discordant ab istis in paucis secundis cuius causa est quia latitudo lune vera et visa differt ab ista aliquando per unum secundum et aliquando per 30 secundos tamen."

15. "Tabula eclipsis solis secundum dyametros Ricardi abbatis de S. Albano ad longitudinem Londonensis per me Lodowycum anno inperfecto 1482 apud Londonie." Tables for 1483 follow.

BMr 12G.1, fol.3r–4r;

BMsl 1697, fol. 27r–v;

CUsj 41(B.19), fol.3r–4v, "facta per me Lodowycum . . . anno Christi 1483." On the inside flyleaf of this manuscript are listed the following items: "Tabula eclipsium cum omnibus requisitis noviter facta per me Lodowycum Caerlyon, in medicinis doctorem et militem, cum suis canonibus;" and

"Tabula et tractatus quidam astrologici per Richardum Abbatum de Sancto Albano et Ludovicum Carlion. Circa annum domini 1482."

16. Tabula punctorum eclipsis solaris ad Londoniensis.

CUL 1017 (Ee.3.61), fol.147v, with the following notation: "Nota quod istas tabulas eclipsium et diversitatis aspectus cancellavi quia non calculavi istas tabulas in presenti sicut tabulas quas dedi universitatibus Canteburgensis et Oxoniensis . . ."

17. Tabula semidiametrorum solis lune et umbre et variationis umbre

[inc.] "Si ergo velis scire quantitatem semidiametri solis per tabulas . . . / . . . per me Lodovicum noviter facta anno Christi 1483."

BMr 12G.1, fol.4r–v, 7r;

BMsl 1697, fol.28r, 29r;

CUsj 41(B.19), fol.4r.

18. Tabulae [variae]:

Tabula angulorum casus eclipsium solaris . . . ad Lond. propriorem;

Tabule diversitatis aspectus lune ad latitudinem [pro] Oxon.;

Tabule eclipsium lune . . . Tabule diversitatis aspectus lune in longitudine pro Oxonia "sed non est preciso: Lewys;"

Tabulae (for each of the 12 signs of the Zodiac).

CUL 1017(Ee.3.61), fols.148r–151v. On fol. 151v, at the lower margin is the following note: "Nota quod tabulas precedentes cancellavi quia eas non in presenti calculavi sicut tabulas quas dedi universitatibus Cantebrigensis et Oxoniensis."

19. "Tabulae ad sciendum initium aspectus eclipsis solis vel lune . . ."

BMsl 1697, fol.32v.

20. "Tabule diversitatis aspectus in longitudine et latitudine veri poli elevati 52 gr. 20 min.," with "Canones eclipsium solis secundum easdem tabulas. Pro quo primitus ista sunt requirenda . . ."

BMr 12G.1, fol.5r;

BMsl 1697, fol.29v, containing: "Tabula diversitatis aspectus in longitudine . . . ad modum Anglie;" followed by "Tabula diversitatis aspectus in latitudine in alt. poli 52 gr. 20 min. cuius est latitudo Cantabrigensis et medium Anglie."

Tabulae eclipsium . . . *see* De arte componendi . . .

21. Tabulae et Canones eclipsium solis (from the tables of John Somer?)[42]

[inc.] "Modus operandi pro eclipsi lune per tabulas novas. Intra in tabulam lunaris . . . / . . . et sic completur opus eclipsis lune;" followed by "Canones eclipsium solis secundum easdem tabulas . . . Pro quo primitus ista sunt requirenda . . . / . . . casus inter duas longitudines et sic complebitur opus. Explicit."

BMr 12G.1, fol.5r;

BMsl 1697, fol.29v;

CUL 1017(Ee.3.61), fols.152v–153r;

CUsj 41(B.19), fols.14v–15r.

See also "Canones eclipsium lune et solis."

22. "Tabule nove radicum per me Lodovicum calculate."

Oxford, BL Saville 38, 15th cent., fols. 6r–(8v).

23. "Tabule continentes numeros quadratos et cubitos cum radicibus eorundem. Nota quod medium proportionale in quadratis est numerus . . ."

CUL 1017(Ee.3.61), fol. 125r; followed by tables at fol. 125v.

24. Umbrae. [Extracts?] De Umbris.

[inc.] "Umbram rectam seu extensam. . ."

CUL 1017(Ee.3.61), fols. 179r–181r.

Authors and works contained in manuscripts which Lewis of Caerlyon transcribed or annotated:

25. Arzachel, "Canones ad tabulas Toletanas;" translated by Gerard of Cremona, inc. "Quoniam cuiusque actionis. . ."[43]

CUL 1017(Ee.3.61), fol. 16r.

26. Euclid, "Geometria."[44]

[inc.] "Punctus est cui pars non est. . ."

Oxford, Corpus Christi College 234, 15th cent., fols. 10r–170r, with notes by Lewis of Caerleon at fols. 2r, 13r *et passim*.

27. Franco of Liège, "De quadratura circuli."[45]

[42] For these tables which were said to have been extracted from the astronomical tables of Friar Somer, see item 32 below. See Thorndike and Kibre, *Catalogue of Incipits*, col. 413.

[43] For other MSS of this work see Thorndike and Kibre, *Catalogue of Incipits of Mediaeval Scientific Writings in Latin* (1937), col. 589.

[44] For other MSS see Thorndike and Kibre, *op. cit.*, col. 537.

[45] *Ibid.*, col. 539.

[inc.] "Franco scolasticus Loadicensis ad Hermanum Archiepiscopum. . ."

CUL 1017(Ee.3.61), fols. 176v–177v. At fol. 176r, another tract on the squaring of the circle precedes [inc.] "Proposito circulo quadratum . . ."

28. Humphrey, duke of Gloucester, "Prologus in tabulas. . ."

[inc.] "Effectus planetarum proficientes probitos et futuros pronosticare. . ."

CUL 1017(Ee.3.61), fol. 108v, followed by tables at fol. 109r *et seq.*

29. John Holbrooke

29, i. "Distinctio calculationis eclipsis solis pro anno 1337 in mense martii secundum tabulas [Arzachelis] Alfonsii ad meridiem Parisius."

[inc.] "Ad investigandi eclipsium solis proximam venturam. . ."

CUL 1017(Ee.3.61), fols. 75r–81r, with notes by Lewis of Caerleon on the calculation of eclipses.

29, ii. Figure constructed by John Holbrooke on the "Hora nativitatis"

CUL 1017(Ee.3.61), fols. 161r–162r.

29, iii. Notes on John de Lineriis, Tabulae[46]

[inc.] "Nota quod mensurum grado Saturni et Jovis fuerit ante annum diluvii 280 annis 33 diebus. . .;"

Item diverse tabule eclipsium et tabula equationum dierum. . .

[inc.] "Nota quod a tempore M. Jo. de Lineriis usque ad annum 1428. . ."

CUL 1017(Ee.3.61), fols. 57r–62v, with tables to fol. 63r

29, iv. Opus primum in reductione tabularum Alfonsis ad annos Christi menses dies et horas.

[inc.] "Quoniam celestium motuum calculus. . ."[47]

CUL 1017(Ee.3.61), fols. 56r–57r;

BM Egerton 889, 15th cent., fols. 133v–151r.

29, v. Opus secundum in compositione novarum tabularum mediorum motuum

[inc.] "Si ergo veram anni quantitatem scire cupis. . ."

CUL 1017(Ee.3.61), fols. 64r–70r; with tables and notes at fols. 70v–74. Preceding the work on fol. 63v, are "Canones Jo. Holbrooke ad opus suum secundum. [inc.] Gloriosus atque sublimis. . ." These Canons are also found in BM Egerton 889, 15th cent., fols. 152v–160v.

29, vi. Tabulae et canones

CUL 1017(Ee.3.61), fol. 56r.

30. John Killingworth

30, i. Algorismus.

[inc.] "Oblivioni raro traduntur. . ."[48]

CUL 1017(Ee.3.61), fols. 31v–42v.

30, ii. "Canones tabularum revolutionibus planetarum," with "Unum canonem de correctione radicum Saturni et Jovis quod ego Ludovicus Caerlion superaddidi."

[inc.] "Multum conferre dinoscitur non solum astronomis. . ."[49]

Oxford, BL Savile 38. fols. 2v–5v.

31. John de Lineriis

31, i. Algorismus, De minutiis vulgaribus[50]

[inc.] "Modum representatis minuciarum. . ."

CUL 1017(Ee.3.61), fols. 26v–29r.

31, ii. Ars operandi per probas in speciebus algorismi

CUL 1017(Ee.3.61), fols. 30r–31r.

31, iii. Canones eclipsium;[51] together with "De calculatione eclipsium extractus de canonibus suis."

[inc.] "Eclipsis solis et lune in quocumque anno. . .;" followed by "Alie generationes de canonibus eiusdem M. Joh. de Lineriis."

[inc.] "Cuiuslibet archus propositi sinum rectum invenire archum. . ."

CUL 1017(Ee.3.61), fol. 82r–86v; 86v–96r.

31, iv. Quedam extracta super canones M. Joh. de Lineriis per M. Johannem de Saxonia (incomplete).

[inc.] "Quia plures astrologorum diversos libros fecerunt. . ."[52]

CUL 1017(Ee.3.61), fol. 178r-v.

32. John Somer: "Quidam bone notule extracte de copia fratris Sommer. . ."[53]

CUL 1017(Ee.3.61), fol. 152r. The tables indicated under item 21 above are said to have been extracted from the astronomical tables of Friar Somer which Lewis of Caerleon transcribed, corrected, and provided with canons for their use: CUL 1017(Ee.3.61), fol. 152r–153r.

33. John Walter or Fitzwalter: "Tabula diversitatis ascensionis signorum pro omni terra habitabili secundum declinationem Almansoris et dicitur esse tabula M. Johannis Walteri sed cum certus sum quod non potest esse vera. . ."

CUL 1017(Ee.3.61), fol. 47r; and see also
Oxford, BL Digby 97, fol. 50v; and
BM Egerton 889, fols. 69r–70v.

34. Richard of Wallingford

34, i. Ars componendi instrumentum rectanguli[54]

[inc.] "Rectangulum in remedium. . ."

---

[46] See Gunther, *Early Science in Oxford*, vol. II, p. 165; and cf. Thorndike and Kibre, *Catalogue of Incipits*, col. 2.

[47] See Thorndike and Kibre, *op. cit.*, col. 588.

[48] See L. C. Karpinski, "The Algorism of John Killingworth," *English Historical Review*, 1914, *29*, pp. 707–717; Gunther, *Early Science in Oxford*, vol. II, p. 66; and Thorndike and Kibre, *Catalogue of Incipits*, col. 455.

[49] See L. C. Karpinski, *loc. cit.*, p. 713; Thorndike and Kibre, *op. cit.*, col. 419, for additional MSS.

[50] See *Ibid.*, col. 412. See also Gunther, *op. cit.*, vol. II, p. 46; and Thorndike, *History of Magic and Experimental Science*, vol. III, 253 ff.

[51] See note 12 above and cf. Thorndike and Kibre, *Catalogue of Incipits*, cols. 126, 228.

[52] See *Ibid.*, col. 570.

[53] See *Ibid.*, col. 18, 24, 123, 322; and Gunther, *Early Science in Oxford*, vol. II, pp. 60–62.

[54] Cf. Thorndike and Kibre, *Catalogue of Incipits*, col. 620; and see Gunther, *Early Science in Oxford*, vol. II, pp. 32–34; and 337–348, where the work is edited. Another MS of the work is: Erfurt, Amplon. Q. 361, 14th cent., fols. 154–156v.

CUL 1017(Ee.3.61), fols. 8r–12r

34, ii. Quadripartitum[55]

[inc.] "Quia canones non perfectem tradunt notitiam sinus. . ." Oxford, BL Digby 178, fols. 15r–38v, with marginal notes and figures by Lewis of Caerleon.

34, iii. De sinubus et arcubus

[inc.] "Arcus dicitur pars circumferentie circuli. . ."

Oxford, BL Digby 178, fols. 39r–41v.

35. Simon Bredon

35, i. Arsmetrica continens sententiam arsmetrice Boetii[56]

[inc.] "Quantitatum alia continua que magnitudo. . ."

CUL 1017(Ee.3.61), fols. 96v–105v.

35, ii. Expositio super quedam capitula *Almagesti* Ptolomei

[inc.] "Nunc superest ostendere quanta sit. . ."

CUL 1017(Ee.3.61), fols. 43r–46v, with the date 1440 on fol. 46r;

Oxford, BL Digby 178, fols. 42r–86v, "Commentum super aliquas demonstrationes Almagesti," with annotations by Lewis of Caerleon.

36. Trutina Hermetis per calculatione nativitatum.

CUL 1017(Ee.3.61), fol. 74r-v, with notes by Lewis of Caerleon.

Index of Incipits

	Item
Ad investigandi eclipsium. . . .	29,i
Ad opus eclipsium. . .	10
Ad sciendum longiorem cum. . .	14
Altitudo capitis arietis. . .	12
Altitudo lune in arcu. . .	note 12
Arcus dicitur pars. . .	34,iii
Ars operandi per probas. . .	31,ii
Circa calculationes eclipsis. . .	4
Circa compositionem tabularum elevationum. . .	2
Circa compositionem tabularum umbrarum. . .	note 12
Cuiuslibet archus propositi. . .	31,iii
Eclipsis solis et lune. . .	31,iii
Eclipsium solis, quantitatem. . .	note 12
Effectus planetarum proficientes. . .	28
Franco scolasticus loadicensis. . .	27
Gloriosus atque sublimis. . .	29,v
Intra in tabulam. . .	21
Intra tabulam eclipsis. . .	4
Invenias primo gradum ascentem. . .	5
Modum representatis minuciarum. . .	31,i
Modus operandi pro eclipsi. . .	21; note 12
Multum conferre dinoscitur. . .	30,ii
Nota quod a tempore M. Jo. de Lineriis. . .	29,iii
Nota quod medium. . .	23
Nota quod mensurum. . .	29,iii
Nota quot requiruntur. . .	12
Nunc superest ostendere. . .	35,ii
Oblivioni raro traduntur. . .	30,i
Paucas premittam suppositiones. . .	11
Postquam novas tabulas. . .	4
Pro diversitate aspectus. . .	11
Pro quo primitus ista sunt. . .	20,21
Proposito circulo quadratum. . .	27
Punctus est cui pars. . .	26
Quantitatum alia continua. . .	35,i
Quia canones non. . .	34,ii
Quia plures astrologorum. . .	31,iv
Quicumque voluerit quantitatem. . .	7
Quoniam celestium motuum. . .	29,iv
Quoniam cuiusque actionis. . .	25
Restangulum in remedium. . .	34,i
Si ergo velis scire. . .	17
Si ergo veram anni. . .	29,v
Si volueris componere. . .	1,10
Tempus vere. . .	3
Umbram rectam seu. . .	24

[55] Cf. Thorndike and Kibre, *op. cit.*, col. 565.

[56] For other MSS see *Ibid.*, col. 547.

XVI

HITHERTO UNNOTED MEDICAL WRITINGS OF DOMINICUS OF RAGUSA (1424-1425 A.D.)

An interesting illustration of the information to be gleaned from manuscript texts for the history of medicine is provided by a fifteenth century manuscript at the New York Academy of Medicine.[1] Although the codex was catalogued in the recent *Census of Medieval and Renaissance Manuscripts in the United States and Canada,* as anonymous " Recipes," [2] the name Dominicus de Ragusia appears as author for all but the first treatise. No other manuscripts or printed copies of the works in this collection appear to be extant, and their author has not hitherto been brought forth from the records of the university of Bologna, where he was professor intermittently between 1395 and 1427, to lay claim to their composition. The manuscript is a paper quarto volume (28 x 21 cm) of 105 leaves, in 2 columns of 33 lines each, and is written in a neat Italian hand. The first leaf is badly torn and the volume is waterstained throughout. On the first leaf are border and initial illuminations in purple, gold, and blue. Initials in red and blue are scattered throughout. The volume is rebacked in brown morocco and was presented in 1921 to the New York Academy of Medicine by the heirs of the late Dr. Abraham Jacobi (1830-1919). Of the earlier provenance of the manuscript nothing is known.

The writings included in this collection were composed as is stated at the opening and close of the volume between December 1424 and April 3rd, 1425, while the author, Dominicus de Ragusia, was lecturing at Siena. Earlier he appears to have been enrolled in medicine and philosophy at the university of Bologna, where he was in 1395-1396 morning lecturer on astrology. In 1397 he lectured on moral

[1] The study of this manuscript was made while I was associated with the Library of the New York Academy of Medicine, as a temporary member of the staff for the historical section, in the Spring of 1939. I am indebted to Dr. Archibald Malloch, Librarian, for helpful suggestions, and to Miss Gertrude Annan, Curator of the Rare Book Room, for the external description of the manuscript.

[2] *Census of Medieval and Renaissance Manuscripts in the United States and Canada* by Seymour de Ricci with the assistance of W. J. Wilson, New York, 1937, p. 1312, no. 9: (166860). Recipes etc. " Incipiunt recepte. . . ."

philosophy and between 1398 and 1399 on medicine. Apparently absent from the university of Bologna for a period of some fifteen years, Dominicus returned in 1415 as morning lecturer on medicine with an annual stipend of L. 300. This was one of the highest salaries received by any member of the medical faculty at that time and may be taken as an indication of Dominicus' prominence at the university. His stipend fluctuated, however, between L. 300 and L. 140 during the years 1415 to 1421 when his name appeared continuously on the records as lecturer in medicine. In 1421 Dominicus probably again left Bologna, possibly for Siena where we find him in the years 1424 to 1425 lecturing on the practice of medicine, according to the present manuscript. He then returned to Bologna in 1426 as lecturer on the practice of medicine until 1427.[3] Further details relating to Dominicus de Ragusia are not forthcoming. A recent account of the physicians of Ragusa identifies him with a Domenico Galeotti Rollandino from Ragusa on the Dalmatian coast.[4] Although Domenico Galeotti was also enrolled at the university of Bologna, his name does not, however, appear on the rolls until 1438, when he is listed as "Galeottus Dominici de Ragusa." He thus appears to have been more likely the son of Dominicus.[5] It is possible that our author may be the Domenico da Bologna who composed a brief prescription against the plague which Sudhoff noted.[6]

There are few biographical details to be gleaned from the text

[3] *I Rotuli dei lettori legisti e artisti dello studio Bolognese dal 1384 al 1799.* Pubblicati dal Dottor Umberto Dallari, Bologna, 1888, IV, 19, 22, 24, 36, 38, 40, 41, 43, 44, 52. The name is variously spelled: *M. Dominichus de Rayghoxa, de Raigoxa, de Raygosa,* or *de Raigosa.* See also G. Zaoli, "Lo studio Bolognese e Papa Martino V (anni 1416-1420)," in *Studi e memorie per la storia dell' università di Bologna,* 1912, III, 141, 143, 147, 149; and G. Zaoli, "Di alcuni 'Rotuli' dello studio della prima metà del secolo XV (Contributo alla storia dello studio dal 1420 al 1455)," *loc. cit.,* 1920, IV, 228.

[4] Georges Koerbler, "Les médecins de Raguse pendant la renaissance," *Janus,* 1927, *31,* 444. Chevalier lists separately Dominicus de Raguse, and Galeotti (Rollandio-Dominique) de Raguse, although following Gliubich, *Uom. ill. Dalmazia,* 1856, p. 138, he describes Galeotti as 'profes. d'astrologie et médecine à Bologne 1394-1422.' I have not had access to a copy of Gliubich.

[5] *I Rotuli . . . dello studio Bolognese,* 1888, I, 12, 13, etc. Galeottus appears on the rolls until 1453.

[6] MS of the R. Bibl. Casanatense at Rome, Cod. 46 (d. VI. 2) from the end of the fourteenth century, fol. 39 recto (lxviii). 'Lattouare [Electuarium] di M[aes-

itself, and there is no mention of contemporary physicians at Bologna or Siena. But Dominicus does provide a brief glimpse of the possible cooperation between the famous artists of the quattrocento and the physicians who utilized their talents to provide accurate charts or drawings of medical subjects. Thus in his tract on urines in the section on diagnosis from color, Dominicus states that he had tried to persuade the famous Venetian painter, Gentile da Fabriano (c. 1370-c. 1450), to illustrate his text by depicting the several colors in drawings of urinal glasses in order to make easier the task of those wishing to learn how to diagnose from the color of the urine. Gentile, however, left the city because of the plague and did not provide Dominicus with the needed drawings.[7]

Aside from the brief second tract on poisons derived from the Latin author, Peter of Abano (c. 1250- c. 1316-19), the writings in this manuscript are chiefly based on Arabic authorities. In addition to the commentaries on Rhazes' *Liber Almansoris* (Lib. IX), and on Avicenna's *Canon* (Lib. III, fen 1-6), the last tract or Compendium on urines makes use of Arabic writings in Latin translation. Thus according to the list of references provided by Dominicus himself at the close of the work, he has utilized in addition to Hippocrates and Galen, Avicenna's *Canon,* Lib. I; Isaac Judaeus, *De urinis*; Haly Abbas, *Theorica* (Lib. regalis), Lib. VII; and Rhazes, *Continens.*

The contents of the manuscript are as follows:

fols. 1r-50v, Incipiunt recepte ordinate secundum experientias mei . . . de . . . usque ad 1424 de mense decembris super nono Almansoris. Et primo de dolore capitis a materia . . . / . . . (fol. 50v, col. 2) ad membra illa appositum. Et sic finivi hoc opus super nono Almansoris die 3a Junii 1425 senis cum auxilio omnipotentis dei eiusque virginis matris marie totiusque curie triumphantis. Amen. Deo gratias.

fols. 50v, col. 2-51v, col. 2, De venenis. Cum enim diis parentibus et magistris pretium equiponderans reddi non potest ut ex nono ethicorum habetur hinc est quod ego Dominicus de Ragusia de Bononia querens virtutem ac nomen magistri mei s. Petri de Ebano

tro] Domenico da Bologna contra a pistolencia.' *Archiv. f. Gesch. d. Medizin,* 1912-1913, *6,* 333.

[7] fol. 96v, "Deliberaveram cum illo summo pictore magistro Gentile de Fabriano facere pingi multos colores in urinalibus correspondentes hiis meis dictis ad meliorem notitiam et faciliorem volentium adiscere vere practicam incipiendo a colore predicto sed propter pestem aufugit et non suffeci."

dicti conciliatoris unici luminaris magni ad omnia tempora cui . . . . . . (fol. 51v, col. 1) cum modico pulveris smiraldi facit exire venenum per seccessum. Deo gratias.

fols. 52r, col. 1-93r, col. 1, Super prima tertii Canonis Avicenne. Cum materiam evacuare voluerimus etc. Ab universalibus incipiendo . . . (fol. 86r, col. 1) Et sic est finis receptarum supra 4a fen tertii A. per me Dominicum de de [*sic*] Raygosa de Bononia physicum . . . (fol. 90v, col. 2) Complete sunt recepte super 5a fen tertii Avicenne per me Dominicum de Raygosa . . . (fol. 93r, col. 1) Menti semper habeas premittere canones universales in evacuationibus etc. Deo gratias Amen. Complete sunt recepte super 6a fen.

fols. 93r, col. 2-101v, col. 2, Tract on urines begins without heading or title: Quia enim multa de urinis a multis pertractata sunt nec tamen distincte adeo ut possimus habere scientiam determinatam ab eis ut signum certis explicitum tam in substantia quam in colore quam in contentis. Ideo ego Dominicus de Raygosa de Bononia physicus rogatu quorundam sociorum scolarium meorum hoc compendium urinarum decrevi ordinare et componere volens votis eorum satisfacere . . . / . . . (fol. 101v, col. 2) cum consimili ypostesi ut supra habitum est. Deo gratias. Hec sunt quelibet ex usu practice et experientiis meis collecta per me Dominicum de Raygosa de Bononia aprobavi tamen primo sententiis auctorum infra scriptorum s. Ypo. et Ga. 2° pronosticorum (fol. 102r, col. 1) et Galeni primo de crisi capitulo 12 et primo de differentiis febrium capitulo 5° et Avicenne 2ª primi et Ysaach suo de urinis et Aliabatis septima particula sue theorice ac Rasis 28 Continentis 2°. Amen. Hunc tractatum compillavi cum legerem practicam senis 1425 complevique 3a die aprilis cum laude et gratia omnipotentis dei Yhesu Christi sueque virginis matris beate marie adiutricis mee in omnibus totiusque curie celestis triumphantis. Amen.

fols. 103r-105r, List of chapter headings for all the treatises in the volume. In the right margin on fol. 103r opposite the heading, De sanguine fluente ex naribus, is written: Pro magistro D. Marco Antonio de Raigusia; on fol. 103v, beside De emissione sanguinis per os, is written Pro idem Raigusia; and on 104v, opposite De aqua descendente in oculis: Pro Ex. Andr. Matteo de Dunalibus (?).

The first treatise in the volume from its close association with the others assigned to Dominicus is doubtless also by him. Its title,

Recepte for the ninth book of Rhazes' *Liber Almansoris,* was used for a similar work by Pietro Curialti da Tossignana (d. about 1407), who preceded Dominicus at the university of Bologna.[8] The two texts are, however, not the same. The *Liber Almansoris* (Kitab-al-Mansuri) so-called after Abu Salih Mansur ibn Ishaq, the patron to whom Rhazes (d. 923-24 A. D.) dedicated the work, contains in ten tractates or books a compendium of medical practice which in the Latin translation from the Arabic by Gerard of Cremona (1114-1187 A. D.), had a considerable vogue among Latin medical authors. The ninth book of the *Liber Almansoris* served as a standard textbook on therapeutics and an examination on it was required by some universities along with Avicenna's *Canon* and Johannitius' *Isagoge* before a candidate could be granted the license in medicine. Like Avicenna's *Canon,* the ninth book especially served for numerous commentaries and expositions. The present commentator follows closely Rhazes' order of subjects beginning with the diseases of the head and proceeding downward to the diseases of the limbs and joints. The author has, however, as he states at the beginning of the commentary drawn largely from his own experience and practice for the particular remedies that he describes. He makes several references to the famous baths of Porretta situated near Bologna.[9] The range of subjects or regions of the body for which treatments and cures are outlined are: (fol. 1r-9v) on the head, including paralysis, melancholy, etc.; (fol. 10r-14r), on the eyes; (14r-15r), the ears; (15v), the nose; (16r), the teeth; (17r), the mouth and tongue; (18v), diseases of the chest; (22r) of the heart; (22v), of the stomach; (26r), of the liver; (28r), on jaundice;

[8] In the edition of Venice, Bernardinus Stagninus de Tridino, 30 March, 1483, bound with Syllanus de Nigris (NYAM 103; Klebs, *Incunabula scientifica et medica,* Bruges, 1937, 946.2), the heading reads: *Incipiunt recepte magistri Petri de Tussignano super nono Almansoris.* It begins: " In descriptione receptarum convenientium . . ." See also G. Mazzini, *Vita e opere di Maestro Pietro da Tossignano,* Rome, 1926, pp. 145 *et seq.*

[9] fol. 5v, col. 2: " Balnea vero della Poretta de comitatu bononie in quibus balneatur que etiam potatur ac etiam si cum dura recipiatur supra caput sunt optima. Similiter balnea de pitriolo et sancti philippi de comitatu senarum . . ."; fol. 6r, col. 1, " dicam loco sui addendo nostrum balneum dictum della poretta "; fol. 32r, col. 2, " Balnea nostra de comitatu bononie dicta della Poretta aut comitatus senarum dicta de aqua burra sunt mirabilia (fol. 32v, col. 1) ad curam et preservationem nec inveni aliquid citius et efficatius "; fol. 36v, " efficatissimum expertum et citum ad curam apud me est balneum ex aqua balnei de la poretta de comitatu bononie . . ."

(30v), on the spleen; (36r), diseases of the bladder; (37v), on stone; (39r), on kidneys and bladder; (41v), on worms; (43r), on hemorrhoids; (44r), on the uterus; (48v), on hernia; (49r), diseases of the joints; (50r), on varicose veins; (50v), on elephantiasis, and other diseases of the skin.

The second treatise in the collection, that on poisons, is extracted from Peter of Abano's *De venenis.* Dominicus refers to Peter of Abano, otherwise known as 'Conciliator,' from his work of that title, as his master, although Peter lived more than a hundred years earlier. He describes him as the great and unique lightgiver of all times, and states that he has set forth a few excerpts from Peter of Abano's treatise, the contents of which Dominicus himself has tested, in order to gratify the wishes of his colleagues. There is repeated the tale of the horn of the serpent (horned-toad?) that sweats in the presence of the plant napellus (i. e. aconite), or before the venomous snake tyre (tyrus), or of leopard's bile indicating that these contain poison; also Dominicus tells of the green and white stone, prase (prasius), on which sometimes appear red drops and which loses its green color in the vicinity of poison. Dominicus states that the stone, hematite (haematites), engraved with the figure of a kneeling man holding a snake, when set in a gold ring preserves the wearer from poisoning; and he further describes several antidotes for poison.[10]

The commentary or *Recepte* on Avicenna's *Canon* covers the first six of the twenty-two fen of the third book dealing with the individual diseases common to particular parts or organs of the body, arranged in the descending order from head to foot. The subjects covered by the first six fen are (1) the head, (2) the nerves, (3) the eyes, (4) the ears, (5) the nose, and (6) the tongue and mouth, ending with the chapter on abscesses of the mouth.

The last treatise, the compendium on urines, was composed, Dominicus states, at the request of several of his students and colleagues. It is concerned chiefly with the analysis of color, substance, and content of urine, as a means of diagnosis.

[10] Fol. 50v, col. 2—51r, col. 2. Cf. Peter of Abano, *De venenis,* ed. Paris, 1515, sig. b3 verso; English translation from the Latin by Dr. H. M. Brown, "De venenis of Petrus Abbonus, Edition of MCDXCVIII," in *Annals of Medical History,* New York City, 1924, *6,* 35. See also Lynn Thorndike, *History of Magic and Experimental Science,* New York, 1923, II, 908.

XVII

DOMINICUS DE RAGUSA, BOLOGNESE DOCTOR OF ARTS AND MEDICINE

Several items of biographical and bibliographical interest relating to Dominicus de Ragusa and throwing further light on his career and medical writings have come to my attention since the publication of my previous article on him.[1] For example, an earlier date is available than that of 1395-1396, when he was giving the ordinary or morning lectures on astrology at Bologna.[2] He had apparently completed his studies the previous year, that is in 1394, when he was " laureato " at Bologna.[3] As noted earlier, he continued until 1399 to be named each year on the faculty rolls as lecturer on moral philosophy and medicine respectively, but was presumably absent from 1400 until 1415.[4] His absence from the city was specifically noted in 1410.[5] In 1415, he returned to Bologna and, from 1415 to 1421, continued to be named as lecturer in medicine in the statutes of the Bolognese studium.[6] In 1417, he delivered an oration on the occasion of the inauguration of the Podestà at Bologna, Ludovicus de Coreto. This oration is now preserved in the Archivio de Stato at Bologna[7] and is a good example, in this type of literary exercise, of the tendency on the part of professors of arts and medicine to exhibit their knowledge of non-medical writers as well as of medical authors. Dominicus de Ragusa particularly cited Aristotle's *Politics*, and *Ethics*, two works that he would of course have been using for his lectures in moral

[1] " Hitherto unnoted medical writings by Dominicus de Ragusa (1424-1425 A. D.)," *Bull. Hist. Med.*, 1939, *7*: 990-995. See below XVIII.

[2] *I rotuli dei lettori legisti e artisti dello Studio Bolognese dal 1384 al 1799*. Pubblicati dal Dottor Umberto Dallari. Bologna, 1888, vol. IV, p. 19.

[3] *Statuti delle università e dei collegì nello Studio Bolognese*, ed. C. Malagola, 1888, p. 498, note 3.

[4] *Bull. Hist. Med., loc. cit.*, pp. 990-991. See below XVIII 990-991.

[5] *Statuti . . . , op. cit.*, p. 521: for the year 1410, " Magister Dominico de Ragosia . . . (et alii) qui ab uno anno et citra non residerunt nec residentiam fecerunt in civitate et comitatu Bonon."

[6] *Bull. Hist. Med., loc. cit.*, p. 991. See below XVIII 991.

[7] Archivio di Stato, No. 57, item 2, 1417, " Dissertaz. scientifica di Domenico da Ragusa." I now have a photostat of the oration.

philosophy, as well as Virgil, Cicero's *De officiis,* Seneca, particularly the *Epistolae ad Lucillum,* and of the more recent writers, Petrarch. He placed special emphasis on the rule of law and on justice as one of the highest virtues. At the same time Dominicus did not neglect to bring in a direct reference to at least one author in the medical field, namely Johannes Mesue, whom he calls the most Christian of medical authors.[8]

Evidence for Dominicus' absence from Bologna in 1421 and for his stay from 1421 to 1425 in Siena is now available. For the three years before 1424, namely, for 1421-1423, there is the assertion, in a manuscript containing a " Consiglio sopra l'acqua Borra di Messer Domenico de Rasii (*sic*) Bolognese," that in the year 1421 to the end of 1423, he was in Siena.[9] Moreover, as noted earlier, the text in the manuscript at the New York Academy of Medicine indicates his stay in Siena between 1424 and 1425.[10] Dominicus returned to Bologna in 1426 and last appeared in the faculty rolls from 1426 to 1427.[11] It is very probable that his death occurred in 1427, since there is a reference to the widow of a " Dominici Galeotti de Ragusa, residing in Bologna," dated 26 June, 1427.[12]

The first of the manuscripts, other than those already noted, containing tracts by Dominicus de Ragusa is that in the British Museum in London: Harley 4087, a fifteenth century manuscript in paper.[13] The folios of the manuscript have been renumbered, suggesting that, in all probability, they have been separated from another codex. However, for convenience the present foliation will be followed. The first five folios (1r-5v) contain the work of John Mesue on medicinal simples, with incipit: " Quoniam quidam de melioribus amicis quos habere videor rogavit ut in scriptis ei regigerem breviter medicinas digestivas . . ." [14] The text is incomplete

[8] *Ibid.,* " illius nostri christianissimi medicorum Johannis Mesue."

[9] MS Florence, Riccardiana 165 (N. 1. XXX), see below. " Consiglio sopra l'aqua Borro di Messer Domenico de Rasii (*sic*) Bolognese nell'anno 1421 per fino all'anno 1423 essendo in Siena io M. Domenico. . . ."

[10] *Bull. Hist. Med., loc. cit.,* p. 990. See below XVIII 990.

[11] *Ibid.,* p. 991.

[12] *Chartularium studii Bononiensis* (Commissione per la storia dell'università di Bologna), vol. I, Bologna, 1909, p. 313: " Honesta domina domina Caterina filia quondam magistri . . . et uxor olim egregii artium et medicine doctoris magistri Dominici Galeottii de Raygoxa vidua Bononie moram trahens. . . ."

[13] This and the following manuscript were called to my attention by the late Professor Lynn Thorndike several years ago. But preoccupation with other tasks prevented my examining them until fairly recently.

[14] For this incipit cf. L. Thorndike and P. Kibre, *A Catalogue of Incipits of Medieval Scientific Writings in Latin,* new edition, Cambridge, Mass.: Mediaeval Academy of America, 1962, col. 1295, where it is indicated as John of Parma, " Practicella ex dictis Mesue abbreviata."

and ends (f. 5v, old number 37v), with the words: " endiva lactuca viola epl'ata et sciantearunt (?)." Recipes and notes in Latin and Italian follow (ff. 5v-10r). The work of Dominicus on fevers is at folio 11 recto (ff. 11r-22v, old numbers 43r-53v). It is entitled: " Introductorium breve utille ad curandas febres compillatum per famosem artium et medicine doctorem magistrum Dominicum de Rayola de Bononia," and opens: " Primo circa effimeram prenotatis et cognitis signis: signis pulsu et urina ac tactu caliditatis et accidentalibus ac tempora durabilitatis. Dico ergo quod conscivens occissum talis febris esse cum levitate et paucitate. . . ." Discussions of the various kinds of fevers follow, including tertiary (ff. 12v, 13v); sinochal (f. 14r), flegmatic (f. 14v); sincopal *humorosa* (f. 16r); and sincopal *minuta* (f. 16v); quartana (f. 16v); ethica (f. 17v) and *ethica senectutis* (f. 18v); pestilential (f. 18v); *appostemata* (f. 21v); and composite and enutric fevers (f. 21v); ending with an account of smallpox (*variola et morbillos*) (f. 22r-v). The text ends on folio 22 verso (old 54v): ". . . ex mixtura prima abluatur autem intingatur per totam noctem. Postea abluatur condictam decoctionem aut aqua mellis est expertissimum mundificans et subtillians cutorem. Deo gratias Amen. Explicit tractatus de febribus compilatus per famosissimum artium et medicine doctorem M. Dominicum de Raygola de Bononia. Amen."

The second manuscript, referred to above, is at the Riccardiana in Florence.[15] It is a miscellany which may have belonged to Dominicus de Ragusa himself. The contents of the codex are as follows:

1. " Dominicus de Rasii medicus Bononiensis. Liber definitionum medicinalium Galeni ordine apphabetico degestus.

(Tit.) " Claudii Galeni librum Diffinitionum medicalium ordine alphabetico in codicum hunc referemus, ac nonnulla ad libitum inseremus, quae operi nostro subservire videbuntur.

(Inc.) " Ars est similium comprehentionum congeries quae ad quendam finem vitae commodum referre possunt . . ." (f. 116r)

2. " Pars Grammaticae Graecae. Lexicon Graecum et Latinum nominum partium corporis humani (f. 128r *et seq.*) et earumdem morborum."

3. " Consilium medicum " (ff. 137r-138r).

4. " Consiglio sopra l'aqua Borra, Bagno vicino a Siena (f. 141r-v).

(Inc.) " Consiglio sopra l'aqua Borra di Messer Domenico de Rasii Bolognese. Nell'anno 1421 per fino all' 1423, essendo in Siena, io M. Domenico me venne nella mente voler recercare, esaminare, et intendere, le qualitadi, effetti et virtù de bagni nel dominio di detto città situati li quali trovai efficacissimi et potentissimi contra cathari et passio di nervi . . . / . . ." (ending on f. 141v).

[15] Riccardiana 165 (N. 1. XXX), fifteenth century in paper of 20 × 28 cent.

Mention might also be made of other notices of Dominicus de Ragusa. He is named with such well-known doctors of medicine as Arnold of Villanova, Gerard de Solo, and Petrus de Tossignano, in a collection of " Verissima experimenta," by Godefridus de Moscendis in a Vatican Palatine manuscript dated in the year 1448.[16] There are doubtless other manuscripts of his works. Indeed, I was informed several years ago by Dr. Mirko Dražen Grmek of Zagreb, that he was planning to edit the text of a " Consilium ad curam lapidis et podagre " written by Dominicus de Ragusa (November 2nd, 1421). But this edition has not come to my attention.[17] The preceding instances will, however, have served to demonstrate how much biographical information there is to be derived from a careful examination of manuscript sources.

[16] Vatican Palatine 1177, a. 1448, ff. 39r-51v. " Hic incipiunt verissima experimenta certissimorum medicine doctorum Dominici de Raygosa, Arnoldi de Villanova, Gherardi de Solo, Petri de Tussianano et quorundam aliorum in medicinis magis expertorum collecta per Godefridum de Moscendis. (Inc.) Fili in tua infirmitate non despicies te ipsum . . ." (Eccl. 3)

[17] A recent communication from Dr. Grmek from Paris informs me that he has not yet published this text. He has, however, prepared a brief sketch of Dominicus in Croatian, with references to his works in Zagreb, which is now in press.

XVIII

CRISTOFORO BARZIZZA: PROFESSOR OF MEDICINE AT PADUA

Less well known today than his uncle,[1] the humanist and grammarian, Gasparino Barzizza,[2] Cristoforo, the nephew was one of a circle of distinguished physicians and professors at the university of Padua in the first half of the fifteenth century. His colleagues included the so-called monarch of the physicians of the day, Antonio Cermisone, in whose footsteps Cristoforo professes to follow, Galeazzo da Sancta Sofia, member of one of the most celebrated families of physicians in Italy, Bartolomeo da Montagnana, whose *Practica* provided the best clinical manual or case-book of the time, also the less well known Stefano de' Dottori, and Gasparino Barzizza, the grammarian and uncle of Cristoforo. Paolo Veneto (d. 1429), the noted logician and philosopher who in the last years of his life taught at Padua, is also said to have been one of Cristoforo's teachers.[3] In the heading and colophon of the incunabulum edition of his works,

[1] There is some confusion regarding the relationship between Cristoforo and Gasparino. Thus in the *Biographisches Lexikon der hervorragenden Ärzte aller Zeiten und Völker*, edited by Dr. August Hirsch, 2nd edition, 1929, I, 367, Cristoforo is listed as the brother of Gasparino. For biographical details I have followed Roberto Cessi, "Cristoforo Barzizza, medico del secolo XV," in *Bollettino della civica Biblioteca di Bergamo*, III (1909), 1-18, with an appendix containing several documents relating to Cristoforo, among them his last will and testament, together with the list of books in his library. It seems clear from the documents adduced by Cessi that Cristoforo was the son of Antonio, a brother of Gasparino. See also Roberto Cessi, "Nota genealogica sui Barzizza," *loc. cit.*, II (1908), 135-39. The periodical containing these two articles was borrowed for my use from the Harvard College Library (which apparently owns the only copy in the United States) by the Columbia University Library. I wish to take this opportunity to express my appreciation especially to the members of the Columbia University Library Reference Staff for their kindly assistance.

[2] The studies on Gasparino (d. 1431) are numerous. From 1422 on he was in the service of the Visconti in Milan. See *Mitteilungen aus der Hamburger Staats- und Universitats-Bibliothek*, neue folge, II (1927), 5 *et seq.*

[3] Roberto Cessi, *loc. cit.*, III (1909), 2, and note 6; 4, citing especially F. Momigliano, *Paolo Veneto e le correnti del pensiero religioso e filosofico nel suo tempo*, Torino, 1907. On pages 139-146, Momigliano reproduces the funeral oration in honor of Paolo Veneto delivered by Cristoforo Barzizza.

Cristoforo is himself dubbed monarch of the physicians and another Hippocrates,[4] while the documents always refer to him as the celebrated (*famosus*) doctor of arts and medicine.[5] Cristoforo's writings are therefore of interest historically since they reflect the nature of the accepted medical instruction at one of the leading Italian universities of the fifteenth century.

It is also noteworthy that although in daily contact with Gasparino, a distinguished humanist of his day,[6] Cristoforo had apparently little interest in humanistic studies. The only volume on that subject among the several medical and logical tracts in his library was a copy of Virgil which it has been suggested may have come from Gasparino's library.[7] Cristoforo appears to have leaned instead toward the teachings of the earlier medieval schoolmen in the fields of ethics and philosophy.[8] This aspect of his interests is further reflected by the books listed in his will. There were copies of Peter of Mantua's *Logica*,[9] of the commentary on Aristotle's *Posterior Ana-*

[4] The edition of Pavia, 1494, is at the New York Academy of Medicine. It is there bound with the commentary on Avicenna's *Canon* by Hugh of Siena. The heading reads: "Incipit Introductorium sive ianua ad opus practicum medicine compillatum per eximium artium et medicine monarcham magistrum Christoforum de Barziziis de Pergamo alterum ipocratem ad laudem omnipotentis dei felici sidere inchoatum. (Praefatio) Antonius Cermesonus nostro tempore primus ex mente Abohali. . . ." The work ends on folio [29]r, col. 2: "Explicit Introductorium sive ianua ad opus practicum medicine compilatum per eximium artium et medicine monarcham magistrum Cristoforum de barziziis de Pergamo alterum Ipocratem. Ad laudem domini nostri iesu Cristi et gloriosissime eius matris Marie Virginis." Some manuscript notes follow in the copy at the Academy of Medicine.

The *Introductorium* was also printed separately at Augsburg, by Sigismund Grim and Marcus Wersung, 14 December, 1518 (Proctor II, 10889). This edition is also at the New York Academy of Medicine (E. C. Streeter Collection).

[5] Cessi, *loc. cit.*, III (1909), 3, note 6.

[6] Cristoforo was a member of Gasparino's household at Padua until the latter's removal to Milan. Roberto Cessi, *loc. cit.*, III (1909), 1 *et seq.*

[7] Roberto Cessi, *Bollettino della civica Biblioteca di Bergamo*, III (1909), 4-5, and the list of Cristoforo's books on pp. 13-14. It seems clear that the humanist, Cristoforo Barzizza of Brescia was different from the physician of Padua, since the former was still living in 1492, while the latter died in 1445. Cf. *Gesamtkatalog der Wiegendrucke*, nos. 3670-71.

[8] Cessi, *loc. cit.*, III (1909), 3-4, and the letter reproduced in the appendix (pp. 15-16), from Cristoforo to his cousin, Guiniforte.

[9] Petrus Mantuanus (ca. 1400), *Logica*, Pavia, 1483; [Venice], 1492: Hain *12854-*12855.

lytics by Aegidius Romanus, and of two other commentaries on Aristotle; also the theological tract entitled *De homine* [10] by Albertus Magnus. Another volume under Albert's name is entitled *Super parvis ritualibus,* which does not correspond with any of the usual titles assigned to the thirteenth century Dominican scholar.

This adherence to standard medieval interests is also reflected in the books on medical subjects listed among Cristoforo's possessions. Included were three volumes relating to the *Aphorisms* of Hippocrates, one of them containing the commentary of Marsiglio da Sancta Sofia (d. 1405); a copy of what was quite probably that handy volume of medical tracts, the *Articella*; [11]; and by Galen, the *Ars Parva* or commentary on it, also a volume containing the seventh book of the *De ingenio sanitatis.* This seventh book in the translation by Burgundio of Pisa, made in the year 1305 A. D., frequently appeared separately.[12] Relating to Hippocrates and Galen too was a work of Gentile entitled, *Contra Ipocratem et Galienum.* It is not clear which Gentile is intended since no work of this title is elsewhere attributed to the fourteenth century physician, Gentile da Foligno, who died during the Black Death of 1348. There was also a copy of the popular medieval *Pantegni* of Constantinus Africanus.

In the pharmaceutical sphere were copies of Dioscorides, Serapion, an anonymous tract on the virtues of herbs, the ever popular *Antidotarium* of Nicolaus of Salerno, and the treatise on medicinal simples completed in 1385 by Aggregator, that is Jacobus de Dondis. Other fourteenth century medical authors named in the list are William of Varignana, by whom were indicated two copies of the *Practica medicinalis,*[13] Christophorus de Honestis, Gentile [da Foligno], and probably Petrus de Tussignano, or Pietro Torrignano de' Torrignana.[14]

[10] That is the *Summa de quatuor coaevis et de homine,* of which Part I is the "Summa de creaturis," and Part II, "Summa de homine": GW 778a-779; A. Borgnet, Albertus Magnus, *Opera omnia,* volumes 34 and 35.

[11] It would seem that this is intended by the book entitled, "Arteylo (*sic*)" in the list, Cessi, *loc. cit.*, III (1909), 13.

[12] Cf. Thorndike and Kibre, *Catalogue of Incipits of Mediaeval Scientific Writings in Latin,* 1937, col. 718; and Galen, *Opera omnia,* Venice, 1490 (Surgeon's General Library 167; Klebs 432.1), II, 405r.

[13] The first copy is indicated as "Practica Guilelmi de Veriana," the second is identifiable by its incipit: "Cunctis militaribus. . . ." Cessi, *loc. cit.*, III (1909), 13. Cf. Thorndike and Kibre, *Catalogue of Incipits,* 1937, cols. 125, 166.

[14] See the item "unus liber qui incipit "Ordinationes receptarum conferentinus,'"

Of thirteenth century medicine there was the the tract on urines and the pulse by Bernard Gordon. The well known physician, Peter of Abano, was represented only by his commentary on the *Problemata* attributed to Aristotle.[15] It is also quite probable that the copy of the *Thesaurus pauperum* listed was the popular medieval handbook by Petrus Hispanus, although the title was a common one.[16]

The most frequently occurring name on the list is, however, that of Avicenna, parts of whose *Canon* occupied at least ten items. These include commentaries by Gentile [da Foligno], and Jacobus de Forlivio, the latter identifiable by the opening words.[17] There was also a copy of Rasis, *De divisionibus,* and of Marsilius [de Sancta Sophia]'s commentary on the ninth book of Rasis, *Liber ad Almansorem.* In addition to the works noted above the list indicates several anonymous tracts, among them one which appears to be on the virtues of the magnet,[18] while another deals with the luminaries (De luminibus). It is curious, however, that there is no mention of works by Cristoforo's contemporaries or colleagues at the university of Padua, although Cristoforo's own works are apparently included.[19] According to the terms of his will, Cristoforo stipulated that the collection of books was to be kept intact until his son, Battista had attained the age of fifteen in case he should wish to devote himself to the study of medicine.[20] That the son did follow in his father's footsteps is indicated by the fact that some twenty-three years later, he is referred to as " the notable doctor of arts and medicine, dominus Joh. Baptista, son of the late Christoforus de Barziziis of Bergamo, distinguished doctor of arts and medicine. . . ." [21]

Cessi, *loc. cit.*, III (1909), 14; which corresponds with the title of a work by Petrus de Tussignano, Thorndike and Kibre, *Catalogue of Incipits*, 1937, col. 515.

[15] " Commentus Problematum Petri de Abbano," Cessi, *loc. cit.*, III (1909), 14; which may possibly refer to the commentary by Jean de Jandun on Abano's work. Cf. Thorndike and Kibre, *Catalogue of Incipits*, 1937, col. 354.

[16] Cf. *Ibid.*, col. 331, 528, and in the index under *Thesaurus pauperum.*

[17] The incipit is " Omissis nootionibus (*sic*) superfluis," Cessi, *loc. cit.*, III (1909), 13, which in general corresponds with the incipit: " Omissis superfluis narrationibus," for Jacobus de Forlivio, *Expositio in primum librum canonis Avicennae,* Thorndike and Kibre, *Catalogue of Incipits,* 1937, col. 458.

[18] " Tractatus de magnatis[sic] virtutibus," Cessi, *loc. cit.*, III (1909), 13.

[19] At least that is what might be inferred from the citation: " Item tres librete tractationum ipsius quondam domini Cristofori. . . ." Cessi, *loc. cit.*, III (1909), 14.

[20] Cessi, *loc. cit.*, III (1909), 6-7.

[21] Roberto Cessi, " Nota genealogica sui Barzizza," *Bollettino della civica Biblio-*

Despite his conservatism and scholastic leanings or possibly for them Cristoforo won recognition at the university of Padua, where he passed his entire academic career in the study and teaching of arts and medicine from about 1415 to 1444.[22] His death occurred in 1445 at Pavia, where he had gone late the preceding year.[23] As early as August 22, 1417, Cristoforo was already master and vice-rector of the faculty of arts at Padua.[24] Three years later, October 24, 1420, he took the examination for the doctorate.[25]

Cristoforo's interest in the standard medieval medical theories and practices, especially as represented by Avicenna, is clearly demonstrated by his chief medical treatise, the *Introductorium*, which was largely based on Avicenna, as well as by the tract on the recognition and cure of fevers which follows closely Avicenna's discussion in the fourth book of the *Canon*. Besides these two works there is also in print a commentary by Cristoforo on the ninth book of Rasis, *Liber ad Almansorem*. Further medical tracts are assigned to Cristoforo by Jöcher who lists a *Commentaria in Prognostica* [of Hippocrates?], also *Declarationes de febribus humidis*, and an *Interpretatio Antidotarii Joh. Mesue, Arabis*.[26] These last named works have not, however, turned up thus far in library catalogues.

The *Introductorium*, as was probably true of the other works, was composed as a part of Cristoforo's teaching program in medicine. It was primarily intended to provide a general introduction and guide

teca di Bergamo, II 1908), 138; "1467. Spect. artium et medicine doctor d. Jo. Baptista qu. clarissimi artium et medicine doctoris d. Christofori de Barziziis de Pergamo civis et habitator Padue."

[22] Roberto Cessi, *loc. cit.*, III (1909), 2, note 5; 3, note 8; *Acta graduum academicorum Gymnasii Patavini*, 1406-1450, ed. C. Zonta et Ioh. Brotto, 1922, nos. 430, 547, 844, 968, 1367, 1855. The last date at which he is named is 16 July, 1444 (*Ibid.*, no. 1855).

[23] Roberto Cessi, *loc. cit.*, III (1909), 6, note 1.

[24] *Acta graduum*, 1922, no. 430.

[25] *Ibid.*, no. 547; Cessi, *loc. cit.*, III (1909), 2. Although Cessi gives the date as October 13, 1420, in the text, the document which he cites in note 7 is clearly "die iovis xxiiii octubris."

[26] C. G. Jöcher, *Allgemeines gelehrten Lexicon*, Leipzig, 1750, I, 836, lists these under Barzizius, Christoph., whom he designates as the eldest son of Gasparino, the grammarian. It is quite possible that there is some confusion here since the physician is also credited with the grammatical writings now usually assigned to Christophorus de Barziziis of Brescia (d. after 1492).

for those youths who were approaching the practice of medicine. The medical doctrines contained in it are Galenic as transmitted through Johannitius' *Isagoge*, which was available to every student of medicine through its inclusion in the *Articella*, and more especially through Avicenna's *Canon*, which was required as a part of the reading program for prospective physicians by the leading medical faculties of Europe. Such general surveys of the field as here presented in the *Introductorium* were common both in Cristoforo's day and in the preceding centuries. Indeed the work before us may well be compared with the thirteenth century mirror of medicine composed by the noted Catalan physician and cleric, Arnald of Villanova (d. 1311). Cristoforo was not concerned with specific cases in the *Introductorium* but dealt rather with the general features of medical practice, and of diseases and their cures. In one instance, however, he does make reference to a specific case that of Petrus Barbo, then aged fourteen, the nephew of Pope Eugenius IV (1431-1447), and the future Pope Paul II.[27]

In the preface to the *Introductorium*, Cristoforo states that he is following in the footsteps of his master, Antonio Cermisone, an indication that there was a continuous tradition for the study and teaching of Avicenna, since the work proceeds according to the order and general plan of Avicenna's *Canon*.[28] The first section of the treatise relates to the general fundamentals with which the physician must be acquainted. Considered first are natural things and their correlatives (res naturales et annexa eis), that is the physiological

[27] Barzizza, *Introductorium*, Pavia, 1494, fol. 3v, col. 1-2: "Pro hoc pono exemplum quod ego vidi fuit Petrus Barbo nepos domini Eugenii pape quarti febriens a collera rubea . . . et erat annorum quatuordecim in autumno de mense septembris . . ." Since it is generally agreed that the Venetian Petrus Barbo became Pope Paul II, August 31, 1464, at the age of forty-eight, this would indicate that Barzizza composed the *Introductorium* not earlier than 1430.

[28] Cf. Arnald of Villanova, *Speculum introductorium medicinae*, Opera, 1505, fol. 1r; Incunabulum edition, Klebs, 106.1. After a definition of medicine the *Speculum* takes up Res naturales: with separate sections devoted to: elementa, complexiones, humores, membra, virtutes, operantes, spiritus. Then follow the Res non-naturales: motus vel exercitus et quies, somnus et vigilia, inanitio et repletio, passio mentis (passio cordis s. accidens animi), consequentes: tempus, regio, coitus, ars ludus, balneum, et consuetudo. Finally there follows: Res contra naturam: diseases arranged according to whether they are simple or complex, the causes and symptoms of diseases, prognostic signs of future diseases and critical days.

constituents of the body which are concerned with the maintenance of health. Of these seven are said to be of importance, first the elements, that is air, fire, earth, water, the male sperm and female menstrual blood; second, the complexions and those things closely allied, such as age, sex, form, and habitude, or profession; third, the four humors; fourth, the organs both simple and complex; fifth, the natural virtues; sixth, the spirits; and seventh, their functions. Next follows the consideration of the six non-naturals, or those things involved in the curing of diseases and the maintenance of health which are unnatural or artificial.[29] These include first the consideration and regulation or conditioning of the air according to its prime qualities, warmth and cold, as well as to its secondary qualities or effects, both occult and manifest; second, of food and drink, considered according to quantity, quality, hour of taking, origin, preparation, and the like; third, of motion or exercise and rest; fourth, of sleep and waking; fifth of emptiness and repletion; and finally sixth, the consideration of the accidents or emotional states of the mind, all according to Avicenna.

The next section of the work relating to those things which are contrary to nature (De rebus preter naturam), treats of diseases. Here are considered the various kinds of diseases, their causes, course and accidents, as well as the outward signs of diseases.[30] Special attention is given to the method of discovering the location or region of the body in which the disease is established. Emphasis is placed at this point upon the necessity of a knowledge of anatomy on the part of the physician.[31] Considerable space is devoted to the exposition of the signs or symptoms of diseases, how they may be recognized and distinguished, the similarities between diseases as to time, place, and the like, and the methods of diagnosis and prognosis. Cristoforo then enumerates the signs of crises and gives a tabulated list for young physicians beginning with those of the head and descending downward to the feet.[32] Methods of care for the sick are next set forth, their diet and the regulation of the air. The physician, Cristoforo states, should be acquainted with the diversities of the

[29] Barzizza, *Introductorium*, 1494, fol. 1v, col. 2-2r, col. 2.
[30] Barzizza, *Introductorium*, 1494, fol. 2r, col. 2 *et seq.*
[31] *Ibid.*, fol. 5r, col. 1.
[32] *Ibid.*, fol. 8r, col. 1 *et seq.*

seasons and climates; he should also prescribe as to the amount of exercise and rest.[33] Careful directions are given for the use of the bath,[34] also on the amounts of sleep and rest,[35] emptiness and repletion, and for the control of the accidents or emotional states of the mind.[36] Then follow instructions for evacuation, including vomiting and phlebotomy,[37] with general canons for the use of clysters, pessaries, and other medicinal aids, as well as for the use of narcotic and other sedative medicines, and finally rules for the application and doses of medicinal simples. In this section reference is made to the works of Serapion and Mesue.

Like frequent other professors of medicine in the fourteenth and fifteenth centuries, Cristoforo also composed a commentary on the ninth book of Rasis' *Liber Almansoris.* This manual of special pathology and therapeutics along with Johannitius' *Isagoge,* and Avicenna's *Canon* was a required textbook in the leading medical faculties of Europe. The commentary which was printed with the *Introductorium* in 1494 [38] follows the general order of subjects of Rasis' text, although in a few instances some changes have been made. The regional distribution of diseases according to their location in the human body is followed. The first section deals with the diseases of the head beginning with cephalaea, then the nerves, beginning with paralysis (fol. 50v),[39] the eyes, beginning with ophthalmia (obtalmia, fol. 64v), the ears (fol. 83r, col. 2), nose (fol. 90v), teeth (fol. 95v, col. 2), gums (fol. 99r), mouth (fol. 98r), tongue (fol. 98r, col. 2, 99r, col. 2-100r), lips (fol. 98r, col. 2),

[33] *Ibid.*, fol. 13v, col. 1.

[34] *Ibid.*, fol. 13v, col. 2-14r, col. 2.

[35] *Ibid.*, fol. 14r-14v, col. 2.

[36] *Ibid.*, fol. 15r, col. 1.

[37] *Ibid.*, fol. 15r *et seq.*

[38] The foliation of this edition is defective throughout especially throughout this commentary, which follows immediately after the *Introductorium* on fol. [31r]. The incipit of Rasis' text precedes: "Quando rubedo et tensio et gravedo. . . ." Then follows the commentary [fol. 31v]: Incipit solempnis expositio super nono Almansoris clarissimi doctoris magistri Cristofori de Barziziis Pergamensis. Permissis puerilibus consueti queri circa principia librorum. . . ." The work ends with the 173rd chapter (fol. 251v) De dolore qui fit in membris manifestis. Then follows the list of chapter headings for both the *Introductorium* and the commentary on the ninth book of Rasis, *Liber Almansoris.*

[39] The numbers given are those of the volume itself. Although these are frequently erroneously enumerated in the volume they will here serve to indicate the general sequence of topics.

and throat (fol. 101v). The second section on the diseases of the spiritual organs, that is of the chest and heart, includes accounts of coughing (fol. 106r), asthma (fol. 108v), pleurisy (fol. 111v), pneumonia (peripleumonia, fol. 117r), tuberculosis (fol. 121r, col. 2), heart murmur (fol. 123v), and fainting. The third part is on diseases of the natural organs, that is of the stomach, with accounts of bilious disorders (fol. 132r, col. 2 *et seq.*), of diseases of the liver (fol. 156r, col. 2), spleen (fol. 171r, col. 2), and other organs of digestion and elimination (fol. 180v, col. 2 *et seq.*), including stone in the kidneys (fol. 207v, col. 2-215r) and bladder. In the fourth section are discussed diseases of the generative or reproductive organs (fol. 225v). Included also is a discussion of gonorrhoea (gomorea, fol. 224r) which was not treated of by Rasis. Considerable attention is given over to the subject of parturition and obstetrics. The final section is brief compared to the preceding and is given over to the account of the diseases of the extremities. It comprises an account of hernia (fol. 244r) or rupture, arthritis (fol. 245v), diseases of the back (fol. 249r), varicose veins (fol. 250v), elephantiasis (fol. 251r), and other external affections. The detailed description of each disease is followed by the rules for its treatment and cure.

The third work in print by Cristoforo is that pertaining to fevers. Although frequently said to have been printed in an edition of Pavia, 1494,[40] there is no mention of this edition by bibliographers of incunabula nor does it appear to have been included with the two preceding works in the edition of Pavia, 1494.[41] Its first appearance in print appears rather to have been in 1517 at Lyons, where it was included in a collection of tracts on fevers by Marsilius de Sancta Sophia, Galeatius de Sancta Sophia, Richardus Anglicus (or Parisiensis), and Anthonius de Gradis.[42] Another edition which I have consulted at the New York Academy of Medicine was published at Basle,

[40] Cf. *Biographisches Lexikon der hervorragenden Arzte*, I, 367; and Neuburger, *Geschichte der Medizin*, Stuttgart, II, 1 (1911), 470; etc.

[41] See *Gesamtkatalog der Wiegendrucke*, no. 3672; Hain *2666; Pellechet 1975 (Klebs, *Incunabula scientifica et medica*, Bruges, 1938, 159.1).

[42] The work is listed in the British Museum Catalogue of Printed Books as Sancta Sophia (Marsilius de), Opus aureum ac preclarum . . . Signa causas et curas febrium complectens, etc. [Edited by Gondisalvas Toledo], Lugduni, 1517, 4to. (1166. f. 1). The work of Cristoforo is indicated as: "Intentiones habende in febribus C. Barsisii. . . ."

1535.[43] The work circulated, however, in manuscript form during the fifteenth century, since manuscripts of it are extant in libraries of Paris and Vienna.[44] A second tract on pestilential fevers is also listed for Barzizza in the Sloane collection of manuscripts at the British Museum in London.[45] The printed tract on the recognition, causes and care of fevers is largely based on Avicenna's *Canon* (Book IV, Fen 1).[46] Among the fevers considered are various forms of tertian, synochal, phlegmatic, syncopal, quartan, quintan, and sextan fevers; also pestilential, small-pox (variola), measles, and semi-tertian (hemitritaeus). The tract devotes less attention to the symptoms of the fevers than to their treatment and cure. Careful directions as to the regime to be followed are given. Besides Avicenna, Cristoforo cites Gentile da Foligno, the fourteenth century author who also wrote on fevers.

The foregoing survey of the intellectual interests and medical compositions of Cristoforo Barzizza illustrates the conservative character of medical teaching in the first half of the fifteenth century. It reveals its close adherence to traditional models; and its lack of deviation from or advance beyond the confines of the teaching of a century or two earlier. Thus may be seen side by side with the so-called modernism of the humanists the persistence of traditional lines of medieval thought which in the medical sphere clung tenaciously to well thumbed authorities like Galen, Avicenna, and Rasis, whom time and use had sanctioned as the *sine qua non* of medical teaching.

[43] The copy at the New York Academy of Medicine is bound with Marcellus (Empiricus), De medicamentis empiricis, Basle, 1536. The collection includes Clemente Clementino, Lucubrationes . . . (pp. 1-187); Richardus Anglicus, De signis febrium liber (pp. 188-200); Antonius de Gradis, Liber de febribus (pp. 201-251); and Christophorus Barzizius, De febrium cognitione et cura (pp. 251-283). The titulus reads: De febrium cognitione et cura per clarissimum doctorem medicum Christophorum Barsisium Pergomen. in laudem domini Ieus Christi cuius nutu factum est omne quod est in inferioribus. The work begins: "De tertiana pura interpollata. In cholerica interpollata pura sunt intentiones. Prima est administratio regiminis rerum sex non naturalium, aeris, scilicet, et qui conservet res naturales et removeat praeter naturales. . . ."

[44] Although the title varies, the incipit identifies it. See Thorndike and Kibre, *Catalogue of Incipits*, 1937, col. 316.

[45] *Ibid.*, col. 518.

[46] Cf. Avicenna, *Canon*, Lib. IV, fen 1, tract 2, cap. xxxv: "De sermone febris cholerice. . . ." I have used the edition of Venice, 1486, printed together with the *De viribus cordis* (Hain *2205; New York Academy of Medicine, E. C. Streeter Collection; Klebs 131.9).

ADDENDUM

Since the publication of the preceding article, I have had an opportunity to examine several manuscripts relating to Cristoforo Barzizza in European (English and Continental) libraries. They have for the most part been included under Cristoforo's name in the new and augmented edition of the *Catalogue of Incipits of Mediaeval Scientific Writings in Latin*, by the late Professor Lynn Thorndike and Pearl Kibre, Mediaeval Academy of America, Cambridge, Mass., 1963. For the corrected references see below.

For note 1, additional information on Cristoforo (here called of Pergamo) and his colleagues may be found in Padua Archivio Antiquo 673, fols. 8r-v, and 20r; and Munich CLM 265, ff. 171r-191v, dated 1431-34.

In regard to note 4, the 'Introductorium sive Ianua' is also contained in the two Munich manuscripts: CLM 182, fifteenth century, fols. 300r (without heading) -331, and CLM 184, fols. 211r-247r. Cap. 1 in CLM 182, fol. 300r begins: 'Circa ergo opus practicum sic procedendam [est] ut primo considerentur fundamenta super quibus medicus edificat rationem ...' In CLM 184, fol. 247r, the work ends: 'Explicit Introductorium compilatum per famosissimum artium et medicine doctorem magistrum Cristoferum de Barziziis de Pergamo finitum 1440 die ultima mensis Marcii (Padue) ad laudem Ihesu Cristi et gloriose matris eius benedicte. Amen.'

On p. 391, line 14 should be corrected to read: [trans]lation from the Greek by Burgundio of Pisa, of the fourteen book text, which was later completed by Peter of Abano and frequently appeared separately.

Note 12 should be changed to read for 1937, col. 1187: 1963, col. 1563.

Note 13, line 1, should be changed to read for 1937, cols. 125, 166: 1963, cols. 273, 359.

On p. 392, cont. of note 14; line 2 should be changed to read for 1937, col. 515: 1963, col. 1105.

Note 15, line 3 should be changed to read for 1937, col. 354: 1963, cols. 749, 804.

Note 16 should be changed to read for 1937, cols. 331, 528: 1963, cols. 698, 1132.

Note 17, last line of note should be changed to read for 1937, col. 438: 1963, col. 981.

Note 44 should be changed to read for 1937, col. 316: 1963, col. 667, where four manuscripts are listed, namely Paris BN 6993, 15th cent., fols. 260-269r; Vienna 5269, 15th cent., fols. 87r-99r; Munich CLM 205, a. 1430, fols. 129r-141v; CLM 184, a. 1440, fols. 150v-161v; also printed 1535, with Clementino Clemente, *Lucubrationes*, pp. 251 et seq.

XIX

GIOVANNI GARZONI OF BOLOGNA (1419-1505), PROFESSOR OF MEDICINE AND DEFENDER OF ASTROLOGY

AN INTERESTING COLLECTION of manuscripts once owned, copied, and written by Giovanni Garzoni,[1] the distinguished professor of medicine in the University of Bologna from 1466 to 1505, deserves greater attention than it has so far received.[2] The manuscripts are not only fairly numerous but also relate to a diversity of subjects that should arouse and engage our interest. They include treatises on medicine, humanistic and literary studies, history, political theory, the usual subjects of the arts curriculum, saints' lives and other traditional themes, and especially astrology. The following account is intended therefore to call attention to these codices now preserved in the University Library at Bologna and, in particular, to provide a brief analysis of Garzoni's views on astrology and medicine as revealed in his own writings.

Before turning to the manuscripts, however, it may be of interest to review briefly the salient facts of Garzoni's career.[3] He was born in Bologna in 1419, the

[1] See Ludovico Frati, "Indice dei Codici Latini Conservati nella R. Biblioteca Universitaria di Bologna," *Studi Italiani di Filologia Classica*, 1908–1909, *16–17*; the index, *ibid.*, *17*:151, mentions some 27 codices containing works by Giovanni Garzoni, that he was the amanuensis of 4, and that he owned some 37 or 39. The following MSS should be added to Frati's list: Bologna University MSS 284 (478) and 500 (876). In this double-number notation for MSS in the Bologna University Library, the number outside the parentheses represents the number in the catalogue and that inside is the shelf mark of the MS.

I should like to express appreciation for the courtesy and attention to my numerous requests accorded me by the members of the Bologna University Library staff, and especially Sig. Luigi D'Aurizio.

[2] Although Albano Sorbelli (*Storia della Università di Bologna,* Bologna: Nicola Zanichelli, 1944, Vol. I, p. 252) suggested that Garzoni's works merited collecting, nothing seems to have been done about it. Garzoni's name does not appear in the *Biographisches Lexikon der hervorragenden Ärzte aller Zeiten u. Völker* (2nd ed., Berlin/Vienna: Urban u. Schwarzenberg, 1929–1935).

[3] For biographical details see the references indicated by Ulysse Chevalier, *Répertoire des sources historiques du Moyen Âge* (Paris: Alphonse Picard et Fils, 1905–1907), Vol. I, p. 658; also Sorbelli, *op. cit.*, pp. 251–252; and D. Umberto Dallari, *I Rotuli dei Lettori Legisti e Artisti dello Studio Bolognese dal 1384 al 1799* (Bologna: Regia Tipographia dei Fratelli Merkini, 1888–1891), Vol. I, pp. 73 *et passim* (see index). Garzoni's name first appears on the rolls of the *Artisti* for the years 1466–1467: "Ad lecturam Practice medicine in tertiis (Legitur tertius Avicenne, nona fen decima

son of Bernardo Garzoni, also a professor of medicine in the University. Giovanni Garzoni accompanied his father to Rome when the latter became personal physician to Pope Nicholas V. In Rome, Giovanni Garzoni directed his attention to humanistic studies. He himself named as his preceptor the noted humanist educator Guarino of Verona.[4] After his father's death in 1456, Giovanni Garzoni returned to his native city, and in 1457, at the age of thirty-eight, he began to study medicine. He achieved the doctorate in 1466, at the age of forty-seven, and was appointed that same year to teach medicine. Thereafter, every year from 1466 to 1505, the year of his death[5] at the age of eighty-six, his name appeared on the teaching rolls for the teaching of "Medicina in practica," that is, for lectures on Avicenna's *Canon*, "Book three, *Fen* nine, ten, eleven, and twelve."[6] In this third book—which deals with the individual diseases that afflict the human body, arranged in the usual order, from the head to the feet—the sections, or *Fen*, nine through twelve relate to the throat, lungs and chest, heart, and breasts, respectively.[7]

In all likelihood, Giovanni Garzoni's earlier training in literary studies accounts for the large proportion of codices formerly in his possession that contain tracts on grammar and classical authors, in addition to his own addresses and *epistolae* on these subjects. Eight of the codices are specifically on grammar;[8] several others contain texts of Cicero, Virgil, together with Guarino of Verona's excerpts from Servius' commentary on Virgil,[9] also Horace,[10] and Juvenal.[11] Excerpts from the

---

undecima, decima secunda)," and thereafter each year through 1504–1505 (*ibid.*, pp. 73 ff.).

In the following details of Garzoni's career I have chiefly followed Serafino Mazzetti (*Repertorio di tutti i Professori Antichi e Moderni della Famosa Università, e del Celebre Istituto delle Scienze di Bologna*, Bologna: Tipographia de S. Tommaso d'Aquino, 1848, pp. 62, 142), who corrects Giovanni Fantuzzi (*Notizie degli Scrittori Bolognesi*, Bologna: Stamperia di S. Tommaso d'Aquino, 1781–1784, Vol. IV, p. 78) on several points of dating.

4 MS 500 (876), fol. 2r: "Ego a disertissimo omnium Veronensium Guarino praeceptore meo. . . ."

5 He died on 28 Jan. 1505 (Mazzetti, *op. cit.*, p. 142; Sorbelli, *op. cit.*, p. 252).

6 Dallari, *op. cit.*, pp. 73 ff. The last time his name appears on the rolls of the *Artisti* is for 1504–1505 (*ibid.*, p. 188).

7 *Cf.* Avicenna, *Liber Canonis in medicina*, trans. from the Arabic into Latin by Gerard of Cremona (Basel, 1556), pp. 465–523: "Liber tertius, De aegritudinibus particularibus quae fiunt in membris hominis a capite usque ad pedes manifestis et occultis." In 22 *fen* and 52 tractates, of which *Fen* IX treats "De dispositionibus gutturis"; *Fen* X, "De dispositionibus pulmonis et pectoris et sunt tractatus quinque"; *Fen* XI, "De dispositionibus cordis," in 2 tractates; and *Fen* XII, "De mamilla et dispositionibus eius." It would appear from the codices in Garzoni's collection that he also discussed other sections from the Avicenna *Canon*. See, e.g., the description of MS 423 (731), below.

8 See, e.g., MS 424 (732), item 17; MS 435 (743); MS 438 (746); MS 441 (749), item 3; MS 455 (794); MS 456 (795); MS 842 (1896 and 1622); MS 928 (1793); and MS 207 (313), item 1, "Iohannis Bonandreae, De modo conscribendi epistolas et alia opuscula." The above MSS are described by Frati, *op. cit.*

9 MS 276 (465); MS 277 (466), "cum notis autographis Baptistae Guarini" (Frati, *op. cit.*, 1908, *16*:217); MS 278 (467), "cum notis autographis Baptistae Guarini Veronensis"; MS 279 (468), "Scriptus per me Ioh. Garzonem 1476, 27 Aprilis in studio Bononie" (Frati, *16*:218); MS 280 (469); MS 281 (476); MS 284 (478) (Frati, *16*: 218–219); MS 440 (748), *a.* 1475, "cum notis marginalibus Baptistae Guarini Veronensis autographis" (Frati, *16*:262); MS 441 (749); MS 834 (1610), *a.* 1468, "Guarini Veronensis. Per ordinem litterarum super Virgileo ex Servio excerpsit" (Frati, *16*: 365).

10 MS 441 (749), item 2, "Horatii Flacci Epistolae" (Frati, *16*:262).

11 MS 500 (876), "D. Iunii Iuvenalis satirae, cum glossis," probably autographed by Garzoni.

last-named author contain notes, made possibly by Garzoni himself from the lectures on Juvenal, that he comments he had heard his preceptor Guarino, "that most eloquent of all Veroneseans," give in the year 1449.[12] There is also a copy of Macrobius' *Saturnalia*[13] among the codices.

Further codices bearing Giovanni Garzoni's name, either as former owner or composer, contain works on history and political theory as well as accounts of important contemporary events. Among such works are found the ancient histories of the classical Greek historian Diodorus Siculus in the Latin translation by Poggio, Garzoni's own history of the legendary Polyphemus,[14] and a collection of histories of Bologna. These include Garzoni's *History of Bologna* from its origins to his own time, his account of the *Deeds of Taddeo Pepoli* (the 14th-century ruler of Bologna), addressed to Guido Pepoli,[15] and his treatise on the Bentivoglio (the rulers of Bologna in the late 15th century).[16] A further historical work by Garzoni, his *History of Saxony,* which is one of the few works by him in print,[17] does not appear among the collection of his works in the University Library. Other codices in the Library do, however, contain further unpublished treatises:[18] *On the Office or Duty of the Prince, On the Instruction of Princes,* and *On the Governing of a City,* besides his essays or orations: *Against Tyrants* and *On Liberty.*[19] The Library also has his accounts of *The Taking of the City of Granada,* or *On the Moorish War,* and *On the Descent of Charles VIII of France into Italy.*[20]

12 *Ibid.*, fol. 2r: "Audivi hunc librum ego a disertissimo omnium Veronensium Guarino praeceptore meo sub anno domini 1449." ("Ex bibl. Bernardi primum, deinde Ioannis Garzoni Bonon." Frati, *16*:279).

13 MS 542 (982), 15th century, "Macrobi Saturnaliorum libri V" (Frati, *16*:291).

14 MS 377 (619) (Frati, *16*:244); MS 426 (734), "Io. Garzoni Poliphemi hist." (Frati, *16*:255–256).

15 MS 445 (753), 15th century; MS 446 (754), 18th century (Frati, *16*:263–264); MS 444 (752), 15th century; MS 443 (751) 15th century (Frati, *16*:263).

16 MS 434 (742), 15th century.

17 In addition to the *De rebus Saxoniae, Thuringiae, . . . ,* written *c.* 1486, with a preface by Erasmus Stella (Basel: J. Frobenius, 1518 and thereafter), his printed works include: *De laudibus legum oratio foeliciter* (s.l.n.d.: now at Paris, Bibliothèque nationale Rés F 2157); *Gloriosissimi martyris Christophori Canonei vita, . . . ,* ed. by M. Fromüth (Leipzig: Per Martinum Herbipolensem, 1510); *De miseria humana. Epistole consolatorie Epigrammata et Epithaphia* (Strasburg: J. Grüninger, 1505); *De rebus Ripanis libellus* (Ancona: A. de Grandis, 1567 and thereafter); "De dignitate urbis Bononiae commentarius . . . ," publ. by L. A. Muratori, *Rerum Italicarum scriptores . . . ,* ed. by F. Argellati (Milan: Typographia Societatis Palatinae, 1723–1751), Vol. XXI, pp. 1141–1168; "D. Joannis Bentivoli senioris gestis ad Joannem Bentivolum juniorem libellus," publ. by F. Ant. Zaccaria, *Iter litterarum per Italiam ab anno 1753 ad 1757* (Venice, 1762), p. 541.

18 See the long list of his unedited works in Fantuzzi, *op. cit.*, Vol. IV, pp. 78–100; Vol. IX, pp. 115–128. Moreover, in addition to the volumes in the Bologna University Library indicated in the following note, an additional tract by Garzoni may be found in a Prague MS: "ad Nicolexium(?) poetam de iudicio communi" (Prague MS 502, paper, 15th to 16th centuries, fols. 47r–60v (Proemium incipit) "Vehemens me cepit admiratio . . . ."

19 MS 427 (735), 15th century, 25 fols.; MS 437 (745), "De eruditione principum libri tres" (Frati, *16*:261); and see Lynn Thorndike, "Giovanni Garzoni on Ruling a City," *Political Science Quarterly,* 1931, *46*: 277–280, based not on the Bologna MS but the MS at Paris, Bibliothèque nationale 6694, 15th century, fols. 1r–17v; and also Thorndike, "Giovanni Garzoni on the Office of the Prince," *Polit. Sci. Q.*, 1931, *46*:589–592, based on a Vatican MS: Urbin. 996, membrane, fols. 1r–25v.

20 MS 433 (741), 15th century, item 31, "Declamatio adversus tyrannos"; item 32, "Oratio pro libertate" (Frati, *16*:258–259);

Other codices formerly in Garzoni's possession contain his own addresses and *epistolae* as well as tracts by other authors on medicine, law, theology, logic, music, natural philosophy, and astrology.[21] These suggest Garzoni's interest in the entire spectrum of subjects comprised in the university curriculum. His concern with logic, in particular, appears in both his addresses in praise of the discipline and in the several books that he owned, among them a well-known medieval textbook, the *Summa logicae* of Petrus Hispanus (Pope John XXI),[22] and two works of later medieval mathematical logic—the *De proportionibus* of Albert of Saxony[23] and the *De latitudinibus formarum*, sometimes assigned to Jacobus de Sancto Marino (or Florentia, or Napoli), and, more frequently, to Nicole Oresme, under whose name it was printed.[24] In addition, the Library has Garzoni's copies of Jean Buridan's commentary on the *Ethics* of Aristotle and the commentary of Friar Antonius Andreas, O.M., on the *Metaphysics* of Aristotle.[25]

Also indicative of Garzoni's adherence to the interests of earlier medieval scholars are the codices, which he had formerly owned, that contain accounts of the lives of saints and other traditional themes. These include individual accounts by Garzoni himself of the lives of St. Peter Martyr, St. Augustine, St. Gregory the Great, and St. Dominic;[26] a copy of Thomas de Wales and Nicholas Traucht, *Expositio librorum S. Augustini de civitate dei*;[27] other tracts by Garzoni on graces (*Gratiarum actio post disputationem*) and on the variability of fortune (*De variatate fortune*);[28] and his addresses to the pope against dice players and gamblers.[29]

Turning now to the works of his collection which relate more directly to science or pseudo-science and to Garzoni's profession, we may take note of the several works pertaining to astrology, the study of which was deemed essential for a physi-

---

MS 424 (732), 15th century, item 1, "Io. Garzoni expugnatio urbis Granatae sive de bello Mauritano"; also MS 433 (741), 15th century, item 22, "De bello Granatensi ad Bartolomeam Gislardum"; and MS 425 (733), "Io. Garz. Caroli VIII Gallicarum regis ingressum in Italiam."

[21] MS 434 (742), 15th century, especially items 34–38 (Frati, *16*:259–260); also MS 438 (746), item 7, "Oratio in laudem logice et physice"; item 8, "Amplissima laus theologiae" (Frati, *16*:261–262); also MS 1391 (2648), *a.* 1500, fol. 118r, "De laudibus legum; fol. 121v, "Laudatio theologiae"; fol. 123, "De laudibus musicae"; fols. 195v–196v, "Oratio de laudibus logicae et philosophiae naturalis." For further items relating to logic, see below.

[22] MS 840 (1619), *a.* 1450 (Frati *16*:366–367).

[23] MS 520 (921), *a.* 1458, fols. 31v–36r (incipit), "Proportio communiter. . . ." For other copies of this work see Lynn Thorndike and Pearl Kibre, *A Catalogue of Incipits of Mediaeval Scientific Writings in Latin*, new and augmented edition (Cambridge, Mass.: Mediaeval Academy of America, 1963), col. 1139.

[24] MS 520 (921), fols. 173r–175ra, "Tract. de latitudinibus formarum multipliciter" (incipit), "Quia formarum latitudinis multipliciter . . ./. . . (desinit) falsitas consequenter probatur." For other copies, see Thorndike and Kibre, *op. cit.*, col. 1218, item 11.

[25] MS 239 (366), *a.* 1395 (Frati, *16*:200); MS 165 (159), *a.* 1464 (Frati, *16*:171).

[26] MS 428 (736); MS 429 (737); MS 431 (739); MS 433 (741); MS 842 (1896 and 1622), 16th century, Vol. III, "Ioh. Garzoni Orationes et vitae sanctorum" (Frati, *16*: 256–258, 367).

[27] MS 809 (1573), *a.* 1456 (Frati, *16*:356–357).

[28] MS 431 (740), item 1; MS 432 (741) (Frati, *16*:257, 258); and in print, his *De miseria humana*, noted above.

[29] MS 442 (750), 15th century, "Orationes aliquot ad summum Pontificem adversus aleatores," "Ex. Bibl. Io. Garzoni autogra." (Frati, *16*:263).

cian. From the evidence of the works formerly in his possession, he was acquainted with such well-known Arabic astrologers and astronomers as Alcabitius, Alfraganus, and Messahala, whose writings had been translated into Latin in the course of the twelfth and thirteenth centuries. He also had tracts on the astrolabe, the *Algorismus*, the *Sphere* of John of Sacrobosco, and works by Gerard of Cremona, Giovanni Campanus, and a calendar by an otherwise unknown Friar Fucus of Ferrara.[30]

Furthermore, although Garzoni himself appears to have written no systematic treatise on astrology, he did, as the collection reveals, set forth his views on the subject in several addresses or orations[31] and in his historical work on Bologna. Among the former group, contained in a collection of his *Opuscula varia*, are two orations in which Garzoni specifically discussed astrology. In the first, addressed to Conrad Nisemanus,[32] he seemingly opposed judicial astrology, or that branch of astrology which makes prognostications on the basis of the position of the constellations at an individual's birth. He thus appears to condemn those who predict by this method man's future from his natal day. He classed this aspect of astrology with magic arts and divination—especially auspices, auguries, and necromancy—all of which he abhorred. To have faith in these arts, he asserted, is the height of madness.[33] However, in the second oration on the praises of astrology, *De laudibus astrologiae,* addressed to Jacobus Petramolaris, Garzoni expressed his high regard for astrology and condemned as imbecilic those who held astrology in contempt.[34] It is his opinion and that of other learned men whom he cites that astrology is of the greatest value and utility. Mankind, he affirmed, derives countless benefits from the foreknowledge that astrology provides on the course of events.[35] Garzoni then reported that he found corroboration for his own high opinion of astrology in Varro, who esteemed it a worthy and salutary science. He also found further historical support for the utility of the science of astrology in the use made of it by the Chaldeans, Egyptians, and Romans.[36] He countered the arguments of those who criticized astrology on the grounds that predicted events did not always come to pass by insisting that such failures were due not to astrology but to the faults of the astrologers (*hoc astrologorum non astrologiae vitium*).[37] To bolster his opinion that astrologers should acquire their skill by training, he cited Crispus for

30 MS 154 (132), 14th century. For an analysis of this MS, see Lynn Thorndike, "Notes upon Some Medieval Astronomical, Astrological, and Mathematical Manuscripts at Florence, Milan, Bologna, and Venice," *Isis*, 1959, *50*:43–45.

31 MS 433 (741); MS 434 (742), both of the 15th century; MS 1391 (2648), written in 1500.

32 MS 433 (741), fols. 105r–107r.

33 *Ibid.*, fols. 106v–107r. "His artibus fidem habere summa fuit dementia" (*ibid.*, fol. 107r).

34 *Ibid.*, fols. 157r–160r:

Ioh. Garzoni Iacobo Petramolari salutem plurima dicat. In non parvam admirationem adducor cum nonnullos videam tanta mentis imbecillitate captos ut astrologiam contempte ac displicere audeant eamque nullum esse arbitrantur. . . .

35 *Ibid.*, fol. 157r:

. . . et mea et omnium sapientum sententia scientie genus quod humano generi tantum afferat utilitatis tantumque ornamenti . . . cum hi quorum ingenium est omni sapientia et doctrina excultum illam esse testentur quae optima est rerum futurorum scientia. . . .

36 *Ibid.*, fols. 157r–158r.

37 *Ibid.*, fols. 158v–159r.

the fact that those astrologers alone have preeminence who have gained their proficiency through observation (*experientia*) and practice (*usu rerum*).[38] Garzoni concluded his discussion at this time by citing Aristotle, Theophrastus, and other Peripatetics on the relation of astrology to other sciences. According to these authorities, he asserted, astrology is the sole science which ministers to other sciences.[39] Its importance is thus unsurpassed. Neither physicians, lawyers, orators, poets, nor philosophers have won such high praise as astrologers have.[40]

In a further oration in praise of astrology, Garzoni again upheld the importance of astrology and the benefits that it conferred.[41] He had no doubt that it belonged with the liberal arts, as was indeed true for the curriculum of the University of Arts and Medicine at Bologna. He repeated his charges against those who condemned astrology, attributing such condemnation to ignorance. And he again turned to the evidence provided by history to demonstrate the merit of astrology. He called attention to Diodorus' predictions of the deaths of princes, of wars, and of pestilence; and he cited Ptolemy for the meritorious proverb, "The wise man will have dominion over the stars" (*sapiens dominabitur astris*).[42] He referred to Hermes Trismegistus, who predicted the eclipses of the stars, also to Thales of Miletus, Callimachus, Sulpitius, Pompeius, Claudius Ptolemy, Strabo, Pomponius Mella, and the thirteenth-century Dominican scholar Albertus Magnus. He added that he had read and marveled at the works of all those experts in astrology.[43] He cited, in respect to its value for poets, the use of astrology by the Greek poet Aratus (of Soli), and he especially took note of the importance of astrology to the physician in determining critical days and in predicting the date of the death of a patient.[44] He also noted that the Phoenicians used astrology for navigation, and the cultivator of the fields derived benefits from it.[45]

Besides the above addresses, two further orations on astrology are contained in the collection *Orationes illustrium virorum*.[46] The first of these, *Oratio in laudem astrologiae*, is a duplicate of the oration described above[47] and can thus be passed over here. The second, *Laus astrologiae*, repeats much that was stated in the previously described addresses. Garzoni again denounced those who disparage astrol-

[38] *Ibid.*, fol. 159r, ". . . teste Crispo . . . astrologi illi dominantur affirmant hi qui usu rerum et experientia docti existunt. . . ."

[39] *Ibid.*, fols. 159r–160r.

[40] *Ibid.*, fol. 160r, "Non medici non jureconsulti non oratores non poetae non philosophi unquam laudis adepti sunt ipsis divini honores tributerentur."

[41] MS 434 (742), 15th century, fols. 108v–112r:

> Ioh. Garz. Laus Astrologiae. Si que nobis beneficia confert astrologia merite agitare voluerimus .../... [explicit] Vale. Quod me de astrologie meritis ac de his que ad illius laudem pertinent (me) satis dixisse puto. Dixi.

The word in parentheses appears only in MS 1391 (2648), *a.* 1500, fol. 127v, which contains the same text.

[42] MS 434 (742), fols. 108v–110r.

[43] *Ibid.*, fols. 110v–111r.

[44] *Ibid.*, fol. 110r–110v.

[45] *Ibid.*, fol. 111r–111v.

[46] MS 1391 (2648), which has a number of Garzoni's other orations. A note on the first leaf, in a fine humanist hand, reads: "Joh. Garzo. seu Garzonius magna nominis fame Bononie floruit nel fine secolo XV et sub initium sec. XVI. Valde celebratus." This volume, together with others by Garzoni, was originally preserved in the Dominican Library in Bologna.

[47] MS 1391 (2648), fols. 125v–127v, which has the same text as MS 434 (742), fols. 108v–112r, described above.

ogy and hold that it is false and deceptive. He insisted that such assertions did not emanate from men of discerning scholarship but rather from men devoid of such perceptiveness.[48] And in support of his own opinions he named some representative learned astrologers—Ludovicus Finetus (?), who appears to be otherwise unknown, and Girolamo Manfredi, the noted astronomer and astrologer of Bologna.[49]

Giovanni Garzoni reiterated his high praise for astrology in his work on the *History of Bologna,* a portion of which, with the title *De dignitate Bononiae,* has been published by Muratori.[50] No other art or science could be compared with astrology, Garzoni asserted, reaffirming that the great merit and significance of astrology lay in the use men could make of it to predict such happenings as the death of princes, political revolutions, wars, pestilence, high prices, and famine. And in providing warnings astrologers might point out the means by which the effects of such predicted happenings might be avoided or mitigated. "What countless calamities would be nullified," he exclaimed, if the counsel and admonitions of astrologers were heeded. One can in fact, he continued, scarcely estimate the extent to which philosophers, poets, and physicians are dependent upon it. And this would be similarly true for the geographer, as Ptolemy and the other geographers would affirm, for navigators, for persons engaged in agriculture, and for military men, all of whom, according to Garzoni, cultivated astrology with the greatest diligence.[51] Garzoni then named some famous Bolognese who were noted as astrologers: he had high praise for Giovanni da Legnano, who combined astrology and oratory with law or jurisprudence;[52] for Giovanni Bianchini;[53] and for Girolamo Manfredi, whom he also named in his *Laus astrologiae*.[54]

In general, it might be concluded, both from the examples that he provides and from his own discussion of the merit and utility of astrology, that Garzoni does not distinguish clearly between what was frequently termed natural astrology, or astronomy, and judicial astrology, or the prediction of events on the basis of the position of the stars. He seemingly likes both indiscriminately and even shows particular favor for the predictive aspect of astrology, despite his abhorrence of divination. He maintained that the foreknowledge that astrology provides is both desirable and essential to mankind.

Giovanni Garzoni's propensity toward astrology is further shown in one of the codices contained in his collection of medical writings.[55] On the verso of the first

48 MS 1391 (2648), fols. 207v–208r: [incipit] Abeant malis omnibus qui de astrologorum dignitate detrahunt atque astrologiam falsam et mendacem esse affirmant. Sunt hii mea sententia non ab eruditorum modi sed ab hominum sensi remoti . . . / . . . [explicit] esse non dubite. Vale.

49 *Ibid.*, fols. 207v–208r, "Ludovicus Finetus(?) Hieronymus Manfredus astrologi peritissimi. . . ." For the latter, see Lynn Thorndike, *History of Magic and Experimental Science* (New York: Columbia Univ. Press, 1934), Vol. IV, pp. 459 ff.

50 Muratori, *op. cit.*, Vol. XXI, pp. 1141–1168.

51 *Ibid.*, pp. 1163 ff.

52 *Ibid.*, pp. 1161. For Giovanni da Legnano, see Thorndike, *History of Magic*, Vol. III, pp. 592 ff.; Vol. IV, p. 94.

53 Muratori, *op. cit.*, Vol. XXI, p. 1163. For Giovanni Bianchini, see Thorndike, *History of Magic*, Vol. IV, pp. 251, 464.

54 Muratori, *op. cit.*, Vol. XXI, p. 1163; and see above, n. 49.

55 MS 423 (731), 15th century, "Garzoni Iohannis scripta medica, autograph."

leaf of this autographed and annotated codex there are two horoscopes, one apparently made by Marsilius of Bologna, whose name appears beneath the horoscope; the second is that of Giovanni Garzoni, as indicated by the explanatory note with the date 1474: "Figura celi tempore interrogationis domini Johannis Garzoni . . . quarti die Marcii post secundam horam noctis . . . in anno . . . 1474." On the second leaf there is another horoscope and interrogation: "Interrogatio circa subiectam . . ." with the names "Iohannes Paxius [?] civis . . . Bononiensis"; "Marsilius Bononiensis 1474 die 15 Marcii"; and "Frater Gabriel Hispanus." Then follows a note: "Quoniam cum secundum astrologorum sententiam iudicium interrogationis vim sumat ex radice. . . ."

The above medical collection, which is in three volumes,[56] was apparently related directly to Garzoni's lectures on Avicenna. In the first volume the table of contents[57] is succeeded by treatises on urine and on the pulse. The tract on urine, which opens "Significationis dispositionum urine (Summa tertie doctrine tertie fen secunda de urina)," coincides with Avicenna's text[58] and is accompanied by numerous marginal notes which define and amplify the text, together with a running commentary. The opening words of the commentary, "Quoniam doctrina significationis dispositionum urine non oportet medicus credere nisi postquam indicationes observationis fuerint . . . ,"[59] suggest Garzoni's empirical approach to the subject by asserting that the physician need not accept the (Avicennian) doctrine of the significance of the disposition of urine until or unless the results of his own observation bear it out. Following the tract on urine is one on the pulse, accompanied also by interlinear and marginal notes: "Summa prima dictionis secunde de pulsu cuius sunt xviii capitula. Capitum primum de pulsu et est sermo universalis anhelitus." It begins: "Pulsus est motus receptaculorum spiritus ex diastole et sistole compositus ad regendum spiritum per aerem attractus. . . ."[60]

Volume two of this collection of *Opera medica* covers a variety of topics relating to therapeutics and medication. The list of thirty-one chapters is indicated on the second flyleaf. The leaves of the manuscript are unnumbered, but the chapter headings are indicated at the upper corner of each recto folio. The opening words of the first treatise in the volume are lacking because of a square cut in the first folio. However, the contents relate to the essential causes of diseases and the utility of medication in their treatment.[61]

56 *Ibid.* These are: Vol. I, *Physiologicus;* Vol. II, *Therapeuticum*; Vol. III, *Therapeuticum.*

57 *Ibid.*, Vol. I, fol. 2v.

58 *Ibid.*, fol. 3r. *Cf.* Avicenna, *Canon, ed. cit.*, Liber III, "Summa tertia doctrinae tertiae Fen secunda."

59 The tract ends in MS 423 (731), Vol. I, at fol. 36r, ". . . reperies expositionis argumentum in re egritudinis de ruine reliquorum. Laus deo 1473 die 4to Septembris."

60 *Ibid.*, fols. 36v–58r. *Cf.* Avicenna, *Canon, ed. cit.*, Liber III, *Fen* 10; and Thorndike and Kibre, *op. cit.*, col. 1150, item 12. Another MS is Vatican 4788, 15th century, fol. 152v. The work ends in MS 423 (731), Vol. I, at fol. 58r (58v is blank, and it is the end of the volume), ". . . que sunt fortis et resolutionis. Finis. Io. Garzonius."

61 MS 423 (731), Vol. II. The work ends: . . . sit quantitas huius nostri sermonis compendiosi de principiis utilibus doctoris medicinalis sufficiens. Deinceps nunc elaboremus et de simplicibus medicinis librum composamus si deus voluerit. . . . Finis 1484 die 17 Novembris.

The third and last volume of this collection is also on therapeutics, particularly on fevers (*Therapeutica sive de cura febrium*). It is dated "Ab anno 1466 ad 1467" and hence coincides with the first year of Garzoni's lectures on Avicenna's *Canon* at Bologna.[62] On the inside cover there is a laudatory statement indicating that Garzoni was placed in the same class with Galen.[63] Preceding the text there is a considerable amount of introductory material which further suggests that this is the notebook in which Garzoni jotted down the items to be discussed in his lectures on Avicenna's *Canon*. The opening words, preceded by the rubric: "Fen prima de febribus et est quatuor tractatus de febre," coincide with those of Avicenna: "Febris est maior extraneus accensus in corde. . . ."[64]

A further medical codex, pertaining to Avicenna and belonging to Garzoni, similarly calls attention to Garzoni's interest in astrology. This codex containing the tract on crises, *De crisibus*,[65] has on the verso of the first flyleaf a citation from Duke Leopold, apparently Leopold of Austria, who wrote on astrology in the thirteenth century.[66] It is possible that there is a page of the manuscript missing since the above fragment is numbered "1" and the tract on crises, which begins abruptly, has a "3" before it. The *De crisibus* itself coincides with Avicenna.[67] As in the previous instances, the work is accompanied by frequent interlinear and marginal notes which serve to clarify the words of the text. Apparently Garzoni also made references in his lectures to actual cases to illustrate his points. For example, in the section dealing with bad signs drawn from sleep and waking, there is in the margin a rubric calling attention to the case of Petrus Antonius.[68]

Also related to medicine is Garzoni's *Questio de causis*. In this tract there is a discussion of the importance of manifest or observable causes, with emphasis upon

So far the work on medicinal simples that Garzoni here suggests that he will write has not yet been located.

[62] MS 423 (731), Vol. III, fols. 1r–139r. The list of chapters is on the verso of the flyleaf. On fol. 2r is the statement: "1466, die prima de Novembris ego Johannes Garzonus de mense et anno supradicto incipit literam primam eius anno."

[63] *Ibid.*:

> Dominum magistrum Johannem Garzonum phisicum egregium oratoremque prestantissimum quem Galienum appellat Johannes Lucas Castellanus Lanificii rector sal. Unde putas Galiene datum quod tolere morbos pestiferi nullus sideris arte queat.

[64] *Ibid. Cf.* Avicenna, *Canon, ed. cit.*, Liber III, *Fen* prima. For other copies of Avicenna's *Canon*, with the same opening words, see Thorndike and Kibre, *op. cit.*, col. 551, item 6. The work in MS 423 (731), Vol. III, ends (fol. 139r) ". . . ut in ea non fiat inceptio ad curandum donec manifestus sit modus egritudinis. . . . Laus deo . . . 1467 die 17 Iulii in studio Bononiensis." On fols. 139r–144v, which follow the close of the tract, are a number of notes or possibly prescriptions.

[65] MS 439 (747), 15th century, leaves unnumbered, "Io. Garzoni de crisibus sive de signis crisis in morbis. Autogr."

[66] The short astrological note from Leopold's tract reads: "1. Io. Garz. Secundum ducis Leopoldi tractatum sententiam spem lucri et prope incrementum in figura interrogationis non aliud conficit (efficit) nisi iupiter." For Leopold of Austria's works on astrology, see Thorndike and Kibre, *op. cit.*, index.

[67] The medical material begins at fol. 2r: "3. De signis crisis quatuor signa motus . . . ," which coincides with Avicenna, *Canon*, Liber IV, *Fen* 2, tract 1, "De prognosticatione et iudiciis crisis." *Cf.* the edition of 1556, pp. 814 ff.

[68] MS 439 (747), "Hoc vidisti in Petro Antonio qui mortuus anno 1453(?), 23 Marcii." The work ends (fol. 72r) with the date 1471, 2nd of May. Notes follow on fol. 72v.

the fact that these should be considered in company with the occult or individual attributes of each humor.[69]

In addition to those already mentioned, a number of other medical codices in the Bologna University Library are associated with Garzoni. One of them, formerly in Garzoni's possession, contains Antonius Guaynerius' *Summarium febrium* (without the author's name, however), under the title *Praxis medica de febribus aliis que morbis,* opening, "Qui amoris gratia me Antoni Magliane. . . ."[70] Others include Garzoni's orations in praise of medicine. For example, his *De laudibus phisicae et medicinae* is found in company with Cicero's *Epistolae et familiares* and other orations;[71] and Garzoni's *On Liberal Arts and Medicine,* addressed to Conrad Nisemanus, is contained in another codex. In the latter oration he insists that medicine does belong with the liberal arts, as was indeed the case in the Bologna studium, and that it does not belong with religion.[72] Still another of Garzoni's orations in praise of medicine is found among his *Opera varia et epistolae*[73] and elsewhere.[74] In this *Laus medicinae* Garzoni traces the history of medicine back to antiquity. He names among its founders Apollonius, Aesculapius, Chiron, Almussa (? Musa), who wrote on herbs, Pythagoras, Democritus, Herophilus of Egypt, as well as the more noted Greek physicians Hippocrates and Galen. Of the latter two, he found Hippocrates the most significant. Among the Romans, he noted that medicine flourished especially well under Antonius Pius, who gave physicians honors beyond all others.[75] Garzoni concluded this discourse with the assertion that medicine brings one from despair to hope, from sickness to health, and from death to life.[76]

Medicine and physicians are also not neglected by Garzoni in his historical account of Bologna. In his *De dignitate Bononiae,* mentioned earlier, Garzoni found a number of physicians among the very worthy learned men of the city who had

69 MS 520 (921), 15th century, fols. 176ra–182rb (182v–191r are blank):

> Questio de causis periodicationis. Utrum pro assignandis causis periodicationis preter causas manifestas sit necessarium ponere in unaquoque humore . . . / . . . [explicit] Et sic dei auxilio est finis huius difficilis questionis quem ego magister Johannes Garzon. scripsi in studio Bon. 1470, die 27 Decembris. Laus deo summo.

70 MS 657 (1222), 15th century, 103 fols. For other copies of the work, see Thorndike and Kibre, *op. cit.,* cols. 318 and 1204.

71 MS 248 (467). The Garzoni work begins: "Non mediocri voluntate . . ." (Frati, *16*:217).

72 MS 433 (741), 15th century, item 20, fol. 96r, beginning, "Cum vero libellum ipsum dicarem tu mihi ante alios occuristi quod non modo liberales disciplinas sed medicinam quoque cum religione coniunxisti. . . ."

73 MS 434 (742), 15th century, item 34, fols. 93v–96r:

> Laus medicinae. [incipit] Frequentia vestrum concioque tanta quantam me vidisse non memini(?) . . . mihi afferet alacritate scientie medicine laudibus . . . / . . . [explicit] per deos immortales id rei magnitudini. Dixi.

74 MS 1391 (2648), *a.* 1500, fols. 116r–117v, "Oratio in laudem medicine." This is a duplicate of the text in MS 434 (742). However, in MS 1391 (2648), there is in addition at fols. 181v–183v an "Oratio in laudem physice. [incipit] Vellem prestantissimi vires . . . / . . . [ending] putabit. Dixi."; and at fols. 195v–196v there is an "Oratio de laudibus logice et philosophie naturali. [incipit] Non est apud me dubium magnifice Rhetor . . . / . . . [ending] ad rem destinatem conservatem."

75 MS 1391 (2648), fol. 116v.

76 *Ibid.*

contributed to many sciences. Among those he named are Mundinus of Bologna, Albertus Zancharius (the noted commentator on Hippocrates and Avicenna), Bartholomaeus Varignana, Petrus Tossignano, Petrus Argellata (the surgeon), Dominicus Ragusius,[77] Michael Bertalia,[78] Christopher Honestus, Jacobus da Forlì, Nicolaus Bertucci, and Jacobus Mons Calvus.[79]

In conclusion, while there appears to be nothing startingly new in the works of Giovanni Garzoni, nevertheless the volumes associated with his name as owner, amanuensis, and author, primarily in the University Library at Bologna, indicate the variety and breadth of his concerns and reveal a happy combination of literary and historical interests with scientific interests. They demonstrate that despite the fact that Garzoni's entire academic career (some 38 years) was devoted to teaching sections of Avicenna's medical *Canon,* he nevertheless found time to pursue and to cultivate his literary, political, and historical interests. His interest in science, it might further be noted, as revealed by his regard for astrology and medicine in his writings and his collected works, was largely traditional. Although there are suggestions in his writings of an interest in the empirical aspect of medicine and in the utilitarian side of astrology, Garzoni's main concern was not with the expansion of frontiers of scientific knowledge through his own efforts and research. His chief contribution was the dissemination of already established knowledge among his contemporaries. Yet because of the esteem in which he was held by these contemporaries, Giovanni Garzoni's writings and the collection of works associated with his name do provide an insight into the intellectual and scientific milieu in which he lived and taught. For this reason as well as for their intrinsic interest they deserve our consideration and study.

77 For works of the physicians, see Thorndike and Kibre, *op. cit.*, index.

78 It is possible that this is intended for "Mercadante de Bertalia," a physician at Bologna in 1309 (Chevalier, *op. cit.*, Vol. II, p. 3199).

79 Muratori, *op. cit.*, Vol. XXI, p. 1162. Jacobus de Mons Calvus (Montecalvi) (d. 1361) was professor of philosophy at Bologna (Chevalier, *op. cit.*, Vol. II, p. 3255).

ADDENDUM

The following additional references on Giovanni Garzoni should be added: Thorndike and Kibre, op. cit. (1963), cols. 107, and 1430 (Prol. inc.: 'Sepe et diu ...'): MS British Library, Harley 3747, 15th century, fols. 2ra-20vb. 'Practica medicinae Joh. Garzoni.' Inc. 'Antequam accedamus ad curam doloris capitis dicentur aliqua spectantia ad dolorem in generali .../... (des.) mixto cum melle. Hec enim cura facie occultare alquassem (?) ad tempus. Laus deo. Et sic est finis practice Iohannis Garconis. Per me Henricum de bergis atque Leonis in anno domini Millesimo et quatuor centum et septuagesima cum septem atque completum.' On the library of Garzoni see Guglielmo Manfre, 'La biblioteca dell'umanista bolognese Giovanni Garzoni (1419-1505),' *Accademie e biblioteche d'Italia*, 27(1959), 249-278; and 28(1960), 17-72; and the more recent article, which contains additional bibliography on Garzoni, by Herbert S. Matsen, 'Giovanni Garzoni (1419-1505) to Alessandro Achillini (1463-1512): An unpublished Letter and Defense,' pp. 518-530 in *Philosophy and Humanism: Renaissance Essays in Honor of Paul Oskar Kristeller*, edited by Edward Mahoney, Leiden, E.J. Brill, 1976.

XX

THE INTELLECTUAL INTERESTS REFLECTED IN LIBRARIES OF THE FOURTEENTH AND FIFTEENTH CENTURIES

Libraries and bibliophiles belong to no particular time or place. Yet the chronological period covered by what is commonly termed the Renaissance, that is roughly the fourteenth and fifteenth centuries, and more particularly the fifteenth century, saw a great increase in the number of private or individual collectors of books.[1] Theodor Gottlieb who published a great many of the catalogues of medieval and renaissance libraries lists some two hundred and nineteen for the fifteenth century, and one hundred and fourteen for the fourteenth, as against sixty for the thirteenth, seventy for the twelfth, and forty-three for the eleventh century.[2] Although these numbers are by no means complete and are particularly inadequate for the Italian libraries of the fifteenth century,[3] they do

[1] Cf. D. Giuseppe Zippel, *Nicolò Niccoli* (Firenze, 1890), 41; C. Frati, *Dizionario bio-bibliografico dei bibliotecari e bibliofili italiani dal sec. XIV al XIX* (Firenze, 1933).

[2] Theodor Gottlieb, *Ueber mittelalterliche Bibliotheken* (Leipzig, 1890), has of course made greater use of German sources than of any other. From his lists the approximate numbers for each country, according to centuries may be summarized as follows: Germanies: about 64 for the 15th, 34 for the 14th, 22 each for the 11th and 13th centuries; 30 for the 12th, 6 for the 10th, and 18 for the 9th century. For France there are 40 for the 15th, 29 each for the 14th and 12th centuries, 18 for the 13th, 14 for the 11th, 5 for the 10th, and 4 for the 9th century. The case is much the same for Italy although the proportion of 15th century libraries is much greater: 65 for the 15th, 23 for the 14th, 11 for the 13th, 6 for the 12th, 4 for the 11th, 2 for the 10th, and none for the 9th century. For British libraries, there are 27 for the 15th, 23 for the 14th, 6 for the 13th, 5 for the 12th, none for the 11th, 2 for the 10th, and none for the 9th century. Of the other countries, the Netherlands including Belgium and Holland had 14 for the 15th century, with only 4 each for the 12th and 14th centuries, 1 each for the 13th and 10th, 2 for the 11th. Spain and Portugal according to Gottlieb's list had 9 for the 15th century, 3 for the 14th, 2 for the 13th, 4 for the 12th, and one each for the 9th and 10th centuries.

[3] Several additional libraries are listed by Gustavus Becker, *Catalogi bibliothecarum antiqui,* Bonn 1885. R. Sabbadini, *Le scoperte dei codici latini e greci ne'secoli XIV e XV,* (Biblioteca storica del rinascimento, II, [Firenze, 1905], especially chapter XI, and *Nuove Ricerche, loc. cit. V,* [1914], adds a number of Italian libraries that are omitted by both Gottlieb and Becker. See also Carlo Frati, *Dizio-*

serve to indicate the extent of the increase. It is of course difficult to determine how much the interest of the humanists in classical texts caused this growth in numbers or what proportion can be credited to the natural tendency for extant records to be more numerous as we approach our own time. Possibly the practice of making and exchanging inventories of their collections, that Pico della Mirandola and other humanists indulged in, resulted in more of them being preserved.[4] The contribution of the printing press to the growth of these libraries is also difficult to evaluate since printed books did not at first find a ready acceptance among the wealthy bibliophiles who preferred the more costly and more finely wrought hand copies. Yet the humanists and other scholars whose chief interest was in the content rather than in the externals of the books welcomed the products of the presses.

The size of these libraries varied considerably both as to the number of codices listed and in the contemporary reports of them. The latter are notoriously exaggerated,[5] and separate items listed give no real index to the actual number of individual treatises, since it was customary to bind several together, even in the case of printed books. A library of about 800 or 900 items might be said to constitute a very fair-sized collection. That of Pico della Mirandola, usually adjudged one of the outstanding private libraries of the fifteenth century numbered some 1190 items.[6] Numbers and size are, however, of much less importance than the nature of the contents for our purpose, which is that of determining the intellectual interests and resources that these libraries reflect. There seems little need for reiterating the importance in this regard of the extant inventories, for despite the brevity and inadequacy of their descriptions these contemporary catalogues do provide tangible evidence for the presence or absence of particular writings.[7]

---

nario bio-bibliografico dei bibliotecari e bibliofili italiani dal sec. XIV al XIX, raccolto e publicato da Albano Sorbelli (Firenze, 1933).

I am indebted to Dr. Paul O. Kristeller, who read the final draft of this paper, for suggestions especially in regard to bibliography on Italian and Spanish libraries.

[4] Cf. P. Kibre, *The library of Pico della Mirandola* (New York, 1936), 15–16.

[5] A. de Hevesy, *La bibliothèque du roi Matthias Corvin* (Paris, 1923), 25, citing Vespasiano and other contemporary authors. Cf. J. Hilgers, S.J., "Zur Bibliothek Nikolaus V," *Centralblatt für Bibliothekswesen,* XIX (1902), 1–2.

[6] P. Kibre, *op. cit.,* introduction.

[7] Joseph Ghellinck, S.J., "En marge des catalogues des bibliothèques médiévales," *Miscellanea Francesco Ehrle,* V (1924), 331–63, has a stimulating discussion on the

And while it may be argued that the mere possession of a work does not mean that its owner has read or assimilated its contents, yet this fact when taken in conjunction with other evidence can do much to throw light on the available resources and mental pabulum of an era. Needless to say a final evaluation of the intellectual interests of the fourteenth and fifteenth centuries must rest upon a careful consideration not only of the resources available but also of the use to which these were put as determined by an analysis of the literary output of those centuries. This paper attempts no such final summing up, it seeks merely to point out various avenues of intellectual interest suggested by the nature of the books that were held in sufficient esteem to be placed on the shelves of many of the libraries of the time.

Considerable attention has already been directed toward these libraries, chiefly, however, from the viewpoint of their external features, or on the basis of special studies of individual collections. Or more particularly they have been examined from the viewpoint of the humanistic revival and the light that they might shed on the currency of Greek and Latin classics.[8] But just as the study of the inventories of the earlier medieval period has tended to dissipate the erroneous conception that the classics of antiquity were entirely lost sight of during the centuries before the fourteenth century,[9] just so must the inventories of these later libraries be studied with regard to their total content, in order to determine not only how many or what Greek and Latin classics they included, but also to determine the relation and proportion of these works to others contained in the collections. Such is the primary purpose of this paper.

---

subject of medieval inventories of libraries, their importance as well as lacunae. Cf. P. Kibre, *The library of Pico della Mirandola,* 9–10, and the bibliography in note 20.

[8] See for example R. Sabbadini, *Le scoperte dei codici Latini e Greci ne'secoli XIV e XV* (Firenze, 1905), especially chapter XI; *op. cit., Nuove Ricerche* (1914); Edward Edwards, *Memoirs of libraries* (London, 1859), Vol. I; W. Wattenbach, *Das Schriftwesen im Mittelalter* (Leipzig, 3rd ed., 1896), 570 ff.; Dorothy M. Robathan, "Libraries of the Italian Renaissance," in J. W. Thompson, *The medieval library* (Chicago, 1939), chapter XVII; also P. Kibre, *The library of Pico della Mirandola.*

[9] M. R. James, *The ancient libraries of Canterbury and Dover* (Cambridge, 1903), pp. xxxi ff.; J. S. Beddie, "The ancient classics in the medieval libraries," *Speculum,* V (1930), 3–20; Max Manitius, "Handschriften antiker Autoren in mittelalterlichen Bibliothekskatalogen, herausgegeben von Karl Manitius," *Beiheft zum Centralblatt für Bibliothekswesen* (Leipzig, 1935), no. 67.

A study of the library catalogues for the fourteenth and fifteenth centuries, reveals first of all that Greek literary texts were slow in making their appearance in these collections before the first half of the fifteenth century. Whatever earlier interest there had been shown in western Europe toward Greek during the twelfth and thirteenth centuries had been directed particularly toward theological and scientific writings,[10] and it was toward Greek books of this nature that such fourteenth century bibliophiles as Richard de Bury and Walter Burley[11] turned their attention. This was also true for the courts of southern Italy especially in that of Robert of Naples, where Greek works were being translated all during the fourteenth century.[12] Only an occasional Greek literary text appears in the inventories of the fourteenth century. Petrarch who had never succeeded in learning the language did treasure the Greek texts of Plato and of Homer that he had obtained;[13] and Boccaccio who not only studied Greek but also, probably at the suggestion of Petrarch, sponsored the first complete, though adjudgedly poor, translation of Homer's *Iliad* and *Odyssey,* appears to have had few Greek texts in his possession.[14] Greek manuscripts were also rare during the first half of the fifteenth century especially in the princely libraries. The famous library of the Visconti in Pavia, one of the richest and most important of the Italian contemporary collections, in 1426 had only four Greek books, despite the fact that Giangaleazzo Visconti had welcomed Manuel Chrysoloras, the leading teacher of Greek, when he came to Pavia in 1400 to help the Byzantine emperor in his appeal for aid against the Turks.[15]

[10] Cf. Louise R. Loomis, *Medieval Hellenism* (Lancaster, Penna., 1906), 29 ff.; R. Sabbadini, *Le scoperte dei codici* (*Nuove ricerche* [Firenze, 1914]), 1 ff.

[11] *Ibid.,* 2 ff.; Loomis, *op. cit.,* 45.

[12] *Ibid.,* 3, 29 ff.; Sabbadini, *op. cit.* (1905), 71, 189, n. 28.

[13] P. de Nolhac, *Pétrarque e l'humanisme* (2nd ed., Paris, 1907), II, 129 ff.; G. Fracassetti, *Lettere di Francesco Petrarca delle cose familiari* (Firenze, 1892), II, 474–75; L. R. Loomis, *op. cit.,* 89 ff., 101.

[14] Fracassetti, *op. cit.,* IV, 96–97; *Lettere senili,* II, 462, lib. xvi, let. 1; I, 173–76, lib. iii, let. 6; I, 267, lib. v, let. 1; I, 321, lib. vi, let. 1; I, 326–27, lib. vi, let. 2; Boccaccio, *De gen. deorum,* xv, cap. 6–7; Loomis, *Medieval Hellenism,* 93 ff.; O. Hecker, Boccacio-Funde (Braunschweig, 1902), 5.

[15] [Girolamo d'Adda], *Indagini storiche artistiche e bibliografiche sulla libreria Visconteo-Sforzesca del Castello di Pavia* (Milano, 1875), nos. 8, 120, 122, 547. For the catalogue of 1459 see G. Mazzatinti, "Inventario dei codici della biblioteca Visconteo-Sforesca redatto da Ser Facino da Fabriano nel 1459 e 1469," *Giornale*

The Florentine humanist, Nicolò Niccoli (d. 1437), was probably the first important collector of Greek books, although he was preceded and aided in this task by the humanists and Greek scholars, Coluccio Salutati, Chrysoloras, probably also by Ciriaco of Ancona, who returned from the Orient in 1400 with a number of Greek manuscripts, and Giovanni Aurispa. Niccoli left his library at his death to the monastery of S. Maria degli Angeli in Florence for the future use not only of the monks but also for the benefit of all studiously inclined citizens. Yet despite his foresight the books were scattered after his death because of his debts. Only about four hundred of a probable eight hundred volumes in the original collection remained to be rescued by Cosimo de'Medici. Of these, one hundred were in Greek.[16] Guarino of Verona (d. 1460), the celebrated educator and grammarian, also collected Greek books. An index of fifty-four of the manuscripts that he had gathered together and that were still at Ferrara in the seventeenth century, represents only a portion of his Greek collection.[17] Probably the most important Greek library in Italy in the fifteenth century was that of Cardinal Bessarion (d. 1472), who had come to Italy in 1438, and was made Cardinal in 1439, after he had affixed his signature to the act of union between the Greek and Latin churches at the council of Florence. A Greek by birth, Bessarion had brought together some five hundred Greek books before his death, when the library according to his bequest went to San Marco in Venice.[18]

---

storico della lett. ital., I (1883), 40–59; D. M. Bueno Mesquita, *Giangaleazzo Visconti, duke of Milan (1351–1402)* (Cambridge, 1941), 183; Legrand, *Bibliographie Hellénique,* I (1885), xxii–iv.

[16] On the search for Greek manuscripts, see D. Robathan, "Libraries of the Renaissance," in J. W. Thompson, *The medieval library,* 515 ff.; Sabbadini, *Le scoperte dei codici* (1905), chap. III et passim; E. Müntz et P. Fabre, *La bibliothèque du Vatican au XVe siècle,* (Bibliothèque des écoles Françaises d'Athènes et de Rome, fasc. 48) (1887), p. iii; Edward Edwards, *Memoirs of libraries,* I, 393; D. Giuseppe Zippel, *Nicoló Niccoli, Contributo alla storia dell'umanismo,* 42 ff.; 66 ff.; *Vite de nomini illustri del secolo XV,* scritte da Vespasiano de Bisticci, ed. by L. Frati (Bologna, 1893) (Collezione di opere inedite o rare, vol. 71), III, 91–92.

[17] Vespasiano, *Vite,* II, (Coll. di op. ined. o rare, vol. 69), 228–32; D. Robathan, "Libraries of the Renaissance," in J. W. Thompson, *The medieval library,* 516. The catalogue of Guarino's Greek books was published by H. Omont, "Les manuscrits grecs de Guarino de Vérone et la bibliothèque de Ferrare," *Revue des bibliothèques,* II (1892), 78–81.

[18] Vespasiano, *Vite,* I, (Coll. di op. ined. o rare, vol. 68), 136 ff.; H. Omont, "Inventaire des manuscrits grecs et latins donnés à Saint-Marc de Venise par le

The rapid increase in the numbers of Greek books in Italian libraries after the first quarter of the fifteenth century is best illustrated by the growth of the collections in the Vatican. Müntz and Fabre report that in 1443 under Eugenius IV out of 340 books only two were in Greek; whereas in 1455, at the death of Nicholas V, there were between 1160 and 1209 volumes of which 353 or 414 were in Greek;[19] and in 1484 at the death of Sixtus IV, there were about 3650 volumes with perhaps 1000 in Greek.[20] This growing interest in Greek is also shown by the collections of the de'Medici family. In 1456 there were no indications of a Greek collection, but in 1495, three years after the death of Lorenzo, the inventory published by Piccolomini lists some three hundred and nineteen volumes in Greek. Several of the books had been added under Pietro, Lorenzo's son, with the continued services of the de'Medici agent for the purchase of such works, Janos Lascaris.[21] The fate of the de'Medici library is illustrative of that of many of these humanist collections which did not long survive their owners. After the expulsion of Pietro de'Medici from Florence, his palace was plundered by the enraged populace and the French troops. The books had, however, been carried to the cloister of San Marco in Florence for safekeeping during the disturbance. Later they were returned to the palace only to be removed shortly afterward to San Marco again. In 1498 as a result of the upheaval over Savonarola the books were brought to the palace of the Signoria, but were returned to San Marco in 1500. In the eventual dispersion of the collection, a part of the books went to Salviati, and the remainder was taken to Rome by Cardinal Giovanni de'Medici, who ascended the papal throne as Leo X. After his death, the remaining books were returned to Florence in 1527.[22]

Cardinal Bessarion, (1468)," *Revue des bibliothèques,* IV (1894), 129–30; Müntz et Fabre, *loc. cit.,* p. iv.

[19] R. Sabbadini, *Le scoperte dei codici* (1905), 56–58; J. Hilgers, S.J., "Zur Bibliothek Nikolaus V," *Centralblatt für Bibliothekswesen,* XIX (1902), 1–11, where the numbers are given as 795 Latin and 414 Greek MSS.

[20] Müntz et Fabre, *La bibliothèque du Vatican au XVe siècle,* (Bibliothèque des écoles françaises d'Athènes et de Rome, fasc. 48) (1887), pp. iii–iv.

[21] Müntz et Fabre, *loc. cit.,* pp. iii–iv; K. K. Müller, "Neue Mittheilungen über Janos Laskaris und die Mediceische Bibliothek," *Centralblatt für Bibliothekswesen,* I (1884), 349; E. Piccolomini, "Delle condizioni e delle vicende della libreria medicea privata dal 1494 al 1508," *Archivio storico italiano,* ser. 3, XIX (1874), 115–16; "Inventario della libreria Medicea privata compilato nel 1495," *loc. cit.,* XX (1874), 51–94.

[22] Müller, *loc. cit.,* I, 349.

Among other conspicuous Greek collections, attention has already been called[23] to Pico della Mirandola's collection of one hundred and fifty-seven Greek books, also to that of George Valla, consisting of some two hundred and twenty Greek books of which seventy were printed. However, the inventory of the library of George Valla, noted encyclopedist and translator, dates from the sixteenth century and may therefore include a number of books added after his death.[24] Attention has been called, too, to the Greek collection of Federigo, duke of Urbino, with ninety-three such manuscripts to its credit.[25]

Only a scattering of Greek books on the other hand is revealed in the inventories of several other humanist collectors. There was only one Greek text in 1467 in the library of the physician and epigrapher, Giovanni Marcanova.[26] Pietro da Montagnana in 1478 had fourteen,[27] and a few are noticeable among the books belonging to Demetrio Guazzelli of Lucca, the first custodian of the Vatican library (1481–1511), and in the collection of Palla Strozzi who left his books at his death to the library of S. Giustina of Padua, where he had gone after his expulsion from Florence.[28] In still other libraries of Italy, Greek authors and writings continued in the fifteenth century to be found only in translations, many of them by contemporary humanists. There was also a host of vernacular translations of Greek works little known in the preceding centuries, which is indicative of the importance of the Greek tradition even to those for whom the barrier of either the Greek or Latin might otherwise have been insurmountable. Such translations were especially conspicuous in the library of the dukes of Este at Ferrara, where the writings of such Greek historians and other authors as Herodotus, Dion Cassius, Diodorus Siculus, Xenophon, Isocrates, Lucian, Procopius, Appian and Strabo are listed among the ver-

[23] P. Kibre, *The library of Pico della Mirandola,* 23–24.

[24] J. L. Heiberg, "Beiträge zur Geschichte Georg Vallas und seiner Bibliothek," *Centralblatt für Bibliothekswesen, Beiheft* XVI (1896), 1–3.

[25] P. Kibre, *op. cit.,* 24, and the references noted there.

[26] Frati, *Dizionario bio-bibliografico,* 331; Sabbadini, *Scoperte dei codici* (1905), 187, note 19.

[27] Sabbadini, *op. cit.* (1905), 187, note 20.

[28] Zippel, *Nicolò Niccoli,* 41; Pietro Guidi, "Pietro Demetrio Guazzelli da Lucca il primo custode della biblioteca Vaticana (1481–1511) e l'inventario dei suo libri," *Miscellanea Fr. Ehrle,* V (1924), 192–218; Sabbadini, *Le scoperte dei codici* (1905), 55; Vespasiano, *Vite,* III (Coll. di op. ined. o rare, vol. 71), 9 ff.

nacular translations.[29] These were made for the most part by the poets and prose writers to whom the house of Este extended hospitality and patronage, among them Battista di S. Paolo better known as Battista Panetti of Ferrara, theologian, orator, and poet; also Matteo Maria Boiardo, the talented author of the chivalrous poem *Orlando Innamorato*. The study and translation of Greek works was at its height in Ferrara during and after the first half of the fifteenth century with the meeting there of the council of Ferrara, and the confluence of a number of humanist scholars of Greek, namely Guarino of Verona, Giovanni Aurispa, Giorgio Valla, Battista Guarini, Pier Candido Decembrio, Niccolò Leoniceno, Theodore Gaza, and George of Trebizond.[30]

The private collection made by pope Julius II before his elevation to the apostolic throne also had Greek works only in translation. These included Herodotus, Thucydides, and Homer, in the renditions into Latin by Lorenzo Valla; Strabo, probably in the version by Guarino of Verona and Gregorio da Città di Castello; Polybius in the translation of Niccolò Perotti; Maximus of Tyre in the recent rendition of Cosimo de'Pazzi, bishop of Arezzo and archbishop of Florence (1508–1513); Appian's history, translated by Pier Candido Decembrio; and Diogenes Laertius, translated probably by Ambrogio Traversari. There were also Aristotle's *Politics,* in the translation by Leonardo Bruni; and the *Ethics,* in the rendition by Johannes Argyropulos.[31] Julius II, whose library was noteworthy for its classical works, was a good example of the typical ecclesiastic of the so-called Renaissance, in his professed interest alike in profane as well as sacred literature.[32]

Outside of Italy, Greek codices were rarely found in any great numbers even in the second half of the fifteenth century, despite the sporadic efforts that had been made during the thirteenth and early fourteenth centuries by princes, popes, the council of Vienne, and the earnest and eloquent pleas of Raymond Lull and Pierre du

[29] G. Bertoni, *La biblioteca Estense e la coltura Ferrarese* (Torino, 1903), 128 ff.; Theodor Gottlieb, *Ueber mittelalterliche Bibliotheken,* no. 547, p. 189; and the inventory published by A. Cappelli, "La biblioteca estense nella prima metà del secolo xv," *Giornale storico della lett. ital,* XIV (1889), 12–30.

[30] G. Bertoni, *op. cit.,* 113 ff., 128 ff.

[31] Léon Dorez, "La bibliothèque privée du pape Jules II," *Revue des bibliothèques,* VI (1896), 99–100. Dorez published the two inventories drawn up after the pope's death.

[32] Dorez, *loc. cit.,* 98–99.

Bois, to encourage the study, for religious or political reasons, of Greek, Arabic, and other eastern tongues. However, Müntz and Fabre indicate that a fair beginning was made at the pontifical library in Avignon, which under Urban V (1369) boasted six volumes in Greek together with a collection on the lives of the Saints, partly in Greek and partly in Latin.[33] There was only an occasional Greek book in the inventories of such ecclesiastical establishments in France as St. Victor, St. Hilary de Poitiers, and St. Denis. Greek texts, especially of the literary works, did not become current until after the sojourn of Georges Hermonymos of Sparta at Paris in 1476.[34] Likewise in Spain, there was no Greek collection of any size until a considerably later period, although here and there individual Greek texts do appear in the catalogues. The first Spanish scholar of Greek who is credited with an interest in Greek texts is don Fernan Nuñez de Guzman of Valladolid, surnamed by his contemporaries, the Greek commander (el Comendador Griego el Pinciano, 1478?–1553). He edited and translated several Greek classics.[35]

Much the same might be said for England, since the English advocates of the "new learning," Thomas Linacre, about 1485–1486, and William Grocyn between 1488 and 1491 were only just being initiated into the study of Greek in Italy.[36] Any Greek work that appeared in an inventory prior to the second half of the fifteenth century, was usually from the field of sacred literature. However, M. R. James noted a twelfth century "Greek Donatus," at Christ Church in Canterbury, as well as a thirteenth century text of the Bible from Genesis to the book of Ruth; also at St. Augustine's in Canterbury a Psalter in Greek and Latin, and a part

[33] L. R. Loomis, *Medieval Hellenism,* 22 ff.; Müntz et Fabre, *La bibliothèque du Vatican au XVe siècle,* v–vi; M. Faucon, *La librairie des papes d'Avignon, sa formation, sa composition, ses catalogues* (1316–1420) (Paris, 1886), I, 81, 191 (no. 1176, not 1179, as indicated by Faucon, p. 81), 217, 253.

[34] Müntz et Fabre, *op. cit.,* pp. v–vi; H. Omont, "Georges Hermonyme de Sparte maître de Grec à Paris et copiste de manuscripts (1476)," *Mémoires de la société de l'histoire de Paris,* XII (1885), 65–98.

[35] Müntz et Fabre, *op. cit.,* p. vi; E. Legrand, *Bibliographie hellénique ou description raisonnée des ouvrages publiée en grec par des grecs au xve et xvie siècles* (Paris, I, 1885), 68, n. 1; C. Graux, *Essai sur les origines du fonds grec de l'escorial* (Paris, 1880) (Bibl. de l'école des hautes études, sciences philol. et hist., 46), 9 ff., 23 ff.; M. Schiff, *La bibliothèque du Marquis de Santillane* (Paris, 1905), (*loc. cit.,* 153), 449 ff.

[36] P. S. Allen, *The Age of Erasmus,* Oxford, 1914, pp. 125–27.

of Roger Bacon's Greek grammar.[37] These were not, however, products of the humanistic resuscitation of Greek in the fourteenth and fifteenth centuries, but in the words of James, "are a monument of that earlier revival of Greek learning in England which Grosseteste initiated and Bacon fostered, but which never attained maturity."[38] Similarly in German libraries, Greek texts were few and far between in the fifteenth century. The large collection of books made at Erfurt by Amplonius Ratinck in the early part of the fifteenth century, although reflecting considerable interest in Latin classical texts, contained not a single volume in Greek. On the other hand Nicholas of Cusa (d. 1464), the learned Cardinal, mathematician, and philosopher, whose interest in humanistic studies and Italian scholars was the result very probably of his long sojourn in Italy, had five Greek books,[39] while the Dominican library at Vienna in the latter part of the century boasted eight, of which three were texts of Homer, one a grammar, and another a hymnal.[40] The university of Erfurt at the same time had only two.[41] In the early sixteenth century, the leading Greek collection was that of the German humanist, John Reuchlin (1455–1522), who in his library had fifty-five Greek works comprising both literary and sacred works.[42]

Of the other learned languages, besides Latin, Hebrew was next to Greek, the most frequently encountered, largely because of its relation to the Bible. In Italy in addition to the collection of Pico della Mirandola which numbered more than a hundred,[43] the library

[37] M. R. James, *The ancient libraries of Canterbury and Dover,* pp. lxxxv–lxxxvii. For the "Greek Donatus," which would appear to correspond with that brought home to England by John of Basingstoke, archdeacon of Leicester, and other works of this period, see L. R. Loomis, *Medieval Hellenism,* 13 ff.; 40–45.

[38] M. R. James, *op. cit.,* p. lxxxvi.

[39] Fr. X. Kraus, "Die Handschriften-Sammlung des Cardinals Nicolaus V. Cusa," *Serapeum* (Leipzig), XXV (1864), 369–83; XXVI (1865), 24–31; 33–42; 49–59; 65–76; 81–89; 97–104; 353–65. Greek texts are listed XXV, 358; XXVI, 98–99.

[40] *Mittelalterliche Bibliotheks-Kataloge Österreichs,* hrsg. von der Kaiserl. Akademie der Wissenschaften in Wien, I. Band Nieder-Österreich, b. von Theodor Gottlieb (Vienna, 1915), I, 307–8. Although the catalogue was written in 1513, it represents the library at the end of the fifteenth century.

[41] H. O. Lange, "Ueber einen Katalog der Erfurter Universitätsbibliothek aus dem 15 Jahrhundert," *Centralblatt für Bibliothekswesen,* II (1885), 279 ff.

[42] K. Christ, "Die Bibliothek Reuchlins in Pforzheim," *Centralblatt für Bibliothekswesen, Beiheft* LII (1924), 51–81.

[43] P. Kibre, *The library of Pico della Mirandola,* 38–39.

of the duke of Urbino had ninety-three Hebrew items,[44] or as many in Hebrew as it had in Greek. Pietro da Montagnana at Padua had ten;[45] and George Valla had some thirty volumes which included Hebrew, Arabic, Aramaic and Syriac texts.[46] Beyond the Alps, the most significant collection was that of the one hundred and twenty Hebrew manuscripts that were preserved at Avignon by Urban V (1369).[47] But elsewhere the situation was much the same as for Greek. In England, Hebrew texts of the Scriptures were to be found scattered here and there in the libraries of various religious houses. M. R. James has pointed out that Psalters in Hebrew and Latin were far from rare and that Hebrew books in general were more commonly available than Greek books.[48] But no collection of any size among Christian scholars is recorded before the close of the fifteenth century. In German lands such collections were also rare. Both Nicholas of Cusa, who had five Hebrew manuscripts,[49] and John Reuchlin, who produced the first Hebrew grammar for Latin scholars, and was interested in the study of the Hebrew texts of the Bible, had had to resort to Italy for the necessary books in that language. Although Reuchlin's library which belongs to the end of the fifteenth and the early sixteenth century is said to have been celebrated for its oriental treasures, only thirty-six such works appear in the inventory published by Karl Christ.[50] Outside of the few texts in Arabic, and Aramaic, listed in the library of Pico della Mirandola, and in that of George Valla,[51] these rarely appear in the inventories.

Much more generally widespread than either Greek or Hebrew books except in the libraries of Italian humanists were the vernaculars.[52] Volumes in French, Provençal, Spanish, Tuscan and other

[44] *Ibid.*, 39, note 11; Vespasiano, *Vite,* I (Coll. di op. ined. o rare, vol. 68, 1892), 301. According to Vespasiano, the Hebrew books included texts of the Bible, and its commentaries; books in medicine, philosophy, and every other possible subject.

[45] R. Sabbadini, *Le scoperte dei codici Latini* e *Greci ne'secoli XIV e XV* (1905), 187.

[46] P. Kibre, *op. cit.,* 39, note 12.

[47] Müntz et Fabre, *La bibliothèque du Vatican au XVe siècle,* p. v; M. Faucon, *La librairie des papes d'Avignon* (Paris, 1886), I, 81, 176 (no. 1177; not 1180 as indicated by Faucon), 191; 217.

[48] M. R. James, *The ancient libraries of Canterbury and Dover,* p. lxxxv.

[49] Kraus in *Serapeum,* XXVI (1865), 99–100.

[50] "Die Bibliothek Reuchlins in Pforzheim," *Centralblatt für Bibliothekswesen,* LII (1924), 36–51. Christ suggests that the inventory is incomplete.

[51] P. Kibre, *op. cit.,* 39.

[52] The paucity of such works in Pico's library has already been noted in my

Italian dialects, accounted for a large number of the books especially in the princely or ducal collections. There were usually more in French than in the Italian dialects, an indication of the prominence of the French language[53] and literature. The library of the dukes of Este at Ferrara, was, however, extremely well provided with books in the Italian dialects. Among the writings in this medium, in addition to the translations from Greek works noted earlier, and translations of Latin authors such as Tacitus, Sallust, Apuleius, Cornelius Nepos, Statius, Valerius Maximus and others, were compositions by Dante, Cecco d'Ascoli, Fazio degli Uberti, Petrarch, Boccaccio, Poggio Bracciolini, Leon Battista Alberti, Antonio (de Becchariis) of Ferrara and Pietro Bembo. There were books by the poet Matteo Maria Boiardo, to whom the dukes of Este had intrusted several missions of diplomatic trust and honor as well as the government of Reggio and Modena; also the works of the poet Lodovico Ariosto, who wherever possible, interwove with his verse panegyrics of the House of Este.[54] Interest in Provençal and other French dialects was manifest in several examples of poetry, romances, and historical chronicles.[55] The interest of the dukes of Este in French writings goes back to an earlier century. Thus the marquis d'Este in the thirteenth century had favored the chivalric literature of Provence and in the first decade of that century, the court of Azzo VI was visited by troubadours, among them Aimeric de Peguilhan, who celebrated in song Azzo's daughter, Beatrice.[56] The library also included several works in Catalan and the other Spanish dialects, a reflection of that close communion between Spain and Italy from early medieval times that Benedetto Croce has discussed.[57] Some such books were intro-

---

study of the latter's library. They were also practically non-existent in Bessarion's collection.

[53] Cf. D. Robathan in J. W. Thompson, *The medieval library,* 533, 534; Bertoni, *La biblioteca Estense,* 70 ff.

[54] Bertoni, *La biblioteca Estense,* 120 ff.; 70 ff.; 91 ff.; 125 ff.

[55] *Ibid.,* 70 ff. Included were tales of King Arthur and his court; also the *favole di Francia.* The dukes of Este showed a particular predilection for French history in the chansons de geste, chivalrous tales and the chronicle of St. Denis: Pio Rajna, "Ricordi di codici Francesi posseduti dagli Estensi nel secolo XV," *Romania,* II (1873), 49–58; P. Breillat, "La Quête du Saint-Graal en Italie," *Mélanges d'archéol. et d'hist., École française de Rome,* LIV (1937), 262–300; 270.

[56] Bertoni, *La biblioteca Estense e la coltura ferrarese,* 4 ff.; 70 ff.

[57] B. Croce, *La lingua spagnuola in Italia* (Rome, 1895), 6 ff.; and B. Croce, *La Spagna nella vita italiana durante la rinascenza* (Bari, 1917), 7 ff.; 22 ff.

duced probably by Eleanor of Aragon, wife of Ercole I, and Lucrezia Borgia. Among these was a copy of the *Siete Partidas*.[58]

About one-third of the contents, or two hundred and ninety-two volumes, in the library of Francesco Gonzaga at Mantua in 1407 was in the vernacular, thirty-three in Italian (lingua vulgari), and seventy-seven in French (lingua francigena).[59] The library of the Visconti, dukes of Milan, in 1426 had some ninety-five of its nine hundred and eighty-eight books in French, some seventeen in Italian, and seven in other vernaculars.[60] For the most part these French vernacular works included the Romances of the Arthurian cycle, of which the quest for the Holy Grail was the most popular, historical chronicles, chansons de geste, or feudal epics, and satirical fabliaux.[61]

In France, as Sabbadini points out, the interest in classical works of antiquity is reflected in the fourteenth and fifteenth centuries by the translation of Latin texts into the vernacular. This is revealed in the reign of John I, and of Charles V, and his brother, John, duke of Berry. At the invitation of John I, the Benedictine Petrus Berchorius translated in 1352 all the books of Livy that were then known. A number of works of Aristotle were translated by Nicholas of Oresme, and several historical tracts were translated by Simon de Hesdin for John, duke of Berry.[62] Charles V, who was celebrated as an ardent book lover by his court historian, the noted feminist and author, Christine de Pisan,[63] had a large number of

[58] Bertoni, *La biblioteca Estense,* 91–93. Bertoni indicates that the spread of the Spanish tongue was rapid as a result of the accession to the papacy of the two Borgias, Calixtus III (1455–1458), and Alexander VI (1492–1503).

[59] Pia Girolla, "La biblioteca di Francesco Gonzaga, secondo l'inventario del 1407," *Accad. Virgiliana, Atti e memorie,* XIV–XVI (1921–23), 33. Cf. Luzio-Renier, "Il Filefo e l'umanismo alla corte dei Gonzaga," *Giornale storico della lett. ital.,* XVI (1890), 121, note 3; W. Braghirolli, "Inventaire des manuscrits en langue française possédés par Francesco Gonzaga I, capitaine de Mantoue, mort en 1407," *Romania,* IX (1880), 497–514; Novati, "I codici Francesi de'Gonzaga secondo nuovi documenti," *Romania,* XIX (1890), 151–200.

[60] Dukas, "La bibliothèque des ducs de Milan," *Bulletin du bibliophile* (Paris, 1876), 379 ff.; [Girolamo d'Adda], *Libreria Visconteo-Sforzesca del Castello di Pavia* (Milan, 1875), nos. 192, 196–98, 202, 227, 229–30, 232–45, 280, 298–317, 320, 401, 404–407, 411, 413, 460, 774–77, 808, 812–16, 829, 841, 848, 851–52, 854, 856, 858, etc.

[61] P. Breillat, *loc. cit.,* 262–300.

[62] Sabbadini, *Le scoperte dei codici* (1914), 34.

[63] L. Delisle, *Cabinet des manuscrits,* I, 18 ff.; 38; On Christine de Pisan, see

translations into French made for his collection, which was regarded as an extremely important one in the fourteenth century. Included were not only such Latin works of antiquity as those by Ovid, Vegetius, Valerius Maximus, and Livy, but also Aristotle's *Ethics* and *Politics,* the Bible and glosses on it, St. Augustine's *Soliloquies* and the *City of God,* Boethius' *Consolation of Philosophy,* John of Salisbury's *Polycraticus,* Petrarch's *Dialogues,* and a host of other works in astrology, chiromancy, and medicine.[64] In the library of John, duke of Berry, who deeded his library to Louis XI, there were not only original compositions in French, but translations as well of such standard Latin classical and medieval favorites as those noted above. The translations of the former were, however, in the ascendency.[65] The library of Charles of Orléans (1391–1465), whose chateau at Blois was the meeting place for the poets Villon, Chastelain, and others, comprised a collection of books almost entirely in French, many of them medieval favorites which had been translated especially for Charles. These included among others, French translations of the Bible, of Vincent of Beauvais' *Speculum historiale,* James of Voragine's *Legends of the Saints,* and Bartholomew of England's treatise on the properties of things, together with the ever present *Consolation of philosophy* of Boethius, the pseudo-Aristotelian *Problems,* Ptolemy's *Almagest,* and a number of Latin classics of antiquity in French translation. There were books by Christine de Pisan, one of them dedicated to Valentine Visconti,[66] and several volumes which comprised French romances, fabliaux, chronicles, and a work on chess. The inventory of Charles' books, some of which had belonged to his father, Louis d'Orléans, and others to his mother, Valentine Visconti, was made while Charles was a prisoner in England.[67] He had been captured at the battle of Agincourt (1415), and was kept in England until he was ransomed in 1440. Fear that the English would capture

---

Marie-Joseph Pinet, *Christine de Pisan, 1364–1430, Étude biographique et littéraire* (Paris, 1927).

[64] Delisle, *op. cit.,* I, 38, 41; Edward Edwards, *Memoirs of Libraries,* I, 388.

[65] Delisle, *Le cabinet des manuscrits,* I, 56 ff.

[66] P. Champion, *La librairie de Charles d'Orléans* (Paris, 1910); Le Roux de Lincy, "La bibliothèque de Charles d'Orléans, à son chateau de Blois en 1427," *Bibliothèque de l'école des chartes,* V (1843–44), 59–82; 71–72, nos. 23, 28; cf. D'Adda, *Libreria Visconteo-Sforzesca del Castello di Pavia* (Milan, 1875), pp. xxxix–xl.

[67] Delisle, *op. cit.,* I, 98 ff.; 105; 114–19.

the city of Blois where the books were housed had led to his request that his secretary, Seigneur de Mortemart, draw up an inventory of the books in 1417, and transport the library and other possessions from Blois to Saumur in Anjou. Ten years later Jean de Rochechomart was authorized to attempt a sale of the books to raise money for the ransom. This was the occasion for drawing up the inventory of 1427 which has been published by Le Roux de Lincy.[68] Another magnificent library chiefly of French books was that of Jacques d'Armagnac, duke de Nemours and Comte de la Marche, one of the members of the nobility in France most interested in arts and letters. He was, however, arrested on charges of conspiracy by Louis XI and his goods were confiscated. A large number of the duke's books were translations from the Latin of works of classical antiquity as well as romances and religious tracts. Included too was a copy of the chronicles of England by Jean de Waurin.[69]

A goodly number of works similar to those found in the collections of Charles of Orléans, John of Berry, and of Charles V, was also included in the inventory of the library belonging to Charlotte of Savoy, the second wife of Louis XI of France in 1451. The catalogue of her books drawn up in 1484 after her death lists as in French, several copies of the Bible, books of sermons, and other religious and devotional manuals, as well as French and Spanish translations of the well known medieval Latin works named above. Among the original works in French were the popular lays of Merlin, Troy, and Alexander, together with "certains laiz et coustumes pour passer temps"; and a book on chess playing.[70] There was a copy of the "Livre des troys vertuz a l'enseignement des dames, bien historie," also "Le debat des quatre dames, petit livre de dames et d'amours," and a copy of *La cité des dames* by Christine de Pisan.[71] This queenly interest in books on her own sex is further revealed in the collection of books made by Anne of Brittany, wife first of Charles VIII and after his death of Louis XII in 1499. Her library, especially celebrated for the famous manuscript of the Book of Hours, illustrated with numerous minia-

[68] *Bibliothèque de l'école des chartes,* V (1843–44), 60 ff.; Delisle, *op. cit.,* I, 108.

[69] Delisle, *Le cabinet des manuscrits,* I, 86–90. For Jean de Waurin's work see C. Gross, The *Sources and literature of English history* (New York, 1915), no. 1863.

[70] Delisle, *op. cit.,* I, 91–94; M. Tuetey, "Inventaire des biens de Charlotte de Savoie," *Bibliothèque de l'école des chartes,* XXVI (1864–65), 338–366; 423–442.

[71] Delisle, *op. cit.,* I, 93; M. Tuetey, *loc. cit.,* 358; and see above note 63.

tures, was made up chiefly of books collected for the most part from Milan and Naples. It contained the "Histoire des femmes célèbres," composed at her request in French by her chaplain, Antoine Dufour.[72] Louis XII acquired the French collection comprising part of the library of Louis of Bruges, powerful lord of Flanders, and an ardent patron of letters who died in 1492.[73]

French books also found a place in the Spanish libraries of Martin of Aragon at Barcelona in 1410, and of Alfonso the Magnanimous of Aragon, according to the inventory made between the years 1412 and 1424. Among the latter's books in addition to original works in French, were translations into French of the Bible, of Boethius', *Consolation of Philosophy,* and of other Latin favorites.[74] Another Spanish library of this century, noteworthy for its French books was that of Don Carlos, prince of Viana (d. 1462), son of John II of Aragon and Blanche of Navarre. Don Carlos, author of a history of the kings of Navarre, was celebrated among the Catalonians particularly for the elegance of his manners, his vast learning, and enthusiasm for letters. His death, which was believed to have been caused by poison administered by his own father, was the occasion for five years of civil war during which time the people of Catalonia sought to avenge Don Carlos' death.[75] In his library, Don Carlos had twenty-four works in French out of a total of one hundred and three volumes. The library of Don

[72] For a description of the work of Antoine du Four, O.P., the fuller title of which is "l'histoire des femmes célèbres depuis la création jusqu'à l'époque de la Pucelle d'Orléans," see *Bulletin du Bibliophile* (1846), 577–80. Le Roux de Lincy, "Détails sur la vie privée d'Anne de Bretagne, femme de Charles VIII et Louis XII," *Bibliothèque de l'école des chartes,* XI (1849–50), 157; [Girolamo d'Adda], *Libreria Visconteo-Sforzesca del Castello di Pavia* (Milan, 1875), xlii ff.; Delisle, *Le cabinet des manuscrits,* I, 124. On the influence of French literature outside France see Léon Gautier, "L'entrée en espagne, chanson de geste inedite," *Bibliothèque de l'école des chartes,* XIX (1857–58), 216 ff.

[73] L. Delisle, *Le cabinet des manuscrits,* I, 140 ff.; M. Van Praet, *Recherches sur Louis de Bruges, seigneur de la Gruthuyse* (Paris, 1831).

[74] J. Massó Torrents, "Inventari dels bens mobles del Rey Martí D'Arago," *Revue hispanique,* XII (1905), 413–590; Ramon D'Alós, "Documenti per la storia della biblioteca d'Alfonso il Magnanimo," *Miscellanea Francesco Ehrle* (Rome), V (1924), 390–422. A similar inventory had been published earlier by E. Gonzalez Hurtebise, "Inventario de los bienes muebles de Alfonso V de Aragon como Infante y como Rey (1412–1424)," *Anuari de l'institut d'Estudis Catalans* (Barcelona, 1907), 148–88. The books are listed on pages 182–85.

[75] Paul Raymond, "La bibliothèque de Don Carlos, Prince de Viane," *Bibliothèque de l'école des chartes* (Paris), XIX (1857–58), 483–87.

Inigo Lopez de Mendoza, first marquis of Santillane at Guadalajara in 1458, also contained a number of works in French, as well as tracts in Castilian and Italian dialects, among them translations of classical authors of Greek and Latin antiquity and of contemporary Italian humanists.[76] English libraries too included works in the romance languages, especially in French, as one might expect. Thus in the libraries of Christ church and of St. Augustine's Abbey at Canterbury as well as in that of the Prior of St. Martin of Dover, translations into French of the Bible and of Latin theological tracts, in addition to French romances, chronicles, and the like were conspicuous in the fourteenth and fifteenth centuries.[77] In general, however, works in the romance tongues were not common in the libraries of German lands. Nicholas of Cusa had one copy each of Italian, French, and Castilian texts.

The vernaculars other than French and Italian were for the most part localized in the collections of their respective countries. Thus although M. R. James, reported several Anglo-Saxon and English books in the fifteenth century catalogues of the libraries of Canterbury and other English centers,[78] they were almost never found outside the British Isles. Likewise German texts were rarely encountered in collections other than in German lands, although they were present in practically every German library.[79] These included both original works in German and translations of Latin texts. However, Charles of Orléans had two German books in his collection which had probably come to him from the collection owned by his mother, Valentine Visconti.[80] Nicholas of Cusa had six German books as against one each of the Italian, French, and Castilian dialects.[81] A particularly large collection of German

[76] M. Schiff, *La bibliothèque du Marquis de Santillane* (Paris, 1905) (Bibliothèque de l'école des hautes études, 153.

[77] M. R. James, *The ancient libraries of Canterbury and Dover,* p. lxxxiv–v; see for example, p. 81, no. 768; p. 103, no. 1137; p. 122, no. 1435; p. 128, no. 1522; p. 129, no. 1552; 1560; p. 140, no. 1753; p. 139, no. 1755; 1724, etc. In St. Augustine's abbey, Canterbury, p. 198, p. 210, 39; p. 224, 20; p. 218, 313–13, pp. 274, 368, 371–74, p. 428, no. 324, 353, pp. 430, 431, 432, no. 390, p. 445, no. 92; p. 455, no. 139; p. 459, no. 160, p. 460, 164, p. 470–71, no. 170; p. 463, no. 195; pp. 482, 484, nos. 364–67, 390; p. 485, 372–73; p. 487, 390; p. 490, 413–14.

[78] M. R. James, *The ancient libraries of Canterbury and Dover,* p. lxxxiv; 374.

[79] W. Wattenbach, *Das Schriftwesen im Mittelalter,* 598–99.

[80] *Bibliothèque de l'école des chartes,* V (1843–44), 76, no. 39; Champion, *op. cit.,* 52, 95.

[81] Dr. Fr. X. Kraus, "Die Handschriften-Sammlung des Cardinals Nicolaus von Cusa," in *Serapeum,* XXV (1864), 356; XXVI (1865), 28, 34–35; 68–69, 73.

works in the fifteenth century was that of Elizabeth von Volkensdorf, who had in her possession fifty of them.[82] Yet for all these Greek, Hebrew and vernacular books, the great bulk of the contents of the libraries of the fourteenth and fifteenth centuries remained true to the Latin tradition. Works composed originally in Greek, Hebrew, and Arabic, continued to circulate chiefly in Latin translations as they had during the earlier middle ages, with additions, to be sure, of a considerable number of new humanistic Latin translations from the Greek of literary, philosophical and scientific works.

In addition to their overwhelming Latinity, many of these fourteenth and fifteenth century collections both cisalpine and transalpine show a remarkable uniformity in subject matter and in arrangement.[83] Although some Italian collections were classified according to languages, as in the case of the Este library, where before the death of Niccolò III in 1436, the Latin books were listed first, then those in Italian, and thirdly those in French,[84] others of the ducal or princely collectors in Italy, followed the canon or rules for a library prepared by Thomas Parentucelli of Sarzana, who later ascended the papal throne as Nicholas V (1447–1455).[85] His canon or list of minimum essentials for a library followed the general outlines of medieval ecclesiastical collections. It was drawn up at the request of Cosimo de'Medici primarily for the library of San Marco in Florence, but was also used for the formation of La Badia at Fiesole, as well as for the libraries of Alessandro Sforza at Pesaro, and of the dukes of Urbino.[86] According to this plan the

[82] Theodor Gottlieb, *Ueber Mittelalterliche Bibliotheken,* 28. But cf. Wattenbach, *op. cit.,* 598, where the number is given as 45.

[83] Sabbadini, *Le scoperte dei codici* (1905), 204; A. de Hevesy, *La bibliothèque du roi Matthias Corvin* (Paris, 1923), 21.

[84] D. Robathan in J. W. Thompson, *The medieval library,* 528 ff.

[85] Vespasiano, *Vite di uomini illustri,* I (Coll. di opere inedite o rare, vol. 68), 35; G. Sforza, *La patria, la famiglia e la giovinezza di papa Niccolò V,* ricerche storiche, *Atti della reale accademia Lucchese di scienze, lettere ed arti,* XXIII (1884), 151–52; App. A, 360–81; K. Löffler, "Papst Nikolaus V als Bücherfreund," *Zeitschrift für Bücherfreunde,* n.F., I (1909–1910), 175; E. Piccolomini, "Ricerche intorno alle condizioni e alle vicende della Libreria Medicea privata dal 1494 al 1506," *Append., Archivio storico italiano,* ser. 3, XXI (1875), 102–106; XIX (1874), 114.

[86] Piccolomini, *loc. cit.,* XXI (1875), 102; G. Sforza, *loc. cit.,* XXIII (1884), 151; Vespasiano, *Vite,* I, 35. For the library at Fiesole, see Vespasiano, III, 50–52; and see below for the Urbino library.

greater portion of the collection was to be devoted to sacred literature, Bibles, missals, psalters, the church fathers, and compositions in theology and philosophy (chiefly Aristotle and his commentators). Next would come treatises in mathematics, especially the arithmetic and tract on music of Boethius, Euclid's *Geometry,* the *Perspective* of Vitelo, Ptolemy's *Almagest* and *Cosmography;* and finally humane literature (de studiis humanitatis), namely grammar, rhetoric, history ("whatever pertains to history, I think should be added"), poetry, and moral philosophy.[87] The set of rules is particularly interesting, as Sabbadini has already pointed out, because it made no provision for works in Greek, a fact that is especially surprising since Nicholas V as pope collected between three or four hundred Greek volumes. It is remarkable too, as Sabbadini has further indicated, that even in the midst of the leading enthusiasts for the humanistic revival, the rule only included five names of classical Latin poets, namely Vergil, Horace, Ovid, Lucan, and Statius, with two works only of Ovid, the *Metamorphoses* and the *Fasti.*[88]

In accordance with this plan, books on the Bible, the works of the church fathers, and other theological writings occupied the position of prominence in the inventory of the private library of Cosimo de'Medici drawn up in 1456. Next came the works of the grammarians, poets, and historians; the books on the art of oratory (Cicero), philosophy (Aristotle), agriculture, architecture, cosmography, military and natural history; and finally books in the vernacular and in fragments or unbound (framentati).[89] A similar arrangement was to be found in the library of the dukes of Urbino before 1482 where the books were arranged under the headings: Scriptures, Church Fathers, Medicine, Law, Cosmography, History, Poets, Grammarians, Orators, and the rest. The completeness of this library is extolled by Vespasiano who says that he compared it with inventories of all the libraries of Italy: that of the Pope, of San Marco in Florence, of Pavia; and even with the

[87] G. Sforza, *loc. cit.,* XXIII (1884), Append. A, 360–81.

[88] *Idem;* Piccolomini, *loc. cit.,* ser. 3, XXI (1875), 106; Sabbadini, *Le scoperte dei codici* (1905), 200; J. Hilgers, "Zur Bibliothek Nikolaus V," *Centralblatt für Bibliothekswesen,* XIX (1902), 1–2.

[89] T. Gottlieb, *Ueber mittel. Bibliotheken,* 193; Vespasiano, *Vite,* III (Coll. di opere inedite o rare, no. 71), 46 ff., 50–53. The inventory is printed by Piccolomini, *loc. cit.,* ser. 3, XXI (1875), 106–112; and in *Bibliotheca Leopoldina Laurentiana,* ed. A. M. Bandini (Florence, 1793), III, 519–24.

catalogue of the university of Oxford which he had sent for, and though these collections frequently contained several copies of the same work they did not have the complete works of an author to the extent that was true for the duke of Urbino's library.[90]

This primacy of the Bible and books in theology, that one might rightfully expect in monastic and other ecclesiastical houses, was likewise a characteristic feature of several other collections of the fifteenth century, among them that of master Ernoldi de Halle in 1427,[91] in the Netherlands, and of the medical doctor Paulico in Dresden in 1459.[92] In the inventory of the library of Francesco Gonzaga in 1407, eighty-six of the two hundred and ninety-two volumes were on sacred literature.[93] The remaining books were classified as works on canon and civil law (30), history (36), chronicles (21), poetry and poetics (24), moral (36) and natural (15) philosophy, medicine (17), grammar and so on; books on astrology (28), geomancy, and *experimentalium.* Then followed books in *lingua vulgari* and in *lingua francigena.*[94] Similarly in the collection of John, duke of Berry (1402–1416), one hundred and thirteen of his two hundred and ninety-seven books were on theology.[95] The same feature is further illustrated in the library of Charlotte of Savoy;[96] in that of Alfonso of Aragon, king of Naples, whose love of letters and delight in the Holy Scriptures is recorded

[90] Vespasiano, *Vite,* I (*loc. cit.,* no. 68), 296–302; Gottlieb, *op. cit.,* 248. The inventory compiled by Federigo Veterano, the fifteenth-century librarian of the duke of Urbino, is printed by C. Guasti, "Inventario della Libreria Urbinate compilato nel secolo xv da Federigo Veterano bibliotecario di Federigo I da Montefeltro duca di Urbino," *Giornale storico degli archivi Toscani* (Florence), VI (1862), 133–47; VII (1863), 46–55, 130–54.

[91] Gottlieb, *Ueber mittel. Bibliotheken,* 257.

[92] *Ibid.,* 61; *Neuer Anzeiger für Bibliographie und Bibliothekswissenschaft,* (1842), 64–67.

[93] Girolla, "La biblioteca di Francesco Gonzaga," *Atti e memorie, R. Accad. Virgiliana di Mantova,* n.s., XIV–XVI (1921–1923), 33, 40–49.

[94] Girolla, *loc. cit.,* 49 ff.; Gottlieb, *op. cit.,* 208–209. The list of French books is given by W. Braghirolli, "Inventaire des manuscrits en langue française possédés par Francesco Gonzaga I, capitaine de Mantoue, mort en 1407," *Romania,* IX (1880), 497–514; the list is on 505–14.

[95] Gottlieb, *op. cit.,* 109. The inventory was published for the first time by M. Hiver de Beauvoir (Paris, 1860). See also L. Delisle, *Cabinet des manuscrits,* III, 171–94, no. xxxiii.

[96] Gottlieb, *op. cit.,* 99; M. Tuetey, "Inventaire des biens de Charlotte de Savoie," *Bibl. de l'école des chartes,* XXVI (1865), 338–66, 423–42; and for a summary of the inventory, Delisle, *op. cit.,* I, 91.

by Vespasiano, the fifteenth century bookseller;[97] as well as in the books owned by Martin of Aragon,[98] and in the well-stocked collection of the Visconti-Sforza at Pavia,[99] and in many others, where the Bible, Books of Hours, and other devotional and theological tracts formed the nucleus and frequently the most substantial part of the library. Especially worthy of note too in these libraries are the vernacular translations of the Bible.[100]

This numerical prominence of the Bible and of theological writings in the fifteenth century, which has already been demonstrated in my account of the library of Pico della Mirandola, is further emphasized by the fact that about half of the total output of the incunabula presses was in this field.[101] It is also reflected, as one might perhaps expect, in the collection of Nicholas of Cusa, half of whose books were on religious subjects; and in that of Cardinal Bessarion. Of the latter's five hundred Greek codices, thirty-six contained texts of the Bible and its commentaries and some one hundred and sixty-five pertained to the works of the church fathers, theologians, church councils, and canon law. Similarly in the Latin section, there were twenty-four texts and commentaries of the Bible, one hundred and eight books pertaining to the church fathers, theologians, church councils, and canon law.[102] The re-

[97] Ramon D'Alós, "Documenti per la storia delle biblioteca d'Alfonso il Magnanimo," *Miscellanea Fr. Ehrle,* V (1924), 392 ff.; Vespasiano, *Vite,* I (Coll. di opere inedite o rare, no. 68), 65. Vespasiano lists works that Alfonso had had translated from Greek, *loc. cit.,* 97–98. See also E. Gonzalez Hurtebise, "Inventario de los bienes muebles de Alfonso V de Aragón, como infante y como rey (1412–1424)," *Anuari, Institut d'Estudis Catalans* (Barcelona, 1907), 182 ff. Alfonso was ruler of seven kingdoms, Aragon, Catalonia, Valencia, the Balearic Isles, Sicily, Sardinia and Corsica, and Naples.

[98] J. Massó Torrents, "Inventari dels bens mobles del Rey Marti d'Aragó," *Revue hispanique,* XII (1905), 414, 416, 417, etc.

[99] G. Mazzatinti, "Inventario della biblioteca Visconteo-Sforzesca," *Giornale storico della lett. ital.* (Torino), I (1883), 43 ff.; [Girolamo d'Adda], *Libreria Visconteo-Sforzesca del Castello di Pavia.*

[100] Cf. Delisle, *Cabinet,* III, 170–94; Sabbadini, *Le scoperte dei codici* (1905), 200; A. de Hevesy, *La bibliothèque du roi Matthias Corvin,* 87, "Bible hongroise." Cf. S. Berger, "Nouvelles recherches sur les Bibles Provençales et Catalanes," *Romania,* XIX (1890), 505–561; also his "Les Bibles Provençales et Vaudoises," *loc. cit.,* XVIII, 353.

[101] P. Kibre, *op. cit.,* chap. VI; Robert Steele, "What fifteenth-century books are about," *Trans. of the Bibliographical Society, The Library,* 2nd series, no. 16, vol. IV (1903), 337–38.

[102] H. Omont, in *Revue des bibliothèques,* IV (1894), 182.

maining Greek books in the collection related to philosophy (87), Aristotelian and Platonic; poetry (27), of which eleven pertained to Homer and his commentators, and fourteen were on grammar and lexicons; medicine (18); civil and canon law (12); mathematics, astronomy, and music (43); rhetoric including the art of oratory and literary works (42); and history (54). The Latin works in addition to theology covered the subjects of mathematics, astronomy, music (10), philosophy (57); poetry and history (18), oratory, chiefly Cicero (12), and miscellaneous works (25).

The earlier fifteenth century collection of Amplonius Ratinck or Ratinger of Rheinberg, doctor of medicine and master of arts, whose books now form the basis of the Stadtbücherei at Erfurt, also illustrates this predominance of theological writings. According to the inventory of 1412,[103] drawn up by Amplonius himself, the books were classed under grammar (36); *poetria* or poetics (37); logic, chiefly Aristotelian (27); rhetoric, "the third subject of the trivium," (12); *mathematica* (73), here including arithmetic, geometry, music, astronomy, astrology, geomancy, magic arts, and nigromancy, in addition to perspective; also natural philosophy (60), under which are included four tracts in alchemy; metaphysics, "that is that science which is divine or which transcendes nature," (15); moral philosophy (35); medicine (101); jurisprudence (23), of which seven were on civil and sixteen on canon law; and finally the largest group of all, theology, which numbered two hundred and thirteen works. These comprised Biblical texts, commentaries, and glosses (51), as well as the *Sentences* of Peter Lombard and his commentators.

In the private collections of popes Gregory XII (1406–1415), Calixtus III (1455–1458), and Julius II (1503–1513), consisting chiefly of books acquired before mounting the papal throne, the large number of legal texts, chiefly canon law, testified to the particular emphasis laid upon juristic studies by papal candidates.[104] Treatises in law, especially canon law, were, however, also promi-

[103] Wilhelm Schum, *Beschreibendes Verzeichnis der Amplonianischen Handschriften-Sammlung zu Erfurt* (Berlin, 1887), 785–867.

[104] Angelo Mercati, "La biblioteca privata e gli arredi di cappella di Gregorio XII," *Miscellanea Fr. Ehrle,* V (1924), 128–65; Francesco Martorell, "Un inventario della biblioteca di Calisto III," *loc. cit.,* 166–91; and Léon Dorez, "La bibliothèque privée du pape Jules II," *Revue des bibliothèques,* VI (1886), 97–124. Julius II at the age of 24 when he was at Perugia for study in 1468, bought a copy of the *Institutes* for the price of five gold ducats (Dorez, *loc. cit.,* 98, note 3).

nent in several other fifteenth century collections. Nicholas of Cusa owned fifty-eight in canon and fourteen in civil law, while the Gonzaga library at Mantua contained thirty-two legal texts, divided between eighteen in canon law and fourteen in civil law. Chiefly noteworthy for its books in canon law was the collection of Professor John Polzmacher, dean of the faculty of law and rector of the university of Vienna in 1438. His entire library which he donated to the Monastery dedicated to the Blessed Virgin (alias Scotorum), at Vienna in 1453, comprised in addition to the legal tracts, other works by Latin authors both ancient and medieval, such as Valerius Maximus, Lucan, Sallust, Ovid, Plautus, Vergil, Cicero, Sedulius, Claudianus, Boethius, Isidore of Seville, Gaufridus (de Vino Salvo), Egidius Romanus, John Beleth, John of Salisbury, Peter Lombard, and Petrarch.[105] Polzmacher's will provided that these books were to be loaned by the monastery to the doctors and students at the University of Vienna in return for an adequate fee according to the length of time and character (?) of the borrower (qualitatem personis). The loan was to be made free, but with adequate safeguards, to those too poor to pay the fee.

The persistent regard for many of the favorite writings of the earlier medieval period is reflected in the inclusion in many of the libraries of the works of the church fathers, with a particular leaning toward St. Augustine, bishop of Hippo. The latter's *City of God* is found not only in its original Latin in most of the libraries but also in the vernacular translations in several of the French ducal collections. Even Petrarch, so-called father of the humanists, reported that with his first money after leaving the parental roof, he purchased St. Augustine's *City of God;* and he effusively thanked Boccaccio for giving him an enormous volume containing St. Augustine's *Commentary on the Psalms.*[106] In most libraries there were copies of the *Dialogues* and *Homelies* of Gregory the Great,[107] and of Boethius' *Consolation of Philosophy.* Vernacular

[105] *Mittelalterliche Bibl. Kat.,* I (1915), 438–42; Gottlieb, *Über mittelalterliche Bibliotheken,* 390; Putnam, *Books and their makers,* I (1898), 157.

[106] D. Robathan, in J. W. Thompson, *The medieval library,* 525; B. L. Ulman, "Petrarch's favorite books," *Transactions of the American Philological Association,* LIV (1923), 31; L. Delisle, *Le cabinet des manuscrits,* I, 138–39. For the works of the church fathers in Petrarch's library and his interest in them, see especially, Pierre de Nolhac, "De patrum et medii aevi scriptorum codicibus in bibliotheca Petrarcae olim collectis," *Revue des bibliothèques,* II (1892), 241–79.

[107] Cosimo de'Medici is said to have spent six months reading the *Moralia* of St. Gregory, Vespasiano, *Vite,* III (Coll. di op. ined. o rare, no. 71), 58.

translations of the latter were included in the library of the Visconti Sforza; in that of the duke of Berry and in that of Charles of Orléans, as well as in other French libraries. Accompanying these works were usually such popular medieval treatises as the *Legends of the Saints* by James of Voragine, the *Rationale of the Divine Office* by William Durandi and, especially in the German libraries, the work on the same subject by the twelfth century author, John Beleth.

Compositions of the leading ecclesiastics and schoolmen of the twelfth and thirteenth centuries appear frequently in the inventories, among them works of St. Anselm, St. Bernard of Clairvaux, Hugh of St. Victor, Peter Lombard, and from the thirteenth century William of Auvergne, Bonaventura, Albertus Magnus, and Thomas Aquinas. More recent writers of the fourteenth and fifteenth centuries on scholastic themes were also not neglected. The works of John Duns Scotus, John of Turrecremata, Jean Gerson, Pierre d'Ailly, and many others, found their way into these libraries and testify to the continued interest in the subjects and themes of scholasticism even in the midst of the humanistic revival.

Fifteenth century libraries also reflected the continuity as well as the blending of medieval interests with those of the humanists in other fields. The first two subjects of the trivium, that is grammar and rhetoric, which had formed the basic pillars of the medieval interest in the liberal arts, now provided the focal points for humanistic interests and achievements. Under these classifications the older grammatical favorites, Donatus, and Priscian, along with the twelfth century *Doctrinale* of Alexander of Villadei and the *Graecismus* of Eberhard of Bethune held their place beside the more recent humanist grammars by Guarino of Verona, Giovanni Tortelli of Arezzo, Lorenzo Valla, and Niccolò Perotti. The fact that Cicero's rhetorical works and the *Declamations* ascribed to Quintilian were especially conspicuous provides a further link with the interests of the immediate past since these had been the standard guides throughout the entire medieval period. But when we turn to the humanistic literature which had formerly been placed under *poetria* as a subdivision of grammar, there is a sharp contrast between the fifteenth century libraries and those of the preceding centuries. For while writings of the classical Greek and Latin poets had never been entirely absent from representative medieval libraries, they were never found in such profusion as was true especially of the Italian libraries of this era. Greek literary classics, seldom found in the original before the fifteenth century, were represented both in the Greek and in translation by the works of Homer, Aristophanes, Xenophon, Aristides, Sophocles, Plutarch, Lucian of Samosata, Oppian, Hesiod, Apollonius and others. There were also Greek texts as well as translations of the historians Herodotus, Thucydides, Xenophon, Flavius Josephus, and Eusebius. The library of Cardinal Bessarion was particularly favorable to historical works in Greek and had copies of all the above authors. Scientific and philosophical writings were also introduced into the libraries in their original form or in new translations. Some of these works had been known in Latin translations of the fifth and sixth centuries directly from the Greek or in twelfth and thirteenth century translations by way of the Arabic as well as directly from the Greek. This was especially true of the medical works of Galen and Hippocrates,[108] also of Euclid, Ptolemy, Aristotle and so on. To the Roman classical authors, known in whole or in part in the medieval period,[109] were now added especially Propertius, Ausonius, Plautus; and additional works of Cicero, and Quintilian. The Roman historians who had never completely disappeared from their place in medieval libraries, were now found in these fifteenth century libraries along with the ancient writers on military arts, similarly known to the bibliophiles of preceding centuries, and Vitruvius Pollio whose work on architecture was to exercise an influence far beyond the library walls.[110]

The works of contemporary humanists were generally also

[108] For the currency of medieval Latin translations of Hippocrates see my article, "Hippocratic Writings in the Middle Ages," *Journal of the History of Medicine,* XVIII (1945), 371–412.

[109] A fairly complete list of the classical authors found in libraries before 1500 is indicated by Max Manitius, "Handschriften antiker Autoren in mittelalterlichen Bibliothekskatalogen," herausgegeben von Karl Manitius, *Beiheft zum Centralblatt für Bibliothekswesen* (Leipzig, 1935), LXVII; a list of the classical works in the libraries of the Renaissance is given in R. Sabbadini, *Le scoperte dei codici* (*Nuove ricerche,* 1914), 198 ff. See also M. R. James, *The ancient libraries of Canterbury and Dover,* pp. xxxiii–xxxiv; xlii; and cf. L. Delisle, *Le cabinet des manuscrits,* I, 139, for such works in Petrarch's possession; as well as other references noted above, notes 8–9.

[110] Eva M. Sanford, "The Study of Ancient History in the Middle Ages," *Journal of the History of Ideas,* V (Jan. 1944), 21–43; G. Bertoni, *La Biblioteca Estense,* 106 ff.; Vespasiano, *Vite,* I (Coll. di opere inedite o rare, no. 68), 292–302, for such works in the Urbino library.

found in these libraries, together with the compositions in the vernacular by poets and authors of the time. The library of the House of Este at Ferrara, and that of the dukes of Urbino were especially favored in this regard. In the Este collection there were the compositions of the leading humanists, among them works of Petrarch, Boccaccio, Leonardo Bruni, Panormita, Marsilio Ficino, Filelfo, Poggio, Poliziano, Flavio Biondo, Guarino of Verona, Candido and Angelo Decembrio, and Paolo Cortesi.[111] Federigo, duke of Urbino, is reported by Vespasiano to have given generously of his wealth to men of letters, and his library was well provisioned with ("all," according to Vespasiano) the works of modern writers. In addition to the humanists listed above the library contained original compositions and translations by Coluccio Salutati, Traversari, Gianozzo Manetti, Niccolò Perotti, Campano, Maffeo Vegio, Pope Pius II, Nicolò Secundino who acted as interpreter for both Greeks and Latins at the Council of the Greeks in Florence, Pontano, Bartolomeo Fazio, Gasparino Barzizza, Lorenzo Valla, Pietro Paolo Vergerio, John Argyropulos, Giovanni Tortelli and a number of others.[112]

Side by side, however, with these literary and humanistic writings the libraries generally had a large number of works representing the third subject of the trivium, namely dialectics or logic. The continued regard for works in logic demonstrates that the overwhelming victory which that branch of learning had achieved in the battle of the seven arts that had raged at Paris and Orléans in the late twelfth and thirteenth centuries, was still of importance in the fourteenth and fifteenth centuries. In this field Aristotle reigned supreme as he had in the thirteenth century. Indeed the fifteenth century libraries testify to the fact that Aristotle was still "the philosopher," par excellence, and that, however much his critics might berate him in the quarrel over the relative merits of Plato and Aristotle, it was the former, who even in the midst of the humanistic revival required the most defense. Cardinal Bessarion, who wrote in defense of Plato against the attack made by George of Trebizond, was one of the few bibliophiles of the fifteenth century to have in his library the large number of thirty-two

[111] G. Bertoni, *op. cit.*, 95 ff.; 108 ff., et passim. For humanists at the court of the Gonzaga at Mantua see A. Luzio and R. Renier, "I Filelfo e l'umanismo alla corte dei Gonzaga," *Giornale storico della letteratura italiana,* VIII (1890), 119–217.

[112] Vespasiano, *Vite,* I (*loc. cit.*, no. 68), 292–302.

volumes containing works of Plato and of several neo-platonists. He also had, however, some fifty-one Aristotelian texts in Greek and about the same number in Latin.[113] Nicholas of Cusa had several works of Plato and of the neo-platonist, Proclus, but here too, as in the case of Bessarion, the works of Aristotle were present in far greater abundance.[114] In general by the late fifteenth century Plato's *Republic* and other *Dialogues* might be found in Italy in the libraries of Cardinal Bessarion, of the dukes of Urbino, of Pico della Mirandola, of George Valla and of the dukes of Este, as well as in other humanist collections. But they were still far less commonly available than the works of Aristotle despite the efforts of the Platonic academy and the sympathetic interest in neo-platonism. Outside of Italy, Plato's works, other than the *Timaeus,* in the fifth century Latin version of Chalcidius, were comparatively rare even in the late fifteenth century.

This preeminence of Aristotle over Plato was especially marked in the collection of books made by Amplonius Ratinck at Erfurt, where Aristotelian texts and commentaries filled half as many volumes as did those in theology; also in the library of St. Augustine at Canterbury, since a third of its contents were on Aristotle. It was further demonstrated in the library of the Visconti-Sforza at Pavia, a collection rich especially in humanistic compositions, but with some sixty-seven volumes relating to Aristotle and his commentators, a number equal to more than one-third of the classics of antiquity and the writings of the later humanists combined. There were seventeen volumes on Plato and the neo-platonists. This Visconti library goes back historically to Giovanni, uncle of Azzo and bishop of Novara from 1329 to 1349, and lord of Milan from 1349 to 1354. From 1426 to 1499 the books were preserved in the castle of Pavia. But in 1499 the greater part was transported

[113] H. Omont, in *Revue des bibliothèques,* IV (1894), 182, nos. 359–409, Aristotle and his commentators; nos. 410–441, contain Plato's works and commentaries on them. E. Legrand, *Bibliographie hellénique* (Paris, 1885), I, xxxvi; (1903), III, 1 ff.; Vespasiano, *Vite,* I (Coll. di op. ined. o rare, no. 68), 137.

[114] Fr. X. Kraus, "Die Handschriften-Sammlung des Cardinals Nicolaus von Cusa, *Serapeum,* XXV (1864), 353; XXVI (1865), 69–74; under K. Philosophia, two codices contained the *Dialogues* of Plato, namely the *Phaedo, Phaedrus,* and *Crito,* in translations by Leonardo Bruni of Arezzo, also the *Apologia Socratis,* and *Meno;* the *Politiae,* in translation by Candido Decembrio; and the works of the neo-platonist Proclus. There were, however, 10 codices containing works of Aristotle in both new and old translations.

to France and placed at Blois by Louis XII. The books were later transferred by order of Francis I to Fontainebleau and eventually became part of the national library in Paris.[115] The library of the university of Erfurt, a fifteenth century creation, also accorded Aristotle a considerable prominence,[116] and his treatises and their commentaries formed a large part of the collections of both George Valla and Giovanni Pico della Mirandola.[117]

Not only in the extent to which the Scriptures, theology, and Aristotle, were represented did the libraries of the fourteenth and fifteenth centuries show a close relationship with those of the thirteenth and earlier ages, but also in the continued treasuring of other works popular with the schoolmen of the twelfth and thirteenth centuries. The presence in the catalogues of Latin translations of such authors as Algazel, Averroes, and Avicenna, reflected the continued interest in Arabic philosophy. The medieval regard for Pliny's *Natural History* still persisted and was sufficiently strong at the end of the fifteenth century to evoke the famous Pliny controversy between the two humanists, Pandolfo Collenuccio and Niccolò Leoniceno.[118] The *De mirabilibus mundi* of Solinus also enjoyed the esteem of fifteenth century collectors, since they chose to place the work on their shelves along with the *Etymologies* of Isidore of Seville. It was the latter, among medieval encyclopedists, however, who was the most favored among humanists. Petrarch relates that a copy of Isidore's work was given him by his father and he treasured it all his life.[119] Of the several encyclopedic works composed in the twelfth and thirteenth centuries, only Bartholomaeus Anglicus, in the *De proprietatibus rerum,* appears to have triumphed on the continent in the struggle with oblivion over Alexander Neckham, Thomas of Cantimpré, and others. Bartholomaeus' work was found in practically every European collection in the fifteenth century. It was current in Italian,

[115] L. Delisle, *Le cabinet des manuscrits,* I, 125 ff.

[116] H. O. Lange, "Ueber einen Katalog der Erfurter Universitätsbibliothek aus dem 15. Jahrhundert," *Centralblatt für Bibliothekswesen,* II (1885), 279 ff.

[117] P. Kibre, *op. cit.,* 28 ff.

[118] See L. Thorndike, *History of magic and experimental science* (New York, 1934), IV, chap. LXVI; R. Sabbadini, *op. cit.* (1914), 241.

[119] D. Robathan, "Libraries of the Italian Renaissance," in J. W. Thompson, *The medieval library,* 525; Pierre de Nolhac, "De patrum et medii aevi scriptorum codicibus in bibliotheca Petrarcae olim collectis," *Revue des bibliothèques,* II (1892), 261; L. Delisle, *Le cabinet des manuscrits,* I, 139. For the distribution of the work of Isidore of Seville in these libraries, see R. Sabbadini, *op. cit.* (1914), 230.

French and Spanish, as well as in English and Dutch translations from the original Latin. Charles of Orléans had it translated into French at his court, and there appear to have been twenty-four printed editions between 1470 and 1500.[120] In English libraries, however, Alexander Neckham's work, *On the nature of things,* continued to be found in most libraries of any size in the late fifteenth century.[121] The three *Specula,* or mirrors of nature, doctrine, and history by Vincent of Beauvais, also found a place, despite their mammoth proportions, in several of the French, English and Italian libraries. Pico della Mirandola, however, appears to have preferred the later *Speculum divinorum et quorumdam naturalium* by Henry Bate of Malines for his library.[122] More recent encyclopedic works of the fourteenth and fifteenth centuries were also found in these libraries but they appear to have lost the universality of appeal that the earlier compositions had had. Thus the moral compendium or *Sophologium* of the Augustinian, Jacques le Grand of Toulouse, is seldom found outside French libraries,[123] and the "Light of the Soul," or *Lumen animae* of Mathias Farinator, the Carmelite of Erfurt and Vienna,[124] is usually found only in German libraries, of which an example is that of Sigismund Gossembrot, the most active German advocate of humanism in the fifteenth century in Augsburg.[125]

Scientific or pseudo-scientific interests which were represented in the catalogues following the divisions of the trivium, centered about the four basic sciences, astronomy or astrology, arithmetic,

[120] Robert Steele, "What fifteenth century books are about," *The Library,* IV (1903), 338–40; A. C. Klebs, *Incunabula scientifica et medica* (Bruges, 1938), nos. 149.1–12 (Latin); 150.1–8 (French), 151.1 (Netherl.); 152.1 (Spanish); 153.1 (Spanish); 154.1 (English). For the translation of Bartholomaeus' work into Italian by Vivaldo Belcalzer in the late 13th and early 14th century, and its general currency in vernacular translations in the 14th and 15th centuries, see V. Cian, "Vivaldo Belcalzer e l'enciclopedismo Italiano," suppl. V, *Giornale storico della lett. ital.* (Torino, 1902), 35 ff.; and the review of Cian's work by A. Sepulcri, in *Archivio Storico Lombardo,* ser. 3, XX (1903), 219–21.

[121] M. R. James, *The ancient libraries of Canterbury and Dover,* 289 et passim.

[122] P. Kibre, *op. cit.,* 96.

[123] L. Thorndike, *op. cit.,* IV, 278–79. There was a copy, however, in the Dominican House in Vienna in the late fifteenth century, *Mittelalterliche Bibl. Kat.,* I (1915), 346; and in the library of Sigismund Gossembrot, see note 125 below.

[124] L. Thorndike, *op. cit.,* III, Chap. XXXII.

[125] Paul Joachimsohn, "Aus der Bibliothek Sigismund Gossembrots," *Centralblatt für Bibliothekswesen,* XI (1894), 264. For a copy of the *Sophologium* see p. 262.

geometry, and music. Practically every library had its share of treatises on astrology, preferably those of the earlier authors from the *Almagest* and *Quadripartitum* of Ptolemy with its commentary by Haly, to the popular Latin works of the later medieval authors, as well as of the Arabic and Hebrew astrologers in Latin translation, namely, Alchabitius, Albumasar, Alkindi, Abraham ibn Ezra, and Thebit ben Corat. Included in many of the collections was the work of the thirteenth century astrologer, Guido Bonatti (d. after 1282), whom Dante had consigned to the fourth division of the eighth circle of inferno, and whose chequered career had included service at the court of the tyrant Ezzelino, a satellite of Frederick II.[126] Equally popular were the works of Peter of Abano, whose talents extended over the fields of astrology, philosophy, and medicine. Thomas of Sarzana in his canon for libraries asserted that the works of Peter of Abano would be fitting for every library.[127] Of fourteenth century authors, the astrological writings of Cecco d'Ascoli continued to circulate in the libraries despite their condemnation by the courts of inquisition; and the compositions of the English astrologer, John of Eschenden of Merton College, Oxford, found a place in German and Italian libraries as well as in those of England. Generally accompanying these works were the astronomical tables, both the Tables of Toledo and the Alfonsine Tables prepared under the direction of Alfonso X of Castile, together with various calendars, tables of eclipses of the moon, and one or more works on the astrolabe.

The interest of princes, dukes and other potentates in astrology as revealed by their libraries is amply supported by Vespasiano, who reports that Cosimo de'Medici had a complete knowledge of the subject from having practiced it with Master Paolo and other astrologers; also that Federigo, duke of Urbino, had in his library "all the writers on astrology and their commentators." The princes of Ferrara, Borso and Ercole I, not only treasured the prognostications of astrologers, but also followed their capricious council. Among the astrologers associated with them were Pietro Bono Avogario, Giorgio Valla, Pellegrino Prisciano, Carlo di S. Giorgio, and Giovanni Arquati.[128] The collection of the Gonzaga

[126] L. Thorndike, *op. cit.* (1923), II, Chap. LXVII.

[127] *Atti reale accad. Lucchese,* XXIII (1884), 379; Thorndike, *op. cit.,* II, Chap. LXX. For the following 14th-century authors, see Thorndike, *op. cit.* (1934), III, passim.

[128] Vespasiano, *Vite,* III (*loc. cit.,* no. 71), 57; I (*loc. cit.,* no. 68), 299; Bertoni *La biblioteca Estense,* 192,n.5,–194; Appen. II^2, 2, 8, 9, 20, 78, 208, 239, 310.

at Mantua with twenty-eight,[129] and that of the Visconti-Sforza at Pavia, with some twenty-four such tracts are especially outstanding for the number and variety of their books on astrology.[130] The library of the Spanish potentate, Martin V, shows a conspicuous leaning toward astrological tracts. In his collection there were, out of a total of two hundred and ninety-four volumes, some forty-four on astrology and astronomy. Included were four copies of Ptolemy, two of them in Catalan, and a third, the *Quadripartitum,* in a Latin translation. There were five almanachs, the tables of Toledo, and the Alfonsine tables, the work on judicial astrology by Leopold of Austria, and several anonymous treatises on the same subject.[131] Under the classification, mathesis, and astronomy, the library of Nicholas of Cusa had treatises by Haly, Zehel (Zael), Ptolemy, Alkindi, Messahala, Geber, Albumasar, and John de Lineriis, who wrote about 1322.[132] The library of Amplonius Ratinck was especially wealthy in this regard since as far as scientific or pseudoscientific works were concerned those on astrology were surpassed in number only by those on medicine. Also well provided with such writings was the abbey church of St. Augustine at Canterbury, with forty-four relating to astrology. This collection at Canterbury which dates back to the ninth century, according to M. R. James, contained a considerable number of books donated by John of London, whom James would identify with the protégé of Roger Bacon.[133]

Mathematical arts were the subject of a number of books found in various of the Renaissance libraries, despite the aspersion cast on mathematics for theologians by Pico della Mirandola,[134] whose view was not especially representative of his contemporaries.

[129] Pia Girolla, in *Atti e memorie, R. Accad. Virgiliana di Mantova,* N. S., XIV–XVI (1921–23), 67–69.

[130] [Girolamo d'Adda], *Libreria Visconteo-Sforzesca del Castello di Pavia,* nos. 203, 246–53, 287–94, 358, 930–31, 971, 973, 980, 986; G. Mazzatinti, "Inventario dei codici della biblioteca Visconteo-Sforzesca," *Giornale storico della lett. ital.,* I (1883), 42–43.

[131] J. Massó Torrents, "Inventari dels bens mobles del Rey Martí D'Aragó," *Revue hispanique,* XII (1905), 414 ff. See particularly nos. 93, 29, 83, 86, 127, 156, 157, 30, 45, 139, 148, 149, 160, 161, 238, 251, etc.

[132] L. Thorndike, *op. cit.* (1934), III, 253 ff.; Kraus in *Serapeum,* XXV (1864), 353; XXVI (1865), 85–89. See also p. 84, no. 25.

[133] M. R. James, *The ancient libraries of Canterbury and Dover,* lxxiv–lxxv; 305, 319–332, 375–73.

[134] P. Kibre, *op. cit.,* 100.

Federigo, duke of Urbino is described by Vespasiano, his contemporary biographer, as "a skilled geometrician and arithmetician," who had in his household a master Paolo, a German, and a very great philosopher and astrologer.[135] In geometry Euclid's work was the indispensable tool as it had been in the earlier ages and it appears almost universally in the inventories. The more elementary steps in arithmetic or numeration were on the other hand represented by tracts on the abacus, and on the *Algorismus*, as well as by Boethius' *Arithmetic*. In the list of books left by Johannes Gmunden to the university of Vienna,[136] he stipulated that a copy of this last named work was to be chained and was not to be loaned out of the library.[137] The writings of such thirteenth century authors as Jordanus Nemorarius, Giovanni Campani of Novara, and John of Sacrobosco, were usually found on the shelves with the newer mathematical treatises of the fourteenth and fifteenth centuries by Thomas Bradwardine, Richard Suiseth or Calculator, Regiomontanus, Giovanni Marliani of Milan, whom Pico considered "the greatest mathematician of his time," and others; while geometrical works by Dominicus de Clavasio and Jean de Murs, supplemented but did not replace Euclid.[138]

Music, the fourth subject of the quadrivium was represented by far fewer treatises than were arithmetic and geometry. Here too the older works by St. Augustine, Boethius, and Guido of Arezzo of the eleventh century were more frequently encountered than the more recent fifteenth century compositions of Niccolò Burzio or Marsilio Ficino.[139] Music was, however, cultivated with enthusiasm and ardor at the court of the Este in Ferrara, also by Federigo, duke of Urbino. Vespasiano relates that the latter greatly delighted in both vocal and instrumental music.[140] Cosimo de'Medici,

[135] Vespasiano, *Vite,* I (*loc. cit.,* no. 68), 294–95.

[136] Joseph von Aschbach, *Geschichte der Wiener Universität* (Wien, 1865), I, 460–65; R. Kink, *Geschichte der kaiserlichen Universität zu Wien* (Wien, 1854), I, pt. 2, 108–111; and more recently John Mundy, "John of Gmunden," *Isis,* XXXIV (1943), 198.

[137] Aschbach, *op. cit.,* I, 461; Kink, *op. cit.,* I, 110; John Mundy, *loc. cit.,* 198.

[138] See "Canone bibliografico di Papa Parentucelli," *Atti Reale Accad. Lucchese,* XXIII (1884), 379; and cf. R. Steele, "What fifteenth century books are about," *The Library,* IV (1903), 341.

[139] P. Kibre, *op. cit.,* 59–60; R. Steele, *loc. cit.,* 344.

[140] Bertoni, *La biblioteca Estense,* 198–99; 236, no. 24; 247, no. 341; Vespasiano, *Vite,* I, 295.

who had three books on music in his library also accorded musicians his appreciative attention.[141]

Of the more practical arts or sciences, medical treatises, which Richard of Furnival in the thirteenth century had listed along with works on civil and canon law as belonging to the lucrative sciences,[142] were the most prominent. No library appears to have been complete without a number of books on this subject. Even that of Pico della Mirandola whose writings reflected slight interest in the subject had a large number of medical tracts.[143] It is difficult to determine to what extent this popularity of the medical writings was due to the general interest that many laymen had in the subject or was the result of more practical needs. There was a leaning toward collections of hygienic rules for maintaining health as well as toward treatises on preventive medicine. Many of these were recent works which had been composed under the stimulus of the devastating ravages of the Black death in the fourteenth century and its recurrences in the fifteenth. But still others were the older works that had provided the medical reading matter during the twelfth and thirteenth centuries. Particularly prominent in the latter category were the treatises by Hippocrates and Galen in the Latin translations by Constantinus Africanus made by way of the Arabic in the early twelfth century, together with the more recent humanistic renderings directly from the Greek by Theodorus Gaza, Lorenzo Laurenziano, and others. The fifteenth-century libraries also frequently included the medical treatise of the Roman physician, Cornelius Celsus, whose work, although known in the middle ages since the extant manuscripts date from the tenth, eleventh, and twelfth centuries, is seldom listed in inventories of libraries before the fifteenth century. It was "found" by Poggio during his systematic search of the monastic establishments while he was presumably attending the council of Constance.[144] Most of the works of Arabic physicians in Latin dress that had been current in the twelfth and thirteenth centuries are included in these fourteenth- and fifteenth-century libraries, among them Albucasis, Averroes,

[141] Vespasiano, *Vite,* III, 57; Piccolomini, in *Archivio storico ital.,* ser. 3, XXI (1875), 111, for the inventory of 1456.

[142] "Bibliomanie de Richard de Furnival," printed in Delisle, *Le cabinet des manuscrits,* II, 521: "Sequens areola libros continet de quibusdam scientiis lucrativis. . . ."

[143] P. Kibre, *op. cit.,* 101 ff.

[144] P. Kibre, *op. cit.,* 52–53; Vespasiano, *Vite,* II, 203.

Avicenna, Rasis, Mesuë, and the like. Of earlier medieval medical writings, the *Viaticus* of Constantinus Africanus, the *Thesaurus pauperum* of Petrus Hispanus, the *Lilium* of Bernard Gordon, together with medical works and translations by Gerard of Cremona, and the *Conciliator* of Peter of Abano, provided the titles most frequently encountered in the catalogues. Treatises on surgery by Bruno of Longoburgo whose works circulated among the libraries of Europe from Italy to the British Isles, by William of Saliceto, and Guy de Chauliac, were also common in the inventories. The work of the last named was, however, more generally found in French libraries than elsewhere. Few contemporary authors of the fourteenth and fifteenth centuries had so universal a following as those mentioned. Medical antidotaries, or lists of simples, recipes for drugs, and information on herbs and foods which one might expect to find useful only for apothecaries were also to be found in the collections of humanists and other bibliophiles. Particular favor was shown toward the *Antidotary* of Nicholas of Salerno, emanating probably from the twelfth century.[145]

Especially noteworthy for its medical works was the collection of Amplonius Ratinck with one hundred and one tracts including all the aforementioned treatises.[146] Similarly conspicuous for its medical books was the library of the abbey church of St. Augustine at Canterbury. Its more than one hundred volumes on this subject comprised works ranging from compositions of Hippocrates and Galen, to those of contemporary Italian authors. The Arabic physicians, Rasis, Averroes, and so on, as well as the medieval Latin authors and works on medicine named above, indicate the prominence of earlier authorities.[147] There were several tracts on women's diseases and on gynaecology, among them the work circulating under the title or author Trotula, also the work of Muscio, and of Caelius Aurelianus.[148] The library of the Prior of St. Martin at Dover, according to the inventory of 1389 was also well provided with books on medical subjects.[149] The medical portion

[145] G. Sarton, *Introduction to the history of Science* (Baltimore, 1931), II, 239–40. Cf. Robert Steele, "What fifteenth century books are about," *The Library,* IV (1903), 345.

[146] Dr. Wilhelm Schum, *Beschreibendes Verzeichnis der Amplonianischen Handschriften-Sammlung zu Erfurt* (Berlin, 1887), 785–867.

[147] M. R. James, *The ancient libraries of Canterbury and Dover,* especially 332–49; also 369 and 385.

[148] *Ibid.,* 347, no. 1274; 385, no. 1599, etc.

[149] *Ibid.,* 429, nos. 337–63; 455, no. 136; 480; 490, no. 410.

of the collection at the university of Erfurt which between 1480 and 1485 contained some eight hundred volumes, included among others the several works of Galen, Macer, Avicenna, Mesuë, the pseudo-Aristotelian *Problems,* also the *Conciliator* of Peter of Abano, and the work of Gerard of Solo. The library also had one volume containing the popular Bartholomaeus Anglicus, *De proprietatibus rerum,* together with Peter Crescentius on agriculture, and a work of Francesco Petrarch.[150] There were twenty books on medical subjects in the library of Nicholas of Cusa, although he appears never to have touched on the subject in his writings.[151]

In Italian libraries the works of Greek and Arabic physicians in translation were particularly well represented. A considerable number of such tracts was included in the library of George Valla whose interest in translating works of early Greek and Arabic scientific authors, with specific emphasis on medicine, provided a strong incentive toward collecting books of this nature. Valla also utilized his collection for his encyclopedic *De expetendis et fugiendis rebus,* in which were excerpts of many of the volumes in his possession.[152] Greek and Arabic physicians in translation were also particularly well represented in the library of the Visconti-Sforza at Pavia. Valla had been associated with the Sforza family first in his capacity as a teacher of the son of Lodovico Moro, and then through his imprisonment for a time by duke Lodovico Sforza. But the interest of the dukes in Greek and Arabic medicine antedates the appearance of George Valla, at Pavia, since the inven-

150 H. O. Lange, "Ueber einen Katalog der Erfurter Universitätsbibliothek aus dem 15. Jahrhundert," *Centralblatt für Bibliothekswesen,* II (1885), 279 ff.

151 Fr. X. Kraus, "Die Handschriften-Sammlung des Cardinals Nicolaus von Cusa," *Serapeum,* XXV (1864), 353, medical works are listed under letter "I"; *loc. cit.,* XXVI (1865), 69–74. Some idea of the varied interests of Nicholas of Cusa may be gathered from the classification of the books in his library under fourteen headings in the inventory reproduced by Kraus. The first four headings, A, B, C, D, comprise 143 volumes related to theology; then follow Nicholas' own compositions (3); books in canon (58), and civil law (14); general historical and geographical works (15); medicine (20); philosophy (26); *mathesis* and *astronomia* (13); grammar (4); Greek (4), and Hebrew (5) codices.

152 J. L. Heiberg, "Beiträge zur Geschichte Georg Vallas u. seiner Bibliothek," *Centralblatt für Bibliothekswesen, Beiheft,* XVI (1896). A collection of tracts translated by George Valla is at the New York Academy of Medicine (Streeter collection) under the title "Nicephorus logica et al. tractatus, Georgio Valla Placentino interprete" (Venice, Simon Papiensis, 30 Sept. 1498). Klebs, *Incunabula scientific et medica* (Bruges, 1938), 1012.1.

tories come down to a period not later than 1469 when Valla would have attained the age of twenty-two. Of the forty-four medical works in the Visconti-Sforza library about one fourth were by the Arabic authors Albucasis, Rasis, Avicenna, Serapion, and John Mesuë. The Greek tradition was preserved in translations of Galen and Hippocrates both in separate texts and in three copies of the *Articella,* the handy collection of early medical tracts that every physician was presumed to have at his elbow. Marsiglio of Sancta Sofia (d. 1405), one of the leading physicians of his day taught medicine at the university of Pavia and attended duke Giangaleazzo Visconti. In addition to the medieval Latin authors mentioned above, there were added according to the inventory of the library under duke Galeazzo Maria Visconti in 1469, several compositions on the preservation of the health against the pestilence by Antonio Guainerio of Pavia, Petrus Codazzo, and Ugo Benzoi; also tracts on guarding against poisons by M. John Martin of Parma, and Peter of Abano, the latter in the vernacular, and a general regime for the conservation of the health by Benedetto da Nursia.[153] A conspicuous collection of medical books was also contained in the library of the dukes of Este at Ferrara. Their library provides ample evidence of the considerable favor shown to medicine by the House of Este probably for the practical reasons connected with the frightful recurrences of the plague. Borso d'Este in 1461 furnished the cadaver for the anatomical sessions at the university of Ferrara, and as court physician the dukes had the renowned Michael Savonarola whose works were kept in their private library. In addition to most of the usual medical works already mentioned, the library contained by Battista Massa of Argenta, a treatise in the vernacular on poisons, also a tract entitled *De fructibus,* in both Latin and vernacular versions; and in the time of Ercole I, the work of Antonio Benivieni. The Este library also had a copy of Maino de Maineri, "On preservation from the epidemic," dated A.D. 1360.[154]

Among the other practical arts, agriculture was represented by

[153] [Girolamo d'Adda], *Libreria Visconteo-Sforzesca del Castello di Pavia,* nos. 185, 425, 427, 429–37, 443, 449–52, 455–59, 481–91, 701, 762–64, 768, 793, 797, 801–802, 826, 830, 975; G. Mazzatinti, "Inventario della biblioteca Visconteo-Sforzesca," *Giornale stor, della lett. ital.,* I (1883), 40–41, 56–9; Bueno Mesquita, *GianGaleazzo Viscount,* 183.

[154] Bertoni, *La biblioteca Estense,* 184; 187–92, 217, no. 42; 236, 243, 246, 247; Appendix, 343; II^2, 33, 34, 36.

the classical authors of antiquity, Hesiod, Varro, Cato, and Palladius, along with the late thirteenth century Petrus Crescentius (d. 1310). There were also several anonymous tracts on the veterinary art, especially in the Visconti-Sforza library, and a manual on the feeding and regimen for birds and falcons.[155] In architecture, Vitruvius was the leading manual. The Visconti library had six treatises on the game of chess, all but one described as illustrated, as well as a work on singing and dancing. In addition there were others on history, duels, military arts, and biography.[156] Such books were found also in the Este library at Ferrara.[157]

Although interest in geography appears to have been fairly wide-spread, since the fifteenth century, especially in its second half is the age of the great expansion of the geographical horizon, contemporary works on the subject are not generally conspicuous in the libraries of the period. The classical works on geography by Ptolemy and Strabo, in recent fifteenth century translations, and of Pomponius Mela were supplemented by several *mappae mundi,* the *Sfera* of Dati, the work of Toscanelli, and the fifteenth-century versified version of Ptolemy made by the Florentine, Francesco Berlinghieri. Books of travel were, however, included in considerable numbers. These comprised the earlier accounts of travels to the orient by Marco Polo, Friar John of Planocarpini, and other medieval travelers, as well as the contemporary reports by Ciriaco of Ancona, and others who journeyed to the near East in search of classical antiquities. In addition the Este library had two tracts on the newly discovered islands belonging to Spain.[158]

Alchemy representative of a more specialized field of endeavor, though numerically in a minority position as compared with mathematics or astrology, appears to have had a fairly wide-spread audi-

[155] [Girolamo d'Adda], *Libreria Visconteo-Sforzesca del Castello di Pavia,* no. 442, 456, 893, 433; G. Mazzatinti, in *Giornale stor. ital.,* I (1883), 43, 56–59.

[156] G. Mazzatinti, *loc. cit.,* I (1883), 43, 50 ff.; 56–59.

[157] A. Cappelli, "La biblioteca estense," *Giornale storico della lett. ital.,* XIV (1889), 15, 16, 23, etc.; Bertoni, *La bibl. estense,* 108, 198, 199, 110, 221, 224, 245, 249; for Chess, 217, 220, 239, 242, 245; and falconry, 217, 218.

[158] Cf. *Ibid.,* 184–85, 215, 224, 246, 250, 261; and for the tracts on the newly discovered islands, p. 243, nos. 245, 248; G. Zippel, *Nicolò Niccoli,* 50; P. Kibre, *op. cit.,* 109–110; F. Flamini, "Leonardo di Piero Dati poeta Latino del secolo XV," *Giornale storico della lett. ital.,* XVI (1890), 1 ff., for an account of the Dati family. For 15th-century editions of Ptolemy, *Mappae mundi,* and the *Sfera,* see Klebs, *Incunabula scientifica et medica,* 36.1–17; 663.1–2; 812.1–7.

ence. Tracts on the art of transmuting baser metals into gold and silver both on the theoretical and practical side were found in a large number of the libraries, both ecclesiastical and lay. One of the largest collections of works of this nature was housed among the books at the abbey church of St. Augustine at Canterbury. Included were such alchemical tracts as Hermes, "On the fifteen stars, herbs, etc"; "the book of the thirty words"; "the book of riddles"; also several works ascribed to a certain Nicholas; to Michael Scot; to Richard of Furnival; and to a certain Tankard. It also contained other anonymous tracts on the tincture of alchemy and on the twelve waters.[159] The last named work is often ascribed to Rasis, Albertus Magnus, and other well-known authors. Possibly other alchemical works were present since it is difficult to identify such works by their titles. The library of the Visconti-Sforza at Pavia, had some nine alchemical tracts, among them the famous *Turba philosophorum* which contains the assertions of numerous authorities regarding the art; the work of the pseudo-Geber, and others appearing anonymously.[160] In the inventory of the books left at the death of Sforza secondo Sforza, the natural brother of Lodovico il Moro (d. 1491), which later passed to Pavia, there were several on alchemy including the tract on the fifth essence, a reagent capable of realizing, according to its authorities,[161] not only the immediate aims of the alchemist but also of providing a cure-all for bodily ills. This library also had several other works in the field of the occult, namely books on chiromancy, geomancy, necromancy, and astrology, as well as treatises on the practical arts of surgery, veterinary medicine, herbs, and animals.[162]

[159] M. R. James, *The ancient libraries of Canterbury and Dover,* 316, 343, 348–49, 375–76, 385–86, 388. There were two copies of Rasis, *Lumen luminum,* in the library of the Prior of St. Martin at Dover in 1389: *Ibid.,* p. 488, nos. 402, 403. The library of Christ Church, Canterbury, had a "Liber Arthuri de alkimia": *Ibid.,* p. 73, no. 651; and several other works in alchemy: *Ibid.,* pp. 73, 75, 92–94; 124.

[160] G. Mazzatinti, "Inventario della biblioteca Visconteo-Sforzesca," *Giornale storico della letteratura italiano,* I (1883), 42. For the most part these works do not appear in the inventory of 1426 published by Girolamo d'Adda. But see no. 929, de naturis auri argenti, et herbarum historiatus et compilatus per Manfredum de Monte Imperiale; *Libreria Visconteo-Sforzesca del Castello di Pavia,* 85; also no. 144, Hermes on alchemy.

[161] The work on the fifth essence is usually attributed to John of Rupescissa, for whom see L. Thorndike, *op. cit.* (1934), III, chapter XXII.

[162] Emilio Motta, "Documenti per la libreria Sforzesca di Pavia, 1456–1494

Alchemical tracts in the collection of Francesco Gonzaga at Mantua in 1407 comprised works of Hermes; the *Lumen luminum* or "Light of lights," variously attributed to Rasis, Geber, and Aristotle; also a collection of experiments or observations in alchemy; some works on the art ascribed to Raynaldus (Arnaldus?) of Villanova, and Albertus Magnus.[163] George Valla had in his library the work on the fifth essence, also the book of secrets attributed to Raymond Lull, and the *Ars alchimie margarita novella* of master Petrus Bonus of Ferrara.[164] In the library of Nicholas of Cusa, such works attributed to Raymond Lull, Arnald of Villanova, Avicenna, and Geber, as well as chemical recipes in German, and other anonymous works on the subject, were all classified under the headings, medicine and philosophy.[165] At Erfurt, as noted earlier, the Amplonian collection had the four books on alchemy placed after the books on natural philosophy.[166] There were also treatises on alchemy in the Spanish library of Martin V of Aragon.[167]

The occult arts of magic and divination, geomancy, nigromancy, chiromancy, and the like, were represented in several treatises in the libraries of the Visconti-Sforza, of Francesco Gonzaga, and other Italian libraries of the fifteenth century, also in French ducal and royal collections and in the Spanish libraries of Martin V and Alfonso X, as well as in English ecclesiastical libraries. The Visconti library had several works on dreams, an anonymous physiognomy, probably the one ascribed to Aristotle, also the pseudo-Aristotelian *Secret of Secrets,* which was so widely current,[168] and the collection entitled *Picatrix.*[169] Alkindi, *On stellar rays,* and

Aggiunte alle Indagini del Marchese d'Adda," *Il Bibliofilo, anno* VII, no. 9–10 (1886), 129–34. See especially 133.

[163] Pia Girolla, "La biblioteca di Francesco Gonzaga, secondo l'inventario del 1407," *Accad. Virgiliana, Atti e memorie,* XIV–XVI (1921–23), 64 ff.

[164] J. L. Heiberg, "Beiträge zur Gesch. Georg Vallas u. seiner Bibliothek," *Beiheft zum Centralblatt für Bibliothekswessen,* XVI (1896), 113, 117. For Petrus Bonus, see Thorndike, *op cit.* (1934), III, chapter IX.

[165] Kraus in *Serapeum,* XXVI (1865), 69–70, 73, 83.

[166] De alchimia que subalternatur philosophie natuali," nos. 61–(64).

[167] J. Massó Torrents, "Inventari dels bens mobles del rey Marti d'Aragó," *Revue hispanique,* XII (1905), 430 ff.; especially nos. 117, 250.

[168] Cf. Steele, "What fifteenth century books are about," *The Library,* IV (1903), 351–52; Delisle, *Cabinet des manuscrits,* I, 117. For 15th-cent. editions of the *Secret of secrets,* see Klebs, *Incunabula scientifica et medica,* nos. 96.1–9.

[169] G. Mazzatinti, "Inventario della biblioteca Visconteo-Sforzesca," *Giornale*

several other treatises of similar tenor were in the collection of Martin V, which in addition contained the compendium of superstitious practices and medicine entitled Kiranides.[170] The Augustinian library at Canterbury also included a large number of works in this category.[171]

For the most part the private collections made during the fourteenth and fifteenth centuries did not long remain intact after the deaths of their owners. In some cases immediate dispersal followed. In others the libraries were either sold to some other collector as in the case of the sale of Pico's books to Cardinal Domenico Grimani; or were bequeathed to religious or monastic establishments.[172] Where the latter was true, provision was made that the books might be loaned out for the use of lay citizens as well as of the members of the religious community. The library of St. Victor in France was especially fortunate in receiving a large number of bequests. This was also true of the Sorbonne and other establishments connected with the universities.[173] Hence it might be concluded that the fate of many precious early classical manuscripts, rescued from a neglected but probably more permanent haven in monastic establishments, was that of only gracing temporarily the library shelves of a humanist or his patron. Those more fortunate than others often found their way back again by the testaments of their erstwhile guardians to other monastic or ecclesiastical houses; while the less fortunate succumbed to the ravages of fire or war and disappeared among the booty or spoils of conquest.

---

storico della lett. ital., I (1883), 43. The books on dreams were by Leo Justus, Richard of St. Victor, and Solomon. See also [Girolamo d'Adda], *Libreria Visconteo-Sforzesca del Castello di Pavia,* no. 978, 967. These works were also in the library of the Gonzaga at Mantua as well as the treatises on necromancy: Girolla, *loc. cit.,* XIV–XVI (1921–23), 67–68; for such works in the Este library see Bertoni, *La biblioteca estense,* 55, 223, no. 120; 219, no. 64; 244, n. 278. On Picatrix, and the other works in the occult sciences, see L. Thorndike, *History of magic and experimental science,* New York, 1923, vols. I–II, passim.

170 J. Massó Torrents, "Inventari dels bens mobles del rey Marti d'Aragó," *Revue hispanique,* XII (1905), 430 ff.; see no. 259, "Quiranides. . . ."

171 M. R. James, *The ancient libraries of Canterbury and Dover,* 318, 340.

172 Sabbadini, *Le scoperte dei codici* (1905), 188 ff., provides a good many examples of such bequests.

173 L. Delisle, *Cabinet des manuscrits,* II, gives the list of such benefactors to the library of St. Victor, 209 ff.; and to the Sorbonne, 142 ff. For bequests to the university of Vienna, see notes 136, 137 above; also *Mittelalterliche Bibl. Kat.,* I (1915), 281; 415–22; 437 ff.; 447 ff.; 498–501; etc.

In content these libraries of the so-called renaissance of the fourteenth and fifteenth centuries may thus be seen to reveal no sharp line of cleavage between the interests of these centuries from those immediately preceding. The humanistic works (litterae humaniores), products of the enthusiasm for and renewed interest in the classics of Greek and Roman antiquity, supplemented but did not replace the hallowed classics of the more immediate past. The ducal and princely collectors continued to be guided in large part in their choice of books by the traditional tastes of their immediate chronological predecessors. Their libraries adhered to the pattern for earlier ecclesiastical establishments in the formula provided by Thomas of Sarzana. Theology was still the mainstay, and scholastic interests appeared side by side with those of humanism. The Bible and St. Augustine continued to hold first place among the most universally read books; while Aristotle and medieval compendia or encyclopedias retained the venerable regard of the great majority of the reading public. Occult sciences were still as popular as they had been earlier and as they were to continue to be into the succeeding centuries. The bulk of the collections remained Latin in their general makeup although the rehabilitation of Greek studies and the growing interest in textual criticism is reflected in the introduction of Greek, Hebrew, and in rare instances, Arabic and Aramaic codices into a chosen few of the libraries, while the ducal and princely collectors revealed a strong leaning toward the vernaculars of which French and Tuscan were the most favored. In large part the libraries reflect the partiality of their owners for ancient and medieval classics, thus adhering to the dictum of Richard de Bury, that most ardent of fourteenth century bibliophiles, who "loved codices more than florins," that "it is more desirable to investigate the well tested labors of the ancients, than to explore the novelties of the moderns."[174] But most of all these libraries in their commingling of the classics of Greek and Roman antiquity with the revered ecclesiastical treasures of the more immediate past, provide an illuminating example of that "picturesque union of contrasts [the mixture of the two traditions, sacred and profane] that is so characteristic of the art at the close of the fifteenth century."[175]

[174] *Philobiblon,* tr. E. C. Thomas (London, 1925), 56; 65.
[175] Walter Pater, *The Renaissance,* Modern Library, 39.

INDEX

Roman numerals I-XX refer to article numbers; arabic numerals following the Roman numerals refer to pages in the article. According to general usage, personal names are listed either under first or last name.

Abacus I 180-2; II 70; XX 288
Abraham ibn Ezra XX 287-8
Abu Abdallah Mohammed ibn Musa Al Khowarismi I 182
Adam of Francovilla XIII 14
Adam Marsh (de Marisco) I 177
Adelard of Bath I 182, 184
Aegidius Romanus, Commentary on Aristotle's *Posterior Analytics* XVIII 390-1
Agriculture XX 292-3
Aimeric de Peguilham XX 268
Alain de Lille I 184
Albategni I 188
Albert of Cologne *see* Albertus Magnus
Albert of Saxony, his *De proportionibus* XIX 507
Alberti, Leon Battista XX 268
Albertus Magnus II 71, 77-9; XI 261-3, 265, 267-9; 'On Alchemy' III 187-202; 'Alchemical Writings ascribed to Albertus' VII 499-518; 'An Alchemical tract' VIII 303-16; *Alkimia minor* IV 267-300; *De mineralibus* VIII 303-5; *De occultis naturae* V 23-39; (Latin text of) VI 157-83; 'Further manuscripts containing alchemical tracts' IX 238-47; X 169, 172, 175; Astronomical tracts ascribed to Albertus I 189; *De homine* XVIII 391; *Super parvis ritualibus* XVIII 391
Albertus de Zanchariis (Commentator on Hippocrates and Avicenna) XIX 514
Albucasis XX 289, 292
Album, Ad IV 270
Albumasar XX 286-7
Alchabitius XIX 18; XX 286
Alchemy: Alchemical art, best imitator of nature III 194-5; Alchemical experiments III 194; Alchemical gold III 195; Alchemical methods of procedure, operations and processes III 192-200, IV 268-72, 297-8; V 32; VII 501; VIII 304-7; Alchemical miscellanies X 167-76; Alchemists visited by Albertus IV 268
Alcuin II 70
Alembic III 194; IV 271-2
Alessandro Sforza, his library at Pesaro XX 274
Alexander of Hales I 184
Alexander of Neckham I 179, 183, 186; XX 284; *De laudibus divinae sapientiae* I 180; *De Natura Rerum* I 180
Alexander de Villedieu I 183, 190; XII 219; *Carmen de algorismo* I 183; *Doctrinale* I 183; XII 221
Alfarabi I 178; XII 219-20
Alfonsine Tables XX 287
Alfonso the Magnanimous, king of Aragon, his library XX 272, 276
Alfraganus I 188-9; XIX 508
Algazel XX 284
Algebra I 182
Algorisms XII 222
Algorismus XIX 508; XX 288
Algorismus demonstratus I 182; II 72
Alkindi XX 286-7
Almanacs XX 287
Alpetragius I 188-9
Alpharabi *see* Alfarabi
Aludel IV 272
Alum of Yemen IV 274
Aluminibus et Salibus, de VI 160
Alums V 31
Ambrogio Traversari, translator XX 264
Amplonius Ratinck (Ratinger) XII 226; medical collection at Erfurt XX 278, 280, 283, 287-90
Anne of Brittany, wife of Charles VIII and

then of Louis XII, XX 271-2
Antidotaries, medical XX 290
Antonio de Becchariis of Ferrara XX 268
Antonius, Andreas O. M, his Commentary on Aristotle's *Metaphysics* XIX 507
Antonius de Gradis, *Tract on Fevers* XVIII 397
Antonius Guaynerius of Pavia XX 292; *Summarium Febrium* XIX 513
Antonius Haneron XII 221
Antonius Pius XIX 513
Apothecaries and university regulations XIII 14-16
Appian XX 263-4
Apuleius of Madaura, resumed translator into Latin of Nicomachus II 68, 80; translated into Italian XX 268
Arabic and Aramaic texts present in some libraries XX 267, 284ff., 297
Arabic physicians in Latin translation XX 289-90
Archelaus V 26
Archytar II 69
Argentum VIII 316
Argentum vivum VIII 315
Ariosto, Ludovico, in Este library XX 268
Aristotle and Aristotelian Corpus I 175-8 *et passim*; XII 218; XX 297; *Categories* I 178; *Logic* XII 221; *Politics* XX 270; *Posterior Analytics* I 178; XVIII 390-1; *Rhetoric* XII 220; *Treatises on natural science and moral philosophy* I 175; III 187-8; VII 499; XII 222-3; Pseudo-Aristotelian *Epistle to Alexander* IX 240; Pseudo-Aristotelian *Problemata* XVIII 392; XX 270, 290-1
Arithmetic I 175, 178, 180ff.; *see also* Boethius II 67ff.
Arithmetic, elementary XX 288
Arithmetica demonstratus I 183
Ark of Noah I 185
Arnold of Villanova IX 239; XII 226; XVIII 394
Arquato, Giovanni, astrologer XX 286
Articella XVIII 391; XX 292
'Arts and Medicine in the Universities in the Later Middle Ages' XIII 213-27
Arts, License in XII 221-2
Assaying IV 272
Astrology I 180; XIX 508-9; XX 286 *et passim*; Doctrines IV 269; Medicine XIV 133-56; Works on in libraries of Cosimo de' Medici, Federigo, duke of Urbino, and the Princes Borso and Ercole I of Ferrara XX 286
"Astronomia" or "Astrologia" Ypocratis XIV 133-56
Astronomy I 180-90; XII 222; Instruments I 189-90; Tables XV 100ff.
Augustine of Hippo, St. XIX 507; XX 270
Augustine of Trent, Augustinian Friar XIV 139
Aurum VIII 315
Averroes I 178; XX 289-90
Avicenna (Abu Ali ibn Sina) V 31; VI 157, 163, 167, 176; XVIII 393, 398; XX 291; Alchemical tracts III 188-9, 195-201; V 30-1; VI 163; IX 238-9; *Canon* XVI 994; XVIII 393-4, 396; XIX 505; Latin translation of, in Visconti-Sforza collection XX 292; University of Erfurt Library copy XX 291
Avignon, Pontifical library at, under Urban V, XX 265
Azoc for quicksilver V 28
Azzo VI, court of XX 268

Baccalaureate I 176, 180
Bacon, Roger *see* Roger Bacon
Baker's oven (*furnis panis*) IV 272
Bale, John (*Scriptorium illustrium* Catalogue [Basle, 1557, 1559]) XV 100, 475
Bartholomaeus Anglicus: *De proprietatibus rerum* XX 284; in library of University of Erfurt XX 291; Printed editions of (1470-1500) XX 285; Vernacular translations of XX 285
Bartholomaeus Varignana XIX 514
Bartolomeo da Montagnana, colleague of Cristoforo Barzizza at Padua XVIII 389
Bartolomew of Parva, Commentary on Sacrobosco's *Sphere* II 73
Barzizza, Cristoforo: 'Cristoforo Barzizza: Professor of Medicine at Padua' XVIII 389-98;
Barzizza, Gasparino, uncle of Cristoforo, humanist XVIII 389-90
Battista Guarini at Ferrara XX 264
Battista Massa of Argenta: *De fructibus*, in Latin and vernacular XX 292; *Treatise on Poisons*, in vernacular XX 292
Battista di S. Paolo *alias* Battista Panetti, of Ferrara, theologian, orator and poet XX 264
Battista, son of Cristoforo (Dominus Joh. Baptista) XVIII 392
Baur, Ludwig I 181
Bayle, François, his rejection of astrological

tract attributed to Hippocrates (1677) XIV 139-40
Beaujouan, Guy II 72
Bede I 182; II 70
Benedetto da Nursia, *Regimen for Conservation of Health* XX 292
Benivieni, Antonio XX 292
Bentivoglio, rulers of Bologna, treatise on XIX 506
Benzi, Ugo XX 292
Bernard of Gordon: *Tract on Urines and Pulse* XVIII 392; *Lilium* and other works XX 290
Bernard de Loen, professor of Medicine, books deeded to University of Cologne XII 226
Berthelot's dictum: 'Alchemy belongs in the field of positive history' IV 269
Bessarion, Cardinal: Collection of Works of Plato and Aristotle XX 282-3; Greek works bequeathed to San Marco in Venice XX 261
Bible: French translation XX 270; Glosses XX 270; Numerical prominence of, also of theological tracts XX 277, 297
Bishop of Maguelone and *Licentia docendi* XIII 5
Bishop of Paris: Court of XIII 7; Urged by Pope John XXII to enforce provisions *vs.*. illegal practice of medicine XIII 11-13
Bishop of Senlis: Urged to assist in preventing illegal practice of medecine XIII 13-14
Black Death XII 216; XX 286
Boccacio XX 260, 268, 279
Boethius I 178, 181-2; *Arithmetica* I 182-3; II 67-80; XX 275, 285, 288; *Consolation of Philosophy* XX 270, 279-80; *Geometry* I 183-4; *Musica* I 186; XX 275, 288
Boiardo, Matteo Maria, *Orlando Innamorado* XX 264
Boiling or cooking IV 272
Bologna: Histories of XIX 506; University of Arts and Medicine XVI 990; XIX 509
Bonaventura, St., works of II 77; V 27, 31
Bonellus, philosopher of the Turba V 27, 33
Book of Alums and Salts V 31
Book of King Kalid V 31-2
Book of the Furnace V 28
Book of the Perfect Mastery V 32
Borgia, Lucrezia XX 209
Borgnet, A. IV 270
Borzo d'Este, provider of cadaver for anatomical sessions at University of Ferrara XX 292
Bradwardine, Thomas XX 288
Bruni, Leonardo, translator XX 266
Bruno Longoburgo, on surgery XX 290
Bubacar maiorem or *Rasis* VI 164
Bubacarda 12 capitulorum librum artis VI 164
Buridan, John, *Commentary on Aristotle's Ethics* XIX 507
Burley, Walter XX 260

'*Cabusatores et cabusatrices*' XIII 18
Caelius Aurelianus XX 290
Calcination IV 272, 274, 278
Calculi (pebbles) I 182
Calculum, Quomodo Fit IV 293-4
Calendar Reform I 190
Calixtenes or Calixthenes *see* Callisthenes
Callixtus III (pope), collection of legal texts XX 278
Callisthenes (Khalid ibn Yazid) III 188, 191, 201; VII 501; VIII 303-4, 309
Calx (Quick lime) and *Lixivium* (Lye) III 190
Campanus of Novara I 184; XIX 508; XX 288
Canterbury, abbey church of St. Augustine, noteworthy for collection of astrological and medical texts XX 287, 290
Cardinal Conrad, papal legate and medical practice at Montpellier XIII 5
Carlo di S. Giorgio, astrologer XX 286
Cassiodorus XIII 3; *Institutiones* II 70
Cato XX 293
Cecco d'Ascoli, *Commentary on the Sphere of John of Sacrobosco* XIV 138
Celsus, Cornelius, work of Roman physician 'found' by Poggio Bracciolini while attending Council of Constance XX 289
Cementation IV 272
Census of Medieval and Renaissance Manuscripts XVI 990
Ceration (reduction to consistency of wax) IV 272
Cermisone, Antonio, colleague or master of Cristoforo Barzizza at Padua XVIII 389, 394
Chalcidius, preface to his translation and commentary on Plato's *Timaeus* IX 238
Chancellor of cathedral of Notre Dame and License to teach (*Licentia docendi*) XIII 5
Charles V, king of France, and his library XVI 98; XX 269-70

Charles VI, king of France XIII 17
Charles VIII, king of France XIV 139; XIX 506
Charles of Orleans: his library XX 270; Translation of Bartholomaeus into French XX 285
Charlotte of Savoy and her library XX 271, 276
Chartres II 70; *Savants* of I 177; Victorines of, and medicine at University of Paris XII 215-16
Chartularium Universitatis Parisiensis XIII 18
Chemical knowledge, status of IV 269
Chemical substances described III 99
Chemist at Cologne VII 499
Chemistry, laboratories, processes and utensils IV 268
Chenu, M. D., O. P. XII 217
Christine de Pisan, court historian XX 269-71; *La cité des dames* XX 271
Christophorus de Honestis XVI 391; named among learned men of Bologna XIX 514
Chrysoloras, Manuel, Greek scholar XX 260-1
Ciriaco of Ancona: Greek manuscripts XX 261; his contemporaries XX 293
Clarice de Rothomago and unlicensed medical practice XIII 7
Classical Greek and Latin poets in Italian libraries XX 275, 280-1
Clavis Sapientiae VII 502
Clement VI, pope, and supervision of medical practice XIII 13
Coagulation, named synonymously with congelation IV 272
Cologne, chemist III 196 *see also* Chemist at Cologne; Laboratories III 194; University XII 216-17, 219, 221, 227
Coloratione spirituum, de X 285
Comets, studies on I 179
Commission of municipal surgeons at Paris XIII 13
Compendium alchemiae VII 502, 506
Compendium on Urines, and diagnosis XVI 995
Compositio de compositis see Albertus Magnus X 169
Compositione omnium predictorum ad medicinam perfectam, de IV 298-300
Conrad Heingarter of Zurich, writer on astrology XIV 139
Conrad Nisemanus XIX 508, 513
Constantinus Africanus, translator from Arabic XX 289; *Pantegni* XVIII 391; *Viaticus* XX 290
Copernicus, Nicholas XIV 133
Copper vessel (*vase eneo*) for commingling of minerals V 32
Corbett, Dr. James, *Catalogue* VII 503
Cornelius Nepos, in Italian translation XX 268
Cosimo de' Medici XX 261, 275; Interest in Astrology XX 286; Interest in Medicine XX 289; Interest in Music XX 288
Cosimo de Pazzi, bishop of Arezzo and archbishop of Florence, translator XX 264
Council of Constance XX 289
Council of Ferrara, and humanists XX 264
Council of Vienne, and interest in Greek *codices* XX 264
Crisibus, de XIX 512
Croce, Benedetto XX 268
Cucurbite, glass IV 273

Dante XX 268
Dati, *Sfera* XX 293
Deadening (*mortificare*) IV 272
Demetrio Guazzelli of Lucca, first custodian of the Vatican Library XX 263
Democritus III 188-90
Descensory IV 273
Dialectics XII 221; *see also* Logic
Dice players XIX 505
Dicta philosophorum IV 269
Diodorus predictions XIX 509
Diodorus Siculus XX 263; translation from Greek by Poggio Bracciolini XIX 506
Diogenes Laertius XX 264
Dion Cassius XX 263
Dioscorides XVIII 391
Dissolution and resolution or liquefaction IV 272
Dissolution of the atrament IV 274
Dissolution of the greeness of copper IV 274
Distillation III 200; IV 271, 273
Dominic, St. XIX 507
Dominican library in Vienna XX 266
Domenico Galeotti Bollandino, from Ragusa, probably son of Dominicus XVI 991
Dominicus de Clavasio, geometrician XX 288
'Dominicus de Ragusa, Bolognese Doctor of Arts and Medicine' XVII 383-6
'Dominicus de Ragusa, Hitherto Unnoted Medical Writings (1424-1425 A. D.)' XVI 990-5

Dominus Odo de Cornessiaco, friar at Hotel de Dieu at Paris and witness for the defense of Jaqueline Felicie XIII 10
Don Carlos, prince of Viana, son of John II of Aragon and Blanche of Navarre, his enthusiasm for letters XX 272-3
Donatus XII 218-19; Twelfth-century 'Greek Donatus' at Christ Church, Canterbury XX 265
Duke of Buckingham XV 102
Dung bath IV 272
Durling, Dr. Richard XIV 135
Dyeing of metals, red or white, symbolic for transmutation into gold or silver IV 267

Eberhard of Bethune, *Graecismus* (*c.* 1202) XII 219
Ecclesiasticus III 197; Admonition to honor the physician XIII 3
Edinburgh, Advocates Library VII 500-1
Edmund of Abington I 179-80
Edward I, king of England I 175
Edward IV, king of England, XV 101
Eleanor of Aragon, wife of Ercol I, XX 269
Elias Salomon, *De scientia artis musicae* I 186
Elixir (or *Fermentum*, Medicine or the Philosophers' Stone) III 191-3 195, 199; IV 267, 273-5; V 30, 32; VI 167; VII 501-2; VIII 304-7
Elizabeth of York XV 101-2
Elizabeth, daughter of Queen Elizabeth of York XV 102
Elizabeth von Volkers XX 274
Empedocles III 189, 192; Practitioner of alchemy III 189
Empirics, denounced XIII 5
Encyclopedic works of 14th and 15th centuries found in few libraries XX 285
Engelbert of Admont, *Musica* I 186
English advocates of 'New Learning', Thomas Linacre and William Grocyn, initiated into the study of Greek in Italy XX 265
English libraries and works in French, Castilian and Italian dialects XX 263
Epistle to Euthesia V 27-8, 32-3
Erasmus XII 221
Ercole I of Ferrara, his interest in astrology XX 286
Erfurt libraries: Amplonian collection, comprising books on the *trivium* and *quadrivium*, also of magic arts, perspective, natural philosophy, alchemy and theology XX 278, 295; University library, comprising, among others, Greek texts XX 266; several texts devoted to Aristotle XX 284
Ernoldi de Halle XX 276
Este library at Ferrara XX 263-4, 268, 274, 282, 292-3. Contents: works of humanists, poets and prose writers XX 264; chivalric literature of Provence XX 268; translations of Greek works XX 263, 268, 274; tracts in Catalan and other Spanish dialects XX 268; treatises on biography, history and military arts etc. XX 293; tracts on geography and on newly discovered islands XX 293; treatises on medicine (of which several related to the plague), and on poisons XX 292
Euclid, *Elementa geometria*, translation of from Greek by Adelard of Bath I 178-80, 184-5; II 72, XX 275, 288; Commentaries on I 184; importance for demonstration of theological proof I 185
Eugenius IV, pope XVIII 394; XX 262
Euthesia VI 165, 178
Experimenta (alchemical), reports of laboratory observations VII 502
Experiments, brought forward by alchemists III 192
Ezzelino XX 286

Faculty of arts XII 216-23 Relation to Faculty of Medicine XII 222-3
Faculty of Medicine at Paris and elsewhere: Basis and foundation in arts XII 217-24; Curriculum at Universities of Louvain and Cologne (Köln) XII 223-7; Program of medical instruction on prescribed texts XII 223-7; Requirement of supervised practice XII 227; Role of the Faculty of Medicine in health care at Paris: Effort to stamp out charlatanism XIII 2-20; Surveillance over apothecaries, herbalists and surgeons XIII 14-19. Effects of the war on medical teaching and practice XII 225; XIII 1
Fazio degli Umberto XX 268
Feces or ash V 32
Federigo, duke of Urbino, "a skilled geometrician and arithmetician" XX 288; Paolo, a German philosopher and astrologer, a member of his household XX 288; reputed to have the works of all the writers on astrology, and their

commentators, in his library XX 286. was generous to men of letters and his library well-provisioned with the works of recent or contemporary authors XX 282; was owner of ninety-nine Hebrew items XX 263, 267
Felicie, Jaqueline, tried and found guilty of illegal practice of medicine XIII 8-9, 12, 20
Fermentum see Elixir
Fernan, Don Nunez de Guzman, of Valladolid, surnamed the Greek commander, editor and translator of several Greek classics XX 265
Ferrara XX 261
Ferrara, Council of XX 264
Ferrara, study and translation of Greek works in XX 264
Fevers XVIII 397; tracts on, by Cristoforo Barzizza and by Galeatus de S. Sophia XVIII 397
Fichet, Guillaume XII 220
Ficino, Marsilio, *On Music* XX 288
Fiesole, library of XX 274
Filter IV 271
Fixation or solidification, either of liquid or gaseous substances IV 272, 275
'*Flores etymologiarum*' V 28, 30; VI 160, 170
'Flower of the lily', attributed to Arnald of Villanova V 34
Francesco Gonzaga, library of, at Mantua, large number of vernacular holdings XX 269
Franciscus Florentinus or Paduanus, minorite and inquisitor XIV 139
Franco of Cologne I 186
Franco de Polonia, *On the construction of the Torquetus*, astronomical instrument I 190
French translations of classical works of antiquity XX 269
French works in English libraries XX 273
French works in Spanish libraries XX 272-3
Friar de Cordelis, Herman, Manfred and others, physicians named in case of Jaqueline Felicie XIII 10
Friar Fucus of Ferrara, Calendar XIX 508
Friar John of Plano Carpini, and other medieval travellers XX 293
Furnace of reverberation IV 272
Furnaces IV 272
'Further manuscripts containing alchemical tracts attributed to Albertus Magnus' IX 238-47
Gabriel, A. L. XII 218
Galeazzo (Galeatius) da Sancta Sofia, colleague of Christoforo Barzizza at Padua XVIII 389; *On Fevers* XVIII 397
Galen XII 214-15, 219, 224; XVIII 398; XIX 513; XX 291-2: *Ars parva* XVIII 391; Copy of in Erfurt University Library, and in Visconti Sforza library XX 272; *De ingenio sanitatis*, translation by Burgundio of Pisa, book 7 XVIII 391; *Opera* XX 291; Authority of XII 219; Named among the founders of medicine XIX 513; *On Lunar Prognostications in Medicine*, attibuted to Galen XIV 135
Garzoni, Bernardo, professor of medicine at Bologna, father of Giovanni Garzoni, personal physician to Pope Nicholas V, XIX 505
Garzoni, Giovanni, professor of medicine at Bologna, defender of astrology XIV 133; XIX 504-14; Lectured on Avicenna's *Canon*, book three, fen 9-12 XIX 505; made various addresses against gamblers and dice players XIX 507; wrote in praise of medicine, and named physicians among the very worthy and learned men of the city in his 'De dignitate Bononiae' XIX 507, 513-14; His other works XIX 506
Geber III 201; V 25, 31-3; VI 157, 163-5, 168, 170; VIII 303-5; X 172-6; *Book of the Perfect Mastery*, attributed to Geber V 25; Excerpts from X 172; *Liber Septuaginta* X 170-1; Nicholas of Cusa's library and Geber XX 287
Generation of heat I 179
Generation of stones III 189
Gentile da Fabriano, famous Venetian painter, asked by Dominico to illustrate medical subject XVI 992
Gentile da Foligno, *Commentary on Avicenna's Canon* XVIII 391-2; *Contra Ipocratem et Galienum* XVIII 391; Works cited by Cristoforo XVIII 398; Works deeded to University of Cologne XII 226
Geography, works in XX 293; *see also* Dati; *Mappae mundi*; Pomponius Mela; Ptolemy; Strabo; Toscanelli
Geometry I 175, 180-1; Euclid's *Geometry* XII 222; Importance of to explain Scriptures I 183-4; Scientific understanding of nature impossible without mathematics and especially

geometry I 185; The study of Nature or natural phenomena I 185
George of Trebizond, at Ferrara XX 264
Gerard of Cremona, works and translations I 182; XIX 508; XX 290
Gerard of Solo, work in library of University of Erfurt XX 291
German libraries and general lack of works in Romance languages XX 273
Gigil, *Book of Secrets* III 188, 191-2
Giovanni de' Medici (Cardinal, later Pope Leo X) XX 262
Glorieux, Mgr. Palemon XII 217
Gold III 191, 194
Gonzaga library in Mantua, works on alchemy, astrology, Hermes, law (canon and civil) XX 279, 286-7, 295
Gottlieb, Theodor XX 257
Grabmann, Mgr. I 181; XII 217
Grammar I 178, 184, 187; XX 275; Schools (preparatory) XII 219
Granada, city of XIX 506
Greek texts in European libraries XX 260-1, 264-6, 281; Literary texts in Italian libraries of the 15th century, in Greek and in translation XX 260, 281; Philosophical and scientific writings introduced in Greek form or in translation XX 281
Gregorio da Città di Castello XX 264
Gregory the Great, St. XIX 507; *Homilies* XX 279
Gregory IX, pope I 186
Gregory XII, pope, collector of legal texts XX 278
Grocyn, William XX 265
Guarino of Verona, humanist, collector of Greek works XX 261; Preceptor of Giovanni Garzoni XIX 506; stay at Ferrara XX 264
Guido of Arezzo, *On Music* XX 288
Guilliem VII, lord of Montpellier, declaration on teaching of medicine at Montpellier XIII 5
Guy de Chauliac, works in French libraries XX 290
Gynaecology, tract on XX 290

Haly I 186; XIV 136, 138; XX 287
Harmony I 187
Hasen (or Hazen), king III 188-9
Hebrew texts XX 266-7
Helias, Fr., *Vade mecum* ascribed to him X 174-5
Helperic II 70
Henry V, king of England XIII 19
Henry Bate of Maline, *Speculum* XX 285
Henry Tudor, earl of Richmond XV 101
Herbs, properties of XIII 18; XVIII 391
Hermes, legendary or mythical founder of alchemy III 188-90, 192-3, 195, 201; IV 270; V 28-33; VI 157, 180-1; VIII 303, 316; XIX 509; alchemical tracts attributed to him: *Emerald Tables; Liber Hermetis; Liber Mercurialis; Liber de transmutationibus* V 26
Hermonymos, George of Sparta, sojourn at Paris and interest in Greek XX 265
Herodotus XX 263-4
Hesiod XX 293
Hildesheim II 70
Hindu art of reckoning I 182
Hippocrates, most significant founder of medicine XII 214-15; XIX 513; *Acute Diseases* XII 224; *Airs, Waters and Places* XIV 134; *Aphorisms* XII 215-16, 224; XVIII 391; *Astronomia* or *Astrologia Ypocratis* XII 222; XIV 133-56; *Epistle to King Maecenus* XII 215; *Oath* XIII 2-3; *Prognostics* XII 224; XVIII 393; Works in Latin translation in Visconti-Sforza library XX 292; Works in library of abbey church of St. Augustine, Canterbury XX 290
Histoire Littéraire I 186
Historical chronicles XX 268
History XX 275
Homer, works of XX 260, 264; Greek text of Homer held by Petrarch XX 260
Honorius of Autun II 70
Honorius III, pope, and medical practice of clerics III 4
Horace XX 275
Hroswitha II 70
Hugh of England III 196
Hugh of St. Victor I 184
Hugues, the physician I 179
Humanism XX 258, 275
Humanists XII 221; XX 258, 281
Humphrey, duke of Gloucester *see* Lewis of Caerleon
Hundred Years War XII 216
Hygienic rules for maintaining health XX 286, 289

Iamblichus II 68
Illegal/or Illicit practices in medicine XIII 12-13, 19
Imbrasius of Ephesus XIV 135
Index of Manuscripts VII 517

Interest in classical works reflected in translations into vernacular XX 269
Isidore of Seville, *Etymologies*, favoured by humanists XX 284
Isocrates XX 263
Italian dialects, compositions in, and translations from Latin authors, and Este library XX 268

Jacobi, Dr. Abraham, and *Mss.* of Dominican works XVI 990
Jacobus de Dondis, *Treatise on Medicinal Simples* XVIII 391
Jacobus de Forlivio (da Forli), *Commentary on Canon of Avicenna* XVIII 392; named among learned men of Bologna XIX 514
Jacobus de (of) Mons Calvus, named among learned men of Bologna XIX 514
Jacobus de Palermo X 174
Jacobus de Sancto Marino (Florentia, or Naples) or Nicole Oresme, *De latitudinibus formarum* XIX 507
Jacobus de Voragine, *Legends of the Saints* XX 270, 280
Jacques d'Armagnac, library primarily of French books XX 271
Jacques le Grand of Toulouse, Augustinian, his *World Compendium* or *Sophologium* seldom found outside of French libraries XX 285
Janos Lascaris XX 262
Jars (flasks, vessels) IV 272
Jean de Domremi, without official authorization designated self physician, surgeon, and visitor of surgeons of kingdom of France XIII 19
Jean de Rochechomart XX 271
Jerome de Moravia, *Musica* I 186
Johanna, wife of a certain Dionysius, named in the case of Jaqueline Felicie XIII 10
Johanna de Monciaco, storekeeper, named in the case of Jaqueline Felicie XIII 10
Johannes, *Congelatio* X 173
Johannes Argyropulos, translator XX 264
Johannes Gmunden, mentioned in alchemical tract X 173; books donated to University of Vienna XX 288
Johannes Stockelpot, doctor of medicine and master and professor of Arts XII 217
Johannes van Eel (or de Neele) de Breda, master of Arts and doctor of medicine from Paris XII 217
Johannitius (Hunain ibn Ishaq), translator of Greek works into Syriac and Arabic XII 215; *Isagoge* XVIII 394, 396
John Beleth, twelfth century author, *Rationale of Divine Office* XX 280
John Davys, gave as bond for astronomical tables a certain 'book of letters of Seneca' XV 104
John, duke de Berry, library of, deeded to King Louis XI, XX 269-71, 276
John II, duke of Bourbon XIV 139
John Faber, witness for defense in case of Jaqueline Felicie XIII 9
John 'the Good', king of France, denounced continued presence of charlatans in medical practice and in dispensing of drugs XIII 15-16
John Halifax (Sacrobosco) XX 288; *Algorismus vulgaris* I 183; II 72-3; Astrolabe I 188; *Computus (Treatise on Calendar)* I 188, 190; Quadrant I 188; *Sphere* I 188; II 73; XII 222
John Holbrooke, Master of Peterhouse, Cambridge, astronomer and chaplain to Henry V, XV 103
John Killingworth, astronomical tables of, at Merton College, Oxford XV 103
John Langton, of Oxford and Cambridge, Master of Pembroke and Chancellor of the Exchequer XV 104
John de Lineriis, work of in the library of Nicholas of Cusa XX 287
John of London, protegé of Roger Bacon XX 287; Donated books to abbey church of St. Augustine, Canterbury XX 287
John Martin of Parma, on guarding against poisons XX 292
John Mesue, *On Medicinal Simples* XVII 384-5; Latin translation in Visconti-Sforza library XX 292
John (Jean) Michel, physician of Charles VIII of France XIV 139
John de Murs, *Geometry* XX 288
John of Padua, physician of Philip IV of France XIII 8
John Polzmacher, professor and dean of faculty of law and rector of University of Vienna XX 279
John Reuchlin, collector of Greek and Hebrew texts XX 266-7
John of St. Omer, witness for defense in case of Jaqueline Felicie XIII 9
John of Salisbury, *Policraticus* XX 270
John of Seville I 182
John Somer of Oxford, astronomical table

XV 103
John Somerset, Oxford and Cambridge Fellow, physician to Henry V and Chancellor of the Exchequer XV 104
John de Turre, probably son of a physician of Montpellier, named in case of Jaqueline Felicie XIII 10n.
John Walter (or Fitzwalter), Fellow of Worcester College, Oxford XV 103
Jordanus Nemorarius XX 288; *Algorismus demonstratus* I 182; *Arithmetica demonstratus*, expansion and alteration of Boethius' earlier work I 183; II 74; *De numeris datis* I 183
Julian the Apostate, Roman emperor XII 214
Julius II, pope; Collection of Greek works in Latin translation XX 264; Collection of legal texts XX 278
Juvenal, excerpts from XIX 806

Khalid ibn Yazid *see* Callisthenes

La Badia at Fiesole, library of XX 274
Laboratories III 194-5, 199
Laboratory experiments III 195-6
Laboratory manual IV 267
Laboratory observations VII 502
Laboratory procedure and apparatus III 199; IV 272; V 34
Lambruschini, cardinal X 171
Laon II 70
Lapide aurea et marchasita aurea, de IV 270
Latin language XII 218
Latin poets taught at Paris (Virgil, Horace, Terence, Ovid, etc.) XII 220
Law XIX 507
Legislation relating to examination and licensing of prospective physicians in Southern Italy XIII 4
Leon Battista Alberti *see* Alberti
Leonardo Bruni *see* Bruni
Leonardo Fibonaci de Pisa, *Liber abaci* I 182, 184
Leoniceno, Nicolo, humanist, and Pliny controversy XX 284
Leopold of Austria, on astrology XIX 512; XX 187
'Lewis of Caerleon, Doctor of Medicine, Astronomer and Mathematician (d. 1494?) XV 100-108
Libellus de alchemia (Semita recta) IV 198, 200; VII 501
Liber abaci I 182
Liber de aluminibus et salibus VI 164
Liber Archilae VI 162
Liber Bubocre Hermetis VI 162
Liber Duodecim Aquarum VI 164
Liber Duodecim Verborum VI 164
Liber Fiducie X 171
Liber Fornacis VI 164n.
Liber Triginta Preceptorum VI 163
Liber Lumen Luminum V 30; VI 164n.
Liber Maiori Habohaly Avicenna VI 164n.
Liber Mappae Clavicula, translated into Latin by Robert of Chester V 27; VI 161
Liber Mercurialis VI 161
Liber Perfecti Magisterii (Geber) VI 163, 164n., 176; VII 502
Liber Rebis X 171
Liber Regis Calith (Khalid) XX 162
Liber Septuaginta Preceptorum (Verborum) VI 163
Liber Trium Preceptorum (Verborum) VI 164
Liberal arts and medicine, 'hoary antiquity of association' XII 216-17
Libraries of the fifteenth century, exhibiting mixture of sacred and profane traditions XX 297
Library of Cardinal Bessarion, favored Greek texts and translations of historians XX 281
Library of dukes of Este, at Ferrara XX 263, 268
Lilium velut ex spinis evulsum see 'Lily torn from the thorns'
Linacre, Thomas XX 265
'Lily torn from the thorns' V 28; VI 164, 167, 169
Liquefaction IV 272
Literary subjects, large number of codices of XIX 305
Little, A. G. X 169-70
Livy XII 220
Logic, first in order of learning (Albertus Magnus) II 79; Mathematical XIX 507; New logic XII 221; Old logic XII 221; Third subject of *trivium* I 178, 180, 184; XII 221; XX 282
Lorenzo Laurenziano, translator from Greek XX 289
Lorenzo de Medici XX 262
Louis of Bruges, patron of letters, his books sent to Louis XII of France XX 272
Louis XI, king of France, received library of John, duke de Berry XX 270-1
Louis XII, king of France, received books of Louis of Bruges XX 272

Louvain, University of XII 216-17, 219, 221, 225. Hippocratic Oath to be recited at licensing and emphasis on texts of ancients XII 226
Ludovico Moro XX 291
Ludovicus de Coreto, Podesta of Bologna XVIII 383
Luminibus, De XVIII 392

Macer, in library of University of Erfurt XX 291
Macrobius, *Saturnalia* XIX 506
Magnet, virtue of XVIII 392
Maino de Maineri, *On Preservation from the Epidemic of the Year 1360*, copy in Este library, at Ferrara XX 292
Mallet or hammer IV 273
Manual operators at Paris, denounced XIII 6
Mappae mundi XX 293
Marble slab IV 272
Marchetus of Padua, *Ars musicae* XII 186; *Commentary on work of Franco of Cologne* XII 186; *Musicae mensuratae* XII 186
Marco Polo, *Travels to the Orient* XX 293
Margaret, countess of Richmond XV 102
Maria, the alchemist VI 167, 169
Maria degli Angeli, S., in Florence XX 261
Maria, the prophetess V 27, 32
Marsilius of Santa Sophia, physician and professor of medicine at Padua XX 292; *Commentary on Aphorisms of Hippocrates* XVIII 391; *On Fevers* XVIII 397; *On Ninth Book of Rasis, Liber ad Almansorem* XVIII 392
Martianus Capella I 181; II 68
Martin V, pope, alchemical and astrological works in library of XX 287, 294-6
Martin of Aragon, large collection of French and theological works in library of, at Barcelona XX 272, 277
Martin, Herman, and others named as physicians in the case of Jaqueline Felicie XIII 10
Martin, R. J., O. P. XII 218
Mathematica (concerning subjects of the *quadrivium*) XII 221-2
Mathematical arts I 175-6, 178
Mathematical works in Renaissance libraries XX 287-8
Mathematics I 177-9
Matheolus of Perugia, on importance and necessity of practical experience XII 216
Mathesis and astronomy XX 287
Mathias Farinator, *Lumen animae* XX 285
Maximus of Tyre XX 264
Medici, de', family of XX 262; Cosimo XX 274
Medicine (alchemy), synonym for elixir or transmuting agent III 199; IV 270; *De medicina ad album et ad rubeum* (alchemical) IV 285-7
Medicine, art of XII 221; Faculty of at Paris, and required competence in practical experience XII 227; Treatises on in Renaissance libraries XX 289-90
Medicines, preventive XX 289
Medieval encyclopedias in Renaissance libraries XX 280, 297
Medieval works favored in Renaissance libraries XX 279-80
Melting IV 272
Mercury (Quicksilver) III 189, 192, 195, 199; VII 502
Merlan, Professor II 69
Merton College, Oxford, and study of Astronomy I 190; Interest there in works of Lewis of Caerleon XV 103
Messahala XIX 508; Works in Nicholas of Cusa's library XX 287
Mesue, John XX 290-2; *Antidotarium* XVIII 393; Works in library of University of Erfurt XX 291
Metal workshops III 194
Metaphysics I 180
Michael Bertalia XIX 514
Michael Scot, characterized by Lynn Thorndike as leading intellectual during first third of thirteenth century III 80
Milleius, geometrician I 185
De mineralibus IV 268
Miners III 194
Mining districts III 194
Mirko Drazen Grmek of Zagreb, Dr. XVII 386
Modo compositionibus medicine, De IV 290
Montpellier and license to teach (*Licentia docendi*) XIII 5
Morigenes (Morienus) V 28; VI 165n., 177
Moral philosophy XX 275
Moslem astronomers (Alfraganus and Albategni) I 188-9
Mundinus of Bologna XIX 514
Mundus V 27, 32
Muntz and Fabre XX 262, 265
Music II 69; XII 222; fourth subject of the *quadrivium* XX 288; one of the mathematical arts I 175, 178, 180, 186-7; tracts on XIX 507; tracts on, in

Renaissance libraries XX 288-9
Musico XX 290

Naples, imperial regulations and licensing of physicians XIII 5
Natural astrology XIV 134
Natural philosophy I 178, 180; XII 221; XIX 507; tracts on XIX 507
Natural science III 191
Nature of spirits (*spiritus*), substance (*corpora*), and of sulphur and mercury VIII 304
Naudé, G., *Apology for all great personages who have been falsely suspected of Magic* III 196; VII 499
Niccoli, Nicolò, humanist, his collection of Greek texts left to monastery of S. Maria degli Angeli, in Florence XX 261
Niccolò III, XX 274
Nicholas V, pope XIX 505; XX 262, 274, 297
Nicholas Abrein, bishop of Trent, and Pseudo-Hippocrates, *On the Influence of the Moon on the Course of Diseases* XIV 139
Nicholas of Clemanges XII 220
Nicholas of Cusa, library of XX 266-7, 277, 279, 283, 291
Nicholas of Salerno, *Antidotarium* (or *Antidotary*) XIII 14; XVIII 391; XX 290
Nichomachus of Gerasia I 181; *De institutione arithmetica* II 68-70
Numerical prominence of Biblical and theological works in Renaissance libraries XX 277

Occult arts, tracts on, in Renaissance libraries XX 295, 297
Occultis naturae, de (alchemical tract) V 23ff.; VI 157ff; VII 500; Latin text reproduced VI 159-83
Oleo auri ad opus solis, de (Alkimia minor) IV 287-8
Oleo fermenti, de (Alkimia minor) IV 289
Oleo lapidus maioris, de (Alkimia minor) IV 289
Oleo martis, de (Alkimia minor) IV 288
Oleo sulphuris, de (Alkimia minor) IV 288
Oleo vitroli Romani, de (Alkimia minor) IV 288
Operations similar to those of alchemist (drying of mercury) III 194
Opus Regis ungarie X 173
Oresme, Nicholas, *De latitudinibus formarum* XIX 507; Translator of several works of Aristotle into French XX 269
Oribasius, commentator on Hippocratic *Aphorisms* XII 214-15
Oronce Fine, copyist VII 301
Orpiment III 199
Ostrogothic Italy II 70
Ovid XX 270; *Fasti* XX 275; *Metamorphoses* XX 275
Oxford, University I 175, 179-80, 182, 184; Libraries of XIV 135; XX 276-7; Statute requirements XII 219, 221

Padua, University of XVIII 392
Paetow, L. J. XII 217
Paladius XX 293
Palatine, Vatican collection V 23
Pandolfo Collenuccio and Pliny controversy XX 284
Paolo, German philosopher and astrologer in household of Federigo, duke of Urbino XX 288
Paolo Veneto, noted logician and philosopher at Padua XVIII 389
Papal dispensations from prohibition against clerical medical practice XIII 4
Paquet, J. XII 218
Parapsis, glazed IV 273
Paris II 70; VII 500-1, 503; University of I 175-6, 179-83, 184ff.; II 71; III 194; XII 216; University of, medical faculty, provisions for licensing of prospective physicians XIII 5; University of, measures against illegal practice of medicine XIII 5-20
Parlement of Paris, considers case of Perretta Petonne XIII 17-18
Partington, J R. III 195; VII 499
Patch, H.R. II 70-1
Pepoli, Guido and Taddeo XIX 506
Perfect gold and silver, production of by artisan VIII 305
Perotti, Nicolò, translator of Polybius XX 264
Peter of Abano, professor and physician at Paris and Padua XII 219-20, 222; XIV 135, 138; XX 286; *Astrologia* of Pseudo-Hippocrates translated from Greek XIV 138; *Commentary on Problemata*, attributed to Aristotle XVIII 392; *Conciliator* XX 290-2; Tract on poisons, *De venenis*, cited XVI 992
Peter of Mantua, *Logica* XVIII 391
Peter Martyr, St. XIX 507

Petonne, Perretta, arrested for illegally operating as a surgeon XIII 17
Petrarch, works of in Renaissance libraries XX 260, 268, 279, 291
Petrus Antonius XIX 512
Petrus Hispanus (Pope John XXI), *Summa logicae* XIX 507; *Thesaurus pauperium* XVIII 393; XX 290
Petrus Tossignano XIX 514
Pharmacy, practices common to III 271
Philip VI, king of France XIII 15
Philosophers VII 501
Philosophers' Stone III 199; V 30
Philosophers of the Turba (Bonellus, Mundus and Zenon) V 27
Philosophy, Moral I 180; Natural I 180-1; Rational I 180; XII 218; Speculative I 180
Physicians, at Bologna XIX 514
Physicians, named in case of Jaqueline Felicie XIII 10
Physics I 180
Pico della Mirandola, library of XX 258, 263, 266, 287-9
Pier Candido Decembrio, humanist, collection of Greek works in Ferrara XX 264
Pierre d Auvergne, professor of theology at Paris, and role of harmony I 186-7
Pierre of Blois I 184; Interest in Greek XX 264-5
Pierre de Maricourt, *De Magnete* X 170n.
Pietro de' Medici XX 262
Pietro da Montagnana, library of XX 263
Pius IX, pope X 171
Planets and minerals IV 270
Plato, works of in Middle Ages II 68-9; XII 213-14; works of, in Renaissance libraries XX 260, 283
Pliny, on physicians XIII 3; Controversy in Renaissance between Pandolfo Collenuccio and Nicolò Leoniceno XX 284; *Natural History* in Renaissance libraries XX 284
Poetry, works on, in Este library XX 268
Poggio Bracciolini XX 268; Brought to light work of Cornelius Celsus XX 289
Polybius, in translation of Nicolò Perotti XX 264
Polyphemus, legendary history of, by Garzoni XIX 506
Porretta, baths of, near Bologna XVI 994
Printing press and growth of libraries XX 258
Priscian XII 219-20
Prisciano, Pellegrino, astrologer XX 286
Proclus XX 283
Procopius XX 263
Prohibitions against clerical practice of medicine outside monasteries XIII 4
Propositions VII 502
Ptolemy I 178, 187-9; *Almagest* I 187-9; XX 270, 275; *Canons* I 188, 270, 275, 286; *Cosmography* (Geography) XX 275, 286; *Quadripartitum* XX 287; Versified version by Francesco Berlinghieri XX 293
Pythagorean or Neo-Pythagorean II 68

Quadrivium I 175-191; II 67-9, 71, 73, 75, 79
Questiones disputatae I 176
Quicksilver *see Argentum vivum* and Mercury
Quid pro quo for apothecaries XIII 14
Quodlibeta I 176

Rabanus Maurus II 70; *Commentary on Book of Ecclesiasticus* XIII 3-4; *De universo* XIII 3-4
Rainbow I 179
Rasis VII 502; X 172; Commentaries on *Liber Almansoris* XVIII 392-3, 396; *De Divisionibus* XVIII 392; *Liber Almansoris* XVI 994; *Liber aluminum et salium* (attributed to Rasis) V 26, 30-1; VI 176-8; *lumen luminum* (attributed to Rasis) V 26, 30-31; VI 176-8; Works in Renaissance libraries XX 290, 292
Raymundus frater Guanfredi, minister (sic) generalis ordinis minorum 'ad solem et ad lunam' X 173
Recipes for *crocus ferri* IV 276; for treating golden stone or gold marcasite IV 275; of various individuals VII 502; X 173-5; *Sal ammoniacum* X 175
Regimen for birds and falcons XX 293
'Regimen for the work on the stone' VII 502
Regiomontanus (mathematician) XX 288
Regulations against unlicensed medical practice XIII 6
Reichenau II 70
Reuchlin, John, humanist, library of XX 267
Rhazes *see* Rasis
Rheims II 70
Rhetoric of both Aristotle and Cicero, lectured on in Paris XII 219-21; Works on in Renaissance libraries XX 275
Richard de Bury XX 260, 297

Richard of Furnival XX 289
Richard Suiseth or Calculator XX 288
Richard of Wallingford, abbot of St. Albans, astronomer at Merton College, Oxford XV 103
Richardus Anglicus (or Parisiensis), *Tract on Fevers* XVIII 397
Robert of Chester, translations I 182; V 27
Robert Grosseteste, bishop of Lincoln I 176-8, 185-6, 189-90; II 71, 74-5
Robert of Naples XX 260
Roger Bacon, Franciscan, master of arts in Oxford and Paris I 176-9, 181ff.; II 71; III 196; Criticized work of Jordanus in arithmetic II 74-5; On need for geometry in biblical interpretation I 185; On use of triangle to explain Trinity I 185; Physicians and study of astrology and astronomy XIV 138; Physicians and study of music I 186; Theologians and study of music I 187; Works of: *Commentary on Euclid's Elements* I 184; *De arte experimentale* X 169; *De magnete see* Pierre de Maricourt; *De multiplicatione specierum* I 185; *De naturis metallorum* or *Breve breviarum* X 172; *De potestate artis et naturae* X 169-70; *De retardande senectute* X 169-70; *De secretis operibus et naturae* X 170n.; *Greek grammar* XX 265-66; *Libri magici et fraudes eorum* X 170; *Opus Maius* I 176-9, 181-2; *Opus Tertian* I 185
Royal restrictions for pharmaceutical establishments in Paris XIII 15
'*Ad rubeum*' or '*ad album*' IV 270
Rubifaction of gold making, and whitening or silver making IV 272, 274, 279

Sabbadini XX 269
Sacrobosco *see* John Halifax
St. Augustine of Canterbury *see* Canterbury
St. Gall II 70
St. Martin of Dover, library of XX 290
Sal alkali IV 274
Sal ammoniac IV 274
Sal communis IV 274
Sale armoniaco et eius preparatione, de IV 280
Salerno, imperial legislation on prospective physicians XIII 5
Salerno, medical school in eleventh century XIII 4
Sallust, in Italian XX 268
Salmasius, or Saumaise, Claude, held that 'tract on astrological medicine should not be assigned to Hippocrates' (1648) XIV 140
Salts V 32
Salutati, Coluccio, humanist XX 261
Salviati XX 262
San Marco, Florence XX 262; Library of XX 274
San Marco, Venice, library of XX 261
San Procolo, Benedictine monastery at Bologna V 24
Savonarola, Michael XX 262; Works of in private library of dukes of Este in Ferrara XX 292
Schism XII 216
Scholastic interests and themes continued in fourteenth and fifteenth centuries XX 280, 297
Scientific and philosophical writings introduced in original form or in new translations XX 281
Scientific or Pseudo-Scientific interests centered about four basic sciences XX 285-6
Secret operations (alchemy) VII 502
Secreta philosophorum VII 502
Secreta secretorum or *Practica Alkimiae* VII 502
Secundo modo fixationis, de IV 284
Seigneur de Mortemart, secretary to Charles of Orleans XX 270-1
Semita recta III 199-200; IV 267, 270; V 23, 25, 33; VII 500-1, 511-15; IX 238-43; X 172
Senior V 27, 39
Septuaginta V 27-8
Serapion XVIII 391; In Latin translation in Visconti-Sforza library XX 292
Seven liberal arts I 175
Sforza, *see* Visconti-Sforza
Sigismund Gosembrot, German humanist, owner of copy of *Lumen animae* XX 285
Simon Bredon, astronomer, works of utilized by Lewis of Caerleon XV 103
Simon de Hesdin, translator of several classical historical tracts into French for John, duke de Berry XX 269
Simon de Phares, owner of *Astrologia Ypocratis* XIV 139
Simples, lists of XX 290; *see also* Antidotaries, medical
Singer, Dorothy Waley, *Catalogue* VII 503
Sixtus IV, pope XX 262
Skeat, T. C., deputy keeper of manuscripts

in British Museum IX 239
Smeltermen III 194
Solinus, *De mineralibus mundi* XX 284
Solomon's temple I 185
Spanish libraries containing French works XX 272-3
Stars, as agencies influencing chemical operations III 193
Statius XX 275; Translated into Italian dialect XX 268
Stefano de' Dottori, colleague of Cristoforo Barzizza at Padua XVIII 389
Stoppers (glass or cloth) IV 273
Stowe manuscripts III 196
Strabo XX 263-4, 293
Strozzi, Palla XX 263
Sublimation of Arsenic IV 275, 283; Mercury III 200; IV 275; Sulphur IV 275
Sublimatione arsenici, de IV 283
Sublimatione mercurii, de IV 281
Sublimatione sulphuris, de IV 282
Sulphur III 188, 192, 194-5, 199; Important for the preparation and production of alchemical or philosophers' stone V 31-2; VI 157; Productive spirit VII 502; Theory of composition of metals VIII 303
Surgeons, bound by oath XIII 6
Surgery, regulations on practice at Naples, Paris and Salerno XIII 17; Treatises on XX 290
Suthwell, Thomas, court astrologer to Henry VI of England XV 103

Tables of Toledo XX 287
Tartar and its preparation IV 271, 275
Thales XIX 509
Thebet ben Corat XX 189, 286
Theodore, Gaza, at Ferrara, translator from Greek XX 264, 289
Theodosian Code, regulations of physicians XIII 3
Theodosius, geometrician I 185
Theology I 178-80; prominence of XIX 507; XX 279
Theory of gold as representing perfection VIII 304
Therapeutica sive de cura febrium (Galen) XIX 512
Thesaurus X 169
Thesaurus pauperum, probably the handbook by Petrus Hispanus XVIII 392
Thomas Aquinas, St. I 176, 178, 180-1, 187; his works XI 261-2; the order of learning: logic, then quadrivial arts II 69, 71, 79; alchemical works ascribed to IV 268
Thomas of Cantimpré XX 284
Thomas de Garbo, works by at Cologne XII 226
Thomas Parentucelli of Sarzana XX 297; *see also* Nicholas V, pope
Thorndike, Lynn I 183; IV 267; VII 499; IX 238, 240-1; XIV 135, 139
Thorndike and Kibre, *Catalogue of Incipits*: List of abbreviations VII 503
Thucydides XX 264
'*Torquena perfecta probata per Magistrum Rugerium de Brandellis* X 173
Torquetus, astronomical instrument I 190
Toscanelli XX 293
Tower of London XV 102
Translation of Greek literary works XX 260
Translation of Latin works into French XX 268
Translations into Italian XX 268
Transmutation of metals III 189, 191, 195, 198; IV 268; VII 499; VIII 304
Transmutation, theories of and the philosophers' stone V 25
Travel books XX 293
Triangle, use as the illustration of the Trinity I 185
Trivium (grammar, rhetoric, logic or dialectic) I 175, 180; II 69; XII 218
Trotula XX 290
Tullius (Grecus) V 33
Turba philosophorum V 27, 32-3; VI 157, 160, 164-5, 168-73, 178-82
Turks XX 260

Universities established on Parisian model (Cologne and Louvain) XII 216
University of Erfurt, medical collection XX 291
Urban IV, pope I 184
Urban V, pope, at Avignon, library of XX 267
Urbino, library of duke of XX 275-6
Urina, de, et eius preparatione IV 280-1
Urine, of boys IV 275

Valens, emperor XIII 3
Valentinian I, emperor XIII 3
Valentinus, magister X 168-9
Valerius Maximus XX 270; Translated into Italian XX 268
Valla, George, humanist, collection of books

XX 263-4, 267, 284, 286, 291, 295; *De expetendis et fugiendis rebus* XX 291
Valla, Lorenzo, humanist XX 264
Van Steenberghen, F. XII 217
Varro I 181; XX 293
Varronean II 70
Vatican, library of XX 262-3; Manuscripts IX 239-40
Vegetius XX 270
Venice IV 273; *see also* San Marco
Vergil, Polydore, historian XV 102
Vermillion, preparation of III 202
Vernacular texts in Renaissance libraries XX 266-8, 273
Vespasian, fifteenth century XX 275-7
Veterinary art, anonymous tracts on, in Visconti-Sforza library XX 293
Vienna, University of XX 288
Vincent of Beauvais, cited Boethius on primacy of arithmetic II 80; *Speculum doctrinale* and mathematics II 79-80; *Speculum historiale* XX 270; Works of, in Renaissance libraries XX 285
Virgil XVIII 390; XIX 505; XX 275
Visconti, Giangaleazzo XX 260-1
Visconti-Sforza library, XX 260, 269, 274, 277, 283-4, 293-5
Visconti, Valentine XX 270
Visio Belini VI 171n.
Vitelo, *Perspective* XX 275
Vitruvius, tract on architecture XX 293
Vivarium, monastic retreat and medicine XIII 3

Weisheipl, J. A., O. P. XII 218
Whitening or silver making IV 272
William of Auvergne, bishop of Paris, *De universo* I 188
William Durandi, *Rationale of the Divine Office* XX 280
William of Moerbeke, archbishop of Corinth, translator from Greek XIV 135-6
William of Saliceto, tract on surgery XX 290
William Stocton XV 103
William of Varignana of Bologna, *Practica medicinalis* III 391; Works of, at Cologne XII 226
Women's diseases XX 290
Works in ancient languages circulating in Latin translations XX 274

Yvo Tueleu, witness for defense of Jaqueline Felicie XIII 9

Xenophon XX 263

Zael XX 287
Zenon V 27, 32
Zetzner VII 500-02